HEALTH AND HUMAN DEVELOPMENT

PUBLIC HEALTH YEARBOOK 2016

HEALTH AND HUMAN DEVELOPMENT

JOAV MERRICK - SERIES EDITOR

NATIONAL INSTITUTE OF CHILD HEALTH
AND HUMAN DEVELOPMENT,
MINISTRY OF SOCIAL AFFAIRS, JERUSALEM

Adolescent Behavior Research: International Perspectives
Joav Merrick and Hatim A. Omar (Editors)
2007. ISBN: 1-60021-649-8

Complementary Medicine Systems: Comparison and Integration
Karl W. Kratky
2008. ISBN: 978-1-60456-475-4 (Hardcover)
2008. ISBN: 978-1-61122-433-7 (eBook)

Pain in Children and Youth
Patricia Schofield and Joav Merrick (Editors)
2008. ISBN: 978-1-60456-951-3 (Hardcover)
2008. ISBN: 978-1-61470-496-6 (eBook)

Challenges in Adolescent Health: An Australian Perspective
David Bennett, Susan Towns, Elizabeth Elliott and Joav Merrick (Editors)
2009. ISBN: 978-1-60741-616-6 (Hardcover)
2009. ISBN: 978-1-61668-240-8 (eBook)

Obesity and Adolescence: A Public Health Concern
Hatim A. Omar, Donald E. Greydanus, Dilip R. Patel and Joav Merrick (Editors)
2009. ISBN: 978-1-60692-821-9 (Hardcover)
2009. ISBN: 978-1-61470-465-2 (eBook)

Poverty and Children: A Public Health Concern
Alexis Lieberman and Joav Merrick (Editors)
2009. ISBN: 978-1-60741-140-6 (Hardcover)
2009. ISBN: 978-1-61470-601-4 (eBook)

Living on the Edge: The Mythical, Spiritual, and Philosophical Roots of Social Marginality
Joseph Goodbread
2009. ISBN: 978-1-60741-162-8 (Hardcover)
2013. ISBN: 978-1-61122-986-8 (Softcover)
2011. ISBN: 978-1-61470-192-7 (eBook)

Alcohol-Related Cognitive Disorders: Research and Clinical Perspectives
Leo Sher, Isack Kandel and Joav Merrick (Editors)
2009. ISBN: 978-1-60741-730-9 (Hardcover)
2009. ISBN: 978-1-60876-623-9 (eBook)

Children and Pain
Patricia Schofield and Joav Merrick (Editors)
2009. ISBN: 978-1-60876-020-6 (Hardcover)
2009. ISBN: 978-1-61728-183-9 (eBook)

Chance Action and Therapy: The Playful Way of Changing
Uri Wernik
2010. ISBN: 978-1-60876-393-1 (Hardcover)
2011. ISBN: 978-1-61122-987-5 (Softcover)
2011. ISBN: 978-1-61209-874-6 (eBook)

Bone and Brain Metastases: Advances in Research and Treatment
Arjun Sahgal, Edward Chow and Joav Merrick (Editors)
2010. ISBN: 978-1-61668-365-8 (Hardcover)
2010. ISBN: 978-1-61728-085-6 (eBook)

Behavioral Pediatrics, 3rd Edition
Donald E. Greydanus, Dilip R. Patel, Helen D. Pratt and Joseph L. Calles, Jr. (Editors)
2011. ISBN: 978-1-60692-702-1 (Hardcover)
2009. ISBN: 978-1-60876-630-7 (eBook)

Rural Child Health: International Aspects
Erica Bell and Joav Merrick (Editors)
2011. ISBN: 978-1-60876-357-3 (Hardcover)
2011. ISBN: 978-1-61324-005-2 (eBook)

International Aspects of Child Abuse and Neglect
Howard Dubowitz and Joav Merrick (Editors)
2011. ISBN: 978-1-60876-703-8 (Hardcover)
2010. ISBN: 978-1-61122-049-0 (Softcover)
2010. ISBN: 978-1-61122-403-0 (eBook)

Environment, Mood Disorders and Suicide
Teodor T. Postolache and Joav Merrick (Editors)
2011. ISBN: 978-1-61668-505-8 (Hardcover)
2011. ISBN: 978-1-62618-340-7 (eBook)

Positive Youth Development: Evaluation and Future Directions in a Chinese Context
Daniel T.L. Shek, Hing Keung Ma and Joav Merrick (Editors)
2011. ISBN: 978-1-60876-830-1 (Hardcover)
2011. ISBN: 978-1-62100-175-1 (Softcover)
2010. ISBN: 978-1-61209-091-7 (eBook)

Understanding Eating Disorders: Integrating Culture, Psychology and Biology
Yael Latzer, Joav Merrick and Daniel Stein (Editors)
2011. ISBN: 978-1-61728-298-0 (Hardcover)
2011. ISBN: 978-1-61470-976-3 (Softcover)
2011. ISBN: 978-1-61942-054-0 (eBook)

Advanced Cancer Pain and Quality of Life
Edward Chow and Joav Merrick (Editors)
2011. ISBN: 978-1-61668-207-1 (Hardcover)
2010. ISBN: 978-1-61668-400-6 (eBook)

Positive Youth Development: Implementation of a Youth Program in a Chinese Context
Daniel T.L Shek, Hing Keung Ma and Joav Merrick (Editors)
2011. ISBN: 978-1-61668-230-9

Social and Cultural Psychiatry Experience from the Caribbean Region
Hari D. Maharajh and Joav Merrick (Editors)
2011. ISBN: 978-1-61668-506-5 (Hardcover)
2010. ISBN: 978-1-61728-088-7 (eBook)

Narratives and Meanings of Migration
Julia Mirsky
2011. ISBN: 978-1-61761-103-2 (Hardcover)
2010. ISBN: 978-1-61761-519-1 (eBook)

Self-Management and the Health Care Consumer
Peter William Harvey
2011. ISBN: 978-1-61761-796-6 (Hardcover)
2011. ISBN: 978-1-61122-214-2 (eBook)

Sexology from a Holistic Point of View
Soren Ventegodt and Joav Merrick
2011. ISBN: 978-1-61761-859-8 (Hardcover)
2011. ISBN: 978-1-61122-262-3 (eBook)

Principles of Holistic Psychiatry: A Textbook on Holistic Medicine for Mental Disorders
Soren Ventegodt and Joav Merrick
2011. ISBN: 978-1-61761-940-3 (Hardcover)
2011. ISBN: 978-1-61122-263-0 (eBook)

Clinical Aspects of Psychopharmacology in Childhood and Adolescence
Donald E. Greydanus, Joseph L. Calles, Jr., Dilip P. Patel, Ahsan Nazeer and Joav Merrick (Editors)
2011. ISBN: 978-1-61122-135-0 (Hardcover)
2011. ISBN: 978-1-61122-715-4 (eBook)

Climate Change and Rural Child Health
Erica Bell, Bastian M. Seidel and Joav Merrick (Editors)
2011. ISBN: 978-1-61122-640-9 (Hardcover)
2011. ISBN: 978-1-61209-014-6 (eBook)

Rural Medical Education: Practical Strategies
Erica Bell, Craig Zimitat and Joav Merrick (Editors)
2011. ISBN: 978-1-61122-649-2 (Hardcover)
2011. ISBN: 978-1-61209-476-2 (eBook)

Advances in Environmental Health Effects of Toxigenic Mold and Mycotoxins
Ebere Cyril Anyanwu
2011. ISBN: 978-1-60741-953-2

Public Health Yearbook 2009
Joav Merrick (Editor)
2011. ISBN: 978-1-61668-911-7 (Hardcover)
2011. ISBN: 978-1-62417-365-3 (eBook)

Child Health and Human Development Yearbook 2009
Joav Merrick (Editor)
2011. ISBN: 978-1-61668-912-4

Alternative Medicine Yearbook 2009
Joav Merrick (Editor)
2011. ISBN: 978-1-61668-910-0 (Hardcover)
2011. ISBN: 978-1-62081-710-0 (eBook)

The Dance of Sleeping and Eating among Adolescents: Normal and Pathological Perspectives
Yael Latzer and Orna Tzischinsky (Editors)
2011. ISBN: 978-1-61209-710-7 (Hardcover)
2011. ISBN: 978-1-62417-366-0 (eBook)

Drug Abuse in Hong Kong: Development and Evaluation of a Prevention Program
Daniel T.L. Shek, Rachel C.F. Sun and Joav Merrick (Editors)
2011. ISBN: 978-1-61324-491-3 (Hardcover)
2011. ISBN: 978-1-62257-232-8 (eBook)

Adolescence and Chronic Illness. A Public Health Concern
Hatim Omar, Donald E. Greydanus, Dilip R. Patel and Joav Merrick (Editors)
2012. ISBN: 978-1-60876-628-4 (Hardcover)
2010. ISBN: 978-1-61761-482-8 (eBook)

Child and Adolescent Health Yearbook 2009
Joav Merrick (Editor)
2012. ISBN: 978-1-61668-913-1 (Hardcover)
2012. ISBN: 978-1-62257-095-9 (eBook)

Child and Adolescent Health Yearbook 2010
Joav Merrick (Editor)
2012. ISBN: 978-1-61209-788-6 (Hardcover)
2012. ISBN: 978-1-62417-046-1 (eBook)

Child Health and Human Development Yearbook 2010
Joav Merrick (Editor)
2012. ISBN: 978-1-61209-789-3 (Hardcover)
2012. ISBN: 978-1-62081-721-6 (eBook)

Public Health Yearbook 2010
Joav Merrick (Editor)
2012. ISBN: 978-1-61209-971-2 (Hardcover)
2012. ISBN: 978-1-62417-863-4 (eBook)

Alternative Medicine Yearbook 2010
Joav Merrick (Editor)
2012. ISBN: 978-1-62100-132-4 (Hardcover)
2011. ISBN: 978-1-62100-210-9 (eBook)

The Astonishing Brain and Holistic Conciousness: Neuroscience and Vedanta Perspectives
Vinod D. Deshmukh
2012. ISBN: 978-1-61324-295-7

Translational Research for Primary Healthcare
Erica Bell, Gert. P. Westert and Joav Merrick (Editors)
2012. ISBN: 978-1-61324-647-4 (Hardcover)
2012. ISBN: 978-1-62417-409-4 (eBook)

Our Search for Meaning in Life: Quality of Life Philosophy
Søren Ventegodt and Joav Merrick
2012. ISBN: 978-1-61470-494-2 (Hardcover)
2011. ISBN: 978-1-61470-519-2 (eBook)

Randomized Clinical Trials and Placebo: Can You Trust the Drugs are Working and Safe?
Søren Ventegodt and Joav Merrick
2012. ISBN: 978-1-61470-067-8 (Hardcover)
2011. ISBN: 978-1-61470-151-4 (eBook)

Building Community Capacity: Minority and Immigrant Populations
Rosemary M Caron and Joav Merrick (Editors)
2012. ISBN: 978-1-62081-022-4 (Hardcover)
2012. ISBN: 978-1-62081-032-3 (eBook)

Applied Public Health: Examining Multifaceted Social or Ecological Problems and Child Maltreatment
John R. Lutzker and Joav Merrick (Editors)
2012. ISBN: 978-1-62081-356-0 (Hardcover)
2012. ISBN: 978-1-62081-388-1 (eBook)

Treatment and Recovery of Eating Disorders
Daniel Stein and Yael Latzer (Editors)
2012. ISBN: 978-1-61470-259-7 (Hardcover)
2012. ISBN: 978-1-61470-418-8 (eBook)

Human Immunodeficiency Virus (HIV) Research: Social Science Aspects
Hugh Klein and Joav Merrick (Editors)
2012. ISBN: 978-1-62081-293-8 (Hardcover)
2012. ISBN: 978-1-62081-346-1 (eBook)

AIDS and Tuberculosis: Public Health Aspects
Daniel Chemtob and Joav Merrick (Editors)
2012. ISBN: 978-1-62081-382-9 (Softcover)
2012. ISBN: 978-1-62081-406-2 (eBook)

Public Health Yearbook 2011
Joav Merrick (Editor)
2012. ISBN: 978-1-62081-433-8 (Hardcover)
2012. ISBN: 978-1-62081-434-5 (eBook)

Alternative Medicine Research Yearbook 2011
Joav Merrick (Editor)
2012. ISBN: 978-1-62081-476-5 (Hardcover)
2012. ISBN: 978-1-62081-477-2 (eBook)

Building Community Capacity: Skills and Principles
Rosemary M Caron and Joav Merrick (Editors)
2012. ISBN: 978-1-61209-331-4 (Hardcover)
2012. ISBN: 978-1-62257-238-0 (eBook)

Textbook on Evidence-Based Holistic Mind-Body Medicine: Basic Principles of Healing in Traditional Hippocratic Medicine
Søren Ventegodt and Joav Merrick
2012. ISBN: 978-1-62257-094-2 (Hardcover)
2012. ISBN: 978-1-62257-172-7 (eBook)

Textbook on Evidence-Based Holistic Mind-Body Medicine: Basic Philosophy and Ethics of Traditional Hippocratic Medicine
Søren Ventegodt and Joav Merrick
2012. ISBN: 978-1-62257-052-2 (Hardcover)
2013. ISBN: 978-1-62257-707-1 (eBook)

Textbook on Evidence-Based Holistic Mind-Body Medicine: Research, Philosophy, Economy and Politics of Traditional Hippocratic Medicine
Søren Ventegodt and Joav Merrick
2012. ISBN: 978-1-62257-140-6 (Hardcover)
2012. ISBN: 978-1-62257-171-0 (eBook)

Textbook on Evidence-Based Holistic Mind-Body Medicine: Holistic Practice of Traditional Hippocratic Medicine
Søren Ventegodt and Joav Merrick
2013. ISBN: 978-1-62257-105-5 (Hardcover)
2012. ISBN: 978-1-62257-174-1 (eBook)

Textbook on Evidence-Based Holistic Mind-Body Medicine: Healing the Mind in Traditional Hippocratic Medicine
Søren Ventegodt and Joav Merrick
2013. ISBN: 978-1-62257-112-3 (Hardcover)
2012. ISBN: 978-1-62257-175-8 (eBook)

Textbook on Evidence-Based Holistic Mind-Body Medicine: Sexology and Traditional Hippocratic Medicine
Søren Ventegodt and Joav Merrick
2013. ISBN: 978-1-62257-130-7 (Hardcover)
2012. ISBN: 978-1-62257-176-5 (eBook)

Health Risk Communication
Marijke Lemal and Joav Merrick (Editors)
2012. ISBN: 978-1-62257-544-2 (Hardcover)
2012. ISBN: 978-1-62257-552-7 (eBook)

Health and Happiness from Meaningful Work: Research in Quality of Working Life
Søren Ventegodt and Joav Merrick (Editors)
2013. ISBN: 978-1-60692-820-2 (Hardcover)
2009. ISBN: 978-1-61324-981-9 (eBook)

Conceptualizing Behavior in Health and Social Research: A Practical Guide to Data Analysis
Said Shahtahmasebi and Damon Berridge
2013. ISBN: 978-1-60876-383-2

Adolescence and Sports
Dilip R. Patel, Donald E. Greydanus, Hatim Omar and Joav Merrick (Editors)
2013. ISBN: 978-1-60876-702-1 (Hardcover)
2010. ISBN: 978-1-61761-483-5 (eBook)

Pediatric and Adolescent Sexuality and Gynecology: Principles for the Primary Care Clinician
Hatim A. Omar, Donald E. Greydanus, Artemis K. Tsitsika, Dilip R. Patel and Joav Merrick (Editors)
2013. ISBN: 978-1-60876-735-9 (Softcover)

Human Development: Biology from a Holistic Point of View
Søren Ventegodt, Tyge Dahl Hermansen and Joav Merrick
2013. ISBN: 978-1-61470-441-6 (Hardcover)
2011. ISBN: 978-1-61470-541-3 (eBook)

Building Community Capacity: Case Examples from Around the World
Rosemary M Caron and Joav Merrick (Editors)
2013. ISBN: 978-1-62417-175-8 (Hardcover)
2013. ISBN: 978-1-62417-176-5 (eBook)

Managed Care in a Public Setting
Richard Evan Steele
2013. ISBN: 978-1-62417-970-9 (Softcover)
2013. ISBN: 978-1-62417-863-4 (eBook)

Bullying: A Public Health Concern
Jorge C. Srabstein and Joav Merrick (Editors)
2013. ISBN: 978-1-62618-564-7 (Hardcover)
2013. ISBN: 978-1-62618-588-3 (eBook)

Bedouin Health: Perspectives from Israel
Joav Merrick, Alean Al-Krenami and Salman Elbedour (Editors)
2013. ISBN: 978-1-62948-271-2 (Hardcover)
2013: ISBN: 978-1-62948-274-3 (eBook)

Health Promotion: Community Singing as a Vehicle to Promote Health
Jing Sun, Nicholas Buys and Joav Merrick (Editors)
2013. ISBN: 978-1-62618-908-9 (Hardcover)
2013: ISBN: 978-1-62808-006-3 (eBook)

Public Health Yearbook 2012
Joav Merrick (Editor)
2013. ISBN: 978-1-62808-078-0 (Hardcover)
2013: ISBN: 978-1-62808-079-7 (eBook)

Alternative Medicine Research Yearbook 2012
Joav Merrick (Editor)
2013. ISBN: 978-1-62808-080-3 (Hardcover)
2013: ISBN: 978-1-62808-079-7 (eBook)

Advanced Cancer: Managing Symptoms and Quality of Life
Natalie Pulenzas, Breanne Lechner, Nemica Thavarajah, Edward Chow, and Joav Merrick (Editors)
2013. ISBN: 978-1-62808-239-5 (Hardcover)
2013: ISBN: 978-1-62808-267-8 (eBook)

Treatment and Recovery of Eating Disorders
Daniel Stein and Yael Latzer (Editors)
2013. ISBN: 978-1-62808-248-7 (Softcover)

Health Promotion: Strengthening Positive Health and Preventing Disease
Jing Sun, Nicholas Buys and Joav Merrick (Editors)
2013. ISBN: 978-1-62257-870-2 (Hardcover)
2013: ISBN: 978-1-62808-621-8 (eBook)

Pain Management Yearbook 2011
Joav Merrick (Editor)
2013. ISBN: 978-1-62808-970-7 (Hardcover)
2013: ISBN: 978-1-62808-971-4 (eBook)

Pain Management Yearbook 2012
Joav Merrick (Editor)
2013. ISBN: 978-1-62808-973-8 (Hardcover)
2013: ISBN: 978-1-62808-974-5 (eBook)

Suicide from a Public Health Perspective
Said Shahtahmasebi and Joav Merrick
2013. ISBN: 978-1-62948-536-2 (Hardcover)
2014: ISBN: 978-1-62948-537-9 (eBook)

Food, Nutrition and Eating Behavior
Joav Merrick and Sigal Israeli (Editors)
2013. ISBN: 978-1-62948-233-0 (Hardcover)
2013: ISBN: 978-1-62948-234-7 (eBook)

Public Health Concern: Smoking, Alcohol and Substance Use
Joav Merrick and Ariel Tenenbaum (Editors)
2013. ISBN: 978-1-62948-424-2 (Hardcover)
2013. ISBN: 978-1-62948-430-3 (eBook)

Mental Health from an International Perspective
Joav Merrick, Shoshana Aspler and Mohammed Morad (Editors)
2013. ISBN: 978-1-62948-519-5 (Hardcover)
2013. ISBN: 978-1-62948-520-1 (eBook)

India: Health and Human Development Aspects
Joav Merrick (Editor)
2014. ISBN: 978-1-62948-784-7 (Hardcover)
2014. ISBN: 978-1-62948-794-6 (eBook)

Alternative Medicine Research Yearbook 2013
Joav Merrick (Editor)
2014. ISBN: 978-1-63321-094-3 (Hardcover)
2014. ISBN: 978-1-63321-144-5 (eBook)

Health Consequences of Human Central Obesity
Kaushik Bose and Raja Chakraborty (Editors)
2014. ISBN: 978-1-63321-152-0 (Hardcover)
2014. ISBN: 978-1-63321-181-0 (eBook)

Public Health Yearbook 2013
Joav Merrick (Editor)
2014. ISBN: 978-1-63321-095-0 (Hardcover)
2014. ISBN: 978-1-63321-097-4 (eBook)

Public Health: Improving Health via Inter-Professional Collaborations
Rosemary M. Caron and Joav Merrick (Editors)
2014. ISBN: 978-1-63321-569-6 (Hardcover)
2014. ISBN: 978-1-63321-594-8 (eBook)

Alternative Medicine Research Yearbook 2014
Joav Merrick (Editor)
2015. ISBN: 978-1-63482-161-2 (Hardcover)
2015. ISBN: 978-1-63482-205-3 (eBook)

Pain Management Yearbook 2014
Joav Merrick (Editor)
2015. ISBN: 978-1-63482-164-3 (Hardcover)
2015. ISBN: 978-1-63482-208-4 (eBook)

Public Health Yearbook 2014
Joav Merrick (Editor)
2015. ISBN: 978-1-63482-165-0 (Hardcover)
2015. ISBN: 978-1-63482-209-1 (eBook)

Forensic Psychiatry: A Public Health Perspective
Leo Sher and Joav Merrick (Editors)
2015. ISBN: 978-1-63483-339-4 (Hardcover)
2015. ISBN: 978-1-63483-346-2 (eBook)

Leadership and Service Learning Education: Holistic Development for Chinese University Students
Daniel TL Shek, Florence KY Wu and Joav Merrick (Editors)
2015. ISBN: 978-1-63483-340-0 (Hardcover)
2015. ISBN: 978-1-63483-347-9 (eBook)

Mental and Holistic Health: Some International Perspectives
Joseph L. Calles Jr., Donald E Greydanus, and Joav Merrick (Editors)
2015. ISBN: 978-1-63483-589-3 (Hardcover)
2015. ISBN: 978-1-63483-608-1 (eBook)

Cancer: Treatment, Decision Making and Quality of Life
Breanne Lechner, Ronald Chow, Natalie Pulenzas, Marko Popovic, Na Zhang, Xiaojing Zhang, Edward Chow, and Joav Merrick (Editors)
2016. ISBN: 978-1-63483-863-4 (Hardcover)
2015. ISBN: 978-1-63483-882-5 (eBook)

Cancer: Bone Metastases, CNS Metastases and Pathological Fractures
Breanne Lechner, Ronald Chow, Natalie Pulenzas, Marko Popovic, Na Zhang, Xiaojing Zhang, Edward Chow, and Joav Merrick (Editors)
2016. ISBN: 978-1-63483-949-5 (Hardcover)
2015. ISBN: 978-1-63483-960-0 (eBook)

Cancer: Spinal Cord, Lung, Breast, Cervical, Prostate, Head and Neck Cancer
Breanne Lechner, Ronald Chow, Natalie Pulenzas, Marko Popovic, Na Zhang, Xiaojing Zhang, Edward Chow and Joav Merrick (Editors)
2016. ISBN: 978-1-63483-904-4 (Hardcover)
2015. ISBN: 978-1-63483-911-2 (eBook)

Cancer: Survival, Quality of Life and Ethical Implications
Breanne Lechner, Ronald Chow, Natalie Pulenzas, Marko Popovic, Na Zhang, Xiaojing Zhang, Edward Chow and Joav Merrick (Editors)
2016. ISBN: 978-1-63483-905-1 (Hardcover)
2015. ISBN: 978-1-63483-912-9 (eBook)

Cancer: Pain and Symptom Management
Breanne Lechner, Ronald Chow, Natalie Pulenzas, Marko Popovic, Na Zhang, Xiaojing Zhang, Edward Chow, and Joav Merrick (Editors)
2016. ISBN: 978-1-63483-905-1 (Hardcover)
2015. ISBN: 978-1-63483-881-8 (eBook)

Alternative Medicine Research Yearbook 2015
Joav Merrick (Editor)
2016. ISBN: 978-1-63484-511-3 (Hardcover)
2016. ISBN: 978-1-63484-542-7 (eBook)

Public Health Yearbook 2015
Joav Merrick (Editor)
2016. ISBN: 978-1-63484-511-3 (Hardcover)
2016. ISBN: 978-1-63484-546-5 (eBook)

Quality, Mobility and Globalization in the Higher Education System: A Comparative Look at the Challenges of Academic Teaching
Nitza Davidovitch, Zehavit Gross, Yuri Ribakov, and Anna Slobodianiuk (Editors)
2016. ISBN: 978-1-63484-986-9 (Hardcover)
2016. ISBN: 978-1-63485-012-4 (eBook)

Cannabis: Medical Aspects
Blair Henry, Arnav Agarwal, Edward Chow, Hatim A. Omar, and Joav Merrick (Editors)
2017. ISBN: 978-1-53610-510-0 (Hardcover)
2017. ISBN: 978-1-53610-522-3 (eBook)

Palliative Care: Psychosocial and Ethical Considerations
Blair Henry, Arnav Agarwal, Edward Chow, and Joav Merrick (Editors)
2017. ISBN: 978-1-53610-607-7 (Hardcover)
2017. ISBN: 978-1-53610-611-4 (eBook)

Oncology: The Promising Future of Biomarkers
Anthony Furfari, George S. Charames, Rachel McDonald, Leigha Rowbottom, Azar Azad, Stephanie Chan, Bo Angela Wan, Ronald Chow, Carlo DeAngelis, Pearl Zaki, Edward Chow and Joav Merrick (Editors)
2017. ISBN: 978-1-53610-608-4 (Hardcover)
2017. ISBN: 978-1-53610-610-7 (eBook)

Pain Management Yearbook 2016
Joav Merrick (Editor)
2017. ISBN: 978-1-53610-949-8 (Hardcover)
2017. ISBN: 978-1-53610-959-7 (eBook)

Alternative Medicine Research Yearbook 2016

Joav Merrick (Editor)

2017. ISBN: 978-1-53610-972-6 (Hardcover)
2017. ISBN: 978-1-53611-000-5 (eBook)

Public Health Yearbook 2016

Joav Merrick (Editor)

2017. ISBN: 978-1-53610-947-4 (Hardcover)
2017. ISBN: 978-1-53610-956-6 (eBook)

HEALTH AND HUMAN DEVELOPMENT

PUBLIC HEALTH YEARBOOK 2016

JOAV MERRICK
EDITOR

New York

NOTICE TO THE READER

The Publisher has taken reasonable care in the preparation of this book, but makes no expressed or implied warranty of any kind and assumes no responsibility for any errors or omissions. No liability is assumed for incidental or consequential damages in connection with or arising out of information contained in this book. The Publisher shall not be liable for any special, consequential, or exemplary damages resulting, in whole or in part, from the readers' use of, or reliance upon, this material. Any parts of this book based on government reports are so indicated and copyright is claimed for those parts to the extent applicable to compilations of such works.

Independent verification should be sought for any data, advice or recommendations contained in this book. In addition, no responsibility is assumed by the publisher for any injury and/or damage to persons or property arising from any methods, products, instructions, ideas or otherwise contained in this publication.

This publication is designed to provide accurate and authoritative information with regard to the subject matter covered herein. It is sold with the clear understanding that the Publisher is not engaged in rendering legal or any other professional services. If legal or any other expert assistance is required, the services of a competent person should be sought. FROM A DECLARATION OF PARTICIPANTS JOINTLY ADOPTED BY A COMMITTEE OF THE AMERICAN BAR ASSOCIATION AND A COMMITTEE OF PUBLISHERS.

Additional color graphics may be available in the e-book version of this book.

Library of Congress Cataloging-in-Publication Data

ISBN: 978-1-53610-947-4

ISSN: 2164-716X

Published by Nova Science Publishers, Inc. † New York

CONTENTS

In: Public Health Yearbook 2016
Editor: Joav Merrick
ISBN: 978-1-53610-947-4

Chapter 1

NEIGHBORHOODS AND PUBLIC HEALTH ISSUES

Joav Merrick*, MD, MMedSc, DMSc
[1]National Institute of Child Health and Human Development, Jerusalem;
[2]Office of the Medical Director, Health Services, Division for Intellectual and Developmental Disabilities, Ministry of Social Affairs and Social Services, Jerusalem;
[3]Division of Pediatrics, Hadassah Hebrew University Medical Center, Mt Scopus Campus, Jerusalem, Israel;
[4]Kentucky Children's Hospital, University of Kentucky College of Medicine, Lexington, Kentucky, US;
[5]Center for Healthy Development, School of Public Health, Georgia State University, Atlanta, US

INTRODUCTION

Physical activity is important for a healthy lifestyle and for example parks can provide opportunities for physical activity for both children and adults in their neighborhood (1). A study in 20 neighborhood parks in Durham, North Carolina with 2,712 children and adolescents showed that the type of activity area and presence of other active children were positively associated with physical activity, while the presence of a parent was negatively associated (1). Results showed that physical activity of girls was more strongly affected by social effects (likeother active children) whereas physical activity of boys was more strongly influenced by the availability of park facilities (1).

A study from Finland of 37,699 adults looked at childhood adverse psychosocial factors and adult neighborhood disadvantage to understand if there was a link to increased cardiovascular disease (2). They found that combined exposure to high childhood adversity and high adult disadvantage was associated with cardiovascular disease risk factors (hypertension, dyslipidaemia, diabetes, obesity, smoking, heavy alcohol use and physical

* Correspondence: Professor Joav Merrick, MD, MMedSci, DMSc, Medical Director, Health Services, Division for Intellectual and Developmental Disabilities, Ministry of Social Affairs and Social Services, POBox 1260, IL-91012 Jerusalem, Israel. E-mail: jmerrick@zahav.net.il.

inactivity), while exposure to high childhood adversity or high adult neighborhood disadvantage alone was not significantly associated with cardiovascular disease (2).

Another study with 1,842 adults from Brazil looked at the local retail food environment and consumption of fruits and vegetables and sugar-sweetened beverages (3). They found that availability in neighbourhoods was associated with regular fruits and vegetables consumption, but regular fruits and vegetables consumption prevalence was significantly lower among lower-income individuals living in neighbourhoods with fewer supermarkets and fresh produce markets. A greater variety of sugar-sweetened beverages was associated with a 15% increase in regular SSB consumption.

A recent (4) study used data from the Multi-Ethnic Study of Atherosclerosis (MESA), which involve more than 6,000 men and women from six communities in the United States (New York, Baltimore, Chicago, Los Angeles, Twin Cities and Winston Salem) to look at how neighborhood environments may influence the risk for developing type 2 diabetes mellitus (T2DM). They wanted to investigate long-term exposures to neighborhood physical and social environments, availability of healthy food and physical activity resources and levels of social cohesion and safety in relationship to T2DM. During a follow-up period of about ten years of adults aged 45-84 years at baseline 616 out of 5,124 participants (12.0%) developed T2DM and the study found a lower risk for developing T2DM associated with greater cumulative exposure to indicators of neighborhood healthy food and physical activity resources (4).

The studies above are just examples of recent research interest into the interrelation between neighborhood and the effects on health (5). This relationship is complex and also very hard to research, since it is multidisciplinary and multi agency with different community development policies, urban planning, zoning and transportation policies involved.

In order to better understand the role of these environments and identify the most effective interventions in order to improve health will require partnerships between researchers, the neighborhood communities and policy makers.

REFERENCES

[1] Bocarro JN, Floyd MF, Smith WR, Edwards MB, Schultz CL, Baran P, et al. Social and environmental factors related to boys' and girls' park-based physical activity. Prev Chronic Dis 2015 Jun 18;12:E97. Doi: 10.5888/pcd12.140532.

[2] Halonen JI, Stenholm S, Pentti J, Kawachi I, Subramanian SV, Kivimäki M, et al. Childhood psychosocial adversity and adult neighborhood disadvantage as predictors of cardiovascular disease: A cohort study. Circulation 2015 Jun 11. pii: CIRCULATIONAHA.115.015392 [Epub ahead of print].

[3] Duran AC, de Almeida SL, Latorre MD, Jaime PC. The role of the local retail food environment in fruit, vegetable and sugar-sweetened beverage consumption in Brazil. Public Health Nutr 2015 Jun 9:1-10 [Epub ahead of print].

[4] Christine PJ, Auchincloss AH, Bertoni AG, Carnethon MR, Sanchez BN, Moore K, et al. Longitudinal associations between neighborhood physical and social environments and incident type 2 diabetes mellitus: The Multi-Ethnic Study of Atherosclerosis (MESA). JAMA Intern Med 2015 Jun 29. Doi: 10.1001/jamainternmed.2015.2691 [Epub ahead of print].

[5] Diez-Roux AV. Neighborhoods and health: Where are we and were do we go from here? Rev Epidemiol Sante Publique 2007;55(1):13-21.

SECTION ONE - EPIDEMIOLOGY OF ARBOVIRUSES IN ZAMBIA

In: Public Health Yearbook 2016
Editor: Joav Merrick

ISBN: 978-1-53610-947-4

Chapter 2

DISTRIBUTION OF ARBOVIRUSES AND THEIR CORRELATES IN NORTH-WESTERN AND WESTERN PROVINCES OF ZAMBIA: A SYNTHESIS OF PAPERS FROM A 2013 YELLOW FEVER RISK ASSESSMENT SURVEY

***Mazyanga L Mazaba-Liwewe*[1,2,*], *BSc*,**
***Olusegun Babaniyi*[1], *MBBS, MPH, MSc*,**
***Freddie Masaninga*[1], *BSc, MSc, PhD*,**
***Peter Songolo*[1], *MBChB, MPH*,**
Idah Mweene-Ndumba*[1,2], *BSc, MPH
and Seter Siziya*[3,4], *BA(Ed), MSc, PhD
[1]World Health Organization, Lusaka, Zambia
[2]University Teaching Hospital, Lusaka, Zambia
[3]School of Medicine, Copperbelt University, Ndola, Zambia
[4]University of Lusaka, Lusaka, Zambia

ABSTRACT

Arboviruses have caused wide-spread morbidity in sub-Saharan Africa and worldwide. The objective was to present a synthesis of the findings on arboviruses infections determined from a 2013 yellow fever risk assessment survey conducted in North-Western and Western provinces of Zambia. We reviewed published and unpublished papers on prevalence and correlates for arboviruses. Prevalence rates for arboviruses infections were 10.3% for West Nile, 6.0% for Zika, 4.1% for dengue, 0.5% for yellow fever and 11.5% for any arbovirus infection. Persons aged less than 5 years were 63% less likely to have infection compared to persons aged 45 years or older. In-door residual spraying was

[*] Correspondence: Mazyanga L Mazaba, EPI Unit, World Health Organization, Lusaka, Zambia and Virology Unit, University Teaching Hospital, Lusaka, Zambia. E-mail: mazmazli@yahoo.com.

associated with reduced risk for West Nile or Zika viruses infections. Visiting Angola was significantly associated with increased risk for dengue, West Nile and Zika arboviruses infections. Respondents living in grass roofed houses were 2-3 times more likely to have any of the infections compared to those living in houses with asbestos roofs. A total of 1401 adult mosquitoes were collected comprising 28.9% Aedes, 37.0% Anopheles, 471 (33.6%) Culex and 71 (5.1%) Mansonia. The factors: roof type and visiting Angola in addition to arbovirus-specific infection correlates should be considered in developing interventions to control them in North-Western and Western provinces of Zambia.

Keywords: arboviruses, yellow fever, dengue, Zika, West Nile, North-Western and Western provinces, Zambia

INTRODUCTION

Recently the following arboviruses were identified in Zambia: Yellow fever (1), dengue (2), West Nile (Mweene-Ndumba et al., unpublished) and Zika (Babaniyi et al., unpublished). These viruses, all among the group B of arboviruses under the genus Flavivirus, have caused wide-spread morbidity in sub-Saharan Africa and worldwide (3).

Yellow fever

Yellow fever known to occur commonly in certain parts of Africa and South America but absent in Asia (4) is caused by yellow fever virus. It is unclear why yellow fever does not occur in Asia. The typical symptoms in yellow fever infected persons include fever, muscle pains, headache, nausea and vomiting from the third to sixth day of infection. Although up-to 85% of illnesses resolve at this stage, others progress to a severe disease following a brief 2-24 hour remission of symptoms. The symptoms in severe disease include nausea, vomiting, epigastric pain, renal failure, jaundice and haemorrhaging. At this stage of the disease about half of patients die within 10–14 days, and those who survive develop immunity for the rest of their lives (5). There is no cure for yellow fever (6). However, there is an effective vaccine for the prevention of yellow fever (7). About 200 000 people are infected with yellow fever annually in the tropics of Africa and South America (4) and causes about 30 000 deaths each year (8).

Dengue

Dengue virus is the cause of dengue disease. The World Health Organization documents existence of 4 serotypes of dengue virus. Infection by one serotype allows lifelong immunity to only the specific infecting serotype. Re-infection with another serotype can occur and lead to dengue haemorrhagic fever (9). Although, dengue virus infection is often unapparent (10), signs and symptoms for dengue virus infection vary from mild, non-specific symptoms to classic dengue fever, with high fevers and severe arthralgia. The non-specific symptoms include fever, nausea/vomiting, rash, aches and pains, abdominal pain or tenderness, persistent vomiting, clinical fluid accumulation, mucosal bleed, lethargy/restlessness, liver enlargement of 2 cm or more and increase in HCT concurrent with rapid decrease in platelet count. Symptoms associated with severe dengue include severe plasma leakage leading to dengue shock syndrome, fluid accumulation with respiratory distress, bleeding and organ (such as liver, Central Nervous System and heart) involvement (11). About 1–5% of the patients will die if not adequately attended to and less than 1% of the patients will die if adequately clinically managed (12). However, 26% of the severely ill patients will die (13). There is no cure for dengue fever. However, symptomatic treatment can reduce mortality from DHF to less than 1% (14). Dengue vaccine is not available for use (15), although a vaccine trial is underway (16). Dengue disease is globally distributed in both endemic and epidemic transmission cycles. Bhatt et al., (17) estimated that of the 96 million dengue infections globally in 2010, 70% of them were from Asia, 14% from the Americas and 16% from Africa (18-20).

West Nile virus

About 20% of the people who become infected with West Nile virus do not develop any symptoms (21). Those who develop symptoms will have headache, body aches, joint pains, vomiting, diarrhea and rash. Most people with this type of West Nile virus disease recover completely, but fatigue and weakness can last for weeks or months. In its severe form, patients will develop a serious neurologic illness whose symptoms include headache, high fever, neck stiffness, disorientation, coma, tremors, seizures or paralysis. About 10% of people who develop neurologic infection will die (22). There is no treatment or vaccine for West Nile virus infection (23). However, vaccine development is underway (24). West Nile virus infection is the most wide spread flavivirus, covering Africa, Europe, Asia, Australia (Kunjin), North and South America (25).

Zika

The symptoms for Zika virus infection that were based on a limited number of case reports and outbreak investigations (26, 27) are acute onset of fever, non-purulent conjunctivitis, headache, arthralgia, myalgia, asthenia, rash (in general maculo-papular) and, less frequently, retro-orbital pain, anorexia, vomiting, diarrhea and abdominal pain. In the literature, Zika is described as a mild, self-limiting febrile illness lasting 28 days without severe complications, no fatalities and a low hospitalisation rate (28, 29). In a well investigated, 2007 Zika virus infection outbreak on Yap Island in the Federated States of Micronesia (29) the common symptoms were rash, fever, arthralgia and conjunctivitis. The other symptoms were included myalgia, headache and retro-orbital pain. There is no specific anti-viral treatment for Zika virus infection and there is no vaccine (26). Zika virus infection has been reported in Africa (Nigeria, Sierra Leone, Ivory Coast, Cameroon, Senegal, Central Africa Republic, Uganda (26) and Kenya (30) and in Asia (Malaysia, Pakistan, Cambodia, Thailand, Indonesia, French Polynesia and Federated States of Micronesia (27).

Vectors

The vectors for yellow fever include Aedes africanus (in Africa) or Haemagogus species (in the Americas) (31, 32), Aedes simpsoni and Aedes albopictus (33). Yellow fever virus is primarily transmitted by Aedes (Stegomyia) aegypti and Aedes (Stegomyia) africanus (34). Dengue virus is transmitted between people by mosquito species Aedes aegypti and Aedes albopictus (35). The main vector associated with Dengue virus is Aedes aegypti (36). West Nile virus (WNV) is transmitted through the bites of infective Culex mosquitoes (37-39). Zika virus is spread by the Aedes species of mosquito including the Aedes aegypti mosquito (40). In summary, Aedes aegypti is the main vector for yellow fever, dengue and Zika viruses, while Culex mosquitoes is a vector for West Nile virus.

The objectives for this study is to present a synthesis of the findings from a yellow fever risk assessment in terms of the prevalence rates for the arboviruses and factors associated with the infections.

METHODS

Studies on arboviruses in Zambia were based on a cross sectional survey conducted in 2013 for yellow fever risk assessment.

Study site

Zambia was administratively, divided into ten provinces. Each province was in turn subdivided into districts. Each district was further subdivided into constituencies and wards. For statistical purposes each ward was subdivided into Census Supervisory Areas (CSAs) and these were in turn subdivided into Standard Enumeration Areas (SEAs). The 2008-2010 census mapping exercise in preparation for the 2010 census of population and housing, demarcated the CSAs within wards, wards within constituencies and constituencies within districts. In total, at the time of constructing the 2010 census frame, Zambia had 74 districts, 150 constituencies, 1,421 wards. Wards were further divided into Census Supervisory Areas (CSAs), which were in turn divided into Standard Enumeration Areas (SEAs). The SEAs were also stratified by urban and rural strata. The listing of SEAs had information on number of households and the population.

The study sites, North-Western and Western provinces (see Figure 1), were conveniently selected being the provinces that were classified as areas of low potential risk of Yellow fever. Western province borders with Angola. Western province had 7 districts with a total of 1,902 SEAs. Fishing was the main occupation in the province. The population of the province was 854,890 (41). Meanwhile, North-Western province had borders with Angola in the west and DR Congo in the north. A total of 1,178 SEAs had been demarcated in North-Western province in the 6 districts of the province. Peasantry farming (mainly cultivating maize, cotton and groundnuts) was the major economic activity in North-Western province. It had a population of 695,599 (41).

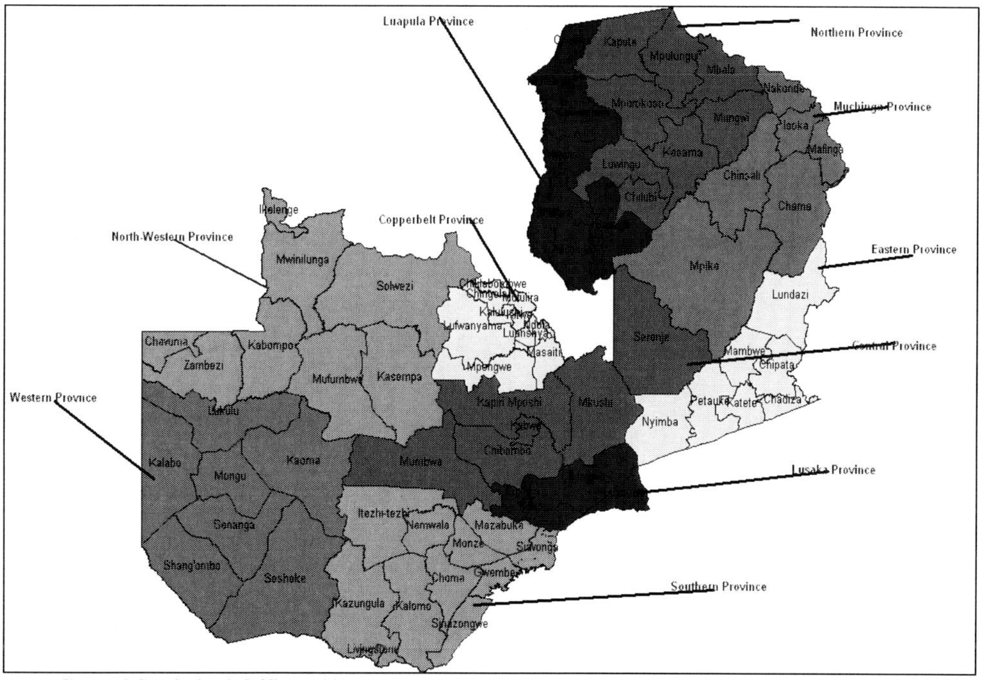

Source: Central Statistical Office (40).

Figure 1. Map of Zambia showing the locations of provinces and districts.

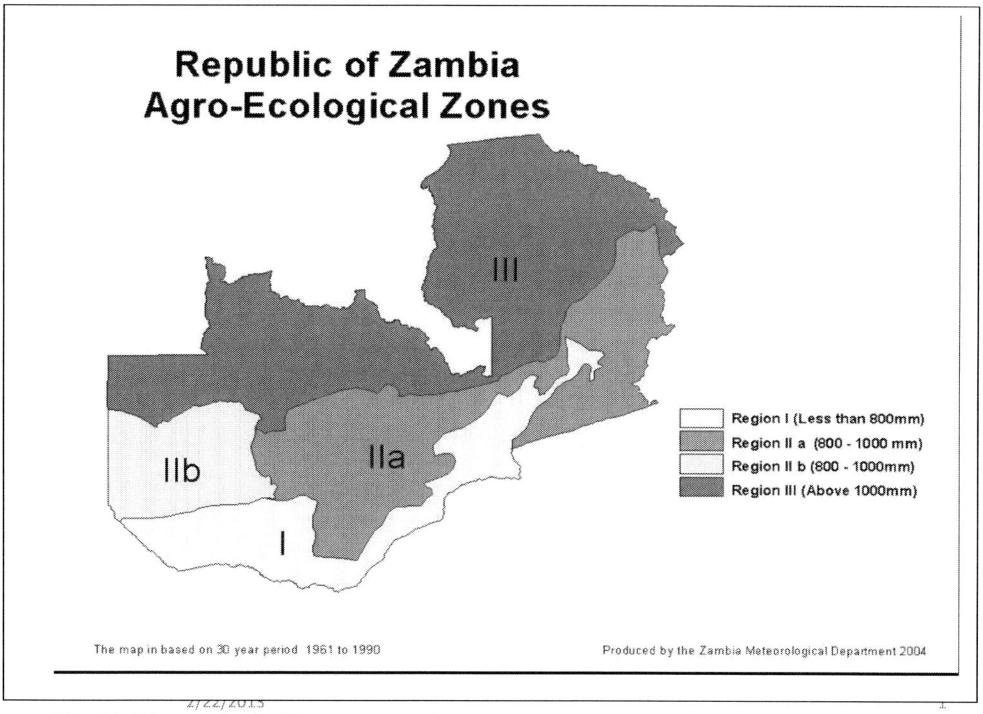

Source: Zambia Meteorological Department (41).

Figure 2. Agro-ecological zones in Zambia.

The study area was divided into three main agro ecological zones (42) that were classified based mainly on the rainfall patterns. Zone I was characterized by low rainfall, short growing season, high temperatures during the growing season, and a high risk of drought. Zone III was characterized by high rainfall, long growing season, low probability of drought, and cooler temperatures during the growing season. Zone II fell in between Zones I and III for most climatic variables. There were great variations in the agro-ecological features (rainfall, elevation, mean temperatures, vegetation and soils) of the three zones and within zones themselves. The location of the ecological zones is shown Figure 2. Agro-ecological Zone I covered the Northern part of the country, Zone III was furthest South and Zone II was intermediate between zones I and III. Our study area was covered by Agro-ecological Zones I, IIb and III.

In a demographic health survey, Central Statistical Office et al., (43) reported that 46.9 and 53.2% of the population slept under an insecticide treated net in the previous night to the survey in Western and North-Western Provinces respectively.

Human seroprevalence study

Study population

This assessment was carried out among individuals aged nine months or older located within households sampled in the selected study sites.

Sample size, inclusion/exclusion criteria and sampling

Sample size

The sample size calculation was based on the assumption that the seroprevalence was 7% based on the study conducted by Robinson (44). In order to design an efficient study to compare the findings with those obtained in that study, the sample size for the current proposed study was comparable to the sample size done by Robinson (44).

Persons aged 5 years or older

In estimating the sample size for persons aged 5 years or older, the following parameters were considered: a prevalence of 7%, desired precision or confidence interval (d) of $\pm 3\%$, and a design effect (DE) of 2 and an 80% response rate.

$$n_{min} = 2 \times \frac{1.96^2 \times 7 \times (100 - 7)}{3^2} = 556$$

and applying the response rate $n_{min} = 556/0.8 = 695$.

Considering sex, we aimed to recruit 700 male and 700 female participants in each province. Assuming an average of 4 persons aged 5 years or older in each household, a total of 12 households in each of the 30 cluster was to be recruited in the survey. The total number of persons that would be recruited from each province was 1,806, totaling 3,612 from both provinces.

Persons under the age of 5 years

The seroprevalence of children was about half that for older children, and in estimating the sample size for persons aged below 5 years, the following parameters were considered: a prevalence of 3.5%, desired precision or confidence interval (d) of ±3.4%, and a design effect (DE) of 2 and an 80% response rate.

The total number of persons aged less than 5 years that would be surveyed was computed as follows:

$$\text{Formula: } n_{min} = DE \times \frac{Z^2 \times p \times (1-p)}{d^2}$$

where Z = 1.96

$$n_{min} = 2 \times \frac{1.96^2 \times 3.5 \times (100 - 3.5)}{3.4^2} = 225$$

and applying the response rate $n_{min} = 225/0.8 = 282$. Therefore, in each province 406 children would be recruited for the survey.

Inclusion/exclusion criteria

Any individual aged 9 months or older and who was a member of a sampled household and resident in the study site for at least seven days. Individuals who received yellow fever vaccination in the last ten years would be eligible to participate in the survey.

Any person, who was either less than 9 months of age, or any person regardless of age, who resided in the study site for a period of less than seven days prior to the survey was excluded from the study. Determining the seroprevalence in children under the age of nine months raises the risk of false positive results as children under this age may still carry maternal antibodies from immunized or exposed mothers.

Sampling

The sample was drawn using a two-stage cluster sampling technique using probability proportional to size. A list of SEAs in each province constituted the sampling frame. The sampling was designed to achieve fairly good estimates at the provincial level of analysis, and not representing the subdivisions of the province.

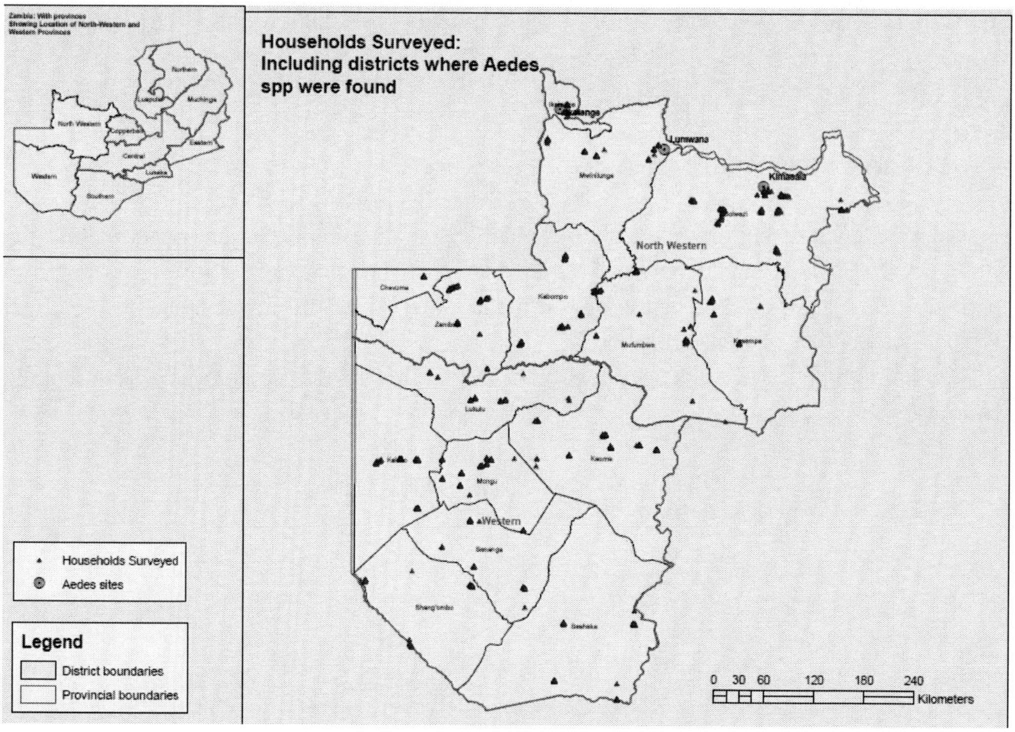

Figure 3. Distribution of surveyed households.

First stage selection

At the first sampling stage, the sampled SEAs were selected with probability to size (PPS) from the ordered list of SEAs on the census 2010 sampling frame. The measure of size for each SEA was based on the household size identified in the 2010 Census (41). In order to ensure representation from all administrative areas, the frame was sorted by district, constituency, region, CSA and SEA.

Second stage selection

In each selected cluster, the first household that was selected was located in the middle of the cluster. The direction that followed from the middle of the cluster was selected at random. The remaining participants were selected in that direction. If the number of participants was not met, the team got back to the middle of the cluster and selected a direction at random and went in that direction until the required number of participants was surveyed. Figure 3 shows the distribution of the surveyed households.

Study variables

Dependent variables

A case with evidence of yellow fever exposure was defined as any individual aged 9 months or older whose blood sample was confirmed to have yellow fever exposure through any of the following: Detection of yellow fever virus-specific IgG and IgM antibodies with yellow fever virus-specific neutralizing antibodies at least four-fold higher than neutralizing antibodies against other flaviviruses. Yellow fever exposure status was therefore determined by way of laboratory testing as 'positive' for a respondent with laboratory evidence of yellow fever exposure or as 'negative' for a respondent who did not have laboratory evidence of yellow fever exposure or as "indeterminate" for a respondent with a less than a four-fold difference in titters between yellow fever and other flaviviruses.

Independent variables

The independent variables included demographic data: age, sex, occupation, history and time of yellow fever vaccination, and use of mosquito preventive measures. For the purposes of the sero-survey, a vaccinated person against yellow fever was defined as a person with a valid yellow fever vaccination certificate.

Laboratory procedure

Each study participant was assigned a study number and the corresponding blood sample was labeled with the same study number. The study number was linked to the laboratory result and questionnaire. About 3 to 5 millilitres of blood was collected from each participant by venepuncture and collected in an EDTA tube (see Figure 4). The samples were transported to a field laboratory on ice, where plasma was separated into labelled cryovials (see Figure 5). At the close of the field work, the samples were transported to the University Teaching Hospital Virology Laboratory (UTHVL) for testing.

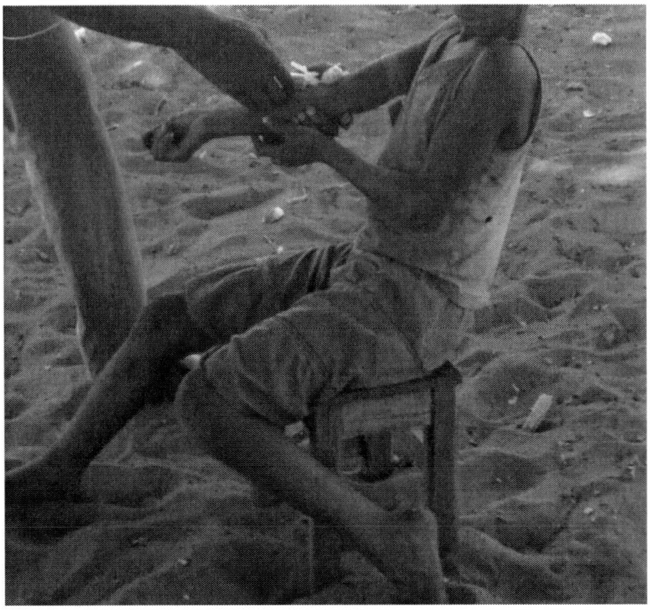

Figure 4. Blood collection from a participant by venepuncture.

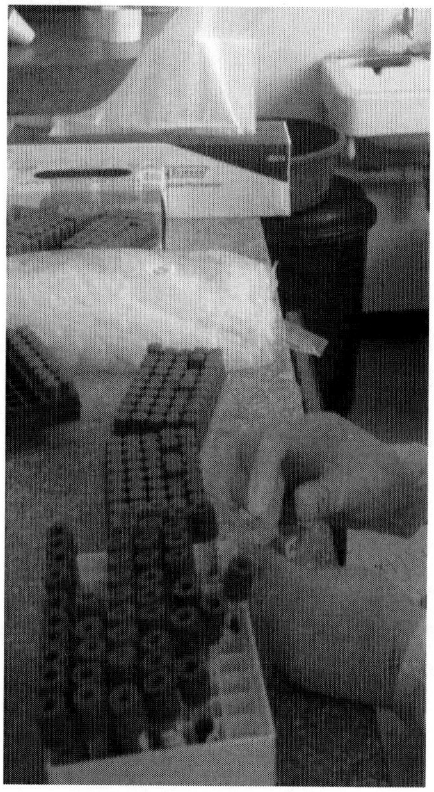

Figure 5. Separation of plasma into labelled cryovials.

Each plasma sample was tested for both yellow fever virus-specific IgG and IgM antibodies by the ELISA method described in the (45) at the UTHVL. All yellow fever virus IgG positive and IgM positive specimens were referred to the Institute Pasteur in Dakar, Senegal which serves as the World Health Organization Africa region reference laboratory for yellow fever. In Dakar, the specimens were subjected to repeat yellow fever virus-specific IgG and IgM Enzyme Linked Immunoassay (ELISA) testing in order to reconfirm the primary results. They were also assessed for IgG and IgM antibodies against other flaviviruses known to cause haemorrhagic fever-like disease including Dengue, Zika and West Nile viruses that are also known to elicit cross-reactivity in antibody ELISA tests. All samples giving a yellow fever virus-specific antibody positive result either in Lusaka or Dakar, were analysed for yellow fever virus neutralising antibodies by Plaque Reduction Neutralisation Testing (PRNT) using standard methods.

Interpretation of laboratory results

Participants with PRNT titres ≥1:10 were considered as being yellow fever seropositive, while those having PRNT titres ≥1:20 were considered to have seroprotective levels of antibodies against yellow fever virus either through natural infection or through vaccination. Those participants who were found to have Immunoglobulin (Ig) M or G antibodies to dengue, West Nile and Zika viruses were considered as having had the respective diseases.

Data collection and quality control

A detailed semi structured questionnaire was used to collect information. The questionnaires were pre-tested to validate the appropriateness of the questions to capture the required information. During the data collection process, questionnaires were checked for inconsistencies and completeness on a daily basis. All data were entered in an Epi-Info data entry screen that had consistency and range checks embedded in it. Further editing was conducted by running frequencies during the analysis stage. Epi data files were exported to SPSS for data analysis.

Data analysis

The data was summarized to describe the occurrence of arboviruses infected individuals in absolute numbers and percentage by place (residence, travel or work) and person (age, sex, occupation). Further analysis was conducted to determine independent factors associated with arboviruses seropositivity. Odds ratios were used to estimate the magnitude of associations.

Ethical considerations in the human seroprevalence study

Ethical clearance was sought from the Tropical Diseases Research Centre Research Ethics Committee, and ethical standards were adhered to throughout this study. Information obtained from the study participants was treated as confidential through the use of anonymous identifiers and restricting the access to collected data only to people directly involved in the study. Respondents were provided with information on possible study risks, for example pain and swelling at the venous-puncture site. In addition information on study benefits like: providing information on yellow fever and its prevention was also provided. Further, the collective benefit of the study of informing the national yellow fever policy was highlighted to the study participants. Informed consent was sought from study participants. Guardians provided assent for the participation of persons under the consenting age. They were asked to read or have read to them, understand and sign/thumbprint an informed consent form. Responsible adults in the household were identified to give proxy consent on behalf of minors. Study participants were informed that their individual test results were not to be relayed to them since the results were not linked to individual participants due to use of unique identifiers and in addition, past exposure to YF carries no future risk.

Socio-mobilisation and community engagement

Before data and specimen collection in any cluster, the community leaders and members were engaged to explain the nature and intention of the study (see Figure 6). It was emphasized that participation was voluntary.

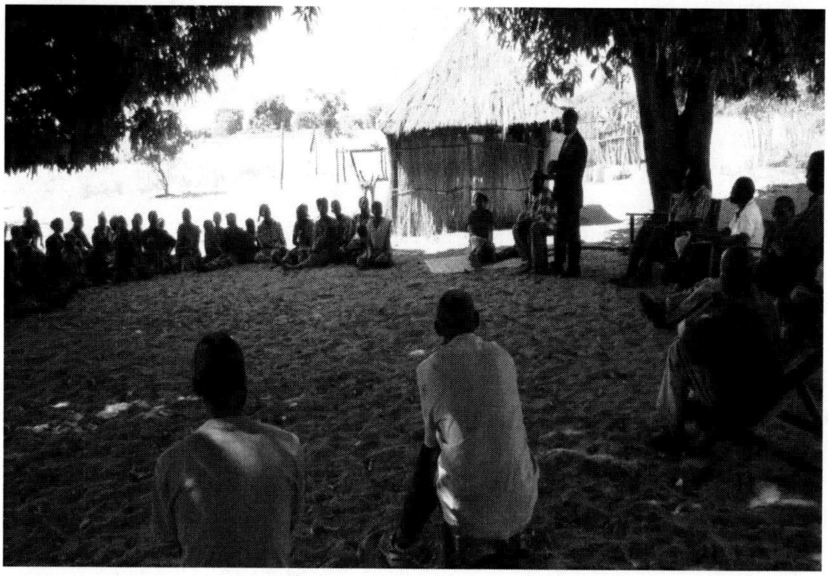

Figure 6. Social mobilization and community engagement.

Mosquitoes study

All three agro-ecological zones were considered for mosquito sampling. Each zone had unique features which affected the types and abundance of mosquitoes present. Attempts were made to collect mosquitoes in all zones with a preference for collecting mosquitoes from at least two distinct areas within each zone. Mosquitoes were identified and sorted in mono-specific batch and, if appropriate, tested for the presence of yellow fever virus by RT-PCR. In addition to sampling adult mosquitoes, larvae was sampled especially in urban centers but also in forested and intermediate areas to the towns, in order to identify more clearly the types of mosquito species in the environment.

Sample size and sampling in the mosquito survey

Attempts were made to collect mosquitoes in all zones since each selected zone contained unique features that could affect types and abundance of mosquitoes present in the area. Eight sampling sites from each province were selected. Adult and larval forms of mosquitoes were sampled in various sites in urban and peri-urban, forest and along plains and on island of the study areas in order to identify the types of mosquito species that occurred in the sampled areas. In order to obtain current information on the level of yellow fever viral circulation in the selected provinces, different sampling techniques were used to sample the mosquito populations. Mosquitoes were sampled around all the 12 selected households in the human survey in each Cluster.

Adult mosquito sampling

Adult mosquitoes were sampled by three groups of researchers (three to four persons per team), who were vaccinated against yellow fever virus and received prior chemoprophylaxis against malaria. Sampling methods that were used were backpack aspirators, aspiration using a mouth aspirator tube, CDC light trap and the Gravid Light traps. Mosquito collections were made inside and outside households.

Indoor adult: Resting mosquitoes were collected by an aspirator (back pack or the use of a mouth aspirator tube) using a torch to locate them. Knockdown spray catch with a pyrethroids insecticide in randomly selected dwellings were also done commencing at 06.00 hours.

Outdoor: Mosquitoes were captured using backpack aspirator; CDC light trap and Gravid light trap for collecting gravid (egg-laying) females to increase the chance for virus isolation. Sampling outdoor with back pack aspirator was done between 16.00 and 19.00 hours.

Larvae/pupae sampling

Larval sampling was done in selected premises in each locality visited. Containers holding water located outside (such as the ones displayed in Figure 7) and inside households (domestic and peri-domestic) were inspected for larvae/pupae in each cluster visited in order to estimate risk indices.

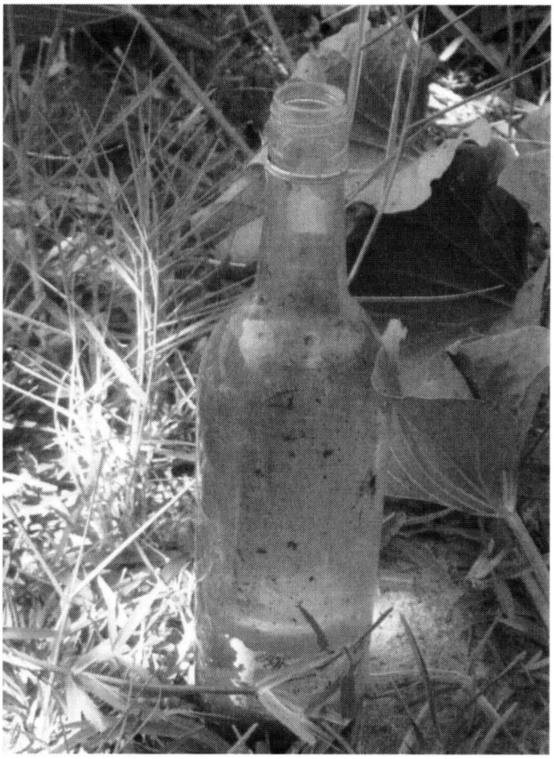

Figure 7. Containers holding water located outside house.

Scoops were used to collect/transfer mosquito larvae from large water bodies onto white trays (see Figure 8) from where larvae were pipetted into bottles labelled with information on date, province, cluster name, site of collection in order to identify the source of the larvae. In the domestic environment, artificial and natural mosquito breeding site were inspected.

An attempt was made to count larvae and pupae in each container found positive to estimate absolute population density per habitation unit. Larvae were counted directly for small quantity and estimated using a correlation between the mean number of larvae in deeper and the total volume of the water in the container.

Specific entomological activities conducted in the assessment

Containers with at least one larva or pupa were considered as positive and these larvae were sent to the insectary at the Tropical Diseases Research Centre for rearing and identification of the emerging adult stages. Samples reared in the insectary allowed an estimation of the population sex ratio and the density of mosquito females in relation to human population density. The following observations were made: (a) Mosquito species breeding inside/outside houses, (b) The proximity of the houses to potential vector breeding sites i.e., how far the houses were located from forests/woodlands, or any plantations where vectors could be breeding, (c) Eggs of any possible vectors breeding in the vicinity of houses and also in forests/woodlands/plantations, (d) Adult mosquitoes resting in vegetation around houses and at the periphery of woodlands/forests and in plantations, (e) Adult mosquitoes flying in the evening, dawn and at night in and outside households and in woodlands/forests and (f) Any possible animals that could serve as reservoirs of yellow fever virus.

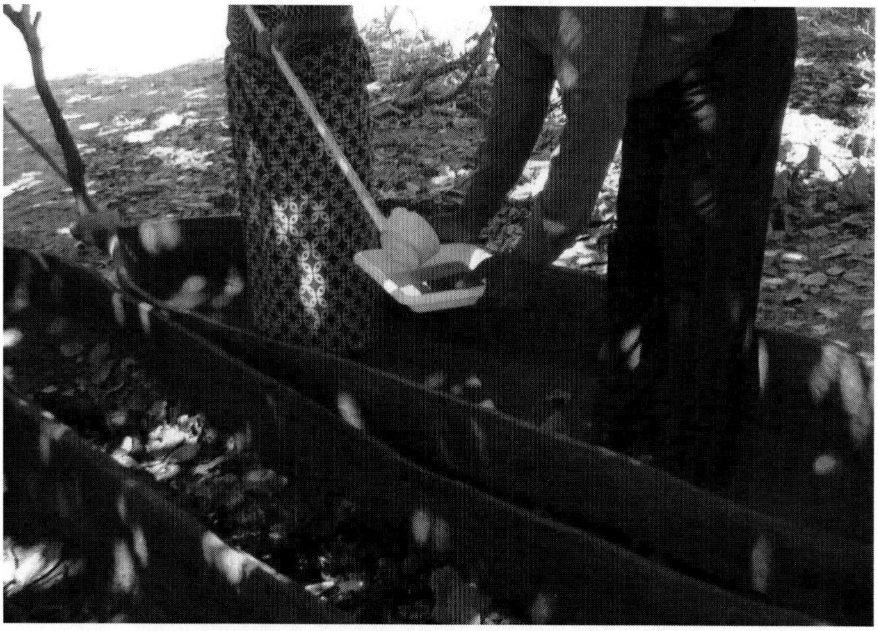

Figure 8. Scooping mosquito larvae from large water bodies onto white trays.

Investigating viral infection in yellow fever mosquito vectors

Assessment of mosquitoes involved the determination of mosquito species around the selected 12 households per cluster in the same households where human survey was conducted. A record was kept of each mosquito in order to determine overall number of each species captured. Special focus was placed on mosquitoes involved in yellow fever viral transmission. Sixty adult Aedes species mosquitoes were airfreighted at -80°Con dry ice to Institute Pasteur in Dakar, Senegal to test for the presence of yellow fever virus by Reverse Transcriptase Polymerase Chain reaction technique.

Sample treatment, processing and testing for yellow fever mosquito vectors

Mosquito species collected as either larvae or pupae were reared to the adult stage and identified using various morphological keys. This meant that larvae and pupae collected in the field were kept at least for 4-6 days to obtain emerging adults. All adult mosquitoes collected from the field were sorted and pooled according to the selected clusters, sex and stored in liquid nitrogen. Adult mosquitoes emerging from the larvae/pupa were sorted accordingly and stored at -80°C until virological tests were completed. For testing of mosquitoes for yellow fever virus, similar species identified were chilled and pooled in maximum 10 mosquitoes per vial and sent to Institute Dakar where they were analysed.

Questionnaire of indoor residual spraying

The human seroprevalence questionnaire contained two questions related to vector control: "Have you slept under a mosquito net the past two weeks?" and "Has your house been sprayed just before the current rainy season?"

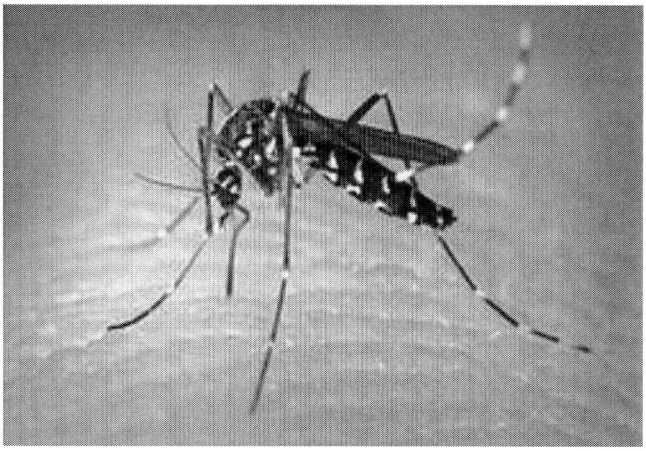

Figure 9. Aedes species.

Training

Training of field staff was conducted in Ndola in Copperbelt province for a week before the commencement of the main study in North-Western and Western Provinces. The training was facilitated by epidemiologists and medical entomologists, experts from the World health Organisation and Inter-Country Support Team (IST) Harare, Zimbabwe, WHO country office/Zambia, Tropical Diseases Research Centre and Institute Pasteur of Dakar, Senegal facilitated through IST/West Africa.

Entomologic data management and analysis

Vector identification was done using entomological keys (46). Data were stored in Excel software. To assess the entomological epidemic potential of yellow fever disease in Zambia in each selected site we calculated Aedes aegypti (Figure 9) larval density or Breteau index (BI) in domestic environments. The BI (% container positive with larvae/habitation unit) was an indirect measure of vector density which helps to infer an epidemic risk (BI > 5% indicates epidemic risk). We calculated House Index (HI) and Cluster Index (CI). The parameter of container index, which is the percentage of containers where larvae were found, was used to find out the presence of disease-causing mosquitoes. Container index above 10% was considered high and problematic.

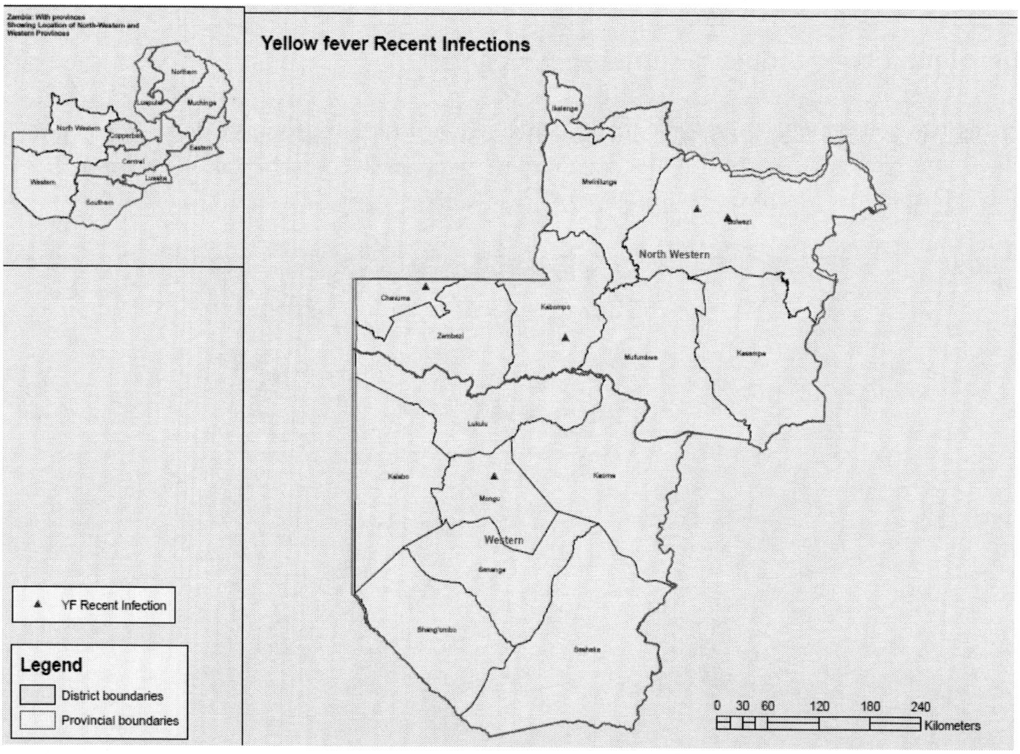

Figure 10. Distribution of recent yellow fever virus infection.

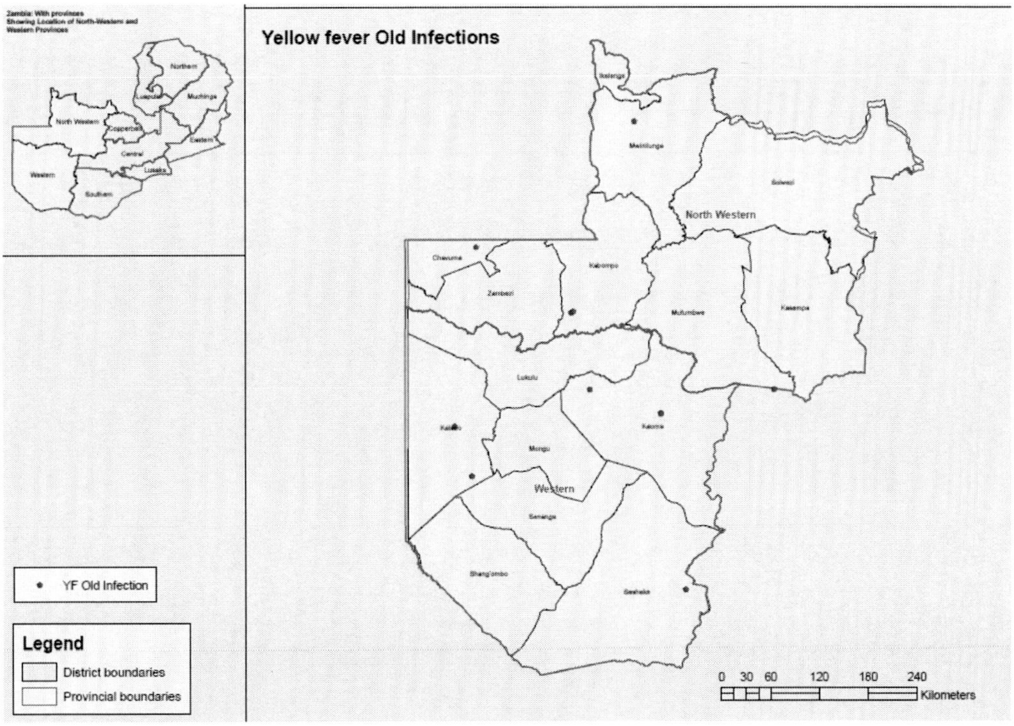

Figure 11. Distribution of old yellow fever virus infection.

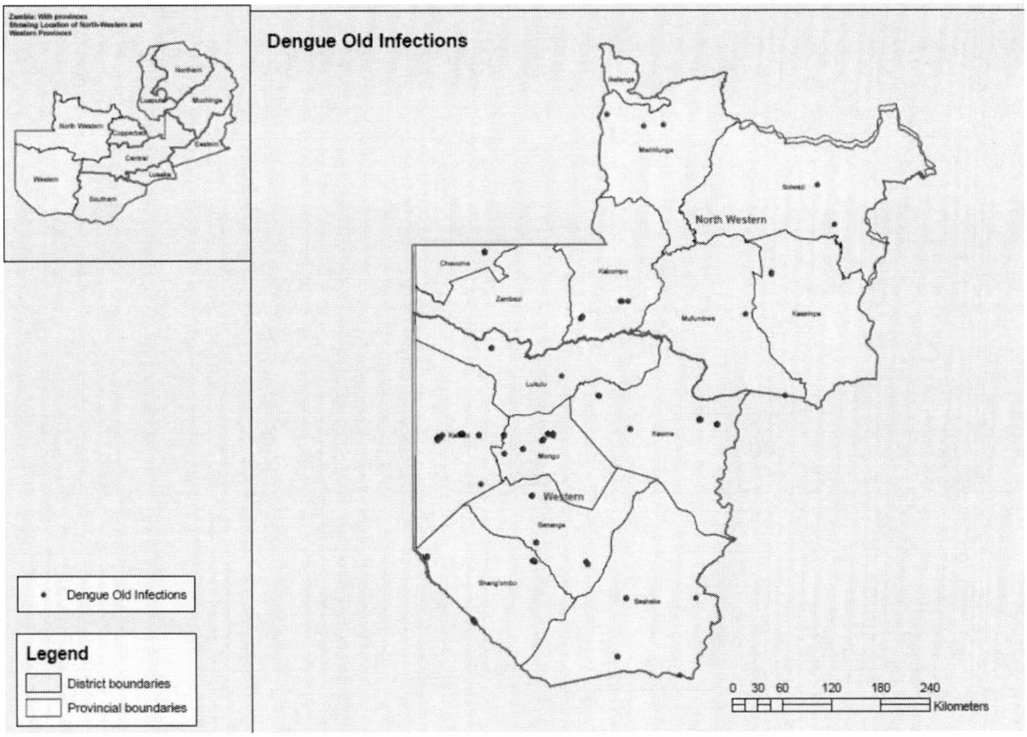

Figure 12. Distribution of old dengue virus infection.

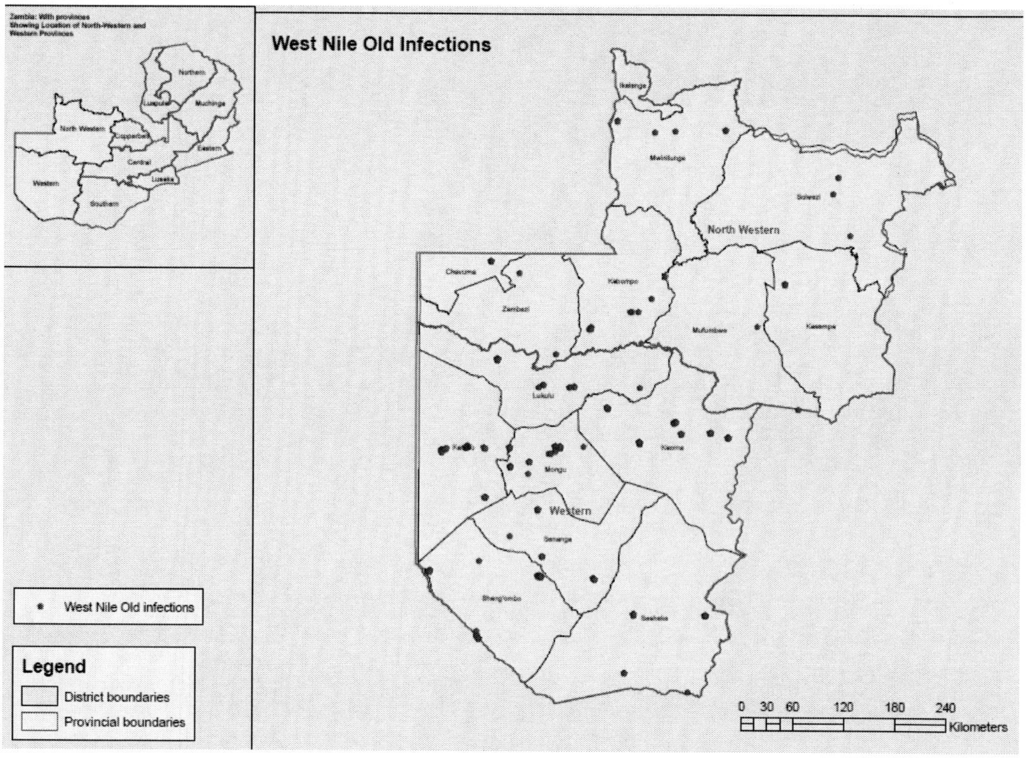

Figure 13. Distribution of old West Nile virus infection.

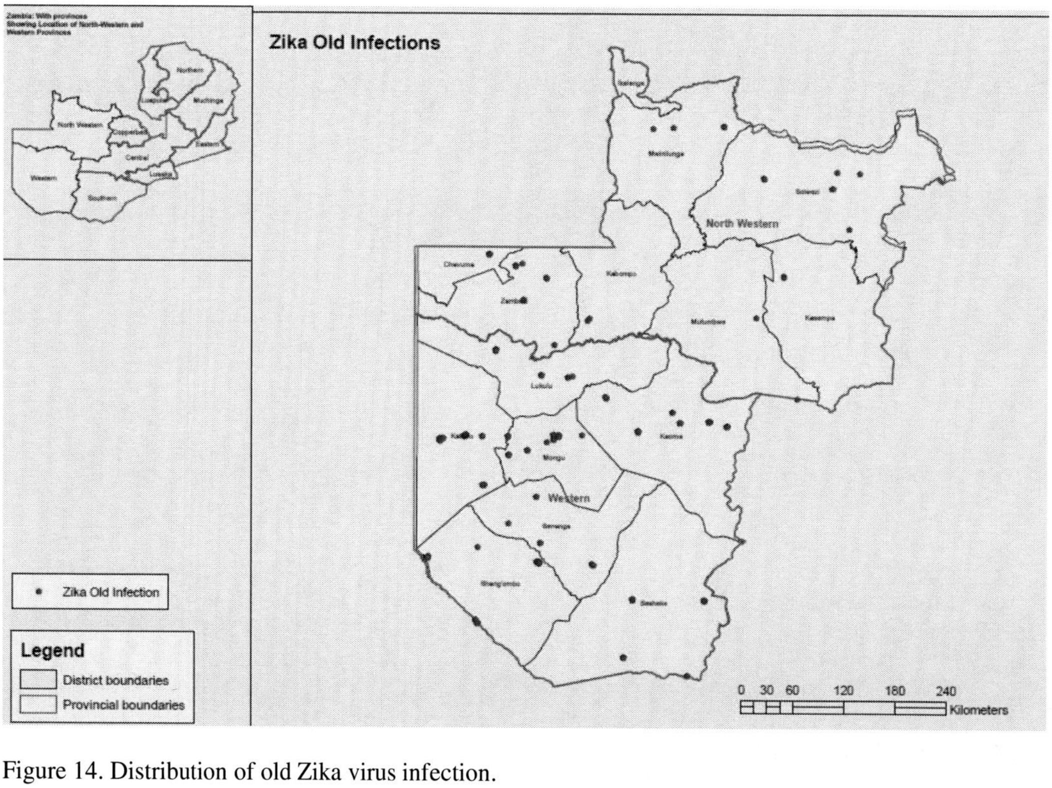

Figure 14. Distribution of old Zika virus infection.

Ethical considerations for sampling mosquitoes

Ethical clearance to conduct the survey was granted by the Tropical Diseases Research Centre, Research Ethics Committee. Ethical standards were adhered to throughout this study. All team members involved with the mosquito survey and collection were trained and vaccinated against yellow fever and had prophylactic anti-malarials according to national guidelines. Oral informed consent was obtained from heads of the households in which larval and adult mosquito collection was undertaken. Also, consent was obtained from field collectors participating in entomological assessment. Thus, written informed consent was obtained from all team members and local personnel involved in the mosquito survey and collection.

Table 1. Prevalence of arboviruses in North-Western and Western provinces in Zambia

Arboviruses	Total n (%)	Male n (%)	Female n (%)	p value
Yellow fever virus new infections				
Yes	6 (0.2)	4 (0.2)	2 (0.1)	0.427
No	3618 (99.8)	1665 (99.8)	1899 (99.9)	
Yellow fever virus old infections				
Yes	12 (0.3)	8 (0.5)	4 (0.2)	0.246
No	3612 (99.7)	1661 (99.5)	1897 (99.8)	
Prevalence of yellow fever virus infection	**18 (0.5)**	**12 (0.7)**	**6 (0.3)**	**0.101**
Total	3624	1669	1901	
Dengue new infections				
Yes	0 (0)	0 (0)	0(0)	-
No	3624 (100)	1668 (100)	1902 (100)	
Dengue old infections				
Yes	149 (4.1)	69 (4.1)	78 (4.1)	1.000
No	3475 (95.9)	1599 (95.9)	1824 (95.9)	
Prevalence of dengue virus infection	**149 (4.1)**	**69 (4.1)**	**78 (4.1)**	**1.000**
Total	3624	1668	1902	
Total				
West Nile new infections				
Yes	2 (0.1)	2 (0.1)	0 (0)	0.218
No	3623 (99.9)	1667 (99.9)	1902 (100)	
West Nile old infections				
Yes	370 (10.2)	174 (10.4)	195 (10.3)	0.909
No	3255 (89.8)	1495 (89.6)	1707 (89.7)	
Prevalence of West Nile virus infection	**372 (10.3)**	**176 (10.5)**	**195 (10.3)**	**0.817**
Total	3625	1669	1902	
Zika new infections				
Yes	0 (0)	0 (0)	0 (0)	-
No	3625 (100)	1669 (100)	1902 (100)	
Zika old infections				
Yes	217 (6.0)	100 (6.0)	116 (6.1)	0.893
No	3408 (94.0)	1569 (100)	1786 (93.9)	
Prevalence of Zika virus infection	**217 (6.0)**	**100 (6.0)**	**116 (6.1)**	**0.893**
Total	3408 (94.0)	1669	1902	

Table 2. Prevalence rates for combinations of arboviruses in North-Western and Western provinces of Zambia

Combinations of arboviruses*	Positive n (%)
0	3206 (88.5)
1	184 (5.1)
2	132 (3.6)
3	96 (2.6)
4	5 (0.1)

* Combinations were for Yellow fever, Dengue, West Nile and Zika viruses.

RESULTS

The most common arboviruses infections were West Nile (10.3%) and Zika virus infection (6.0%). The prevalence for dengue virus infection was 4.1% and that for yellow fever was 0.5%. No association was observed between sex and arboviruses infection. Both recent and old infections were observed for yellow fever, 0.2% and 0.3%, respectively and West Nile, 0.1% and 10.2%, respectively. No recent infections were noted for both dengue and Zika virus infection. These results are shown in Table 1 and Figures 10-14. Altogether, 5 (0.1%) of the participants were positive for all the four arboviruses, 6.3% of the participants were positive for 2 or more arboviruses and 11.5% were positive for any arboviruses (see Table 2).

The study was not powered to conduct correlates for yellow fever. Table 3 shows correlates for dengue, West Nile and Zika arboviruses infection. Consistently, persons aged less than 5 years were about 63% less likely to have any arbovirus infection compared to persons aged 45 years or older. While persons aged 35-44 years were equally likely to have any arbovirus infection as those aged 45 years or older for dengue and Zika, persona aged 35-44 years were 41% more likely to have West Nile virus infection compared to those aged 45 years or older. Education was only significantly related to West Nile virus infection. Participants who attained primary level of education were 32% (AOR = 1.32; 95%CI [1.01-1.72]) more likely to have West Nile virus infection compared to those who attained tertiary level of education. Respondents who were engaged in farming were 20% (AOR = 0.80; 95% CI [0.64, 0.99] less likely to have West Nile virus infection compared to respondents who were students.

Participants who used ITNs were more likely to have dengue or West Nile virus infection compared to those who did not use ITNs. Respondents who had in-door residual spraying were 19% less likely to have West Nile or Zika virus infection compared to respondents who did not have in-door residual spraying.

Visiting Angola was significantly associated with increased risk for dengue West Nile and Zika arboviruses infections. Respondents who visited DR Congo were 72% (AOR = 0.28; 95% CI [0.10, 0.74]) less likely to have West Nile virus infection compared to those who did not visit DR Congo.

Table 3. Correlates in multivariate analysis for prevalence of arboviruses in North-Western and Western province of Zambia

	Adjusted odds ratio (95% Confidence interval)		
Factor	Dengue	West Nile	Zika
Age (years)			
<5	0.37 (0.16, 0.86)	0.38 (0.20-0.73)	0.36 (0.18, 0.72)
5-14	0.92 (0.62, 1.38)	0.73 (0.50-1.08)	0.76 (0.54, 1.08)
15-24	0.98 (0.65, 1.47)	1.07 (0.82-1.42)	0.91 (0.64, 1.28)
25-34	1.38 (0.94, 2.03)	1.06 (0.77-1.48)	1.20 0.86, 1.68)
35-44	0.94 (0.59, 1.50)	1.41 (1.01-1.97)	1.27 (0.89, 1.82)
45+	1	1	1
Sex			
Male	-	-	-
Female			
Education			
None	-	0.83 (0.60-1.15)	-
Primary		1.32 (1.01-1.72)	
Secondary		0.98 (0.74-1.30)	
Tertiary		1	
Occupation			
House wife/husband	-	1.13 (0.85-1.51)	-
Farming		0.80 (0.64-0.99)	
Other		1.35 (1.02-1.79)	
Student		1	
Use of an insecticide treated net			
Yes	1.21 (1.01, 1.44)	1.13 (1.00-1.27)	-
No	1	1	
In-door residual spraying			
Yes	-	0.81 (0.69-0.95)	0.81 (0.66, 0.99)
No		1	1
Visited Angola			
Yes	1.73 (1.27, 2.35)	1.40 (1.09, 1.81)	1.42 (1.06, 1.90)
No	1	1	1
Visited DR Congo			
Yes	-	0.28 (0.10, 0.74)	-
No		1	
Roof type			
Grass	2.28 (1.15, 4.53)	2.97 (1.81-4.88)	2.03 (1.24, 3.33)
Iron sheet	0.98 (0.49, 1.99)	0.96 (0.58-1.58)	0.85 (0.51, 1.43)
Asbestos	1	1	1

Consistently, participants who stayed in houses that had grass roof were 2-3 times more likely to have any of the arboviruses infection compared to those who lived in houses with asbestos roofs. Participants who lived in houses with iron sheet roof were equally likely to have any arboviruses infection as those who lived in houses with asbestos roof.

A total of 1,401 adult mosquitoes were collected comprising 405 (28.9%) Aedes, 518 (37.0%) Anopheles, 471 (33.6%) Culex and 71 (5.1%) Mansonia. The two main yellow fever vectors found in the study area were Ae. (Stegomyia) aegypti and Ae. (Stegomyia) africanus. Also found in the study area were Aedes (Aedimorphus) mutilus, Ae. (aedimorphus) minutus and Ae. (Finlaya) wellmani.

DISCUSSION

The current study reports a comprehensive distribution of four arboviruses, all of genus Flavivirus, in North-Western and Western provinces. The prevalence rates were 10.3% for West Nile, 6.0% for Zika, 4.1% for dengue and 0.5% for yellow fever. No recent infections were observed for dengue and Zika viruses. In a study conducted in three rural districts of Kenya, Mease et al., (47) reported prevalence rates for West Nile of 9.5%, dengue 14.4% and yellow fever 9.2% in 2004. In the 1966-1968 Kenyan study, the most prevalent arboviruses were West Nile with a prevalence of 23.8%, followed by Zika (17.6%), dengue (17.3%) and lastly yellow fever (14.3%) (30). In another study in rural Cameroon, the prevalence of yellow fever (26.9%) was higher than that for West Nile (6.6%) (48). Dominant arboviruses infections varied in different surveys. Differences in rates may partly be due to different laboratory tests that were conducted and different stages of the epidemic. In the Cameroonian study, the plaque–reduction neutralization test was used. The 2004 Kenyan study used IgG antibodies to test the samples and in the 1966-1968 Kenya study the haemagglu-tination-inhibition test was used. The Zambian samples were subjected to both IgG and IgM antibody tests and PRNT. Differences in the power of the study may partly explain the different rates that have been observed between studies. Since tests for arboviruses cross react with each other, it is important that confirmatory tests be conducted, and it's none use by some studies may have led to different test results. Given that the study design allowed for computation of point prevalence, the observed rates may be an underestimate for the true prevalence because only those who survived the arboviruses infection were considered in the study.

The finding that about 1 in 20 participants were positive for two or more arboviruses indicates the need to test for more than one arbovirus. This will ensure that patients receive comprehensive management of the infections.

Correlates for arboviruses generally differed between arboviruses, indicating the need to design interventions to control arboviruses infections that are arboviru-specific. However consistently across all the arboviruses, visiting Angola was associated with increased risk for arboviruses. Recently, Angola reported epidemics for Dengue (49). Stoddard et al., (50) and Reiter (51) have argued that human movement is an important factor in the transportation of vectors and pathogens.

The finding that participants aged less than 5 years were less likely to have arboviruses infections compared to older participants cut across all infections suggests that these individuals may have had maternal protection. However, Ministry of Health (52) reported that about a third of children of age 24-59 months had malaria parasites in the 2010 Malaria Indicator Survey, suggesting that children in this age group are susceptible to mosquito bites that may transmit arboviruses. Another finding that cut across all infections was that participants who lived in houses with grass roof type were more likely to have infections compared to those who lived in houses with roofs made of asbestos. It is possible that grass roof type offers favourable house environment for mosquitoes in our study area.

The finding of two main vectors for yellow fever (Ae. (Stegomyia) aegypti and Ae. (Stegomyia) africanus) indicates that there is a possibility of sustaining the virus if it was imported into the study area. Interventions mainly placed for malaria control including insecticide residual spraying and insecticide treated nets are in place but with only about half the population in our study sites using insecticide treated nets (43), the other half of the population or more remain susceptible to arbovirus infections. We may assume that factors that could have contributed to the risk of arbovirus infection in the population under study include the activities of the vectors, that of the human host and a possible bias in answering the questionnaire on use of ITNs. Aedes aegypti generally bites during the day (53) and therefore the use of ITNs would not be expected to provide a barrier between the humans and the transmitting vector. Considering the outdoor activities participated in during the day such as farming, fishing, and socialising, the population may be at risk of being bitten by the vector.

Worthwhile to note is that subsequent infections with dengue increases the severity of disease and if interventions are not timely put in place, Zambia risks a dengue outbreak. In conclusion, the factors: roof type and visiting Angola in addition to arbovirus-specific correlates should be considered in developing interventions to control arboviruses in North-Western and Western provinces of Zambia.

REFERENCES

[1] Babaniyi OA, Mwaba P, Mulenga D, Monze M, Songolo P, Mazaba-Liwewe ML, et al., Risk assessment for Yellow Fever in Western and North-Western provinces of Zambia. J Global Infect Dis (Ahead of print).

[2] Mazaba-Liwewe ML, Siziya S, Monze M, Mweene-Ndumba I, Masaninga F, Songolo P, et al., First sero-prevalence of dengue fever specific immunoglobulin G antibodies in Western and North-Western provinces of Zambia: a population based cross sectional study. Virol J 2014;11:135.

[3] Lvov DK, Tsyrkin YM, Karas FR, Timopheev EM, Gromashevski VL, Veselovskaya OV, et al., "Sokuluk" Virus, a new group B arbovirus isolated from Vespertilio pipistrellus Schreber, 1775, bat in the Kirghiz S.S.R. Arch Gesamte Virusforschung 1973;41:170-4.

[4] Vainio J, Cutts F. Yellow Fever. WHO Division of Emerging and other Communicable Diseases Surveillance and Control: Geneva: WHO, 1998.

[5] Monath TP. Yellow fever: an update. Lancet Infect Dis 2001;1:11–20.

[6] Julander JG. Experiment therapies for yellow fever. Antiviral Res 2013;97:169-79.

[7] Monath TP. Review of the risks and benefits of yellow fever vaccination including some new analyses. Expert Rev Vaccines 2012;11:427-48.

[8] World Health Organization. Division of Epidemiological Surveillance and Health Situation and Trend Assessment. Global Health Situation and Projections: Estimates. Geneva: World Health Organization, 1992.

[9] World Health Organization. Media centre. Dengue and severe dengue. Fact sheet N°117. Updated March 2014. Accessed 2014 September 12. URL: http://www.who.int/mediacentre/factsheets/fs117/en/).

[10] Simmons CP, Farrar JJ, van Vinh Chau N, Wills B. Dengue. N Engl J Med 2012;366:1423–32.

[11] Whitehorn J, Farrar J. Dengue. Br Med Bull 2010;95:161–73.

[12] World Health Organization, Special Programme for Research and Training in Tropical. Diseases: Dengue: guidelines for diagnosis, treatment, prevention and control. Geneva: World Health Organization, 2009.

[13] Ranjit S, Kissoon N. Dengue hemorrhagic fever and shock syndromes. Pediatr Crit Care Med 2011;12:90–100.

[14] World Health Organization. Dengue and Dengue Hemorrhagic Fever. Fact sheet No117. Revised April 2002. Accessed 2014 September 11: URL: http://shuidao.cn/factSheets/Health_and_Nutrition/whoHealth/whoFS_dengue.pdf.

[15] Halstead SB. Dengue vaccine development: a 75% solution? Lancet 2012;380:1535-6.

[16] Sabchareon A, Wallace D, Sirivichayakul C, Limkittikul K, Chanthavanich P, Suvannadabba S, et al., Protective efficacy of the recombinant, live-attenuated, CYD tetravalent dengue vaccine in Thai schoolchildren: a randomised, controlled phase 2b trial. Lancet 2012;380;1559-67.

[17] Bhatt S, Gething PW, Brady OJ, Messina JP, Farlow AW, Moyes CL, et al., The global distribution and burden of dengue. Nature 2013;496:504–7.

[18] Endy TP, Anderson KB, Nisalak A, Yoon IK, Green S, Rothman AL, et al., Determinants of inapparent and symptomatic dengue infection in a prospective study of primary school children in Kamphaeng Phet, Thailand. PLoS Negl Trop Dis 2011;5:e975.

[19] Gubler DJ. Dengue and dengue hemorrhagic fever. Clin Microbiol Rev 1998;11:480–69.

[20] Kakkar M. Dengue fever is massively under-reported in India, hampering our response. Br Med J 2012;345:e8574.

[21] Mostashari F, Bunning ML, Kitsutani PT, Singer DA, Nash D, Cooper MJ, et al., Epidemic West Nile encephalitis, New York, 1999: results of a household-based seroepidemiological survey. Lancet 2001;358:261–4.

[22] Centers for Disease Control and Prevention. West Nile Virus: Symptoms & Treatment. Accessed 2014 September 05. URL: http://www.cdc.gov/westnile/symptoms/.

[23] Centers for Disease Control and Prevention. West Nile Virus: Symptoms & Treatment. Accessed 2014 September 05. URL: http://www.cdc.gov/westnile/symptoms/.

[24] Rojahn SY. Few Options in the West Nile Fight: The seasonal and unpredictable nature of the infection makes it difficult to test any potential treatment or vaccine. Accessed 2014 September 16. http://www.technologyreview.com/news/428926/few-options-in-the-west-nile-fight/).

[25] Bakonyi T, Nowotny N. West Nile epidemiology: global situation and recent outbreaks in Europe. Workshop on West Nile virus. Berlin, 13th -17th of February, 2012.

[26] European Centre for Disease Prevention and Control. Rapid risk assessment: Zika virus infection outbreak, French Polynesia. 14 February 2014. Stockholm: ECDC, 2014.

[27] Olson JG, Ksiazek TG, Suhandiman, Triwibowo. Zika virus, a cause of fever in Central Java, Indonesia. Trans R Soc Trop Med Hyg 1981;75:389-93.

[28] Heang V, Yasuda CY, Sovann L, Haddow AD, Travassos da Rosa AP, Tesh RB, et al., Zika virus infection, Cambodia, 2010. Emerg Infect Dis 2012;18:349-51.

[29] Duffy MR, Chen TH, Hancock WT, Powers AM, Kool JL, Lanciotti RS, et al., Zika virus outbreak on Yap Island, Federated States of Micronesia. N Engl J Med 2009;360:2536-43.

[30] Geser A, Henderson BE, Christensen S. A multipurpose serological survey in Kenya: 2. Results of arbovirus serological tests. Bull World Health Organ 1970;43:539-52.

[31] Aitken TH, Tesh RB, Beaty BJ, Rosen L. Transovarial transmission of yellow fever virus by mosquitoes (Aedes aegypti). Am J Trop Med Hyg 1979;28:119–21.

[32] Fontenille D, Diallo M, Mondo M, Ndiaye M, Thonnon J. First evidence of natural vertical transmission of yellow fever virus in Aedes aegypti, its epidemic vector. Trans R Soc Trop Med Hyg 1997;91:533–5.

[33] Gratz NG. Critical review of the vector status of Aedes albopictus. Med Vet Entomol 2004;18:215–27.

[34] Masaninga F, Muleba M, Masendu H, Songolo P, Mweene-Ndumba I, Mazaba-Liwewe ML, et al., Distribution of yellow fever vectors in Northwestern and Western Provinces, Zambia. Asian Pac J Trop Biomed 2014; 4(12):(in press).

[35] Kyle JL, Harris E: Global spread and persistence of dengue. Annu Rev Microbiol 2008, 62:71–92.

[36] World Health Organization: Dengue control: the mosquito. Accessed 2014 September 11. URL: http://www.who.int/denguecontrol/mosquito/en/.

[37] Centers for Disease Control and Prevention. Surveillance for West Nile virus disease—United States, 1999–2008. MMWR Surveill Summ 2010;59:1–17.

[38] Reimann C, Hayes E, DiGuiseppi C, Hoffman R, Lehman J, Lindsey N, et al., Epidemiology of neuroinvasive arboviral disease in the United States, 1999–2007. Am J Trop Med Hyg 2008;79:974–9.
[39] Nash D, Mostashari F, Fine A, Miller J, O'Leary D, Murray K, et al., The outbreak of West Nile virus infection in the New York City area in 1999. N Engl J Med 2001;344:1807–14.
[40] Zika Virus Infection. Accessed 2014 September 2014. URL: http://www.fitfortravel.nhs.uk/advice/disease-prevention-advice/zika-virus-infection.aspx.
[41] Central Statistical Office. 2010 census of population and housing. National analytical report. CSO, 2012.
[42] Aregheore EM. Country pasture/forage resource profiles: Zambia. Accessed 2014 May 19. URL: http://www.fao.org/ag/agp/AGPC/doc/Counprof/zambia/zambia.htm#_Toc131995467.
[43] Central Statistical Office (CSO), Ministry of Health (MOH), Tropical Diseases Research Centre (TDRC), University of Zambia, and Macro International Inc. 2009: Zambia Demographic and Health Survey 2007. Calverton, Maryland, USA: CSO and Macro International Inc, 2011.
[44] Robinson GG. A note on mosquitoes and yellow fever in Northern Rhodesia. East Afr Med J 1950;27:284-8.
[45] World Health Organization. WHO manual for the monitoring of yellow fever virus infection WHO/IVB/04.08. Geneva: World Health Organization, 2004.
[46] Kent RJ. The mosquitoes of Macha, Zambia. Johns Hopkins Malaria Research Institute; Department of Molecular Microbiology and Immunology, Johns Hopkins Bloomberg School of Public Health. Baltimore, MD USA, 2006. Accessed 2014 September 16. URL: http://malaria.jhsph.edu/programs/conferences_workshops/conference_meetings%20archives/2006%20events/The_Mosquitoes_of_Macha-March06.pdf.
[47] Mease LE, Coldren RL, Musila LA, Prosser T, Ogolla F, Ofula VO, et al., Seroprevalence and distribution of arboviral infections among rural Kenyan adults: A cross-sectional study. Virology J 2011;8:371.
[48] Kuniholm MH, Wolfe ND, Huang CY-H, Mpoudi-Ngole E, Tamoufe U, Burke DS, et al., Seroprevalence and distribution of Flaviviridae, Togaviridae, and Bunyaviridae arboviral infections in rural Cameroonian adults. Am J Trop Med Hyg 2006;74:1078–83.
[49] CDC. Ongoing Dengue Epidemic — Angola, June 2013. Morbidity and Mortality Weekly Report (MMWR) 2013;62:504-507. Accessed 2014 September 10. URL: http://www.cdc.gov/mmwr/preview/mmwrhtml/mm6224a6.htm.
[50] Stoddard ST, Morrison AC, Vazquez-Prokopec GM, Paz Soldan V, Kochel TJ, Kitron U, et al., The role of human movement in the transmission of vector-borne pathogens. PLoS Negl Trop Dis 2009;3:e481.
[51] Reiter P. Climate change and mosquito-borne disease: knowing the horse before hitching the cart. Rev Sci Tech 2008;27:383-98.
[52] Ministry of Health. Zambia National Malaria Indicator Survey 2010. Lusaka: Ministry of Health, 2010.
[53] Centers for Diseases Control and Prevention: Dengue and the Aedes Aegytpi mosquito. Accessed 2014 September 16. URL: http://www.cdc.gov/dengue/resources/30jan2012/aegyptifactsheet.pdf.

In: Public Health Yearbook 2016
Editor: Joav Merrick

ISBN: 978-1-53610-947-4

Chapter 3

PREVALENCE OF YELLOW FEVER IN NORTH-WESTERN PROVINCE OF ZAMBIA

Olusegun Babaniyi[1,*], MBBS, MPH, MSc,
Mazyanga L Mazaba-Liwewe[1], BSc,
Freddie Masaninga[1], BSc, MSc, PhD,
Peter Mwaba[2], MBChB, MMed, David Mulenga[3], BSc, MPH,
Peter Songolo[1], MBChB, MPH,
Idah Mweene-Ndumba[1], BSc, MPH,
Emmanuel Rudatsikira[4], MD, MPH, DrPH
and Seter Siziya[3,5], BA(Ed), MSc, PhD
[1]World Health Organization, Lusaka, Zambia
[2]Ministry of Home Affairs, Lusaka, Zambia
[3]School of Medicine, Copperbelt University, Ndola, Zambia
[4]School of Health Professions, Andrews University, Michigan, US
[5]University of Lusaka, Lusaka, Zambia

ABSTRACT

Yellow fever virus infection is a public health problem in Africa. North-Western province of Zambia was reclassified from a no risk to a low risk area for YF in 2010. To ascertain this reclassification, an assessment for the risk of YF was conducted in 2013 in North-Western province. A total of 1,754 persons took part in the survey of which 48.8% were males. Overall, 15.8% of the participants were of age 45 years or older. Significantly more males (37.4%) than females (26.0%) had attained secondary or higher levels of education. Nine (0.5%) out of 1,754 participants had YF virus infection. Of the

* Corresponding author: Olusegun A. Babaniyi, MBBS, MPH, MSc, World Health Organization, Lusaka, Zambia. E-mail: agbagba@yahoo.com.

9 cases, 4 were old infection and 5 were new. There were 6 Male and 3 female cases. The age range of the cases was 37-81 years. None of the cases had jaundice or bled but 3 had fever. Three cases had travelled to Congo DR and 1 case had travelled to Angola. Use of mosquito net was reported by 4 cases and another 4 cases reported that their houses were sprayed with IRS. The prevalence of YF virus infection among participants of ages 45 years or older (2.9%) was significantly ($p < 0.001$) higher than that for participants aged less than 45 year (0.1%). North-Western province was experiencing an epidemic for YF virus infection. With a low prevalence, the area qualifies to be classified as a low risk for YF. Efforts to curb the epidemic are urgently needed. Yellow fever surveillance and the capacity of laboratories to diagnose YF should be strengthened.

Keywords: yellow fever, prevalence, Western province, Zambia

INTRODUCTION

Yellow fever virus infection is a public health problem in Africa. Epidemics of YF have spread from West Africa (1, 2) where 13 of 14 west African countries reported YFV infection from 2000 to 2006 (3, 4, 5) to North Africa (6), East Africa (7), Central Africa and Southern Africa (8).

Yellow fever affects about 200000 people annually in the tropics of Africa and South America (9). Symptoms for YF virus infection includes: fever, chills, severe headache, back pain, general body aches, nausea, vomiting, fatigue and weakness to severe liver disease with bleeding. About 15% of cases progress to a more severe form of the disease that is characterized by high fever, jaundice, bleeding, and eventually shock and failure of multiple organs (10). There is no treatment for yellow fever and only symptoms can be alleviated. YF virus infection can be prevented by using insect repellent, wearing protective clothing, and getting vaccinated.

Although by 2005, Yellow fever was endemic in Congo DR, the area of Congo DR bordering North-Western was classified as a low risk area for YF (11). North-Western province of Zambia was reclassified by WHO from a no risk area to a low risk area for YF in 2010 (8). To ascertain this reclassification, an assessment for the risk of YF was conducted in 2013 in North-Western province.

METHODS

The study was conducted in North-Western province of Zambia. North-Western province borders with Angola on the western side and Democratic Republic of Congo (DRC) on the northern side with 6 districts divided into 1,178 Standard Enumeration Areas (SEAs). The 2010 census reveals a population of 706,462 with population density of 5.6 (12). The main economic activity was pineapple growing, with fast growing mining activities. Zambia Demographic Health Survey, 2007 reports 46.9 and 53.2% of the population sleeping under a net in the past night in Western and North Western Provinces respectively (13).

Study population, sample size and sampling

This assessment was carried out among individuals aged nine months or older. The sample size calculation was based on the assumption that the sero-prevalence was 7% based on the study conducted by Robinson (14).

In estimating the sample size for persons aged 5 years or older, the following parameters were considered: a prevalence of 7%, desired precision or confidence interval (d) of ±3%, and a design effect (DE) of 2 and an 80% response rate. Considering sex, we aimed to recruit 700 male and 700 female participants in each province. Assuming an average of 4 persons aged 5 years or older in each household, a total of 12 households in each of the 30 clusters was to be recruited in the survey. The total number of persons that would be recruited was 1806.

The sero-prevalence of children was about half that for older children, and in estimating the sample size for persons aged below 5 years, the following parameters were considered: a prevalence of 3.5%, desired precision or confidence interval (d) of ±3.4%, and a design effect (DE) of 2 and an 80% response rate. The computed sample size was 282. Therefore, 406 children would be recruited for the survey.

The sample was drawn using a two-stage cluster sampling technique using probability proportional to size. A list of the standard enumeration areas (SEAs) in each province constituted the sampling frame.

Data management and analysis

Data were entered in an Epi-Info data entry screen that had consistency and range checks embedded in it. Further editing was conducted by running frequencies during the analysis stage. Epi data files were exported to SPSS for data analysis. The chi-square test was used to determine associations between qualitative factors. The cut off point for statistical significance was set at the 5% level.

Ethical considerations

Ethical clearance was sought from the Tropical Diseases Research Centre Research Ethics Committee, and ethical standards were adhered to throughout this study. Informed consent was sought from study participants. Guardians provided assent for the participation of the persons under the consenting age. They were asked to read or have read to them, understand and sign/thumbprint an informed consent form. Responsible adults in the household were identified to give proxy consent on behalf of minors.

RESULTS

A total of 1,754 persons took part in the survey of which 48.8% were males. Overall, 15.8% of the participants were of age 45 years or older. Significantly more males (37.4%)

than females (26.0%) had attained secondary or higher levels of education. These results are shown in Table 1.

Nine (0.5%) out of 1754 participants had YF virus infection. Of the 9 cases, 4 were old infection and 5 were new. There were 6 Male and 3 female cases. The age range of the cases was 37-81 years. None of the cases had jaundice or bled but 3 had fever.

Three of the cases had no formal education, 4 attained primary level of education and 2 attained secondary level of education. Three cases lived in houses that had roofs made of grass, 5 had roofs made of iron sheets and 1 lived in a house that had a roof made of asbestos. Walls for houses for the cases were made of mud (2), cement plastered (10 and unburnt bricks (6).

Three cases had travelled to Congo DR and 1 case had travelled to Angola. Use of mosquito net was reported by 4 cases and another 4 cases reported that their houses were sprayed with IRS.

None of the factors considered in the analysis was significantly associated with YF virus infection except age. The prevalence of YF virus infection among participants of ages 45 years or older (2.9) was significantly ($p < 0.001$) higher than that for participants aged less than 45 year (0.1%).

Discussion

Yellow fever virus was circulating in North-Western province with a prevalence of 0.5%. Both new and old cases were identified in the study area. All the cases of Yellow fever were adults and none of the cases had been vaccinated against YF virus. This survey was conducted 50 years after the last survey of YF virus risk assessment was conducted.

Table 1. Sample description for the participants in yellow fever risk assessment, 2013

Factor	Total	Male	Female	p value
	n (%)	n (%)	n (%)	
Age (years)				
<45	1476 (84.2)	703 (82.4)	2769 (85.7)	0.067
45+	278 (15.8)	150 (17.6)	128 (14.3)	
Sex				
Male	854 (48.8)	-	-	
Female	897 (51.2)			
Education				
None or primary	1182 (68.4)	525 (62.6)	654 (74.0)	<0.001
Secondary or higher	545 (31.6)	314 (37.4)	230 (26.0)	
Yellow fever				
Yes	9 (0.5)	6 (0.7)	3 (0.3)	0.459
No	1745 (99.5)	848 (99.3)	893 (99.7)	

The prevalence of the infection in the current study is less than the 7% that was reported by Robinson (14). The difference in the prevalence could partly be due to differences in the stages of the epidemic at the time of the survey. It might be that North-Western province was in the early stage of the epidemic, while 50 years ago when that study was conducted the area was at an advanced stage of the epidemic. Another possibility for the difference could be that Western province that is not part of the current study could have had a higher proportion of the 7% prevalence.

All the cases of YF in the current study were adults. This finding contradicts the observation that children are more affected than adults because adults could have acquired immunity in a Yellow fever endemic area (15). However, the finding in the current study that adults were more affected is in agreement with the finding by Geser et al. (16) which suggests that stable rates of transmission in the population.

In conclusion, North-Western province was experiencing an epidemic for YF virus infection. With a low prevalence, the area qualifies to be classified as a low risk for YF. Efforts to curb the epidemic are urgently needed. Yellow fever surveillance and the capacity of laboratories to diagnose YF should be strengthened.

ACKNOWLEDGMENTS

We are grateful to the interviewers for their dedicated work to successfully complete the survey. The survey could not have been successful without the cooperation of the participants and the virology laboratory staff both in Lusaka, Zambia and Dakar, Senegal for in testing samples. The survey was funded by the Ministry of Health [Zambia] and the World Health Organization.

REFERENCES

[1] Nasidi A, Monath TP, DeCock K, Tomori O, Cordellier R, Olaleye OD, et al. Urban yellow fever epidemic in western Nigeria, 1987. Trans R Soc Trop Med Hyg 1989; 83: 401–6.

[2] Robertson SE, Hull BP, Tomori O, Bele O, LeDuc JW, Esteyes K. Yellow fever: a decade of reemergence. JAMA 1996; 276: 1157-62.

[3] World Health Organization. Yellow fever vaccine: WHO position paper. Wkly Epidemiol Rec 2003; 78: 349-59.

[4] Nathan N, Barry M, Van Herp M, Zeller H. Shortage of vaccines during a yellow fever outbreak in Guinea. Lancet 2001; 358: 2129-30.

[5] Anonymous. The yellow fever situation in Africa and South America in 2004. Wkly Epidemiol Rec 2005; 80: 249-56.

[6] Gould LH, Osman MS, Farnon EC, Griffith KS, Godsey MS, Karch S, et al. An outbreak of yellow fever with concurrent chikungunya virus transmission in South Kordofan, Sudan, 2005. Trans R Soc Trop Med Hyg 2008; 102: 1247-54.

[7] Sanders EJ, Marfin AA, Tukei PM, Kuria G, Ademba G, Agata NN, et al. First recorded outbreak of yellow fever in Kenya, 1992-1993. I. Epidemiologic investigations. Am J Trop Med Hyg 1998; 59: 644-9.

[8] Jentes ES, Poumerol G, Gershman MD, Hill DR, Lemarchand J, Lewis RF, et al. The revised global yellow fever risk map and recommendations for vaccination, 2010: consensus of the Informal WHO Working Group on Geographic Risk for Yellow Fever. Lancet Infect Dis 2011; 11: 622-32.
[9] Vainio J, Cutts F. Yellow fever. In: World Health Organization. Expanded Programme on Immunization. Global Programme for Vaccines and Immunization: Expanded Programme on Immunization. Geneva: Global Programme for Vaccines and Immunization, Expanded Programme on Immunization, World Health Organization, 1998.
[10] Centers for Disease Control and Prevention. Symptoms and treatment. Accessed 2014 August 28. URL:http://www.cdc.gov/yellowfever/symptoms/index.html.
[11] Barnett ED. Yellow fever: epidemiology and prevention. Clin Infect Dis 2007; 44: 850-6.
[12] Central Statistical Office. 2010 census of population and housing. National analytical report. Lusaka, Zambia: CSO, 2012.
[13] Central Statistical Office (CSO), Ministry of Health (MOH), Tropical Diseases Research Centre (TDRC), University of Zambia, and Macro International Inc. 2009. Zambia Demographic and Health Survey 2007. Calverton, Maryland, USA: CSO and Macro International Inc.
[14] Robinson GG. A note on mosquitoes and yellow fever in Northern Rhodesia. East Afr Med J 1950; 27: 284-8.
[15] Monath TP, Craven RB, Adjukiewicz A, et al. Yellow fever in the Gambia, 1978-1979: epidemiologic aspects with observations on the occurrence of Orungo virus infection. Am J Trop Med Hyg 1980; 29: 912-28.
[16] Geser A, Henderson BE, Christensen S. A multipurpose serological survey in Kenya: 2. Results of arbovirus serological tests. Bull World Health Organ 1970; 43: 539-52.

In: Public Health Yearbook 2016
Editor: Joav Merrick

ISBN: 978-1-53610-947-4

Chapter 4

TRAVEL TO ANGOLA ASSOCIATED WITH DENGUE IGG SEROPREVALENCE IN NORTH-WESTERN PROVINCE OF ZAMBIA

***Mazyanga L Mazaba-Liwewe*[1,2,*], *BSc*,**
***Olusegun Babaniyi*[1], *MBBS, MPH, MSc*,**
***Mwaka Monze*[2], *MBChB, PhD*,**
***Idah Mweene-Ndumba*[1,2], *BSc, MPH*,**
***Freddie Masaninga*[1], *BSc, MSc, PhD*,**
***Peter Songolo*[1], *MBChB, MPH*,**
Muzala Kanyanga*[3], *MBChB, MPH
and Seter Siziya*[4,5], *BA(Ed), MSc, PhD
[1]World Health Organization Country Office, Lusaka
[2]University Teaching Hospital, Lusaka, Zambia
[3]Ministry of Health, Lusaka, Zambia
[4]School of Medicine, Copperbelt University, Ndola, Zambia
[5]University of Lusaka, Lusaka, Zambia

The factors associated with Dengue fever may not be well understood but documentation cites an association with demographic and societal changes over the past 50 years. Information on dengue virus infection in North-Western province is lacking. The objective of the study was to determine the prevalence and correlates for dengue virus infection in the province. Secondary data obtained in a yellow fever risk assessment was used in the study. Logistic regression analysis was used to determine magnitudes of associations. A total of 1,755 participants had both laboratory results and filled in the questionnaires. The results indicated that 1.0% of participants had previous dengue infection with no sex difference ($p = 0.729$). Visiting Angola was significantly associated with previous dengue infection (OR = 2.73; 95% CI [1.55, 4.83]). This study provides

* Correspondence: Mazyanga L Mazaba, EPI Unit, World Health Organization, Lusaka, Zambia and Virology Unit, University Teaching Hospital, Lusaka, Zambia. E-mail: mazmazli@yahoo.com

evidence of dengue virus circulation and its association with travel to Angola. There is need for active surveillance and adequate diagnostic systems.

Keywords: dengue, IgG sero-prevalence, North-Western, travel, Angola

INTRODUCTION

Dengue fever caused by dengue virus of genus *Flavivirus* and family *Flaviviridae* is a leading cause of morbidity and mortality in the tropics and subtropics posing a risk to one third of the world's population living in these areas (1, 2). The virus is transmitted to humans through the bite of a mosquito, primarily Aedes Aegypti and Aedes albopictus (2). Until the middle of the 20th century, dengue was relatively minor, geographically restricted disease (3-4). Pandemic Dengue begun in Southeast Asia in the mid 1940's after the second World War and has intensified in the last 15 years, (5) and has become endemic in more than 100 countries in Africa, the Americas, the Eastern Mediterranean, South-east Asia and the Western Pacific with the American, South-east Asia and the Western Pacific regions affected most seriously (6-8). Based on data submitted by WHO member states mostly affected by dengue indicates cases exceeding 1.2 million in 2008 and 2.3 million in 2010 (9). In Africa, documentation indicates dengue epidemics occurring as far back as 1927 (10) and increasing activity since 1980 (11). Angola and Kenya continued to experience dengue outbreaks in 2013 (12).

The factors associated with Dengue fever may not be well understood but documentation cites an association with demographic and societal changes over the past 50 years (13, 14). Factors including sex, age, urbanization and mobility of people have been associated with increased dengue fever. The difference in incidence of dengue fever in relation to sex is attributed exposure to the vector (mosquito) (15). Most studies indicate risk of dengue fever increasing with age, urbanization and travel (9, 16-20). Older children and adults are more disposed to dengue fever (6). WHO documents that the increased mobility of people has contributed to the increase in the number of epidemics and circulating viruses (9). Persons with chronic diseases including diabetes and asthma are likely to encounter complicated disease which is life threatening (21). Once infected with dengue, IgG antibodies and detectable after 10 to 14 days of onset and one acquires life time immunity to the specific serotype. Infection with another serotype also increases chances of severity (22). This paper describes the association if any of factors including age, sex, education and travel with dengue fever in North-Western province of Zambia.

METHODS

North-Western province borders with Angola on the western side and Democratic Republic of Congo (DRC) (see Figure 1) on the northern side with 6 districts divided into 1,178 Standard Enumeration Areas (SEAs). The 2010 census reveals a population of 706,462 with population density of 5.6. The main economic activity was pineapple growing, with fast growing mining activities in one of the districts, Solwezi (23). Central Statistical Office (CSO) (24) reported in 2007 that 53.2% of the population slept under a net in the past night in North-Western province (24).

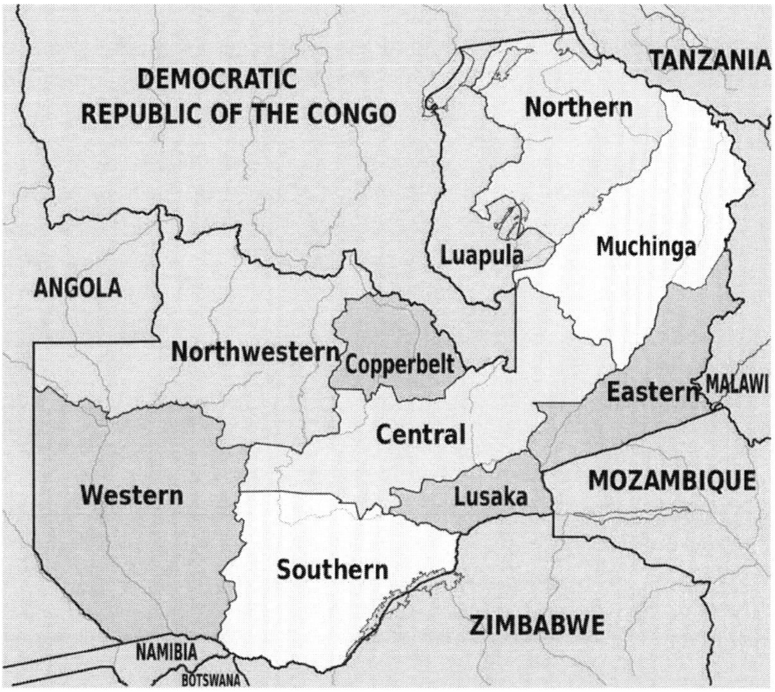

Figure 1. Map of Zambia showing provinces and bordering countries.

Study population, sample size, inclusion/exclusion criteria and sampling

This assessment was carried out among individuals aged nine months or older. The sample size calculation was based on the assumption that the sero-prevalence was 7% based on the study on Yellow fever conducted by Robinson, 1950 (25). For persons aged 5 years or older the following parameters were considered in estimating the sample size, a prevalence of 7%, desired precision or confidence interval (d) of ±3%, and a design effect (DE) of 2 and an 80% response rate. The study aimed to recruit 700 male and 700 female participants in each province. A total of 12 households in each of the 30 clusters, assuming an average of 4 persons aged 5 years or older in each household, were to be recruited in the survey. The total number of persons that would be recruited from each province was 1,806, totaling 3,612 from both provinces.

The sero-prevalence of children below five years was about half that for older children, and in estimating the sample size for persons aged below 5 years, the following parameters were considered: a prevalence of 3.5%, desired precision or confidence interval (d) of ±3.4%, and a design effect (DE) of 2 and an 80% response rate. The computed sample size was 282. A total of 406 children would be recruited in each province for the survey.

Any individual aged 9 months or older and who was a member of a sampled household and resident in the study site for at least seven days. Individuals who received YF vaccination in the last ten years would be eligible to participate in the survey. Exclusion criteria left out any person, who was either less than 9 months of age, or any person regardless of age, who resided in the study site for a period of less than seven days prior to the survey. Children under the age of nine months raises the risk of false positive results as children under this age may still carry maternal antibodies from immunized or exposed mothers.

A two-stage cluster sampling technique using probability proportional to size was used to draw the sample. A list of the standard enumeration areas (SEAs) in each province constituted the sampling frame. The sampling was designed to achieve fairly good estimates at the provincial level of analysis, and not representing the subdivisions of the province.

Study variables

Dependent variable

A case with evidence of Dengue infection exposure was defined as any individual aged 9 months or older whose blood sample was confirmed to have Dengue virus exposure through the detection of Dengue virus-specific IgG and IgM antibodies.

Independent variables

The independent variables included age, sex, occupation, history of travel to Angola and/or DRC, and use of mosquito preventive measures.

Laboratory procedure

About 3 to 5 millilitres of blood was collected by venepuncture into an EDTA vacutainer tube and transported on cold chain to the local laboratories for serum separation and storage. Samples were subjected to primary testing (YFV specific IgG and IgM) at the University of Teaching Hospital in Zambia virology unit and Institute Pasteur, Dakar. All presumptive YFV-specific IgG and IgM samples were subjected to IgG and IgM antibodies against other flaviviruses known to cause haemorrhagic fever-like disease including dengue.

Data management and analysis

Data were entered in an Epi-Info data entry screen that had consistency and range checks embedded in it. Further editing was conducted by running frequencies during the analysis stage. Epi data files were exported to SPSS for data analysis. The data was summarized to describe the occurrence of dengue virus exposed individuals in absolute numbers and percentage by place (residence, travel or work) and person (age, sex, occupation). Further analysis was conducted to determine independent factors associated with yellow fever sero-positivity. Odds ratios were used to estimate the magnitude of associations.

Ethical considerations

Ethical clearance was sought from the Tropical Diseases Research Centre Research Ethics Committee, and ethical standards were adhered to throughout this study. Informed consent was sought from study participants. Guardians provided assent for the participation of the persons under the consenting age. They were asked to read or have read to them, understand and sign/thumbprint an informed consent form. Responsible adults in the household were identified to give proxy consent on behalf of minors.

Table 1. Sample description for North-Western provinces for dengue virus infection

Factor	Total	Male	Female
	n (%)	n (%)	n (%)
Age (years)	[$x^2 = 7.79$, $p = 0.168$]		
<15	533 (30.4)	267 (31.3)	265 (29.5)
15-24	348 (19.8)	164 (19.2)	182 (20.3)
25-34	348 (19.8)	151 (17.7)	197 (22.0)
35-44	247 (14.1)	121 (14.2)	125 (13.9)
45+	278 (15.8)	150 (17.6)	128 (14.3)
Sex			
Male	854 (48.8)	-	-
Female	897 (51.2)	-	-
Education	[$x^2 = 26.22$, $p < 0.001$]		
None	370 (21.4)	160 (19.1)	209 (23.6)
Primary	812 (47.0)	365 (43.5)	445 (50.3)
Secondary or higher	545 (31.6)	314 (37.4)	230 (26.0)
Dengue virus infection	[$x^2 = 0.12$, $p = 0.729$]		
Yes	18 (1.0)	10 (1.2)	8 (0.9)
No	1737 (99.0)	844 (99.8)	889 (99.1)

RESULTS

A total of 1755 participants had both laboratory results and filled in the questionnaires. The sample comprised 48.8% females. Overall, 30.4% of the participants were aged less than 15 years. Male participants tended to have attained higher education levels than females ($p < 0.001$). The results indicated 1.0% previous dengue infection amongst the participants in North-Western province. No significant association was observed between sex and dengue infection ($p = 0.729$). These results are shown in Table 1.

Of the factors considered in bivariate analyses (Table 2), only visit to Angola was significantly associated with previous dengue infection (OR = 2.73; 95% CI [1.55, 4.83]).

DISCUSSION

This study reveals that 1.0% of the study population in North-western had dengue IgG antibodies, indicating having past exposure to dengue infection. A retrospective study on German expatriates who worked in endemic countries for an average of 10 years revealed 4.3% dengue IgG response (26). A prospective study on 104 long term Israel travelers to dengue endemic areas indicated a dengue seroprevalence of 6.7% (27).

Of the factors investigated including age, sex, education and travel to Angola and or Democratic Republic of Congo (DRC), only travel to Angola was positively associated with exposure to dengue infection. Various studies have indicated travel as a significant factor in dengue infection. Wilder-Smith and Gubler (28) described travel as having the most impact for the spread of dengue from one region to another. They documented that epidemics of dengue, its seasonality and oscillations over time are reflected in the epidemiology of dengue in travelers (29). In a study on travelers returning from endemic countries, dengue infection was associated with 7-45% of cases of fever (30).

Table 2. Factors associated with Dengue virus infection in logistic regression analysis for Western province

Factor	OR (95% CI)
Age (years)	
<15	0.61 (0.21, 1.71)
15-24	0.31 (0.06, 1.55)
25-34	1.24 (0.48, 3.19)
35-44	2.21 (0.91, 5.33)
45+	1
Sex	
Male	1.15 (0.72, 1.83)
Female	1
Education	
None	0.81 (0.35, 1.87)
Primary	1.11.(0.59, 2.11)
Secondary or higher	1
Use of mosquito net	
Yes	1.41 (0.84, 2.37)
No	1
Insecticide Residual Spraying	
Yes	1.30 (0.8, 2.09)
No	1
Visited Angola	
Yes	2.73 (1.55, 4.83)
No	1

Among the countries with evidence of on-going dengue outbreaks including Angola, Democratic Republic of Congo, Mozambique, Tanzania and Seychelles, all except Seychelles neighbour Zambia. The North-Western province of Zambia shares the border with Angola and DRC (Figure 1). This boundary, like most in Africa tends to divide villages, with inhabitants of the same family living on either side of the border. Small scale trade, and search for medical facilities necessitates frequent travels across the border and this could be a contributing factor to spread of disease including dengue.

It is safe to assume the continued circulation of dengue in Angola is associated with sero-prevalence in North-Western province of Zambia, considering its proximity to Angola and a significant association of Dengue infection with travel to Angola. Mazaba et al. indicated presence of dengue IgG antibodies in Western province of Zambia, which borders North-Western province on the southern side and also borders with Angola (31). There may also be transmission of dengue virus between the two provinces of Zambia.

Limitations in this study lie in the fact that plaque reduction neutralization tests (PRNTs) to increase the specificity of ELISA testing and reduce potential cross reactivity were not performed. Although the IgG capture-ELISA test used is a suitable tool to detecting Dengue IgG antibodies in large epidemiologic surveys (32), caution must be taken considering that cross-reactivity may occur with other Flavivirus antibodies (33).

Conclusion

This study provides evidence of dengue virus circulation in North-Western provinces of Zambia. It also elaborates on an important factor of association with travel to Angola which is a dengue endemic area. Dengue is a disease of public health importance especially that subsequent infection with other serotypes mya lead to more severe cases and fatalities. There is need for active surveillance and adequate diagnostic systems considering how porous the borders with the endemic countries are.

Acknowledgments

We acknowledge the laboratory support received from Virology laboratory staff (Cynthia Mubanga-Phiri, Julia Chibumbya and Hope Nkamba), University Teaching Hospital, Lusaka, Zambia and Institute de Pasteur, Dakar, Senegal. We are grateful to the interviewers for their dedicated work to successfully complete the survey. The survey could not have been successful without the cooperation of the participants. The survey was funded by the Ministry of Health [Zambia] and the World Health Organization for field activities.

All authors have approved the submission and declare that they have no competing interests.

References

[1] US Centers for Disease Control (CDC). Accessed February 2014. URL: http://www.cdc.gov/dengue/.

[2] US Centers for Disease Control (CDC). Accessed February 2014. URL: http://www.nc.cdc.gov/travel/yellowbook/2014/chapter-3-infectious-diseases-related-to-travel/dengue.

[3] US Centers for Disease Control (CDC). Accessed February 2014. URL:http://www.cdc.gov/Dengue/epidemiology/index.html.

[4] Bhatt S, Gething PW, Brady OJ, Messina JP, Farlow AW, Moyes CL, et al. The global distribution and burden of dengue. Nature 2013;496(7446):504-7.

[5] Gubler DJ, Clark GG. Dengue/Dengue hemorrhagic fever: The emergence of a global health problem. Emerg Infect Dis 1995;2: 55-7.

[6] Gubler DJ. Dengue and Dengue hemorrhagic fever. Clin Microbiol Rev 1998;11(3):480.

[7] Hayes EB, Gubler DJ. Dengue and dengue hemorrhagic fever. Pediatr Infect Dis J 1992;11:311–7.

[8] Ranjit S, Kissoon N. Dengue hemorrhagic fever and shock syndromes. Pediatr Crit Care Med 2011;12(1):90–100.

[9] World Health Organization. Dengue and severe dengue fact sheet. Accessed 4 February 2014. URL:http://www.who.int/mediacentre/factsheets/fs117/en/index.html.

[10] Sang RC. Dengue in Africa. Accessed 28 February, 2014.URL: http://www. tropika. net/svc/review/061001-Dengue_in_Africa. Tropika.net 2007.

[11] Gubler DJ. Dengue. In: Monath TPM, ed. Epidemiology of arthropodborne viral disease. Boca Raton, FL: CRC Press, 1988:223-60.

[12] Schwartz E, Meltzer E, Mendelson M, Tooke A, Steiner F, Gautret P, et al. Detection on four continents of dengue fever cases related to an ongoing outbreak in Luanda, Angola, March to May 2013. Euro Surveill 2013;18(21): pii-20488.

[13] Gubler DJ. Dengue and dengue hemorrhagic fever in the Americas. P R Health Sci J 1987;6:107–11.

[14] Gubler DJ. Dengue and dengue hemorrhagic fever. Semin Pediatr Infect Dis 1997;8:1.

[15] Anker M, Amina Y. Male-female differences in the number of reported incident dengue fever cases in six Asian countries. Western Pac Surveill Response J 2011;2(2):17-23.
[16] Egger ER, Coleman PG. Age and clinical dengue illness. Emerg Infect Dis 2007;13(6):924-5.
[17] Hayes EB, Gubler DJ. Dengue and dengue hemorrhagic fever. Pediatr Infect Dis J 1992;11:311–7.
[18] Teixera MG, Costa Mda C, Barreto ML. Dengue: twenty-five years since reemergence in Brazil. Cad Saude Publica 2009;25(suppl 1):S7-18.
[19] Cavalcanti LP, Vilar D, Santos RS, Teixeira MG. Change in age pattern of persons with Dengue, northeastern Brazil [letter]. Emerg Infect Dis 2011;7(1):132-4.
[20] Blackburn NK, Rawat R. Dengue fever imported from India: A report of 3 cases SAMJ 1987;71: 386-7.
[21] Guzman MG, Halstead SB, Artsob H, Buchy P, Farrar J, Gubler DJ, et al. Dengue: a continuing global threat. Nature Rev Microbiol 2010;8(12Suppl):S7–S16.doi:10.1038/nrmicro246.
[22] Gubler DJ. Dengue and dengue haemorrhagic fever. Clin Microbiol Rev 1998;11(3):480-96.
[23] Civil Society for Poverty Reduction. 2013 report. Accessed February 2014. URL: http://www.csprzambia.org/.
[24] Central Statistical Office (CSO), Ministry of Health (MOH), Tropical Diseases Research Centre (TDRC), University of Zambia, and Macro International Inc. Zambia Demographic and Health Survey 2007. Calverton, MD: CSO, Macro International, 2009.
[25] Robinson GG. A note on mosquitoes and yellow fever in Northern Rhodesia. East Afr Med J 1950;27(7):284-8.
[26] Potasman I, Srugo I, Schwartz E. Dengue seroconversion among Israeli travelers to tropical countries. Emerg Infect Dis 1999;5(6):824-7.
[27] Groen J, Koraka P, Velzing J, Corprac, Osterhaus AD. Evaluation of six immunoassays for detection of dengue virus specific immunoglobulin M and G antibodies. Clin Diagn Lab Immunol 2000;7(6):867-71.
[28] Wilder-Smith A, Gubler DJ. Geographic expansion of dengue: the impact of international travel. Med Clin North Am 2008;92(6):1377-90.
[29] Cobelens FG, Groen J, Osterhaus AD, Leentvaar-Kuipers A, Wertheim-van Dillen PM, Kager PA. Incidence and risk factors of probable dengue virus infection among Dutch travellers to Asia. Trop Med Int Health 2002;7(4):331-8.
[30] Jänisch T, Preiser W, Berger A, Niedrig M, Mikulicz U, Thoma B, et al. Emerging viral pathogens in long-term expatriates (II): Dengue virus. Trop Med Int Health 1997;2(10):934-40.
[31] Mazaba-Liwewe ML, Siziya S, Monze M, Mweene-Ndumba I, Masaninga F, Songolo P, et al. First sero-prevalence of dengue fever specific immunoglobulin G antibodies in Western and North-Western provinces of Zambia: a population based cross sectional study. Virol J 2014;11:135.
[32] Groen J, Koraka P, Velzing J, Copra C, Osterhaus AD. Evaluation of six immunoassays for detection of dengue virus-specific immunoglobulin M and G antibodies. Clin Diagn Lab Immunol 2000;7: 867-71.
[33] Ha DQ, Huong VTQ, Loan HTK, Thang DQ, Duebel V. Seroprevalence of dengue antibodies, annual incidence and risk factors among children in southern Vietnam. Trop Med Int Health 2005;10:379-86.

In: Public Health Yearbook 2016
Editor: Joav Merrick

ISBN: 978-1-53610-947-4

Chapter 5

Correlates of Zika Virus Infection Specific IgG in North-Western Province of Zambia: Results from a Population-Based Cross-Sectional Study

Olusegun Babaniyi*[1], *MBBS, MPH, MSc,
Peter Songolo*[1,*], *MBChB, MPH,
Mazyanga L Mazaba-Liwewe*[1], *BSc,
Idah Mweene-Ndumba*[1], *BSc, MPH,
Freddie Masaninga*[1], *BSc, MSc, PhD,
Emmanuel Rudatsikira*[2], *MD, MPH, DrPH
and Seter Siziya*[3,4], *BA(Ed), MSc, PhD
[1]World Health Organization, Lusaka, Zambia
[2]School of Health Professionals, Andrews University, Michigan, US
[3]School of Medicine, Copperbelt University, Ndola, Zambia
[4]University of Lusaka, Lusaka, Zambia

Abstract

Arthropod-borne viruses (arboviruses) have become significant public health problems, with the emergency and re-emergency of arboviral diseases nearly worldwide. The objective of this study was to determine the prevalence and the risk factors for Zika virus infection in North-Western Province of Zambia. A cross-sectional study using a standardised questionnaire was used. Bivariate logistic regression analyses were conducted to obtain odds ratios and their 95% confidence intervals. In total, 1,755 survey participants were recruited. Overall, 48.8% of the survey participants were males. Males tended to have higher education levels than females, with 37.4% of males and 26.0% of

* Correspondence: Peter Songolo, MBChB, MPH, World Health Organization, Lusaka, Zambia. E-mail: songolop@who.int.

females having attained secondary or higher levels of education ($p < 0.001$). Altogether, 1.8% of participants had Zika virus infection, with no sex difference (2.1% of males and 1.4% of females, $p = 0.957$). Visiting Angola was the only factor that was significantly associated with Zika virus infection. Participants who visited Angola were 2.82 (95% CI [1.82, 4.38]) times more likely to have Zika virus infection compared to participants who had not visited Angola. Zika virus infection is prevalent among residents of North-Western Province in Zambia. Strengthening of disease surveillance, clinical management of cases and laboratory diagnostic capacities are necessary to curb the infection.

Keyword: Zika virus infection, prevalence, correlates, North-Western province, Zambia

INTRODUCTION

Zambia is undergoing rapid developmental changes particularly in infrastructure. The opening up of new mines in recent years in North-Western province means that mining has become a major occupation for the province. This has resulted in population movement especially from the 'traditional' Copperbelt province, creating a sudden increase in the total population of the province with resultant challenges for the health sector. Sudden population increase has resulted in over-crowding making a suitable environment for disease spread including the arboviruses.

Among the emerging infectious diseases, the arboviral diseases group has particularly warranted attention in the global health landscape with its potential for epidemics and its unprecedented spread (1). Despite the significance and increasing public health impact on individuals worldwide, arboviruses remain poorly understood and controlled. While increasingly well characterised in industrialised countries, the epidemiology of the these viruses is a major challenge to developing countries and surveillance often is usually in the form of reports during outbreaks due to the poor population-based surveillance systems (2). The majority of the surveillance systems were designed to detect known pathogens (61.5%), while 19.9% were for both known and unknown pathogens and only a small proportion were designed to detect unknown pathogens (3).

The diagnosis of Zika virus infection is based on detection of specific antibodies (4) or virus isolation from animals or mosquitoes which is time consuming; however, rapid diagnostic methods have been developed for the African and Asian strains (5). Several serological surveys have been carried out in Africa and notable among these is the Portuguese Guinea survey which demonstrated frequent antibodies to group B viruses particularly Yellow Fever, Zika and Wesselbrons; a finding similar to previous surveys in the same region (6). Based on serological analyses, flaviviruses were classified into eight antigenic complexes; however, many viruses including the prototype of the group Yellow Fever and many new viruses could not be affiliated to any complex partly due to extensive geographical distribution, diversity of arthropod vector or vertebrate hosts and also confusion in virus nomenclature (7).

No information on Zika virus infection has been reported in Zambia. The objective of the study was, thus, to determine the prevalence and correlates for Zika virus infection in North-Western province of Zambia in order to contribute to the body of knowledge on the epidemiology of Zika virus infection in Zambia.

METHODS

North-Western Province borders with Angola in the West and Democratic Republic of Congo (DRC) in the North. North-Western Province was one of Zambia's nine provinces at the time of the survey before the creation of the tenth province. It covers an area of 125,826 km² and had a population of 695,599 (8).

A total of 1,178 Standard Enumeration Areas (SEAs) were demarcated in North-Western province in the eight districts of the province. North-Western province is located in Agro-ecological zone III which is suitable for cultivating rice, cassava, pineapples and bananas (9).

Sample size

The data was obtained from a survey on Yellow fever. The sample size calculation was based on the assumption that the sero-prevalence for Yellow fever was 7% based on the study conducted by Robinson (10). A Statcal program in Epi Info v6.04 was used to estimate the sample size. After adjusting for 80% response rate, a sample size of 3600 was obtained. The sample size was equally divided into the two provinces and powered to avoid chance findings, that is, 1,800 participants from each province.

Sampling

A multi-stage sampling technique was used for participants in all districts. Firstly, wards were randomly selected from each constituency. In the second stage of sampling, standard enumeration areas (SEAs) proportional to the ward size were systematically sampled. All survey participants aged nine months or older in a selected household were eligible to be enrolled in the study.

Ethical approval

The study protocol was reviewed and approved by the Tropical Diseases Research Centre Research Ethics Committee, and permission to conduct the study was obtained from the Ministry of Health, Zambia. Informed consent was obtained from survey participants after the interviewer had explained the benefits and risks of participating in the study. Entry forms were viewed only by those approved to be part of the survey.

Data collection

A detailed semi structured questionnaire was used to collect information. During the data collection process, questionnaires were checked for inconsistencies and completeness on a daily basis.

Table 1. Sample description for North-Western Province for Zika virus infection

Factor	Total n (%)	Male n (%)	Female n (%)	p value
Age (years)				
<15	533 (30.4)	267 (31.3)	265 (29.5)	0.102
15 – 24	348 (19.8)	164 (19.2)	182 (20.3)	
25 – 34	348 (19.8)	151 (17.7)	197 (22.0)	
35 – 44	247 (14.1)	121 (14.2)	125 (13.9)	
45+	278 (15.8)	150 (17.6)	128 (14.3)	
Sex				
Male	854 (48.8)			
Female	897 (51.2)			
Education				
None	370 (21.4)	160 (19.1)	209 (23.6)	<0.001
Primary	812 (47.0)	365 (43.5)	445 (50.3)	
Secondary or higher	545 (31.6)	314 (37.4)	230 (26.0)	
Zika virus infection				
Yes	31 (1.8)	18 (2.1)	13 (1.4)	0.957
No	1724 (98.2)	836 (97.9)	884 (98.6)	

Data management and analysis

All data were entered in Epi-Info data entry screen that had consistency and range checks embedded in it. Epi data files were exported to SPSS for data analysis. Further editing was conducted by running frequencies during the analysis stage. Odds ratios and their 95% confidence intervals were used to estimate magnitudes of associations.

RESULTS

In total, 1755 survey participants were recruited. Overall, 48.8% of the survey participants were males. Males tended to have higher education levels than females, with 37.4% of males and 26.0% of females having attained secondary or higher levels of education ($p < 0.001$). Altogether, 1.8% of participants had Zika virus infection, with no sex difference (2.1% of males and 1.4% of females, $p = 0.957$). Table 1 below describes the sample population.

Visiting Angola was the only factor that was significantly associated with Zika virus infection. Participants who visited Angola were 2.82 (95% CI [1.82, 4.38]) times more likely to have Zika virus infection compared to participants who had not visited Angola. Age, sex, education, use of mosquito net and in-door residual spraying were not significantly associated with Zika virus infection.

DISCUSSION

Information concerning the distribution of Zika virus in North-Western Province was non-available until after the risk assessment was conducted in April/May 2013 by the Ministry of

Health with the support of World Health Organization. The risk assessment carried out in North-Western Province was conducted to respond to the re-classification of the province as a low-risk area for arboviruses particularly Yellow Fever. There was no assessment carried out in the province since 1950 when the last sero-survey was conducted during the colonial era. The sero-survey of 1950 concentrated in Barotseland (Western), Balovale (North-Western) and Ndola in present day Copperbelt Province (10).

Zika virus which had not been previously reported in North-Western Province appeared to be an important flavivirus affecting 1.8% of the survey participants. Our finding indicates that Zika virus was circulating among people of North-Western Province. Our finding is much lower than those reported in Kainji lake basin of Nigeria of 56% (11), Oyo State of Nigeria of 31% (12), Yap island of Federated States of Micronesia of 73% (13). Differences in rates of infection may partly be due to different laboratory tests, power of the studies and epidemiological stages of the infection in study areas.

The risk assessment revealed that international travel especially outside of the province was highly associated with acquisition of infection for Zika virus. The survey participants with a history of travel to neighbouring countries especially to the Republic of Angola had twice as much risk of acquiring Zika infection than their counterparts without history of travel (Table 2). However, travel to the Democratic Republic of Congo was not found to be significant probably due to host ecology and host behaviour (14). Stoddard et al, using mathematical models, illustrated the importance of human movement in the transmission of pathogens especially for populations most at risk to vector-borne diseases such as Zika virus (15).

Table 2. Factors associated with Zika virus infection in North-Western Province in bivariate logistic regression analysis

Factor	OR (95% CI)
Age (years)	
<15	0.37 (0.14, 0.99)
15 – 24	0.38 (0.12, 1.21)
25 – 34	1.15 (0.54, 2.47)
35 – 44	1.19 (0.93, 3.96)
45+	1
Sex	
Male	1.21 (0.84, 1.73)
Female	1
Education	
None	0.82 (0.43, 1,58)
Primary	1.36 (0.84, 2.22)
Secondary or higher	1
Use of mosquito net	
Yes	1.27 (0.87, 1.86)
No	1
In-door residual spraying	
Yes	0.96 (0.64, 1.43)
No	1
Visited Angola	
Yes	2.82 (1.82, 4.38)
No	1

Despite the fact that 1.8% of samples collected during the risk assessment tested positive for Zika virus infection, no human case of Zika disease has been reported from North-Western Province. This may be due to the lack of knowledge by the medical personnel and also due to the absence of case definition in the Integrated Diseases Surveillance and Response (IDSR) guidelines which are widely used for syndromic diseases surveillance in health facilities. Furthermore, the symptoms of Zika infection apart from being sub-clinical in presentation could be mimicking malaria which has been known to be prevalent in the province. Therefore, suspected malaria cases might have continued to mask outbreaks of Zika virus infection.

The other challenge contributing to lack of information on arboviral disease presence or absence is the limitation on availability of diagnostic methods, thereby making it difficult to identify these emerging diseases in the country. Until 2013 in preparation for the risk assessment on Yellow Fever, the laboratory capacity to diagnose arboviruses had not been developed.

In conclusion, Zika virus infection is prevalent among residents of North-Western Province in Zambia. Strengthening of disease surveillance, clinical management of cases and laboratory diagnostic capacities are necessary to curb the infection.

Acknowledgments

We are grateful to the interviewers for their dedicated work to successfully complete the survey. The survey could not have been successful without the cooperation of the participants and the virology laboratory staff both in Lusaka, Zambia and Dakar, Senegal for testing of samples. The survey was funded by the Ministry of Health [Zambia] and the World Health Organization.

References

[1] Dash AP, Bhatia R, Sunyoto T, Mourya DT. Emerging and re-emerging arboviral diseases in South-East Asia. J Vector Borne Dis 2013;50:77-84.

[2] Kuniholm MK, Wolfe ND, Huang CYH, Mpoudi-Ngole E, Tamufe U, Burke DS, Duane J. Gubler DJ. Seroprevalence and distribution of Flaviviridae, Togaviridae and Bunyaviridae arboviral infection in rural Cameroonian adults. Am J Trop Med Hyg 2006;74:1078-83.

[3] Vrbova L, Stephen C, Kasman N, Boehnke R, Doyle-Waters M, Chablitt-Clark A, Gibson B, FitzGerald M, Patrick DM. Systematic review of surveillance systems for emerging zoonoses. Trandbound Emerg Dis 2010;57:154-61.

[4] Causey OR, Theiler M. Virus antibody survey on sera of residents of the Amazon valley in Brazil. Am J Trop Med Hyg 1958;7:36-41.

[5] Faye O, Faye O, Diallo D, Diallo M, Weidman M, Sall AA. Quantitative real-time PCR detection of Zika virus and evaluation with filed-caught mosquitoes. Virol J 2013;10:311.

[6] Pinto MR. Survey for antibodies to Arboviruses in the sera of children in Portuguese Guinea. Bull World Hlth Org 1967;37:101-8.

[7] Kuno G, Chang GJ, Tsuchiya KR, Kabaratsos N, Cropp CB. Phylogeny of the genus flaviviruses. J Virol 1998;72:73-83.

[8] Central Statistical Office. 2010 census of population and housing. National analytical report. Lusaka, Zambia: CSO, 2012.

[9] Country profile-Zambia. New Agriculturist. Accessed 2014 May 19. URL: http://www.new-ag.info/en/country/profile.php?a=2621.

[10] Robinson GG. A note on mosquitoes and yellow fever in Northern Rhodesia. East Afr Med J 1950;27:284-8.

[11] Adekolu-John EO, Fagbami AH. Arthropod-borne virus antibodies in sera of rfesidents of Kainji lake basin, Nigeria 1980. Trans R Soc Trop Med Hyg 1983;77:149-51.

[12] Fagbami AH. Zika virus infections in Nigeria: virological and seroepidemiological investigations in Oyo State. J Hyg (Camb) 1979;83:213-9.

[13] Duffy MR, Chen T-H, Hancock TW, Powers AM, Kool JL, Lanciotti RS, Pretrick M, Marfel M, Holzbauer S, Dubray C, Guillaumot L, Griggs A, Bel M, Lambert AJ, Laven J, Kosoy O, Panella A, Biggerstaff BJ, Fischer M, Hayes EB. Zika virus outbreak on Yap island, Federated States of Micronesia. N Eng J Med 2009;360:2536-43.

[14] Reiter P. Climate change and mosquito-borne disease: knowing the horse before hitching the cart. Rev Sci Tech Off Int 2008;27:383-98.

[15] Stoddard ST, Morrison AC, Vazquez-Prokopec GM, Soldan VP, Kochel TJ, Kitron U, Elder JP, Scott TW. The role of human movement in the transmission of vector-borne pathogens. PLoS PLoS Negl Trop Dis 2009;3:e481.

In: Public Health Yearbook 2016
Editor: Joav Merrick

ISBN: 978-1-53610-947-4

Chapter 6

IS NORTH-WESTERN PROVINCE OF ZAMBIA AT RISK FOR WEST NILE VIRUS INFECTION?

Idah Mweene-Ndumba[1,*], BSc, MPH, Seter Siziya[2], BA(Ed), MSc, PhD, Mwaka Monze[3], MBhB, PhD, Mazyanga L Mazaba-Liwewe[1], BSc, MSc, Freddie Masaninga[1], BSc, MSc, PhD, Peter Songolo[1], MBChB, MPH, Peter Mwaba[4], MBChB, PhD and Olusegun Babaniyi[1], MBBS, MPH, MSc

[1]World Health Organization, Lusaka, Zambia
[2]School of Medicine, Copperbelt University, Ndola, Zambia/University of Lusaka, Lusaka, Zambia
[3]University Teaching Hospital, Lusaka, Zambia
[4]Ministry of Home Affairs, Lusaka, Zambia

ABSTRACT

West Nile virus infection has been reported in Asia, Middle East, Europe, Americas and Africa but there is no documentation about its existence in Zambia. Therefore the purpose of this study was to determine the seroprevalence of WNV infection and its correlates in North-Western province of Zambia. Secondary data collected in a yellow fever risk assessment conducted in Zambia in 2013 was used in this study. Bivariate and multivariate logistic regression analyses were used to determine correlates for WNV infection. Unadjusted odds ratios and adjusted odds ratios with their 95% Confidence Intervals (CI) are reported. Out of a total of 1755 participants in the survey, 51.3% were females. About a third of the participants (30%) were aged 5-14 years. Overall, 2.0% of the participants had WNV infection. Having travelled to Angola was independently

* Corresponding author: Idah Mweene-Ndumba, BSc, MPH, World Health Organization, Lusaka, Zambia. E-mail: idahndumba12@gmail.com.

associated with WNV infection. Participants who visited Angola were 2.58 (95% CI [1.67, 3.98]) times more likely to have WNV infection compared to those who had not travelled to Angola. Instituting an active surveillance for the infection at border post would help in preventing further importation of the virus.

Keywords: West Nile virus infection, correlates, North-Western province, Zambia

INTRODUCTION

West Nile virus (WNV) is an arthropod borne virus from the Flaviviridae family. Humans get infected from a *culex* mosquito bite. Most of the infections are asymptomatic but about 1% show symptoms which sometimes could develop into severe illness (nueroinvasive symptoms) which could also result into death (1).

West Nile fever was first identified in a woman from the west Nile province, Uganda, who presented with influenza like illness in Uganda (2). After the discovery in Uganda the virus became endemic in many African countries, mainly epizootic at that time, with reported seasonal outbreaks in humans (3). The disease was viewed as of very low public health importance till its recognition as an emerging infectious disease as it spread across the globe with reports in Asia, Middle East, Europe and Americas (4-6). In North Africa, a more virulent strain of WNV emerged in 1994 and it caused outbreaks of severe disease symptoms and more deaths than reported previously (5).

Several risk factors for WNV infection emerged from the study in America such as climate and environmental factors. High population density was significantly associated with the viral transmission even after adjusting for other environmental factors (7) and the results were comparable to results obtained in other studies which confirmed an association between urban/sub-urban versus a more rural area (8, 9). However other studies reported significant association when there was less population density and rural. Temperature changes determining human activity and mosquito replication was also significantly associated with risk of infection. It was also concluded that these factors could differ yearly due to changes in bird populations with high bird population as being protective (7). It is possible that when there are more birds the virus could be concentrated in bird mosquito bird cycle whereas if there are fewer birds the mosquito could resort to human meals. Studies have also confirmed that age has a bearing on the severity of the infection with the older age group, 50 years and above, being most at risk (7). In Arizon staying at home and not attending school were found to be risk factors to the WNV infection, although it was argued that the possibility that those who stayed at home were the elderly who were already known to be at high risk of infection with WNV (10).

Although WNV infections have been reported worldwide and furthermore around Zambia's neighboring countries, there is still no information on the extent of the problem in the North-western province of Zambia. Therefore the purpose of this analysis was to determine the seroprevalence of WNV and its correlates in North-western province of Zambia.

METHODS

The study was conducted in North-Western province of Zambia. The province was selected based on the classification as low potential risk areas for yellow fever transmission by World Health Organization (11). North-Western province which borders with Angola on the western side and Democratic Republic of Congo (DRC) on the northern side has a population of 706,462 (12). It is the most sparsely populated province in the country and the provincial capital is Solwezi. The province comprised of 8 districts which were divided into 1178 Standard Enumeration Aras (SEAs) and the main economic activities were mining in one district and general pineapple growing.

Study population, sample size, inclusion/exclusion criteria and sampling

This assessment was carried out among individuals aged nine months or older. In estimating the sample size for persons aged 5 years or older, the following parameters were considered: a prevalence of 7% (13), desired precision or confidence interval (d) of $\pm$3%, and a design effect (DE) of 2 and an 80% response rate.

Considering sex, we aimed to recruit 700 male and 700 female participants in each province. Assuming an average of 4 persons aged 5 years or older in each household, a total of 12 households in each of the 30 cluster was to be recruited in the survey. The total number of persons that would be recruited from each province was 1806, totaling 3612 from both provinces.

The seroprevalence of children was about half that for older children, and in estimating the sample size for persons aged below 5 years, the following parameters were considered: a prevalence of 3.5%, desired precision or confidence interval (d) of +3.4%, and a design effect (DE) of 2 and an 80% response rate. The computed sample size was 282. Therefore, in each province 406 children would be recruited for the survey.

Included in the study were individuals aged 9 months or older who were found in a sampled household at the time of the study and were resident in the study site for at least seven days. Individuals who had received YF vaccination in the last ten years to the survey were also included in the survey. Excluded from the study were persons who were aged less than 9 months, or individuals regardless of age who resided in the study site for less than 7 days prior to the survey. Children under the age of 9 months were excluded based on the fact that at this age children could still carry maternal antibodies from exposed mothers which could pose the risk of false positive results.

The sample was drawn using a two-stage cluster sampling technique using probability proportional to size. A list of the standard enumeration areas (SEAs) in each province constituted the sampling frame. The sampling was designed to achieve fairly good estimates at the provincial level of analysis, and not representing the subdivisions of the province.

Study variables

Dependent variable

A case with evidence of WNV exposure was defined as any individual aged 9 months or older whose blood sample was confirmed to have WNV exposure. WNV exposure status was positive if IgG or IgM antibodies were determined in the serum sample by laboratory testing and negative if the IgG or IgM antibodies were absent by laboratory testing.

Independent variables

The independent variables included demographic data: age, sex, occupation, education, roof type and use of mosquito preventive measures such as insecticide treated nets (ITNs) and indoor residual spray (IRS).

Laboratory procedures

Three to 5 millilitres of blood was collected by venepuncture into an EDTA vaccutainer tube and transported on cold chain to the local laboratories for serum separation and storage.

Subsequently serum samples were transported on cold chain and thereafter subjected to primary testing (YFV specific IgG and IgM) at the University of Teaching Hospital in Zambia virology unit and Institute Pasteur, Dakar. All presumptive YFV-specific IgG and IgM samples were subjected to IgG and IgM antibodies testing against other flaviviruses known to cause haemorrhagic fever-like disease including WNV. The testing was carried out using IgG capture enzyme-linked immunosorbent assay (ELISA).

Table 1. Sample description North-West province

Factors	**Total**	**Male**	**Female**	
	n (%)	**n (%)**	**n (%)**	**p value**
Age (years)				
5-14	533 (30.4)	267 (31.3)	265 (29.5)	0.102
15-24	348 (19.8)	164 (19.2)	182 (20.3)	
25-34	348 (19.8)	151 (17.7)	197 (22.0)	
25-44	247 (14.1)	121 (14.2)	125 (13.9)	
45+	278 (15.8)	150 (17.6)	128 (14.3)	
Sex				
Male	854 (48.8)	-	-	-
Female	897 (51.2)	-	-	
Education				
None	370 (21.4)	160 (19.1)	209 (23.6)	<0.001
Primary	812 (47.0)	365 (43.5)	445 (50.3)	
Secondary/College/University	545 (31.6)	314 (37.4)	230 (26.0)	
West Nile Infection				
Positive	35 (2.0)	19 (2.2)	16 (1.8)	0.625
Negative	1720 (98.0)	835 (97.8)	881 (98.2)	

Data management and analysis

Data collected from the field were entered in an Epi-Info data entry screen that had consistency and range checks embedded in it. Further editing was conducted by running frequencies during the analysis stage. Epi data files were exported to SPSS for data analysis. The data was summarized to describe the occurrence of WNV exposed individuals in absolute numbers and percentage by place (residence, travel or work) and person (age, sex, occupation, education). Further analysis was conducted to determine independent factors associated with WNV sero-positivity. Odds ratios were used to estimate the magnitude of associations

Ethical considerations

Ethical clearance was sought from the Tropical Diseases Research Centre Research Ethics Committee, and ethical standards were adhered to throughout this study. Informed consent was sought from study participants. Guardians provided assent for the participation of the persons under the consenting age. They were asked to read or have read to them, understand and sign/thumbprint an informed consent form. Responsible adults in the household were identified to give proxy consent on behalf of minors.

RESULTS

Out of a total of 1755 participants in the survey, 51.3% were females. Most of the participants (30%) were aged 5-14 years of age. There were more females who had attained primary school than males ($p = 0.001$). On the other hand more males (37.4% males and 26% females) attained secondary or higher education than the females. There was no significant association between WNV infection and sex ($p = 0.625$). Overall, 2.0% of the participants had antibodies to WNV.

The variables in Table 2, age, sex, education, sleeping under a mosquito net, house with IRS and travelled to Angola were analyzed in bivariate and multivariate models. Having travelled to Angola was the only factor that was significantly associated with WNV infection in multivariate analysis. Participants who visited Angola were 2.58 (95% CI [1.67, 3.98]) times more likely to have WNV infection compared with those who had not travelled to Angola.

DISCUSSION

This study presents the first documentation of the prevalence of WNV infection and the contributing factors to the infection in North-western province of Zambia This study has indicated that 2.0% of the participants had antibodies to WNV. This finding is similar to a 2.6% reported in New York during the 1999 epidemic (14), implying that both epidemics might have been at the same stage of the epidemic. A study conducted in Kenya reported varying rates of the infection of 3.2-65.3% within the same country (15). Higher rates of the infection have been reported in Egypt and Sudan of 61% and 40%, respectively (16) and 55%

in South Africa (17) as way back as the 1950s to 1970s. Disease prevalence is dependent upon a wide range of risk factors, climate and the environment affecting the activities of the virus and the humans (7, 8, 9). It is therefore important that surveys be conducted not only in specific regions of a country but the whole country in order to inform the designs of interventions to curtail the spread of the virus.

Travelling to Angola was associated with being infected with WNV. Travel could have been necessitated by visiting relatives across the border in Angola or to conduct trade. While in Angola, one could have been bitten by an infected mosquito. A similar observation was made by Cameron et al. who observed that the continued spread of dengue was supported by global trade and increasing travel within and between countries (18). Furthermore, travel increases the risk of introducing arthropod-borne virus diseases from endemic to non-endemic areas.

In conclusion, surveillance at the border should be strengthened in order to curtail further importation of the virus into the province, assuming that persons who had traveled to Angola did not have the virus before they traveled.

Table 2. Factors associated with West Nile Virus infection in bivariate and multivariate analysis for North-Western province

Factor	OR (95% CI)	AOR (95% CI)
Age (years)		
5-14	0.59 (0.29-1.21)	-
15-24	0.45 (0.17-1.17)	
25-34	0.91 (0.44-1.87)	
35-44	1.96 (1.04-3.69)	
45+	1	
Sex		
Male	1.12 (0.80-1.57))	-
Female	1	
Education		
None	0.74 (0.39-1.40)	-
Primary	1.36 (0.85-2.16)	
Secondary/College/University	1	
Slept under Mosquito Net		
Yes	1.30 (0.90-1.86)	-
No	1	
House with IRS		
Yes	1.41 (1.01-1.99)	-
No	1	
Travelled to Angola		
Yes	2.61 (1.69-4.02)	2.58 (1.67-3.98)
No	1	1

ACKNOWLEDGMENTS

We are grateful to the interviewers for their dedicated work to successfully complete the survey. The survey could not have been successful without the cooperation of the participants and the virology laboratory staff both in Dakar, Senegal and Lusaka, Zambia for testing the samples. The survey was funded by the Ministry of Health [Zambia] and the World Health Organization.

REFERENCES

[1] Smithburn KC, Hughes TP, Burke AW, Paul JH. A neurotropic virus isolated from the blood of a native of Uganda. Am J Trop Med 1940; 20: 471-2.

[2] Petersen LR, Carson PJ, Biggerstaff BJ, Custer B, Borchardt SM, Busch MP. Estimated cumulative incidence of West Nile virus infection in US adults, 1999–2010. Epidemiol infect 2013; 141(03): 591-5.

[3] Stiasny K, Aberle SW, HeinzFX. Retrospective identification of human cases of West Nile virus infection in Austria (2009 to 2010) by serological differentiation from Usutu and other flavivirus infections. Euro Surveill 2013; 18(43). Pii: 20614.

[4] Gubler DJ. The continuing spread of West Nile virus in the western hemisphere. Clin Infect Dis 2007; 45: 1039-46.

[5] Hayes EB, Komar N, Nasci RS, Montgomery SP, O'Leary DR, Campbell GL. Epidemiology and transmission dynamics of West Nile virus disease. Emerg Infect Dis 2005; 11: 1167-73.

[6] Liu A, Lee V, Galusha D, Slade MD, Diuk-Wasser M, Andreadis T, Scotch M, Rabinowitz PM. Risk factors for human infection with West Nile Virus in Connecticut: a multi-year analysis. Int J Health Geogr 2009; 8: 67.

[7] Brown HE, Childs JE, Diuk-Wasser MA, Fish D. Ecological factors associated with West Nile virus transmission, northeastern United States. Emerg Infect Dis 2008; 14: 1539-45.

[8] Gibbs SEJ, Wimberly MC, Madden M, Masour J, Yabsley MJ, Stallknecht DE. Factors Affecting the Geographic Distribution of West Nile Virus in Georgia, USA: 2002–2004. *Vector Borne* Zoonotic Dis 2006; 6: 73-82.

[9] Gibney KB, Colborn J, Baty S, Bunko Patterson AM, Sylvester T, Briggs G, Stewart T, Levy C, Komatsu K, MacMillan K, Delorey MJ, Mutebi JP, Fischer M, Staples JE. Modifiable Risk Factors for West Nile Virus Infection during an Outbreak—Arizona, 2010. Am J Trop Med Hyg 2012; 86: 895–901.

[10] Schweitzer BK, Kramer WL, Sambol AR, Meza JL, Hinrichs SH, Iwen PC. Geographic Factors Contributing to a High Seroprevalence of West Nile Virus-Specific Antibodies in Humans following an Epidemic. Clin Vaccine Immunol 2006; 13: 314-8.

[11] Jentes ES, Poumerol G, Gershman MD, Hill DR, Lemarchand J, Lewis RF, Staples JE, Tomori O, Wilder-Smith A, Monath TP; Informal WHO Working Group on Geographic Risk for Yellow Fever. The revised global yellow fever risk map and recommendations for vaccination, 2010: consensus of the Informal WHO Working Group on Geographic Risk for Yellow Fever. Lancet Infect Dis 2011; 11: 622-32.

[12] Central Statistical Office. 2010 census of population and housing. National analytical report. Lusaka, Zambia: CSO, 2012.

[13] Robinson GG. A note on mosquitoes and yellow fever in Northern Rhodesia. East Afr Med J 1950; 27: 284-8.

[14] Mostashari F, Bunning ML, Kitsutani PT, Singer DA, Nash D, Cooper MJ, Katz N, Liljebjelke KA, Biggerstaff BJ, Fine AD, Layton MC, Mullin SM, Johnson AJ, Martin DA, Hayes EB, Campbell GL. Epidemic West Nile encephalitis, New York, 1999: results of a household-based seroepidemiological survey. Lancet. 2001; 358: 261-4.

[15] Geser A, Henderson BE, Christensen S. A multipurpose serological survey in Kenya: 2. Results of arbovirus serological tests. Bull Wld Hlth Org 1970; 43: 539-52.

[16] Taylor RM, Work TH, Hurlbut HS, Rizk F. A study of the ecology of West Nile in Egypt. Am J Trop Med Hyg 1956; 5: 579-620.

[17] Mcintosh BM, Jupp PG, Dos Santos I, Meenehan GM. Epidemics of West Nile and Sindbis viruses in South Africa with Culex (Culex) univittatus Theobald as vector. South Afr J Sci 1976; 72: 295-300.

[18] Cameron P. Simmons CP, Farrar JJ, van Vinh Chau N, Wills B. Dengue. N Engl J Med 2012; 366: 1423-32.

[19] Blackburn NK, Rawat R. Dengue fever imported from India: a report of 3 cases. S Afr Med J 1987; 71: 386-7/.

In: Public Health Yearbook 2016
Editor: Joav Merrick

ISBN: 978-1-53610-947-4

Chapter 7

LARVAL HABITAT DISTRIBUTION: AEDES MOSQUITO VECTOR FOR ARBOVIRUSES AND CULEX SPPS IN NORTH-WESTERN AND WESTERN PROVINCES OF ZAMBIA

Freddie Masaninga[1,*], BSc, MSc, PhD,
Mbanga Muleba[2], BSc, MSc,
Hieronymo Masendu[3], BSc, MSc, PhD,
Peter Songolo[1], MBChB, MPH, Idah Mweene-Ndumba, BSc, MPH,
Mazyanga L Mazaba-Liwewe[1], BSc, Mulakwa Kamuliwo[6], MD,
Birknesh Ameneshewa[5], BSc, MSc, PhD,
Seter Siziya[4], BA(Ed), MSc, PhD and
Olusegun A Babaniyi[1], MBBS, MPH, MSc
[1]World Health Organization, Lusaka, Zambia
[2]Tropical Diseases Research Centre, Ndola, Zambia
[3]Abt Associates Harare, Zimbabwe
[4]The Copperbelt University, School of Medicine, Zambia/University of Lusaka, Lusaka, Zambia
[5]World Health Organization, Harare, Zimbabwe
[6]Ministry of Health, Lusaka, Zambia

ABSTRACT

Zambia is prone to mosquito-borne diseases: malaria, filariasis and arthropod-borne viruses (arboviruses). There is limited information on the distribution of larval habitats of vectors of arboviruses in Zambia. A study was conducted to determine the distribution of

[*] Corresponding author: Freddie Masaninga, PhD, National Professional Officer, WHO Country Office, Lusaka, Zambia. E-mail: Masaningaf@who.int.

mosquito larval habitats in Western and North-Western provinces of Zambia. Mosquito larval surveys were conducted in rural, urban and peri-urban locations, indoor and outdoor. Altogether, 350 potential breeding habitats were inspected: flower pots, old tyres, banana leaf axils, water storage containers, shallow wells, disused wells, disused bottles, canoes and water pools soaked with cassava tubers. Aedes (stegomyia) aegypti larvae were collected in a disused cooking oil plastic container; 1 (1.9%) out of 52 containers in peri-urban areas of North-Western province was positive for larvae, while no container in Western province was positive for larvae. Culex quiquefasciatus larvae were collected in 12 (3.9%) of 350 containers outdoor in peri-urban, urban and rural areas, in abandoned water wells, discarded plastic containers, canoes and in water pools for processing cassava. Distribution of micro-habitats including those less suspected to be mosquito larval habitats by local communities highlights a need for strengthening vector surveillance to provide real-time entomological data for policy decisions.

Keywords: mosquitoes, larval, habitat, distribution, Zambia

INTRODUCTION

Mosquitoes transmit various mosquito-borne diseases such as malaria, filariasis and arthropod-borne viruses (arboviruses) including, dengue virus, yellow fever virus, West Nile virus and Zika virus (1-8). Zambia is prone to mosquito-borne diseases because it has suitable ecological and climatic conditions for mosquito vector survival throughout the year during the rainy and hot season (November-May) and cool dry season (June-September) (9, 10).

A yellow fever risk assessment survey (11) necessitated a similar entomological survey to obtain a greater understanding on the vector-larval distribution in relation to human settlements. Information on mosquito spatial distribution patterns in Zambia is limited and yet, its use could optimize resource utilization and hopefully contribute towards evidence-based vector control to reduce mosquito-borne diseases (12).

Mosquito breeding sites, areas where immature forms of mosquitoes transform and grow into the adult stage, are an important determinant of the distribution and abundance of adult forms of mosquitoes. Mosquito breeding habitats include containers for species such as Aedes aegypti, pit-latrines, waste water near human habitation for Culex quiquefasciatus mosquitoes and sunlit water pools for Anopheles mosquitoes. Removal of these sources would complement interventions that target adult forms of mosquitoes (13). Regular application of chemical and biological insecticides to malaria mosquito breeding sites, larviciding, is recommended where the sites are few, fixed and findable (14).

Accurate understanding of bionomics, distribution and seasonal changes of mosquito breeding habitats is vital for designing effective interventions for reducing mosquito population. While adult mosquito studies mainly on malaria vectors have been conducted (15), larval habitat distribution of Aedes mosquito vector for arboviruses is limited in Zambia. Therefore, an entomological survey was undertaken to determine the distribution of peridomestic larval breeding habitats for mosquito vectors of arboviruses in North-Western and Western provinces of Zambia bordering countries where arboviruses have been recently reported.

METHODS

North-Western province is located at 1,354 metres above sea level, latitude -13.0 and longitude 25.0 and has a population of 706,462. The province borders with Angola on the western side and Democratic Republic of Congo on the northern side with population movement between countries. It had six districts at the time of the survey. The province receives the highest rainfall in the country, with annual rainfall of 1320 mm. The mean minimum temperature in June and mean maximum temperature in October are 6.8°C and 30.6°C, respectively (16). North-Western province is located within the Central African plateau. Rice, cassava, banana and pineapple cultivation is the main economic activity of the province.

Western province which borders with Angola has a population of 881,524 and had seven districts at the time of the survey (16). It is the driest area of Zambia and located at 1,119 metres above sea level and latitude -15.0 and longitude 24.0. The mean minimum and maximum temperatures of 8.7°C and 34.2°C are in June and October, respectively, and an annual rainfall of 740 mm (17). Western province major valleys extend to the Kalahari sand plateau and lies within the Zambezi flood plains. Crop and livestock production as well as fishing along the available water bodies are the main economic activities in the province.

Rural and urban or peri-urban areas: Classification into rural, urban and peri-urban was based on an analysis by the Department for International Development (DFID) of the United Kingdom, which took into account several parameters including access to basic services-health, education (and other social services) and population density (18).

Household: The term household as used in this study means one or more people who live in the same dwelling and also share meals or living accommodation (19).

Districts sampled

Mosquito sampling – larval and adult sampling were undertaken in North-Western province (Mwinilunga, Mufumbwe, Kabompo, Chavuma, Solwezi and Zambezi districts) and in Western province (in Kaoma and Mongu districts) of Zambia.

Training

Training in field mosquito larval sampling was conducted for a week at the Tropical Diseases Research Center, Ndola, Zambia and was facilitated by experts from the World Health Organization and Pasteur Institute, Dakar, Senegal. The training included larval sampling methods, preservation of entomological specimens and rearing of larvae to adults to enable identification of emerged adult mosquitoes. The training helped to standardize the collection, preservation and analysis of the mosquito larval samples.

Mosquito larval sampling

Three teams of 3-4 research members undertook mosquito larval searches in rural, urban and peri-urban areas of the two provinces (North-Western and Western provinces) of Zambia. The target was to sample mosquito larvae inside and outside houses for each household visited covering at least 10 households per day. All containers kept inside houses were inspected for mosquito larvae (flower-pots and water storage). The following habitats outside houses were inspected: shallow wells, discarded clay-pots, discarded bottles, plastics containers, tyres, banana (Musa sapientum) leaf axils and edges of water canals. A larval scoop was used to collect water for larval inspection on a white tray. The collected mosquito larvae were pipetted and transferred into a bottle labeled with relevant information for identification such as province, district, locality (urban or rural), house number (randomly allocated during sampling), number of habitation units or occupied rooms and date of collection.

Types and characteristics of containers

Information was collected for each breeding habitat where mosquito larvae were collected. The information included type of breeding habitat and its purpose (whether for storage of drinking water or disused/discarded); whether breeding habitat was man-made (plastic containers, bottles, metal buckets, earthen pots, tyres or cement blocks) or natural (such as banana leaf axils and stagnant water pools); presence or absence of plant growth or debris inside or around container habitats; and latitude and longitude which were obtained using a Global Positioning System.

Distribution of larval habitats

To understand the distribution of the mosquito larval sites, different locations were searched in diverse potential mosquito breeding sites in urban and rural areas. The container index (CI) was estimated as percentage of containers found with mosquito larvae to determine the presence of disease-causing mosquitoes. A CI above 10% was considered high and this was the threshold that was used in this study. In the field, adult mosquitoes that emerged from pupae were cryopreserved in liquid nitrogen. Each cryo-tube was labeled with a unique code indicating household number and cluster number where larvae were collected in addition to the province and district codes.

Mosquito larval rearing

Sampled mosquito larvae were transported to the Tropical Diseases Research Centre insectary laboratory in Ndola, Zambia and bred through to the adult stage for species identification using entomological keys (20-22). Larvae were fed on fish flakes Tetramin and maintained at relative humidity of 80 ± 2% and temperature of 23 ± 2°C. All emerged adult mosquitoes were stored at -80°C to preserve their viability prior to airfreighting them to Institute Pasteur in Dakar, Senegal for species identification.

Ethical considerations

Oral informed consent was obtained from heads of households in which larval inspections were undertaken. Written informed consent was obtained from all team members and local personnel who were involved in rearing mosquitoes.

Data analysis

Data were entered into Microsoft Excel 2010, checked for consistency and exported into SPSS version 16.0 for analysis.

RESULTS

Distribution of mosquito larvae habitats: The distribution of mosquito breeding habitats for Aedes species and Culex species in the North-Western and Western provinces are displayed in Tables 1 and 2, respectively.

Types and characteristic of containers: A plastic container was the favoured breeding microhabitat for Aedes aegypti, with a density of at least 15 per larval scoop. Meanwhile, habitats for Culex quiquefasciatus larvae were abandoned water wells, shallow wells and canoes that contained a lot of organic matter. The canoes were overgrown with grass and plant vegetation.

Table 1. Distribution of Aedes species mosquito larvae in North Western and Western provinces, Zambia and percentage of containers positive for larvae, April-May, 2013

	No. houses	Occupied rooms	Number of containers		%
			pos/exam Indoor[1]	pos/exam Outdoor[2]	
North Western					
Peri-Urban	48	277	0/0	1/52	1.9
Urban	24	112	0/0	0/40	0.0
Rural	48	237	0/0	0/98	0.0
Western					
Urban	60	316	0/0	0/117	0.0
Rural	36	171	0/0	0/43	0.0

Indoor[1] containers were drinking-water-storage containers; outdoor[2] containers were flowerpots, discarded plastic, container and shallow wells; pos = positive; exam = examined.

Distribution of Aedes larvae: Aedes (stegomyia) aegypti larvae were collected in a disused cooking oil plastic container. One (1.9%) of the 52 containers in peri-urban locality of North-Western province was positive for larvae and none of the containers in Western province was positive for larvae (Table 1). This discarded plastic container was located at the edge of a village. Aedes larvae were not collected in other habitats such as banana leaf axils, flower pots, cement blocks for house construction and discarded bottles.

Distribution of Culex larvae: Culex quiquefasciatus larvae were collected in 12 (3.9%) of the 350 container habitats outdoor in peri-urban, urban and rural areas, in abandoned water wells, water pools and in discarded plastic containers (data not shown). In North-Western province, Culex quiquefasciatus was also collected in water pools-soaked with cassava tuber to soften it prior to its pounding. The water pool was situated at a forested edge of a village (Figure, 1). Culex quiquefasciatus larvae was also found in disused canoes containing wood fibre to soften it prior to use in house construction (Figure 2) and in Clay-pots (see Figure 3).

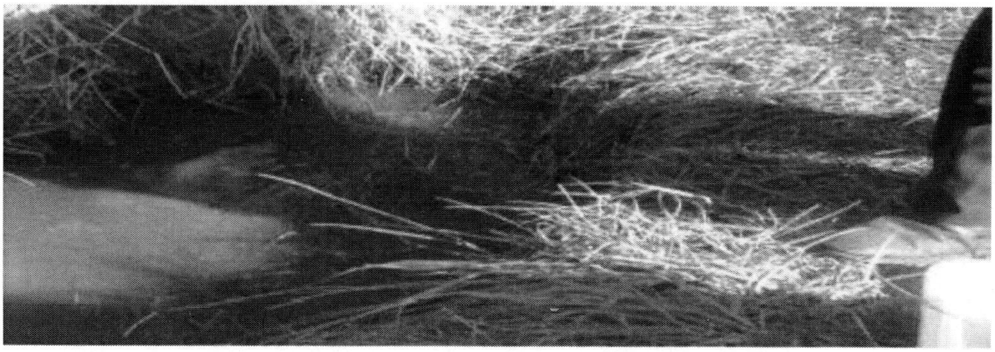

Figure 1. Breeding sites of *Culex quiquefasciatus* larvae in water pools soaked with cassava tubers in North Western province, Zambia.

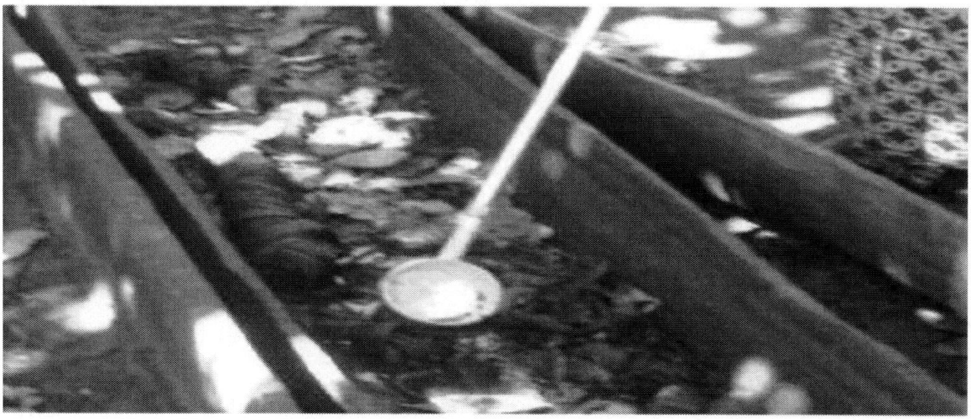

Figure 2. A canoe *Culex quiquefasciatus* was collected; this mosquito larval habitat contained wood fibre soaked in water to soften it before use. The position of the larval scoop (dipper) indicates the sites where the larvae were collected in Western Province of Zambia, Mongu District.

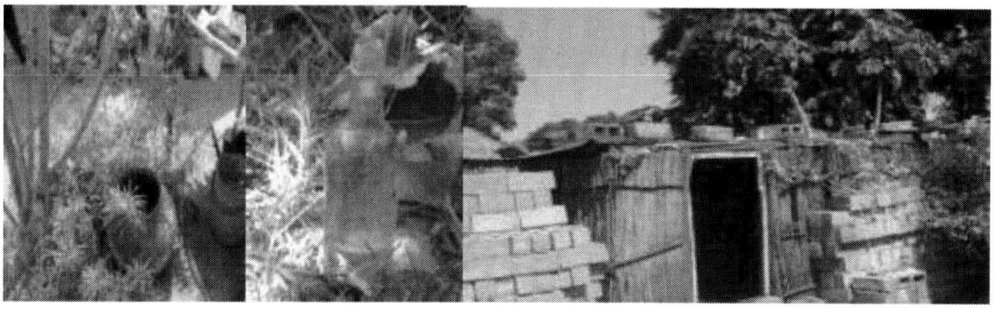

Figure 3. Various habitats searched for mosquito larva including clay pots, disused bottles, cement blocks placed by household owners to stop wind blowing roof tops, and cement blocks stored for future house construction.

Discussion

This study demonstrates Aedes mosquito larvae distribution in limited locations outdoor only in discarded plastic container in peri-urban areas of North-Western province of Zambia. No Aedes or other mosquito larval habitats were found indoor possibly since all water-storage containers were closed with a plastic cap. This is the first study in 64 years on Aedes bionomics during a yellow fever risk assessment survey in North-Western province. In the 1950s, Robinson (23) reported Aedes aegypti and Aedes africanus larvae breeding in tree holes during the wetter months of January-February in Baluvale location, currently called Zambezi, North-Western Province, Livingstone and Ndola. In those studies, only 1% of the 5,267 larvae collected was Aedes aegypti and 1% was Aedes africanus. In addition, Robinson observed that Aedes africanus was the commonest mosquito during the drier parts of the year (May-October). He found Aedes africanus breeding in bamboo (artificially made) pots in Ndola, Copperbelt, but rarely found Aedes aegypti and Aedes simpsoni larvae in other habitats that were searched (23). In addition, Robinson reported Aedes Aegypti larval habitats on rock pools in Livingstone. Our finding of Aedes mosquito larvae in plastic containers corroborates the finding that was reported in a Nigerian study (24) which showed that the most preferred peri-domestic larval habitats were plastic containers (47%) followed by metal containers (35%) and earthen ware pots (14%). The plastic containers in the Nigerian study were mainly used by Aedes species, whereas earthen pots were mainly used by Anopheles species.

The Container Index (CI) reported in this study was 1.9% which is much lower than the 10% threshold above which is considered a problem in as far as yellow fever vector breeding is concerned. Recently, CI ranging from 38.7 to 79.3% have been reported during a yellow fever outbreak in central part of Senegal (25).

The presence of Aedes species in North-Western province and not in Western province despite having used similar sampling techniques could be explained by possible varying microhabitat, ecological and environmental conditions in the two provinces. North-Western province is wetter than Western province, which is occupied by a large water body for approximately half of the year. Better adaptation of Aedes aegypti to arid conditions has been observed in a Cameroonian study but not in the current study (26).

Table 2. Distribution of mosquito breeding sites by location and type of container in North Western and Western Province of Zambia April-May 2014

Location	Container	No. Positive/ Examined
Outdoor	Canoes	1/2
	Discarded plastic containers	2/67
	Discarded wells	2/8
	Flower pots	0/83
	Tyres	0/3
	Claypots	0/3
	Cement blocks	0/50
	Bottles (discarded)	0/1
	Banana leaf axils	0/27
	Water pools for soaking cassava	1/2
	Stagnant water pools	1/9
	Calabash	0/1
	Bucket water storage	0/20
	Subtotal	**7/276**
Indoor	Bucket water storage	0/35
	Butiza (plastic) water storage	0/4
	Clay pot	0/1
	Plastic containers (Discarded)	0/34
	Subtotal	0/74
	Grand total	**7/350**

This study demonstrates more diverse breeding habitats for Culex quiquefasciatus than Aedes. Culex quiquefasciatus larvae were collected in rural, urban and peri-urban locations. Some habitats such as water pools for cassava tubers were less suspected by the community for mosquito breeding. It was perceived that the environment created by the cassava tuber, with its possible cyanide and or/ fermentation products could present a less favorable microhabitat for larval breeding. This finding should be communicated to communities to enhance effective community-based integrated vector control. In a previous study we observed Culex quiquefasciatus mosquito larvae proliferating under water hyacinth in microhabitats located in sewer ponds which led to un precedent increased mosquito densities and biting, attesting further to the remarkable adaptation of Culex quiquefasciatus to different microhabitats (27).

Observations of Culex quiquefasciatus breeding in canoes that are used for soaking wood fibers for house construction calls for community health education on the role of various discarded containers and the activities that create conducive mosquito larval habitats. These observations underscore the increasing importance of Integrated Vector Management and the value of collaboration among researchers, policy makers in health and non-health and communities enshrined within an Integrated Vector Management concept to ensure a holistic approach in addressing challenges of vector control in public health (28, 29).

In conclusion, outdoor breeding habitats for Aedes (stegomyia) aegypti were limited but more abundant for Culex quiquefasciatus in all ecological locations (rural, urban and peri-urban) in water pools, canoes, discarded clay-pots and shallow water pool soaked with cassava. Continuous surveillance is essential to monitor breading sites for potential vectors for arbo-viruses to ensure evidenced-based interventions.

ACKNOWLEDGMENTS

We are grateful to heads of households for agreeing to survey both inside and outside their houses for mosquito larvae. The research assistants are thanked for their effort in making the survey a success. This study was funded by the World health Organization and the Ministry of Health, Zambia as part of a yellow fever risk assessment survey in Zambia.

REFERENCES

[1] Rogers DJ, Wilson AJ, Hay SI, Graham AJ. The Global Distribution of Yellow Fever and Dengue. Adv Parasitol 2006; 62: 18-22.
[2] Mondet B, da Rosa AP, Vasconcelos PF. The risk of urban yellow fever outbreaks in Brazil by dengue vectors. Aedes aegypti and Aedes albopictus. Int J Infect Dis 2012; 16: 27.
[3] World Health Organisation (WHO). Wkly Epidemiol Rec 2013; 88: 201-16.
[4] Gubler DJ. The changing epidemiology of yellow fever and dengue, 1900 to 2003: full circle? Comp Immunol Microbiol Infect Dis 2004; 27: 319-30.
[5] Phoutrides EK, Coulibaly MB, George CM, Sacko A, Traore S, Bessoff K, et al. Dengue virus seroprevalence among febrile patients in Bamako, Mali: results of a 2006 surveillance study. Vector Borne Zoonotic Dis 2011; 11: 1479-85.
[6] De Filette M, Ulbert S, Diamond M, Sanders NN. Recent progress in West Nile virus diagnosis and vaccination. Vet Res 2012; 43: 16.
[7] Kautner I, Robinson MJ, Kuhnle U. Dengue virus infection: Epidemiology, pathogenesis, clinical presentation, diagnosis, and prevention. J Pediatr 1997; 131: 516-24.
[8] Grard G, Caron M, Mombo IM, Nkoghe D, Ondo SM, Jiolle D, et al. Zika Virus in Gabon (Central Africa) - 2007: A new threat from Aedes Albopictus? PLoS Negl Trop Dis 2014; 8: 1-6.
[9] Central Statistical Office. Zambia 2010 Census of population and housing. National Descriptive Tables. Lusaka, Central Statistical Office. Accessed 2014, August 27. URL; www.zamstats.gov.zm.
[10] Ministry of Health (MOH). Guidelines for Epidemic Preparedness, Prevention and Control of malaria in Zambia second Edition. Lusaka: Government Printers, 2007: 3-13.
[11] Mazaba-Liwewe ML, Siziya S, Monze M, Mweene-Ndumba I, Masaninga F, Songolo P, et al. First sero-prevalence of dengue fever specific immunoglobulin G antibodies in Western and North-Western provinces of Zambia: a population based cross sectional study. Virol J 2014; 11: 135.
[12] Van den BH, Mutero CM, Ichimori K. Guidance on policy-making for Integrated Vector Management. Geneva: WHO, 2012.
[13] Orshan L, Bin H, Schnur H, Kaufman A, Valinsky A, Shulma L, et al. Mosquito Vectors of West Nile Fever in Israel. J Med Entomol 2008; 45: 939-47.
[14] WHO. The role of larviciding in sub-Saharan Africa. Interim Position Statement. Global Malaria Programme. Geneva: WHO, 2012.
[15] Masaninga F, Chanda E, Chanda-Kapata P, Hamainza B, Masendu HT, Kamuliwo M, et al. Review of the malaria epidemiology and trends in Zambia. Asian Pac J Trop Biomed 2013; 3: 89-94.
[16] Climate of Zambia. Accessed 2014 August 27. URL: http://www.zambiatourism.com/about-zambia/climate.
[17] Aregheore EM. Country Pasture/Forage Resource, Zambia. Accessed 2014 August 27. URL: http://www.fao.org/ag/AGP/AGPC/doc/Counprof/zambia/zambia.htm#_Toc131995463.

[18] Department for International Development. Urban and rural change. Accessed 2014 August 27. URL: http://eldis.org/vfile/upload/1/document/0901/UR_overview.pdf.

[19] Zambia National Malaria Indicator Survey 2012. Government of the Republic of Zambia. Ministry of Health, Central Statistical Office, PATH, MACEPA, CDC, WHO. Accessed 2014 August 27. URL: http://www.nmcc.org.zm/files/FullReportZambiaMIS2012_July2013_withsigs2.pdf.

[20] Gillies MT, Coetzee M. A supplement to the anophelinae of Africa South of the Sahara (Afrotropical Region). Johannesburg: Publications of the South African Institute for Medical Research, 1987.

[21] Rueda ML. Pictorial keys for the identification of mosquitoes (Diptera: Culicidae) associated with Dengue Virus Transmission. Auckland, New Zealand: Magnolia Press, 2004: 14-22.

[22] Yiau-Min H. A pictorial key for the identification of the subfamilies of Culicidae, genera of Culicinae, and subgenera of Aedes mosquitoes of the Afrotropical region (Diptera: Culicidae). Proceedings of the Entomological Society of Washington 2001; 103: 1-53.

[23] Robinson GG. A Note on Mosquitoes and Yellow Fever in Northern Rhodesia. East Afr Med J 1950; 27: 284-8.

[24] Okogun GRA, Nwoke BEB, Okere AN, Anosike JC, Esekhegbe AC. Epidemiological Implications of preferences of breeding sites of mosquito species in Midwestern Nigeria. Ann Agric Environ Med 2003; 10: 217–22.

[25] Diallo M, Tall A, Dia I, Ba Y, Sarr FD, Ly AB, et al. Yellow fever outbreak in central part of Senegal. Epidemiological findings. J Public Health Epidemiol 2013; 5: 291-6.

[26] Kamgang B, Happi JY, Boisier P, Njokou F, Herve JP, Simard F, et al. Geographic and ecological distribution of Dengue and Chikungunya virus vectors of Aedes aegypti and Aedes albopictus in three major Cameroonian towns. Med Vet Entomol 2010; 24: 132-41.

[27] Masaninga F, Nkhuwa DCW, Goma FM, Shinondo C, Chanda E, Kamuliwo M, et al. Mosquito biting and malaria situation in an urban setting in Zambia. J Public Hlth Epidemiol 2012; 4: 261-9.

[28] Chanda E, Masaninga F, Coleman M, Sikaala C, Katebe C, MacDonald M, et al. Integrated vector management: The Zambian experience. Malar J 2008; 7: 164.

[29] Chanda E, Govere JM, Macdonald MB, Lako RL, Haque U, Baba SP, et al. Integrated vector management: a critical strategy for combating vector-borne diseases in South Sudan. Malar J 2013; 12: 369.

In: Public Health Yearbook 2016
Editor: Joav Merrick

ISBN: 978-1-53610-947-4

Chapter 8

RISK ASSESSMENT FOR YELLOW FEVER IN WESTERN PROVINCE OF ZAMBIA

Olusegun Babaniyi[1,*], MBBS, MPH, MSc, Mazyanga L Mazaba-Liwewe[1], BSc, Freddie Masaninga[1], BSc, MSc, PhD, Peter Mwaba[2], MBChB, MMed, David Mulenga[3], BSc, MPH, Peter Songolo[1], MBChB, MPH, Idah Mweene-Ndumba[1], BSc, MPH, Emmanuel Rudatsikira[4], MD, MPH, DrPH and Seter Siziya[3], BA(Ed), MSc, PhD

[1]World Health Organization, Lusaka, Zambia
[2]Ministry of Home Affairs, Lusaka, Zambia
[3]School of Medicine, Copperbelt University, Ndola, Zambia
[4]School of Health Professions, Andrews University, Michigan, US

ABSTRACT

Western province of Zambia was reclassified from a no risk to a low risk area for YF in 2010. To ascertain this reclassification, an assessment for the risk of YF was conducted in 2013. Altogether, 1824 persons participated in the survey of which 44.8% were males. Overall, 9 (0.5%) of the participants had YF virus infection. Of the 9 cases of YF, 6 were males. The age range for the cases was 20-77 years, with 5 cases aged below 40 years. Eight cases had long term infection and only 1 had recent infection. Two cases had fever, 1 had jaundice and none suffered from bleeding. None of the cases had travelled to Angola or Congo DR. Mosquito net use was reported by 4 cases and only 1 case reported that the house was sprayed with insecticide residual spray. None of the cases had been

* Correspondence: Olusegun A. Babaniyi, MBBS, MPH, MSc, World Health Organization, Lusaka, Zambia. E-mail: agbagba@yahoo.com

vaccinated against YF. Western province was experiencing an epidemic for YF virus infection. With a low prevalence, the area qualifies to be classified as a low risk for YF. Efforts to curb the epidemic are urgently needed. Yellow fever surveillance and the capacity of laboratories to diagnose YF should be strengthened.

Keywords: Yellow fever, prevalence, Western province, Zambia

INTRODUCTION

Yellow fever (YF) is estimated to affect about 200,000 people annually in the tropics of Africa and South America (1) and 30,000 deaths occur worldwide (2). The majority of persons infected with YF suffer from a self-limiting febrile illness. In persons who develop symptoms, symptoms occur 3-6 days after being infected and include fever, chills, severe headache, back pain, general body aches, nausea, vomiting, fatigue and weakness to severe liver disease with bleeding. Most persons who develop symptoms improve after the initial presentation of symptoms. About 15% of cases progress to a more severe form of the disease that is characterized by high fever, jaundice, bleeding, and eventually shock and failure of multiple organs (3). There is no specific treatment for yellow fever; care is based on symptoms. Steps to prevent yellow fever virus infection include using insect repellent, wearing protective clothing, and getting vaccinated (3).

Transmission of YF in Africa has been maintained by a high density of sylvatic and urban vector mosquitoes (4), mainly Aedes aegypti and Aedes africanus (5). Prevention of YF depends on avoiding mosquito bites by using repellent and wearing protective (long-sleeves, long pants and socks when outdoors) clothing and persons aged 9 months or older who live in YF endemic areas or travelling to such areas may be vaccinated to prevent infection (3).

In Africa, Yellow fever was mainly a problem of the sub-Saharan countries of West Africa, but reached as far east as central Sudan and East Africa (6-10). By 2005, Yellow fever was endemic in Angola that borders Western province of the Zambia (4). Zambia as a whole country was classified as a no risk area but Western and North-western provinces of Zambia were classified as low risk areas for yellow fever. The history behind the current classification of Western province as a low risk area for yellow fever is such that before 2005, it was classified as endemic area and in the period 2005-2010 it was removed from the list of areas with risk of transmission of yellow fever virus. The decision to classify Western province as a low potential for yellow fever exposure (11) was based on a suspected case of yellow fever that was described in North-western province of Zambia in 1943 (12), 18% seroprevalence of neutralizing antibodies to Yellow fever (13) and neighbouring areas in Angola and Democratic Republic of the Congo being at risk of yellow fever risk (11). There was no recent evidence that could have been used to classify the area. Thus, a yellow fever risk assessment survey was conducted in 2013 to provide evidence for or against the classification of the area as low risk area for yellow fever.

METHODS

Western province borders with Angola and had seven districts divided into 1902 Standard Enumeration Areas (SEAs). The population stood at 881,524 with a population density of 7.0 (14). Crop and livestock production as well as fishing were the main economic activities.

Study population, sample size and sampling

This assessment was carried out among individuals aged nine months or older. The sample size calculation was based on the assumption that the seroprevalence for yellow fever was 7% based on the study conducted by Robinson (12). In estimating the sample size for persons aged 5 years or older, the following parameters were considered: a prevalence of 7%, desired precision or confidence interval (d) of $\pm$3%, and a design effect (DE) of 2 and an 80% response rate. Considering sex, we aimed to recruit 700 male and 700 female participants in each province. Assuming an average of 4 persons aged 5 years or older in each household, a total of 12 households in each of the 30 clusters was to be recruited in the survey. The total number of persons that would be recruited from each province was 1806, totaling 3612 from both provinces.

The seroprevalence of children was about half that for older children, and in estimating the sample size for persons aged below 5 years, the following parameters were considered: a prevalence of 3.5%, desired precision or confidence interval (d) of $\pm$3.4%, and a design effect (DE) of 2 and an 80% response rate. The computed sample size was 282. Therefore, in each province 406 children would be recruited for the survey.

The sample was drawn using a two-stage cluster sampling technique using probability proportional to size. A list of the standard enumeration areas (SEAs) in each province constituted the sampling frame. The line lists of the SEAs were provided by the Government's Central Statistics Office (CSO). The sampling was designed to achieve fairly good estimates at the provincial level of analysis, and not representing the subdivisions of the province.

Data management and analysis

Data were entered in an Epi-Info data entry screen that had consistency and range checks embedded in it. Further editing was conducted by running frequencies during the analysis stage. Epi data files were exported to SPSS for data analysis. The chi-square test was used to determine associations between qualitative factors. The cut off point for statistical significance was set at the 5% level.

Ethical considerations

Ethical clearance was sought from the Tropical Diseases Research Centre Research Ethics Committee, and ethical standards were adhered to throughout this study. Informed consent was sought from study participants. Guardians provided assent for the participation of the persons under the consenting age. They were asked to read or have read to them, understand

and sign/thumbprint an informed consent form. Responsible adults in the household were identified to give proxy consent on behalf of minors.

RESULTS

Altogether, 1824 persons participated in the survey of which 44.8% were males. Significantly more males (34.3%) than females (27.1%) had achieved secondary or higher levels of education (p = 0.001). Overall, 9 (0.5%) of the participants had YF. These results are shown in Table 1.

Table 1. Description for participants in a 2013 yellow fever risk assessment in Western province

	Total	Male	Female	
Factor	n (%)	n (%)	n (%)	p value
Age (years)				
<45	1503 (82.5)	679 (83.3)	823 (81.9)	0.464
45+	318 (17.5)	136 (16.7)	182 (18.1)	
Sex				
Male	815 (44.8)			
Female	1005 (55.2)			
Education				
None or primary	1256 (69.7)	528 (65.7)	727 (72.9)	0.001
Secondary or higher	546 (30.3)	276 (34.3)	270 (27.1)	
Yellow fever				
Yes	9 (0.5)	6 (0.7)	3 (0.3)	0.314
No	1815 (99.5)	809 (99.3)	1002 (99.7)	

Of the nine cases of YF, six were males. The age range of the cases was 20-77 years, with five cases aged below 40 years. Three cases had attained up to primary level of education, three had not attended school, three attained primary level of education and another three had secondary level of education.

Eight cases had long term infection and only one had recent infection. Two cases had fever, one had jaundice and none suffered from bleeding. None of the cases had travelled to Angola or Congo DR. Mosquito net use was reported by four cases and only one case reported that the house was sprayed with insecticide residual spray. Seven cases had houses with roofs made of grass and two cases house with roofs made of iron sheets. Of the nine cases, two cases had walls of houses made of mud, three had walls of houses made of poles, one had walls made of plastered cement, two had walls made of cement bricks but not plastered, and one had walls made of unburnt bricks. None of the cases had been vaccinated against YF.

DISCUSSION

This study was conducted about 50 years after the last survey on Yellow fever risk assessment was conducted. It was prompted by a reclassification of the area from a no risk to low risk area for Yellow fever. Nine cases of YF (0.5%) were identified of which eight were of long term infection and 1 was a recent infection. None of the cases had been vaccinated against YF.

The yellow fever virus was currently circulating. The prevalence of the infection in the current study is less than the 7% (12) that was reported 50 years ago in the present Western and North-western provinces. The difference in the prevalence could partly be due to differences in the stages of the epidemic. It might be that Western province was in the early stage of the epidemic, while 50 years ago when that study was conducted the area was at an advanced stage of the epidemic. Another possibility for the difference could be that North-western province that is not part of the current study could have had a higher proportion of the 7% prevalence.

All the cases of YF in the current study were adults, indicating that younger participants were less likely to have yellow fever than older participants. This finding accords that of Geser et al. (15) that the prevalence of yellow fever was positively associated with age. The increasing age with increasing seroprevalence suggests more stable rates of ongoing transmission in the population (16).

One of the reasons that were used to classify Western province as an area of low risk for yellow fever transmission was because it bordered with areas designated as having yellow fever in neighbouring Angola and DR Congo (11). Apart from North-western province that was surveyed recently, it is important that other provinces of the country be surveyed, especially Northern province that shares a border with Tanzania that has low potential for yellow fever transmission and DR Congo with most areas regarded as endemic. Resources allowing, a national survey should be conducted to clearly state the status of the country with regard to yellow fever classification.

In conclusion, Western province was experiencing an epidemic for YF virus infection. With a low prevalence, the area qualifies to be classified as a low risk for YF. Efforts to curb the epidemic are urgently needed. Yellow fever surveillance and the capacity of laboratories to diagnose YF should be strengthened.

ACKNOWLEDGMENTS

We are grateful to the interviewers for their dedicated work to successfully complete the survey. The survey could not have been successful without the cooperation of the participants and the virology laboratory staff both in Lusaka, Zambia and Dakar, Senegal for in testing samples. The survey was funded by the Ministry of Health [Zambia] and the World Health Organization.

REFERENCES

[1] Vainio J, Cutts F. Yellow Fever. Geneva: WHO Division of Emerging and other Communicable Diseases Surveilance and Control, 1998.

[2] WHO. Yellow fever. Fact sheet No100. Accessed 2014 August 08. URL:http://www.who.int/ mediacentre /factsheets/fs100/en/. May 2013.

[3] Centers for Disease Control and Prevention. Yellow fever. Accessed 2014 August 08. URL:http:// www.cdc.gov/yellowfever/.

[4] Barnett ED. Yellow fever: epidemiology and prevention. Clin Infect Dis 2007;44:850-6.

[5] Diallo M, Tall A, Dial I, Ba Y, Sarr FD, Ly AB, et al. Yellow feveroOutbreak in central part of Senegal 2002: Epidemiological Findings. J Public Health Epidemiol 2013;5:291-6.

[6] WHO. Yellow fever, Sudan — update. Wkly Epidemiol Rec 2012;87:477-92.

[7] Okello GBA, Agata N, Ouma J, Cherogony SC, Tukei PM, Ochieng W, den Boer JW, Sanders EJ. Outbreak of yellow fever in Kenya. Lancet 1993;341(8843):489.

[8] Haddow AJ. Yellow fever in central Uganda, 1964. I. Historical introduction. Trans R Soc Trop Med Hyg 1965;59:436–40.

[9] Reiter P, Cordellier R, Ouma JO, Cropp CB, Savage HM, Sanders EJ, et al. First recorded outbreak of yellow fever in Kenya, 1992–1993. II. Entomologic investigations. Am J Trop Med Hyg 1998;59:650–6.

[10] Bell H. Frontiers of medicine in the Anglo-Egyptian Sudan, 1899–1940. Oxford Historical Monographs. Oxford; Oxford University Press, 1999.

[11] Jentes ES, Poumerol G, Gershman MD, Hill DR, Lemarchand J, Lewis RF, et al. The revised global yellow fever risk map and recommendations for vaccination, 2010: consensus of the Informal WHO Working Group on Geographic Risk for Yellow Fever. Lancet Infect Dis 2011;11:622-32.

[12] Robinson GG. A note on mosquitoes and yellow fever in Northern Rhodesia. East Afr Med J 1950;27:284-8.

[13] Bonnel PH, Deutschman Z. Yellow fever in Africa during recent years. Bull World Health Organ 1954;11:325-89.

[14] Central Statistical Office. 2010 census of population and housing. National analytical report. Lusaka, Zambia: CSO, 2012.

[15] Geser A, Henderson BE, Christensen S. A Multipurpose Serological Survey in Kenya: 2. Results of Arbovirus Serological Tests. Bull World Health Organ 1970;43:539-52.

[16] Mease LE, Coldren RL, Musila LA, Prosser T, Ogolla F, Ofula VO, et al. Seroprevalence and distribution of arboviral infections among rural Kenyan adults: A cross-sectional study. Virology J 2011;8:371.

In: Public Health Yearbook 2016
Editor: Joav Merrick

ISBN: 978-1-53610-947-4

Chapter 9

DENGUE FEVER AND FACTORS ASSOCIATED WITH IT IN WESTERN PROVINCES OF ZAMBIA

Mazyanga L Mazaba-Liwewe[1,*], BSc,
Olusegun Babaniyi[1], MBBS, MPH, MSc,
Mwaka Monza[2], MBChB, PhD,
Idah Mweene-Ndumba[1], BSc, MPH,
David Mulenga[3], BSc, MPH, Freddie Masaninga[1], BSc, MSc, PhD,
Peter Songolo[1], MBChB, MPH, Francis Kasolo[4], MBChB, MPH
and Seter Siziya[5,6], BA(Ed), MSc, PhD
[1]World Health Organization, Lusaka, Zambia
[2]University Teaching Hospital, Lusaka, Zamia
[3]School of Medicine, Copperbelt University, Ndola, Zambia
[4]World Health Organization, AFRO region, Congo Brazzaville
[5]School of Medicine, Copperbelt University, Ndola, Zambia
[6]University of Lusaka, Lusaka, Zambia

ABSTRACT

Dengue virus infection has become a major public health concern worldwide, although it has not been reported before in Zambia. The objective of the study was to determine the prevalence and correlates for dengue virus infection in Western province of Zambia. Secondary data, obtained in a yellow fever risk assessment survey, was used in the study. A total of 1,823 persons were investigated of whom 55.2% were female and 25.1% were in the 5-14 years age group. Overall, 7.1% (7.2% males and 7.0% females; p = 0.887) were infected with dengue virus. Persons in the age group 25-34 years were 66% (AOR = 1.66; 95% CI [1.09, 2.54]) more likely to have the infection compared to those aged 45

* Corresponding author: Mazyanga Lucy Mazaba, World Health Organization, Lusaka, Zambia. E-mail: mazmazli@yahoo.com.

years or older. Persons who had attained primary education were 37% (AOR = 1.37; 95% CI [(1.05, 1.78]) more likely to have the infection than those who had higher levels of education. Persons who had travelled to Angola were 2.11 times (AOR = 2.11; 95% CI [1.41, 3.15]) more likely to have the infection compared to those who had not travelled to Angola. Surveillance should be strengthened at the border in order to curtail the epidemic.

Keywords: dengue virus infection, prevalence, correlates, Western province, Zambia

INTRODUCTION

Dengue is a mosquito-borne (Aedes aegypti) systemic viral infection found in tropical and sub-tropical regions and has become a major public health concern worldwide (1). The complications of dengue infection (Dengue Haemorrhagic Fever or Dengue Shock Syndrome) are life-threatening in those with chronic diseases and asthma (2). Major epidemics caused by dengue fever occurred from the 17th to early 20th centuries (3). It is estimated that close to 4 billion persons living in 128 countries are at risk of dengue infection (4), with the virus being endemic in over 110 countries. The endemic countries are in Africa, the Americas, the Eastern Mediterranean, South-east Asia and Western Pacific. Severely affected regions including the Americas, the Eastern Mediterranean, South-east Asia and Western Pacific reported more than 1.2 million and 2.3 million cases in 2008 and 2010 respectively.

Dengue epidemics in Africa have increased since 1980 with most activity documented in East Africa (5). Most recently outbreaks have been reported in Angola (6), and Kenya (7). Dengue is now one of most important tropical diseases second to malaria causing approximately 50 to 100 million cases of DF and 500,000 cases of DHF (8). The public health impact of dengue is greatly underestimated because of poor surveillance data (9). Though the factors responsible for the dramatic resurgence of epidemic dengue are not fully understood, it appears it is closely associated with demographic and societal changes over the past 50 years (10).

The relationship between age and risk of dengue fever has not been consistent. According to Egger and Coleman (11), the risk for age in relation to classic dengue fever had never been quantified. Using data from clinical patients, Egger and Coleman showed that the risk of classical dengue after primary dengue increases with age. Another study revealed that classic dengue is primarily common among older children and adults (12, 13). The epidemiologic characteristics of dengue differ by region and the incidence by age (14-16). A study by Anker and Amina indicated a consistent pattern of male predominance in the reported number of dengue cases among 15 years or older in six Asian countries (17). Travel (18) and education (19) have also been documented to be associated with Dengue fever.

Zambia recently (in 2013) carried out a yellow fever risk assessment in Western and North-Western provinces. Positive cases for dengue fever were identified amongst the study population in the survey. This paper documents the prevalence and correlated for dengue fever in Western province.

METHODS

Western province borders with Angola and had seven districts divided into 1,902 Standard Enumeration Areas (SEAs). The population stood at 881,524 with a population density of 7.0. Crop and livestock production as well as fishing were the main economic activities (20).

Study population, sample size, inclusion/exclusion criteria and sampling

The survey was carried out among individuals aged nine months or older. The sample size calculation was based on the assumption that the seroprevalence for yellow fever was 7% based on the study on yellow fever conducted by Robinson (21). For persons aged 5 years or older, the following parameters were considered in estimating the sample size, a prevalence of 7%, desired precision or confidence interval (d) of ±3%, and a design effect (DE) of 2 and an 80% response rate. The study aimed to recruit 700 male and 700 female participants in each province. A total of 12 households in each of the 30 clusters, assuming an average of 4 persons aged 5 years or older in each household, were to be recruited in the survey. The total number of persons that would be recruited from each province was 1806, totaling 3612 from both provinces.

The seroprevalence of children below the age of five years was about half that for older persons, and in estimating the sample size for persons aged below 5 years, the following parameters were considered: a prevalence of 3.5%, desired precision or confidence interval (d) of ±3.4%, and a design effect (DE) of 2 and an 80% response rate. The computed sample size was 282. A total of 406 children would be recruited in each province for the survey.

Any individual aged 9 months or older and who was a member of a sampled household and resident in the study site for at least seven days was requested to participate in the survey. Individuals who received yellow fever vaccination in the last ten years were eligible to participate in the survey. Exclusion criteria left out any person, who was either less than 9 months of age or any person, regardless of age, who resided in the study site for a period of less than seven days prior to the survey. Children under the age of nine months raises the risk of false positive results as children under this age may still carry maternal antibodies from immunized or exposed mothers.

A two-stage cluster sampling technique using probability proportional to size was used to draw the sample. A list of the standard enumeration areas (SEAs) in each province constituted the sampling frame. The sampling was designed to achieve fairly good estimates at the provincial level of analysis, and not representing the subdivisions of the province.

Study variables

Dependent variable

A case with evidence of dengue infection exposure was defined as any individual aged 9 months or older whose blood sample was confirmed to have dengue virus exposure through the detection of dengue virus-specific IgG and IgM antibodies.

Independent variables

The independent variables included age, sex, occupation, history of travel to Angola and/or DRC and use of mosquito preventive measures.

Laboratory procedure

About 3 to 5 millilitres of blood was collected by venepuncture into an EDTA vacutainer tube and transported on cold chain to the local laboratories for serum separation and storage. Samples were subjected to primary testing (yellow fever virus specific IgG and IgM) at the University of Teaching Hospital in Zambia virology unit and Institute Pasteur, Dakar. All presumptive yellow fever virus specific IgG and IgM samples were subjected to IgG and IgM antibodies against other flaviviruses known to cause haemorrhagic fever-like disease including dengue.

Data management and analysis

Data were entered in an Epi-Info data entry screen that had consistency and range checks embedded in it. Further editing was conducted by running frequencies during the analysis stage. Epi data files were exported to SPSS for data analysis. The data was summarized to describe the occurrence of dengue virus exposed individuals in absolute numbers and percentage by place (residence, travel or work) and person (age, sex, occupation). Further analysis was conducted to determine independent factors associated with yellow fever seropositivity. Odds ratios were used to estimate magnitudes of associations.

Ethical considerations

Ethical clearance was sought from the Tropical Diseases Research Centre Research Ethics Committee, and ethical standards were adhered to throughout this study. Informed consent was sought from study participants. Guardians provided assent for the participation of the persons under the consenting age. Participants were asked to read or have read to them, understand and sign/thumbprint an informed consent form. Responsible adults in the household were identified to give proxy consent on behalf of minors.

RESULTS

A total of 1,823 persons were investigated (questionnaires and laboratory tests) for dengue virus in Western province. Overall, 55.2% of the participants were female and 25.1% were in the age group 5-14 years. Altogether, 48.2% of all persons sampled had attained primary education. Males tended to be more educated than females ($p = 0.002$). No significant association was observed between sex and dengue virus infection. Overall, 7.1% of the participants in western province had previous dengue. These results are shown in Table 1.

Of the factors considered in bivariate analysis age, education, and visit to Angola were significantly associated with risk of dengue infection (see Table 2). After adjusting for other factors in multivariate analysis, those in the age group 25-34 years were 66% (AOR = 1.66; 95% CI [1.09, 2.54]) more likely to have dengue infection compared to those aged 45 years or older. Those who had attained primary education were 37% (AOR = 1.37; 95% CI [(1.05, 1.78]) more likely to have dengue infection than those who had attained secondary education or higher. In relation to visitation to Angola, those who visited were 2.11 times (AOR = 2.11; 95% CI [1.41, 3.15]) more likely to have dengue infection.

Discussion

There is no documentation of a previous survey except for a confirmed case of a European traveler/expatriate who was in Zambia between 1987 and 1993 (22). This study reveals a prevalence of dengue infection in Western province at 7.1% with those in the age group 25-34 being more likely to be affected. Respondents with lower than secondary school qualification, as well as those who travelled to Angola were more likely to be associated with dengue infection.

The factors responsible for epidemic dengue as a global public health problem in the past 17 years are complex and not fully understood. However, demographic changes over the past 50 years have been associated with dengue (12). There are inconsistencies in the description of the relationship between age and risk of dengue infection. Some studies cite the younger age as more likely to get dengue infection, others cite increasing infection rate with increasing age (23). Epidemiological data on dengue infection in Brazil indicates changing age group patterns (24).

Travel has been documented to be associated with increase in the spread of Dengue virus from endemic to non-endemic areas. The continued spread of dengue has been supported by global trade and increasing travel within and between countries (25). Travel whether by air, motor vehicles or foot, increases the risk of introducing arthropod-borne virus diseases including dengue fever from endemic to non-endemic areas (23). With small scale cross border trading, want for closer health facilities, and family ties across borders, there is increasing travel between the dengue endemic neighbouring country of Angola and Zambia. Angola is currently having a dengue epidemic (26) and this could have facilitated the introduction of dengue virus and infection in Zambia.

The finding in the current study that education was related to infection was not consistent (no gradient in the odds of being infected among the levels of education) in that while persons who had no formal education were equally likely to have the infection as those who had secondary or higher levels of education, persons who had primary level of education were more likely to have infection compared to those who had higher levels of education. Results from a study in urban areas in Thailand indicated that persons who earned secondary or higher levels of education had a higher risk for being infected than those who earned elementary or lower levels of education (19). Contrary to the explanation of such phenomena by Koyadun et al. (19) that persons who have a high level of schooling may have a higher chance to get skilled careers and seek jobs far away from their community where they would increase their risk of getting infection, it is not clear what factors would put both persons with no formal education and persons with secondary or higher levels of education at equal chances of getting the infection. Further studies are needed to elucidate the relationship between education and dengue virus infection. In order to curtail the epidemic in Western province of Zambia, surveillance at border posts should be enhanced through screening of persons crossing the border and strengthening laboratory capacity to detect infection.

Table 1. Sample description for Western province for dengue virus infection

Factor	Total n (%)	Male n (%)	Female n (%)	p value
Age (years)				
<5	184 (10.1)	81 (9.9)	102 (10.1)	0.131
5-14	471 (25.1)	231 (28.3)	240 (23.9)	
15-24	390 (21.4)	180 (22.1)	210 (20.9)	
25-34	245 (13.5)	94 (11.5)	151 (15.0)	
35-44	213 (11.7)	93 (11.4)	120 (11.9)	
45+	318 (17.5)	136 (16.7)	182 (18.1)	
Sex				
Male	815 (44.8)	-	-	-
Female	1005 (55.2)	-	-	
Education				
None	388 (21.5)	152 (18.9)	235 (23.6)	0.002
Primary	868 (48.2)	376 (46.8)	492 (49.3)	
Secondary or higher	546 (30.3)	276 (34.3)	270 (27.1)	
Dengue virus infection				
Yes	130 (7.1)	59 (7.2)	70 (7.0)	0.887
No	1693 (92.9)	755 (92.8)	935 (93.0)	

* Numbers may not add up due to missing information.

Table 2. Factors associated with dengue virus infection in logistic regression analysis for Western province

Factor	OR (95% CI)	AOR (95% CI)
Age (years)		
<5	0.43 (0.20, 0.91)	0.54 (0.24, 1.24)
5-14	0.71 (0.47, 1.08)	0.63 (0.40, 0.98)
15-24	0.96 (0.63, 1.44)	1.02 (0.66, 1.58)
25-34	1.66 (1.10, 2.50)	1.66 (1.09, 2.54)
35-44	0.83 (0.48, 1.43)	0.76 (0.44, 1.32)
45+	1	1
Sex		
Male	1.02 (0.85, 1.22)	-
Female	1	
Education		
None	0.84 (0.61, 1.16)	0.89 (0.62, 1.29)
Primary	1.31 (1.03, 1.67)	1.37 (1.05, 1.78)
Secondary or higher	1	1
Use of mosquito net		
Yes	1.13 (0.94, 1.36)	-
No	1	
Insecticide residual spraying		
Yes	1.14 (0.90, 1.44)	-
No	1	
Visited Congo DRC		
Yes	1.62 (0.55,4.75)	-
No	1	
Visited Angola		
Yes	2.41 (1.65, 3.52)	2.11 (1.41, 3.15)
No	1	1

ACKNOWLEDGMENTS

The survey could not have been successful without the cooperation of the participants. We acknowledge the laboratory support received from Virology laboratory staff, University Teaching Hospital, Lusaka, Zambia and Institute de Pasteur, Dakar, Senegal. We are grateful to the interviewers for their dedicated work to successfully complete the survey. The survey was funded by the Ministry of Health [Zambia] and the World Health Organization.

REFERENCES

[1] Centers for Disease Control and Prevention. Dengue. Accessed 2010 August 31. URL: www.cdc.gov/dengue/.

[2] Guzman MG, Halstead SB, Artsob H, Buchy P, Farrar J, Gubler DJ, et al. Dengue: a continuing global threat. Nat Rev Microbiol 2010; 8(Suppl 12) S7–16.

[3] Gubler DJ. Dengue and dengue hemorrhagic fever: its history and resurgence as a global public health problem. In: Gubler DJ, Kuno G, eds. Dengue and dengue hemorrhagic fever. London: CAB International, 1997: 1-22.

[4] Brady OJ, Gething PW, Bhatt S. Refining the global spatial limits of dengue virus transmission by evidence-based consensus. Nature 2013; 496(7446): 504-7.

[5] Gubler DJ. Dengue. In: Monath TPM, ed. Epidemiology of arthropodborne viral disease, Boca Raton (FL): CRC Press, 1988: 223-60.

[6] Centers for Disease Control and Prevention. Ongoing dengue epidemic - Angola, June 2013. MMWR 2013; 62: 504-7.

[7] Mease LE, Coldren RL, Musila LA, Prosser T, Ogolla F, Ofula VO, et al. Seroprevalence and distribution of arboviral infections among rural Kenyan adults: a cross-sectional study. Virology J 2011; 8: 371.

[8] World Health Organization. Global alert and response. Impact of dengue. Accessed 2014 August 31. URL: http://www.who.int/csr/disease/dengue/impact/en/index.htm.

[9] Gubler DJ. Resurgent vector-borne diseases as a global health problem. Emerg Infect Dis 1998; 4: 442-50.

[10] Gubler D. The emergence of epidemic dengue fever and dengue hemorrhagic fever in the Americas: a case of failed public health policy. Rev Panam Salud Publica 2005; 17: 221-4.

[11] Egger JR, Coleman PG. Age and clinical dengue illness. Emerg Infect Dis 2007; 13: 924-7.

[12] Gubler DJ. Dengue and dengue hemorrhagic fever. Clin Microbiol Rev 1998; 11: 480-96.

[13] Hayes EB, Gubler DJ. Dengue and dengue hemorrhagic fever. Pediatr Infect Dis J. 1992; 11: 311-7.

[14] Cavalcanti LP, Vilar D, Souza-Santos R, Teixeira MG. Change in age pattern of persons with dengue, northeastern Brazil. Emerg Infect Dis 2011; 17(1): 132-4.

[15] Halstead SB. Dengue in the Americas and Southeast Asia: do they differ? Rev Panam Salud Publica 2006; 20: 407-15.

[16] Teixeira MG, Costa Mda C, Barreto F, Barreto ML. Dengue: twenty-five years since reemergence in Brazil. Cad Saude Publica 2009; 25 Suppl 1: S7-18.

[17] Anker M, Arima Y. Male-female differences in the number of reported incident dengue fever cases in six Asian countries. Western Pac Surveill Response J 2011; 2: 17-23.

[18] Blackburn NK, Rawat R. Dengue fever imported from India. A report of 3 cases. S Afr Med. 1987; 71: 386-7.

[19] Koyadun S, Butraporn P, Kittayapong P. Ecologic and sociodemographic risk determinants for dengue transmission in urban areas in Thailand. Interdiscip Perspect Infect Dis 2012, Article ID 907494, 12 pages. doi:10.1155/2012/907494.

[20] Central Statistical Office (CSO), Ministry of Health (MOH), Tropical Diseases Research Centre (TDRC), University of Zambia, and Macro International Inc. Zambia Demographic and Health Survey 2007. Calverton, MD: CSO Macro International, 2009.

[21] Robinson GG. A note on mosquitoes and yellow fever in Northern Rhodesia. East Afr Med J 1950; 27: 284-8.

[22] Amarasinghe A, Kuritsk JN, Letson GW, Margolis HS. Dengue virus infection in Africa. Emerg Infect Dis 2011; 17: 1349-54.

[23] Blackburn NK, Rawat R. Dengue fever imported from India: a report of 3 cases. S Afr Med J 1987; 71: 386-7.

[24] Cavalcanti LP, Vilar D, Souza-Santos R, Teixeira MG. Change in age pattern of persons with dengue, northeastern Brazil. Emerg Infect Dis 2011; 17: 132-4).

[25] Cameron P. Simmons CP, Farrar JJ, van Vinh Chau N, Wills B. Dengue. N Engl J Med 2012; 366: 1423-32.

[26] Centers for Disease Control and Prevention. Dengue in Angola. Accessed 2013 May 24. URL: http://wwwnc.cdc.gov/travel/notices/watch/dengue-angola.

In: Public Health Yearbook 2016
Editor: Joav Merrick

ISBN: 978-1-53610-947-4

Chapter 10

DISTRIBUTION OF ZIKA VIRUS INFECTION SPECIFIC IGG IN WESTERN PROVINCE OF ZAMBIA: A POPULATION-BASED STUDY

Olusegun Babaniyi[1], MBBS, MPH, MSc, Peter Songolo[1,*], MBChB, MPH, Mazyanga L Mazaba-Liwewe[1], BSc, Idah Mweene-Ndumba[1], BSc, MPH, Freddie Masaninga[1], BSc, MSc, PhD, Emmanuel Rudatsikira[2], MD, MPH, DrPH and Seter Siziya[3,4], BA(Ed), MSc, PhD

[1]World Health Organization, Lusaka, Zambia
[2]School of Health Professionals, Andrews University, Michigan, US
[3]School of Medicine, Copperbelt University, Ndola, Zambia
[4]University of Lusaka, Lusaka, Zambia

ABSTRACT

Zika virus (ZIKV) is a flavivirus that causes disease with similar but milder symptoms to dengue fever. There is no information on Zika virus infection in Zambia. Hence, the objective of the study was to determine the prevalence and correlates for Zika virus infection in Western province of Zambia. A cross-sectional study using a standardised questionnaire was conducted. Logistic regression analyses were conducted to determine factors associated with Zika virus infection. Out of 1824 respondents, 44.8% were males and 36.0% were aged below 15 years. Altogether, 10.2% of the participants had Zika virus infection. Factors associated with the infection were age and education. Participants aged less than 15 years were 53% (AOR = 0.47, 95% CI [0.34, 0.65]) less likely to be infected compared to those aged 45 years or older. Compared to participants who had

* Corresponding author: Peter Songolo, MBChB, MPH, World Health Organization, Lusaka, Zambia. E-mail: songolop@who.int.

attained secondary or higher levels of education, those who had attained primary level of education were 1.28 (95% CI [1.04, 1.58]) times more likely to have the infection. Zika virus infection is prevalent among the residents of Western Province in Zambia. There is need to strengthen strategies to address the emerging challenge of Zika virus infection such as laboratory diagnostic capacities.

Keywords: Zika virus infection, correlates, Western province, Zambia

INTRODUCTION

Zika virus (ZIKV) is a flavivirus that causes disease with similar but milder symptoms to dengue fever. Clinical pictures range from asymptomatic cases to an influenza-like syndrome associated with fever, headache, malaise and cutaneous rash (1). Other less frequent symptoms and signs of ZIKV include myalgia, headache, retro-orbital pain, oedema and vomiting (2). Its natural transmission cycle in Africa involves primarily mosquitoes (*Aedes* species) and monkeys. While serological and entomological Zika virus infection have been reported in different areas in Africa including Burkina Faso, Ivory Coast, Egypt, Central African Republic, Mozambique, Nigeria, Uganda and Senegal, entomological and virological surveillance for arboviruses have been conducted since 1972 in Senegal and revealed presence of Zika virus (3). The virus was first identified in 1947 in rhesus monkey serum from Zika forest in Uganda (4). However ZIKV antibodies have been detected in humans across Africa, and Asia (5, 6). In Cameroon, the infection with Zika virus spread to neighbouring Nigeria resulting in an epidemic with symptoms including jaundice (7), an indicator for potential global spread (8).

Despite the widespread distribution of Zika virus, there have been very few reported human cases until the Yap outbreak in 2007 (9). In particular, there is no documented information on Zika virus infection in Western province of Zambia. Following a risk assessment for Yellow fever in Western province of Zambia resulting from a re-classification of the province by World Health Organization as a low-risk area for Yellow fever, a study was undertaken using data collected from the Yellow fever survey to determine the prevalence and correlates for Zika virus infection in Western province of Zambia.

METHODS

Western Province has a common border with Angola. The geography of the province is dominated by the Barotse Floodplain of the Zambezi river. This floodplain is inundated from December to June; this is important to agriculture as it provides natural irrigation for the grasslands. Much of the province is covered by sand believed to come from the Kalahari Desert, grasslands and woodlands.

Western Province had seven districts with a total of 1,902 Standard Enumeration Areas (SEAs). Fishing and cattle rearing were the main occupation in the province. The population of the province was 881,524 according to national census of 2010 (10).

Western province borders with Angola and had seven districts divided into 1,902 SEAs. The population stood at 881,524 with a population density of 7.0 (10). Crop and livestock production as well as fishing were the main economic activities.

Sample sizes

The sample size calculation was based on the assumption that the seroprevalence for Yellow fever was 7% based on the study conducted by Robinson (11). A Statcal program in Epi Info v6.04 was used to estimate the sample size. The sample size was equally allocated to North-Western and Western provinces and powered to avoid chance findings, that is, 1,800 participants from each province.

Sampling

A multi-stage sampling technique was used for participants in both districts. Firstly, wards were randomly selected from each constituency. In the second stage of sampling, standard enumeration areas (SEAs) proportional to the ward size were systematically sampled. All survey participants aged nine months or older in a selected household were eligible to be enrolled in the study.

Ethical approval

The study protocol was reviewed and approved by the Tropical Diseases Research Centre Research Ethics Committee, and permission to conduct the study was obtained from the Ministry of Health, Zambia. Informed consent was obtained from survey participants after the interviewer had explained the benefits and risks of participating in the study. Entry forms were viewed only by those approved to be part of the survey.

Data collection

A detailed semi structured questionnaire was used to collect information. The questionnaires were pre-tested to validate the appropriateness of the questions to capture the required information. During the data collection process, questionnaires were checked for inconsistencies and completeness on a daily basis.

Data management and analysis

All data were entered into a computer using Epi-Info data entry screen that had consistency and range checks embedded in it. The Epi data file was exported to SPSS for data analysis.

Further editing was conducted by running frequencies during the analysis stage. Odds ratios were used to estimate magnitudes of associations using unadjusted odds ratios (OR) and adjusted odds ratios (AOR) together with their 95% confidence intervals (CI).

RESULTS

A total of 1,824 participants out of which 44.8% were males participated in the survey. The age distribution was similar between sexes with 36.0% of the participants belonging to the under 15 years age group. A significant association between education and sex was observed (p = 0.002) with 34.3% of males and 27.1% of females having attained secondary or higher levels of education.

Altogether, 10.2% of the participants had Zika virus infection with no sex difference (p = 0.957). Table 1 shows the description of the sample. While age, education and visiting Angola were significantly associated with Zika virus infection in bivariate analyses, only age and education remained significantly associated with the infection in multivariate analysis. Participants aged less 15 years were observed to be 53% (AOR = 0.47, 95% CI [0.34, 0.65]) less likely to have the infection compared to participants of age 45 years or older. Meanwhile, participants who had attained primary level of education were 28% (AOR = 1.28, 95% CI [1.04, 1.58]) more likely to have the infection compared to participants who had attained secondary or higher levels of education (Table 2).

Table 1. Sample description for Western province for Zika virus infection

Factor	Total n (%)	Male n (%)	Female n (%)	p value
Age (years)				
<15	655 (36.0)	312 (38.3)	342 (34.0)	0.122
15 – 24	390 (21.4)	180 (22.1)	210 (20.9)	
25 – 34	245 (13.5)	94 (11.5)	151 (15.0)	
35 – 44	213 (11.5)	93 (11.4)	120 (11.9)	
45+	318 (17.5)	136 (16.7)	182 (18.1)	
Sex				
Male	815 (44.8)			
Female	1005 (55.2)			
Education				
None	388 (21.5)	152 (18.9)	235 (23.6)	0.002
Primary	868 (48.2)	376 (46.8)	492 (49.3)	
Secondary or higher	546 (30.3)	276 (34.3)	270 (27.1)	
Zika virus infection				
Yes	186 (10.2)	82 (10.1)	103 (10.2)	0.957
No	1638 (89.8)	733 (89.9)	902 (89.9)	

DISCUSSION

Zika virus which had not been previously reported in Western province of Zambia was prevalent affecting 10.2% of the survey participants. Compared to other findings, the prevalence in the current study is much lower than what has been reported elsewhere in Africa. The findings in Nigeria, reporting rates of 31 and 56% (12, 13) and in Yap island of Federated States of Micronesia reporting a rate of 73% (14) were based on small sample sizes, and this may partly explain the differences in the rates reported.

While age was significantly associated with Zika infection in the current study, no significant association was observed between age and the infection on the Yap Island (14). However, in a study conducted in Kenya, age was significantly associated with the infection. The risk of infection linearly increased with age (15). Older persons may have been more exposed to infection than the younger ones partly due to activities such as social gathering and economic activities such as fishing, crop and livestock production that may predispose them to mosquito bites. Repellents may not be affordable in poor communities. Wearing of long sleeved shorts and trousers for men and wearing of wrappers, traditionally known as *chitenge*, by women may be possible alternatives to minimize man-mosquito contact.

The association between education and Zika virus infection was not consistent. While persons who had never been to school were equally likely to be infected as those with secondary or higher levels of education, persons who had attained primary level of education were more likely to be infected compared to persons with higher levels of education (Table 2). Further analysis is needed to consider possible confounding factors such as the wealth index in the relationship between education and infection. Alternatively, persons with primary level of education may be more engaged in activities, for which we are unable to suggest, that may predispose them to mosquito carrying the infection.

Despite the fact that a high proportion of samples collected during the risk assessment tested positive for Zika virus infection (10.2%), no human case of Zika disease had been reported from Western province. This may be due to the lack of knowledge by the medical personnel and partly due to the absence of a case definition for Zika virus infection in the Integrated Diseases Surveillance and Response (IDSR) guidelines which are widely used for syndromic disease surveillance in Zambia. Furthermore, the symptoms of Zika infection apart from being sub-clinical in presentation could mimic malaria which is prevalent in the province. Therefore, suspected malaria cases may mask outbreaks of Zika virus infection. Grard et al. (16) in their study observed that the number of human cases of Zika virus infection were few compared to Dengue virus infection probably due to the occurrence of sub-clinical form of Zika disease that did not require medical attention.

The other challenge contributing to lack of information on arboviral disease is the limitations on availability of diagnostic methods, thereby making it difficult to identify these emerging diseases in the country. Brady et al. in assessing the distribution of dengue in the entire continent alluded to this challenge in many healthcare settings coupled with scanty information or data on surveillance and research generated reports in many resource poor countries (17).

Table 2. Factors associated with Zika virus infection in Western Province in bivariate and multivariate logistic regression analyses

Factor	OR (95% CI)	AOR (95% CI)
Age (years)		
<15	0.51 (0.38, 0.69)	0.47 (0.34, 0.65)
15 – 24	0.74 (0.53, 1.02)	0.81 (0.57, 1.13)
25 – 34	1.19 (0.85, 1.67)	1.24 (0.88, 1.74)
35 – 44	1.03 (0.71, 1.50)	1.03 0.71, 1.48)
45+	1	1
Sex		
Male	0.99 (0.85, 1.15)	
Female	1	
Education		
None	0.92 (0.71, 1.19)	1.02 (0.77, 1.34)
Primary	1.23 (1.00, 1,51)	1.28 (1.04, 1.58)
Secondary or higher	1	1
Use of mosquito nets		
Yes	0.98 (0.84, 1.15)	–
No	1	
In-door residual spraying		
Yes	0.90 (0.72, 1.14)	–
No	1	
Visited Angola		
Yes	1.67 (1.12, 2.50)	–
No	1	

The discovery of ZIKV in the Western Province of Zambia strongly indicates the need to develop laboratory capacity for diagnosis of flaviviruses and strengthen Integrated Disease Surveillance and Response (IDSR). Strengthening the capacities of the laboratory is key to confirming clinically suspicious cases. There is need to strengthen control measures for malaria as the vector is similar and as such the country should scale-up the use of Insecticide-treated nets (ITNs) and in-door residual spraying to reduce human mosquito contact. Other measures include health education to promote personal protection using long-sleeved clothes and repellents. Furthermore, although research efforts have focused on many of these viruses, other medically important members of the mosquito-borne flaviviruses, such as Zika virus, have received far less attention.

References

[1] Faye O, Freire CCM, Iamarino A, Faye O, de Oliveira JVC, Molecular evolution of Zika virus during its emergence in the 20th century. PLoS Negl Trop Dis 2014; 8: 2636.

[2] Hayes EB. Zika virus outside Africa. Emerg Infect Dis 2013; 15: 1347-9.

[3] Faye O, Faye O, Diallo D, Diallo M, Weidman M, Sall AA. Quantitative real-time PCR detection of Zika virus and evaluation with filed-caught mosquitoes. Virol J 2013; 10: 311.

[4] Whelan P, Hall J. Zika virus disease, The Northern Territory Disease Control Bulletin. 2008; 15: 19-21.

[5] Tappe D, Rissland J, Gabriel M, Emmerich P, Günther S, Held G, et al. First case of laboratory-confirmed Zika virus infection imported into Europe, November 2013. Euro surveill 2014; 19: 1-3.

[6] Faye O, Faye O, Freire CCM, de Oliviera JV, Rubing C, Zanotto PMA, et al. Molecular evolution of Zika virus, an neglected emerging disease in Africa and Asia. BMC Proc 2011; 5: 59.

[7] Fokam EB, Levai LD, Guzman H, Amelia PA, Titanji VPK, Tesh RB, et al. Silent circulation of arboviruses in Cameroon. East Afr Med J 2010; 87: 262-7.

[8] Grard G, Moureau G, Charrel RN, Holmes EC, Gould EA, de Lamballerie X; Genomics and evolution of Aedes-borne flaviviruses. J Gen Virol, 2010; 91: 87-94.

[9] Duffy MR, Chen T-H, Hancock WT, Powers AM, Kool JL, Lanciotti RS, et al. Zika virus outbreak on Yap island, Federated States of Micronesia. New Engl J Med 2009; 360: 2536-43.

[10] Central Statistical Office. 2010 census of population and housing. National analytical report. Lusaka, Zambia: CSO, 2012.

[11] Robinson GG. A note on mosquitoes and yellow fever in Northern Rhodesia. East Afr Med J 1950; 27: 284-8.

[12] Fagbami AH. Zika virus infections in Nigeria: virological and seroepidemiological investigations in Oyo State. J Hyg Camb 1979; 83: 213-9.

[13] Adekolu-John EO, Fagbami AH. Arthropod-borne virus antibodies in sera of rfesidents of Kainji lake basin, Nigeria 1980. Trans R Soc Trop Med Hyg 1983; 77: 149-51.

[14] Duffy MR, Chen T-H, Hancock TW, Powers AM, Kool JL, Lanciotti RS, et al. Zika virus outbreak on Yap island, Federated States of Micronesia. N Eng J Med 2009; 360: 2536-43.

[15] Geser A, Henderson BE, Christensen S. A multipurpose serological survey in Kenya. Bull World Health Organ 1970; 43: 539-52.

[16] Grard G, Caron M, Mombo IM, Nkoghe D, Ondo SM, Jiolle D, et al. Zika virus in Gabon (Central Africa) – 2007: a new threat from Aedes albopictus? PLoS Negl Trop Dis 2014; 8: e2681.

[17] Brady OJ, Gething PW, Bhatt S, Messina JP, Brownstein JS, Hoen AG, et al. Refining the global spatial limits of dengue virus transmission by evidence-based consensus. PLoS Negl Trop Dis, 2012; 6: e1760.

In: Public Health Yearbook 2016
Editor: Joav Merrick

ISBN: 978-1-53610-947-4

Chapter 11

West Nile virus infection in Western province of Zambia: Assessing the contributing factors

Idah Mweene-Ndumba[1,*], BSc, MPH,
Seter Siziya[2], BA(Ed), MSc, PhD,
Mwaka Monze[3], MBhB, PhD,
Mazyanga L Mazaba-Liwewe[1], BSc, MSc,
Freddie Masaninga[1], BSc, MSc, PhD,
Peter Songolo[1], MBChB, MPH,
Peter Mwaba[4], MBChB, PhD
and Olusegun A Babaniyi[1], MBBS, MPH, MSc
[1]World Health Organization, Lusaka, Zambia
[2]School of Medicine, Copperbelt University, Ndola, Zambia/
University of Lusaka, Lusaka, Zambia
[3]University Teaching Hospital, Lusaka, Zambia
[4]Ministry of Home Affairs, Lusaka, Zambia

Abstract

West Nile virus (WNV) infection has been reported worldwide with varying prevalence rates within countries. The purpose of this study was to determine the extent of WNV infection and its correlates in Western province of Zambia. The study used secondary data that was collected in a yellow fever risk assessment survey. Logistic regression analyses were used to determine correlates for infection. A total of 1824 respondents participated in the survey of which 55.2% were females. The prevalence of WNV infection was 18.3%. Participants aged below 15 years were 61% (AOR 0.39 95% CI

* Correspondence: Idah Mweene-Ndumba, BSc, MPH, World Health Organization, Lusaka, Zambia. E-mail: idahndumba12@gmail.com.

[0.30-0.51]) less likely to be infected with WNV compared to those above 15 years of age. Participants who attained primary level education were 44% (AOR 1.44, 95% CI [1.22-1.70]) more likely to be infected than those who attained secondary and higher levels of education. Participants who travelled to Angola were 78% (AOR, 1.78, 95% CI [1.25-2.55]) more likely to be infected with the virus than those who did not travel. WNV infection is common in Western province, and interventions should be designed taking into account the correlates for WNV infection that have been identified in the current study.

Keywords: West Nile virus infection, correlates, Western province, Zambia

INTRODUCTION

West Nile virus (WNV), an arthropod-borne Flavivirus, is transmitted to human beings through a mosquito bite of the *culex* species (1). The life cycle of WNV is primarily between birds and mosquitoes and human beings are infected by mosquito bites when the normal cycle has been broken (1). Of those that are infected by the virus 1:4 become ill and less than 1% develop severe symptoms (nueroinvasive disease) such as meningitis, encephalitis and acute flaccid paralysis. WNV infection has been reported to have a case fatality rate of 10% among the severe cases (1, 2, 5). Most of the infections are usually asymptomatic but those who show symptoms come down with headaches, myalgia, arthralgia and rash (6). Currently no treatment exists for arboviral diseases and there are no licensed vaccines for humans, therefore preventive measures against infection with WNV are encouraged (1, 4).

WNV human infections have been reported worldwide after being first discovered in Uganda in 1937 (5, 6) with reports in Africa, Asia, Australia, Europe and the United States of America (7). The seroprevalence studies in these countries have shown prevalence rate variations within countries with some parts of the country having higher rates than the other (8). At present up to 30,584 cases and 1,214 deaths have been reported to CDC, which is a major health threat and assessment of the factors leading to the disease was needed (2). In America, strategies to identify the risk factors to human infections had been put in place (2). However control measures for WNV infection are not properly defined except the common ones such as mosquito control measures, avoiding exposure to mosquito bites and use of insect repellent which have been reported to have proved to have reduced the disease (1, 4).

Several risk factors for WNV infection such as climate and environmental factors emerged from studies in America. High population density was significantly associated with the viral transmission even after adjusting for other environmental factors (2) and the results were comparable to results obtained in other studies which confirmed an association between urban/sub-urban versus a more rural area (9,10). However other studies reported significant association when there was less population density and rural. Temperature changes determining human activity and mosquito replication was also significantly associated with risk of infection. It was also concluded that these factors could differ yearly due to changes in bird populations with high bird population as being protective (2). It is possible that when there are more birds the virus could be concentrated in bird-mosquito-bird cycle whereas if there were fewer birds the mosquito could resort to human meals. Studies have also confirmed that age has a bearing on the severity of the infection with the older age group, 50 years or older, being most at risk (2). In Arizona, staying at home and not attending school were found to be risk factors for WNV infection, although it was argued that the possibility that those who stayed at home were the elderly who were already known to be at high risk of infection with WNV (1).

There is knowledge gap concerning WNV infections in Zambia and particularly in Western province despite the province being neighbors with countries which are endemic with the disease. The purpose of this analysis was to determine the extent of WNV infection and to assess its correlates in Western province of Zambia.

METHODS

The study was conducted in Western province of Zambia. The selection of the province was based on its re-classification as low potential risk area for yellow fever transmission by World Health Organization in 2010 (11). Western province with a population of 881,524 (12), borders with Angola and has seven districts divided into 1,902 Standard Enumeration Areas (SEAs). The main economic activities were crop farming, livestock production and fishing.

Study population, Sample size, inclusion/exclusion criteria and sampling

This assessment was carried out among individuals aged nine months or older. In estimating the sample size for persons aged 5 years or older, the following parameters were considered: a prevalence of 7%, desired precision or confidence interval (d) of $\pm$3%, and a design effect (DE) of 2 and an 80% response rate. Considering sex, we aimed to recruit 700 male and 700 female participants in each province. Assuming an average of 4 persons aged 5 years or older in each household, a total of 12 households in each of the 30 cluster was to be recruited in the survey. The total number of persons that would be recruited from the province was 1,806.

The seroprevalence of children was about half that for older children, and in estimating the sample size for persons aged below 5 years, the following parameters were considered: a prevalence of 3.5%, desired precision or confidence interval (d) of +3.4%, and a design effect (DE) of 2 and an 80% response rate. The computed sample size was 282. Therefore, in each province 406 children would be recruited for the survey.

Included in the study were individuals aged 9 months or older who were found in a sampled household at the time of the study and were resident in the study site for at least seven days. Individuals who had received YF vaccination in the last ten years to the survey were also included in the survey. Excluded from the study were persons who were aged less than 9 months, or individuals regardless of age who resided in the study site for less than 7 days prior to the survey. Children under the age of 9 months were excluded based on the fact that at this age children could still carry maternal antibodies from exposed mothers which could pose the risk of false positive results.

The sample was drawn using a two-stage cluster sampling technique using probability proportional to size. A list of the standard enumeration areas (SEAs) in each province constituted the sampling frame. The line lists of the SEAs were provided by the Government's Central Statistics Office (CSO). The sampling was designed to achieve fairly good estimates at the provincial level of analysis, and not representing the subdivisions of the province.

Study variables

Dependent variable

A case with evidence of WNV exposure was defined as any individual aged 9 months or older whose blood sample was confirmed to have WNV exposure. WNV exposure status was positive if IgG or IgM antibodies were determined in the serum sample by laboratory testing and negative if the IgG or IgM antibodies were absent by laboratory testing.

Independent variables

The independent variables included demographic data: age, sex, occupation, education, roof type and use of mosquito preventive measures such as insecticide treated nets (ITNs) and indoor residual spray (IRS).

Laboratory procedures

Three to 5 millilitres of blood was collected by venepuncture into an EDTA vaccutainer tube and transported on cold chain to the local laboratories for serum separation and storage.

Subsequently serum samples were transported on cold chain and thereafter subjected to primary testing (YFV specific IgG and IgM) at the University of Teaching Hospital in Zambia virology unit and Institute Pasteur, Dakar, Senegal. All presumptive YFV-specific IgG and IgM samples were subjected to IgG and IgM antibodies testing against other flaviviruses known to cause haemorrhagic fever-like disease including WNV. The testing was carried out using IgG capture enzyme-linked immunosorbent assay (ELISA).

Data management and analysis

Data collected from the field were entered in an Epi-Info data entry screen that had consistency and range checks embedded in it. Further editing was conducted by running frequencies during the analysis stage. Epi data files were exported to SPSS for data analysis. The data was summarized to describe the occurrence of WNV exposed individuals in absolute numbers and percentage by place (residence, travel or work) and person (age, sex, occupation, education). Further analysis using logistic regression was conducted to determine independent factors associated with WNV sero-positivity. Unadjusted Odds ratios (OR) and adjusted odds ratios (AOR) together with their 95% confidence intervals (CI) were used to estimate magnitudes of associations.

Ethical considerations

Ethical clearance was sought from the Tropical Diseases Research Centre Research Ethics Committee, and ethical standards were adhered to throughout this study. Informed consent was sought from study participants. Guardians provided assent for the participation of the persons under the consenting age. They were asked to read or have read to them, understand and sign/thumbprint an informed consent form. Responsible adults in the household were identified to give proxy consent on behalf of minors.

RESULTS

A total of 1,824 respondents participated in the survey of which 55.2% were females. About half (48.0%) of the participants, (46.8% male and 49% females) attained primary school level of education. Of the participants, 30.3% (34.3% males and 27% females) attained higher level of education. Meanwhile the rates of being infected with WNV were 18.3% (19% males and 17.7% females, p = 0.512). These results are shown in Table 1.

Table 1. Sample description Western province

Factors	Total	%	Male	%	Female	%
Age (years) [$x^2 = 7.27$, $p = 0.122$]						
<15	655	36.0	312	38.3	342	34.0
15-24	390	21.4	180	22.1	210	20.9
25-34	245	13.5	94	11.4	151	15.0
25-44	213	11.7	93	11.4	120	11.9
45+	318	17.5	136	16.7	182	18.1
Sex						
Male	815	44.8				
Female	1005	55.2				
Education [$x^2 = 12.83$, $p < 0.002$]						
None	388	21.5	152	18.9	235	23.6
Primary	868	48.2	376	46.8	492	49.3
Secondary	546	30.3	276	34.3	270	27.1
College/University						
West Nile Infection [$x^2 = 0.43$, $p = 0.512$]						
Positive	334	18.3	155	19.0	178	17.7
Negative	1490	91.7	660	81.0	827	82.3

Table 2. Factors associated with West Nile Virus infection in bivariate and multivariate analysis for Western province

Factor	OR	95% CI	AOR	95% CI
Age (years)				
<15	0.42	(0.33-0.53)	0.39	(0.30-0.51)
15-24	0.84	(0.66-1.07)	0.93	(0.72-1,19)
25-34	1.20	(0.92-1.56)	1.25	(0.96-1.63)
35-44	1.24	(0.94-1.64)	1.20	(0.91-1.59)
45+	1	1	1	1
Sex				
Male	1.05	(0.64-0.97)		
Female		1		
Education				
None	0.79	(0.64-0.97)	0.89	(0.71-1.13)
Primary	1.34	(1.14-1.57)	1.44	(1.22-1.70)
Secondary	1	1	1	1

Table 2. (Continued)

Factor	OR	95% CI	AOR	95% CI
College/University				
Slept under Mosquito Net				
Yes	1.05	(0.93-1.19)		
No	1	1		
House with IRS				
Yes	0.92	(0.77-1.09)		
No	1			1
Travelled to Angola				
Yes	2.14	(1.52-3.02)	1.78	(1.25-2.55)
No	1		1	

Variables that were considered in the analysis were age, sex, education level, sleeping under a mosquito net, using IRS and travel to DRC and to Angola (Table 2). Those below the age of 15 years were 61% (AOR 0.39 95% CI [0.30-0.51]) less likely to be infected with WNV compared to those above 15 years of age. Participants who had attained primary level of education were 44% (AOR 1.44, 95% CI [1.22-1.70]) more likely to be infected by the virus than those who had attained secondary or higher levels of education. Travelling to Congo DRC was not associated with acquiring the infection but those who travelled to Angola were 78% (AOR, 1.78, 95% CI [1.25-2.55]) more likely to be infected with the virus than those who did not travel. Meanwhile gender, sleeping under a mosquito net and house with IRS were not associated with WNV infection.

DISCUSSION

This study provides the first evidence of the circulation of WNV and correlates for the infection in Western province of Zambia. The study has indicated that 18.3% of the participants in the yellow fever risk assessment survey had antibodies to WNV. This result is consistent with results from surveys conducted worldwide although in some areas very high seroprevalence was discovered. In Italy, the study conducted in blood donors had lower rates which ranged from 3-33/1000 blood donors (13). The seroprevalence in USA varied across the country with rates ranging from 4.2% to 19.7%. Disease prevalence is dependent upon a wide range of risk factors, climate and the environment affecting the activities of the virus and the humans (2, 9, 10). In Africa higher rates (60-74%) in Egypt, (3-65%) in Kenya and (13-24%) in South Africa, were reported as way back as the 1950s to 1970s (14, 15).

Age, education and travelling to Angola were significantly associated with WNV infection. Participants younger than 15 years old were less likely to be infected with the virus. Activities associated with older age such as working outside homes may increase chances of being exposed to the mosquito vector carrying the virus. A similar finding has been reported by Liu et al. (2) who found that persons above the age of 50 years were more at risk for the disease compared to those below the age of 50 years. An increase in prevalence of WNV antibodies against age may suggest endemic infection (16).

The finding that education was significantly associated with infection was not consistent. While persons with no formal education were equally likely to have the infection as those with secondary of higher levels of education, persons with primary level of education were more likely to be infected. When comparing persons with no formal education with those who had attained primary level of education, the finding in the current study contradicts that found by Gibney et al. (1) who indicated that those who did not attend school and were more often at home were more at risk of the disease than those who were often attending school. It is not clear what exposure factors persons who had attained primary level of education had to have increased risk of infection.

West Nile virus has been active in Angola (17). Movement of people across the border with Zambia and Angola by motor vehicle or on foot may increase the risk of introducing WNV infection from endemic to non-endemic areas (18). However, the fact that there has been no report on the infection in Western province, does not exclude the province from being an endemic area for West Nile infection. In conclusion, WNV infection is common in Western province, and interventions should be designed taking into account the correlates for WNV infection that had been identified in the current study.

ACKNOWLEDGMENTS

We are grateful to the interviewers for their dedicated work to successfully complete the survey. The survey could not have been successful without the cooperation of the participants and the virology laboratory staff both in Lusaka, Zambia and Dakar, Senegal for in testing samples. The survey was funded by the Ministry of Health [Zambia] and the World Health Organization.

REFERENCES

[1] Gibney KB, Colborn J, Baty S, Bunko Patterson AM, Sylvester T, Briggs G, et al. Modifiable risk factors for West Nile virus infection during an outbreak--Arizona, 2010. Am J Trop Med Hyg 2012;86:895-901.

[2] Liu A, Lee V, Galusha D, Slade MD, Diuk-Wasser M, Andreadis T, et al. Risk factors for human infection with West Nile Virus in Connecticut: a multi-year analysis. Int J Health Geogr 2009;8:67.

[3] Nash D, Mostashari F, Fine A, Miller J, O'Leary D, Murray K, et al. 1999 West Nile Outbreak Response Working Group. The outbreak of West Nile virus infection in the New York City area in 1999. N Engl J Med 2001;344:1807-14.

[4] LaBeaud AD, Kile JR, Kippes C, King CH, Mandalakas AM. Exposure to West Nile virus during the 2002 epidemic in Cuyahoga County, Ohio: a comparison of pediatric and adult behaviors. Public Health Rep 2007;122:356-61.

[5] Petersen LR, Carson PJ, Biggerstaff BJ, Custer B, Borchardt SM, Busch MP. Estimated cumulative incidence of West Nile virus infection in US adults, 1999-2010. Epidemiol Infect. 2013;141:591-5.

[6] Smithburn KC, Hughes TP, Burke AW, Paul JH. A Neurotropic Virus Isolated from the Blood of a Native of Uganda. Am J Trop Med 1940;20:471-2.

[7] Stiasny K, Aberle SW, Heinz FX. Retrospective identification of human cases of West Nile virus infection in Austria (2009 to 2010) by serological differentiation from Usutu and other flavivirus infections. Euro Surveill. 2013;18(43):pii=20614.

[8] Schweitzer BK, Kramer WL, Sambol AR, Meza JL, Hinrichs SH, Iwen PC. Geographic factors contributing to a high seroprevalence of West Nile virus-specific antibodies in humans following an epidemic. Clin Vaccine Immunol 2006; 13(3):314-8.
[9] Brown HE, Childs JE, Diuk-Wasser MA, Fish D. Ecological factors associated with West Nile virus transmission, northeastern United States. Emerg Infect Dis 2008;14:1539-45.
[10] Gibbs SEJ, Wimberly MC, Madden M, Masour J, Yabsley MJ, Stallknecht DE. Factors affecting the geographic distribution of West Nile virus in Georgia, USA: 2002–2004.Vector Borne Zoonotic Dis 2006;6:73-82.
[11] Jentes ES, Poumerol G, Gershman MD, Hill DR, Lemarchand J, Lewis RF, et al. The revised global yellow fever risk map and recommendations for vaccination, 2010: consensus of the Informal WHO Working Group on Geographic Risk for Yellow Fever. Lancet Infect Dis 2011;11:622-32.
[12] Central Statistical Office. 2010 census of population and housing. National analytical report. Lusaka, Zambia: CSO, 2012.
[13] Pezzotti P, Piovesan C, Barzon L, Cusinato R, Cattai M, Pacenti M, et al. Prevalence of IgM and IgG antibodies to West Nile virus among blood donors in an affected area of north-eastern Italy, summer 2009. Euro Surveill 2011;16(10):pii=1981.
[14] Darwish M A, Ibrahim AH. Survey for antibodies to arboviruses in Egyptian sera. I. West Nile virus antihemagglutinins in human and animal sera. Egypt Public Health Assoc 1971;46:61-70.
[15] Murgue B, Murri S, Triki H, Deubel V, Zeller HG. West Nile in the Mediterranean basin: 1950-2000. Ann N Y Acad Sci 2001;951:117-26.
[16] Fagbami AH, Monath TP, Fabiyi A. Dengue virus infections in Nigeria: a survey for antibodies in monkeys and humans. Trans R Soc Trop Med Hyg 1977;71:60–5.
[17] Kokernot RH, Casaca VMR, Weinbren MP, McIntosh BM. Survey for antibodies against arthropod-borne viruses in the sera of indigenous residents of Angola. Trans R Soc Trop Med Hyg 1965);59:563-70.
[18] Blackburn NK, Rawat R. Dengue fever imported from India: a report of 3 cases. S Afr Med J 1987;71:386-7.

In: Public Health Yearbook 2016
Editor: Joav Merrick

ISBN: 978-1-53610-947-4

Chapter 12

FIRST RECORD OF AN AEDES SPECIES MOSQUITO IN NORTH-WESTERN PROVINCE OF ZAMBIA? OBSERVATION DURING A YELLOW FEVER RISK ASSESSMENT SURVEY

Freddie Masaninga[1,*], BSc, MSc, PhD,
Mbanga Muleba[2], BSc, MSc,
Osbert Namafente[1], BSc, MSc[2],
Peter Songolo, MBChB, MPH,
Idah Mweene-Ndumba[1], MSc, MPH,
Mazyanga L Mazaba-Liwewe[1], BSc,
Mulakwa Kamuliwo[3], MD,
Seter Siziya[4,5], BA(Ed), MSc, PhD
and Olusegun A Babaniyi[1], MBBS, MPH, MSc
[1]World Health Organization (WHO), Lusaka, Zambia
[2]Tropical Diseases Research Centre, Ndola, Zambia
[3]Ministry of Health, Zambia
[4]School of Medicine, Copperbelt University, Ndola, Zambia
[6]University of Lusaka, Lusaka, Zambia

ABSTRACT

Although records on mosquitoes belonging to *Aedes* date back to 1950s, there is paucity of knowledge on the distribution, species composition and bionomics of arthropod-borne vectors in Zambia. In 2013, during a yellow fever risk assessment survey conducted in North-Western province of Zambia, an entomological survey was conducted to ascertain

* Correspondence: Freddie Masaninga, PhD, National Professional Officer, WHO Country Office, Lusaka, Zambia. E-mail: Masaningaf@who.int

the availability, density and infectivity of yellow fever vectors in the province. We present information on *Aedes* species which was not identified into *Aedes (Stegomyia) aegypti*, *Aedes simpsoni*, or any other previously collected mosquitoes. *Aedes* species were collected in forested and peri-urban locations of North-Western province. Approximately 75% were classified as *Aedes (Finlaya) wellani*, while the rest were classified as *Aedes (Stegomyia) aegypti, Aedes (Stegomyia) africanus, Aedes (aedimorphus) mutilus* and *Aedes (aedimorphus) minutus*. Literature search showed that this is the first collection of *Aedes (Finlaya) wellani* in Zambia. Analysis of *Aedes* species (N = 60) using the Polymerase Chain Reaction (PCR) for viral infection showed no viral activity. Observation of *Aedes (Finlaya) wellani* which has hitherto not been reported in Zambia indicates the importance of strengthened entomological surveillance in Zambia.

Keywords: Aedes (Finlaya) wellani, mosquito, vector, Zambia

INTRODUCTION

Studies on *Aedes* species distribution, bionomics and species composition in Zambia are limited and systematic reports date back to 1950s. Mosquito vector studies have tended to focus on vectors of malaria (1, 2). Malaria is ranked among the top ten common causes of illness in the country. In 2013, during a yellow fever risk assessment survey, an entomological survey was conducted to ascertain the availability, density and infectivity of yellow fever vectors in North-Western province of Zambia.

METHODS

The study was conducted in North-Western province of Zambia in six districts, namely, Mwinilunga, Mufumbwe, Kabompo, Chavuma, Solwezi and Zambezi. North-Western province is located at 1,354 metres above sea level, latitude -13.0 and longitude 25.0 and has a population of 706,462. The province borders with Angola on the western side and the Democratic Republic of Congo on the northern side. Highest rainfall in the country, with annual rainfall of 1320 mm is recorded in this province. The mean minimum temperature in the dry cold month of June is 6.8°C and the mean maximum temperature in dry hot month of October is 30.6°C (3). The province is located within the Central African plateau.

Mosquito sampling

Sampling was conducted in April-May 2013, in the transition from wet to the drier month (3).

Larvae: Larval searches were conducted in rural, urban and peri-urban areas of the province. Both inside and outside house searches for larvae were made. The survey team covered at least 10 households per day. The term household meant one or more people who lived in the same dwelling and also shared meals or living accommodation.

Indoor inspection included flower-pots and water storage, whereas outside inspection included wells, discarded Clay-pots, discarded bottles and plastic containers; banana (*Musa sapientum*) leaf axils, discarded tyres and edges of water canals. The collected mosquito larvae were kept in larval bottles (Figure 1). Mosquito larval data included province, district, locality (urban or rural), house number (randomly allocated during sampling) and date of collection.

Adults: Adult mosquitoes were sampled by three research teams consisting of four persons per team. The following sampling methods were used to collect adult mosquitoes: backpack aspirators, aspiration using a mouth aspirator tube, CDC Light trap and the Gravid Light traps. Mosquito collections were made inside and outside households in different ecological locations: rural, urban, forest and plains. Outdoor mosquitoes were captured using backpack aspirator, CDC Light trap and the Gravid Light trap for collecting gravid (egg-laying) females to increase the chance for virus isolation. Sampling mosquitoes using back pack aspirator was conducted outdoor between 16.00 hours and 19.00 hours. Indoor adult resting mosquitoes were collected by various methods such as a mouth aspirator tube using a torch to locate these resting sites and knockdown spray catch with pyrethroid insecticide in randomly selected dwellings which commenced at 06.00 hours. All adult mosquitoes collected from the field were sorted and pooled by site of collection, sex and stored in liquid nitrogen to maintain mosquito morphological features.

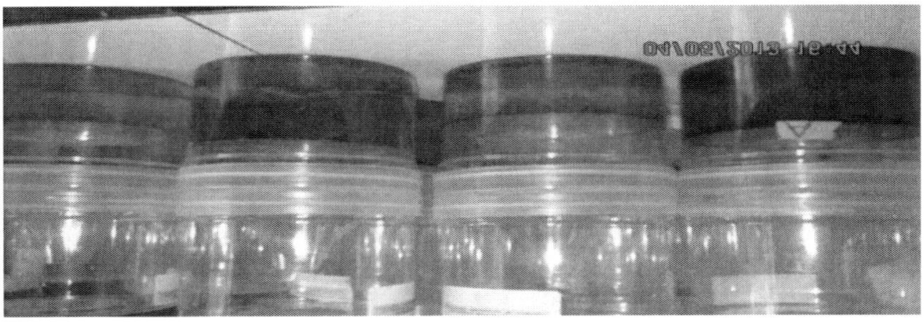

Figure 1. Mosquito larvae kept for emerging into adult in TDRC, Ndola, Zambia.

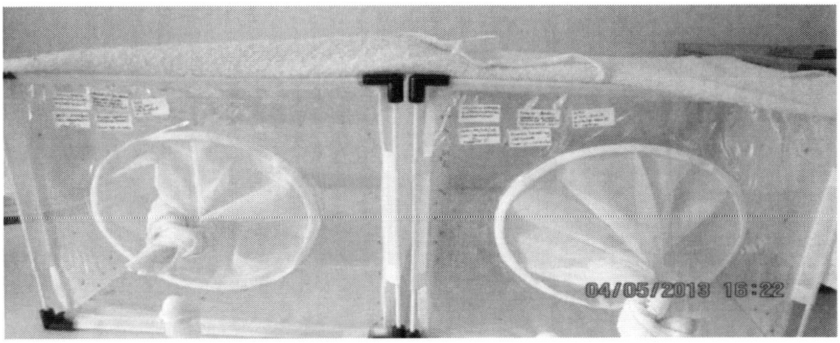

Figure 2. Field collected adult mosquitoes in cages transported to TDRC, Ndola, Zambia.

Mosquito larval rearing

Sampled mosquito larvae were transported to the Tropical Diseases Research Centre (TDRC) Insectary Laboratory in Ndola, Zambia, to rear them into the adult stage for species identification using entomological keys (5-7). At the TDRC Laboratory, the larvae were fed on fish flakes Tetramin and maintained at relative humidity of 80 ± 2% and temperature 23 ± 2°C. Emerged adult mosquitoes were stored at -80°C to preserve their viability.

Shipment, viral tests and vector species identification

Sixty adult *Aedes* species mosquitoes were airfreighted to Institute Pasteur in Dakar (IPD), Senegal to test for the presence of arthropod-borne viral activity in the *Aedes* specimen vector species by Reverse Transcriptase Polymerase Chain reaction (RT-PCR) technique and to identify and/or validate the sub-sample species. In transit to IPD, the mosquito specimens were preserved at -80°C in dry ice to maintain DNA viability.

Ethical considerations

Each participant in the study had earlier been vaccinated against yellow fever virus and received prior chemoprophylaxis against malaria (4). The protocol was approved by the Tropical Diseases Research Centre Research Ethics Committee in Ndola, Zambia. Permission to access houses was sought from heads of houses.

RESULTS

Out of a total of 453 *adult Aedes* species of mosquitoes collected from rural, urban, peri-urban and forest locations, the majority (75.47%) were classified as *Aedes (Finlaya) wellani* (Figures 3 and 4).

Aedes (Finlaya) wellani were collected from Ikelenge, situated near the source of the river Zambezi in the Zambezi district of Zambia. The other Aedes species that were collected are *Aedes (Stegomyia) aegypti, Aedes (Stegomyia) africanus, Aedes (aedimorphus) mutilus* and *Aedes (aedimorphus) minutus.*

None of the 60 female *Aedes* species of *Aedes (stegomia) aegypti, Aedes (stegomyia) africanus, Aedes (aedimorphus) minutus, Aedes (aedimorphus) mutilus* and *Aedes (Finlaya) wellmani* were positive for the yellow fever virus.

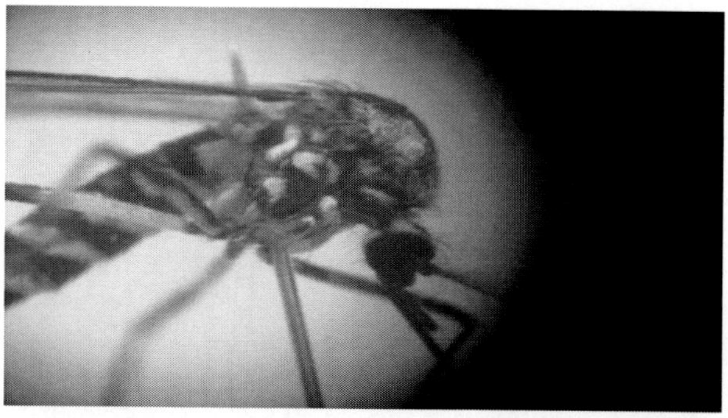

Figure 3. Field collected adult *Aedes (Finlaya) Wellani* side view.

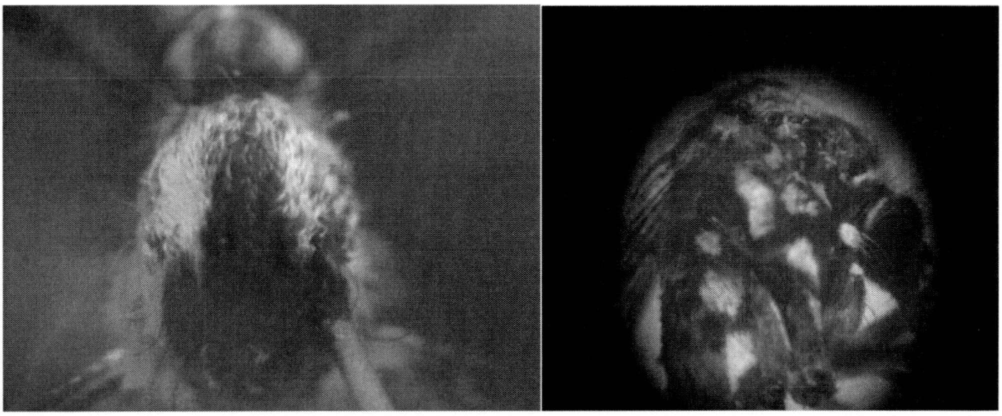

Figure 4. Dorsal head view of *Aedes (Finalaya) wellani;* collected from Ikelenge, Zambezi district Zambia.

DISCUSSION

This study has identified *Aedes* mosquitoes collected from Ikelenge, Zambezi district, which did not belong to the species reported by the previous investigators (8). Independent verification at a WHO accredited, collaboration centre of the mosquito specimens, identified it as *Aedes (Finlaya) wellani.* To our knowledge this is the first report of this *Aedes* species at Ikelenge, Zambezi district in Zambia.

More studies should be conducted to study the behaviour, spatial and geographical distribution of this mosquito in North-Western province and other provinces in Zambia to gain more accurate understanding on the possible role of *Aedes (Finlaya) wellani* in the transmission of arboviruses in Zambia.

Entomological studies on mosquito vector distribution are critical given the increasingly importance of new emerging arthropod-borne infections such as Zika, Dengue and reports of expansion through increased global trade and climatic changes which are being reported in Africa, Asia and other regions (9). Strengthening entomological surveillance becomes imperative in Zambia in order to provide accurate data base for evidenced-based vector control decisions.

In conclusion, collection of *Aedes (Finlaya) wellani* during a yellow fever risk assessment survey in Zambia underpins the increasing need to maintain a strong entomological surveillance in-country for guiding rational vector control programs.

REFERENCES

[1] Littrell M, Miller JM, Ndhlovu M, Hamainza B, Hawela M, Kamuliwo M, et al. Documenting malaria case management coverage in Zambia: a systems effectiveness Approach. Malar J 2013;12:371.

[2] Masaninga F, Chanda E, Chanda-Kapata P, Hamainza B, Masendu HT, Kamuliwo M, et al. Review of the malaria epidemiology and trends in Zambia. Asian Pac J Trop Biomed 2013;3:89-94.

[3] North-Western province, Zambia 2010. Accessed 2014 August 27. URL: http://1worldmap.com/Zambia/North-Western-Province.

[4] WHO. Meeting of the Strategic Advisory Group of Experts on immunization, April 2013 – Conclusions and Recommendations. Weekly Epidemiol Record 2013;88:201–16.

[5] Gillies MT and Coetzee M. A supplement to the Anophelinae of Africa south of the Sahara (Afrotropical Region). Johannesburg: Publications of the South African Institute for Medical Research, 1987.

[6] Rueda ML. Pictorial keys for the identification of mosquitoes (Diptera: Culicidae) associated with Dengue Virus Transmission. Auckland, New Zealand: Magnolia Press, 2004:14-20.

[7] Yiau-Min H. A pictorial key for the identification of the subfamilies of Culicidae, genera of Culicinae, and subgenera of Aedes mosquitoes of the Afrotropical region (Diptera: Culicidae). Proceedings of the Entomological Society of Washington 2001;103:1-53.

[8] Robinson GG. A note on mosquitoes and yellow fever in Northern Rhodesia. East Afr Med J 1950;27:284-8.

[9] Dash AP, Bhatia R, Sunyoto T, Mourya DT. Emerging and re-emerging arboviral diseases in South East Asia. J Vector Borne Dis 2013;50:77-84.

SECTION TWO - SOCIAL WORK AND HEALTH INEQUALITIES

In: Public Health Yearbook 2016
Editor: Joav Merrick

ISBN: 978-1-53610-947-4

Chapter 13

FEDERAL FINANCING FOR THE BRAZILIAN MENTAL HEALTH POLICY

*Maria LT Garcia**
Social Work Department, Espirito Santo Federal University,
Vitoria, Espirito Santo, Brazil

ABSTRACT

This study analyzes the federal funding for mental health care and services in Brazilian Mental Health policy between 2003 and 2012. Social workers and other professionals are included this analysis to show how organized social movements in the mental health field provide support relating to the principles of Psychiatric Reform. Financing for mental health is an important tool in the Psychiatric Reform process because there is a direct correlation between expenditures in the field and direction that public policy values psychiatric treatment. Methods: Bibliographical review of the Brazilian Health Ministry's Mental Health Coordination annual reports between 2001 and 2012. Results: The Brazilian Ministry of Health expenditure on mental health care in 2011 was around one billion eight hundred and twelve million reais (R$522 million on hospital care and R$1290 million on out-of-hospital care). The Brazilian mental health policy proposes the organization of a full care network of diversity of resources to provide psychosocial care to people with mental disorders. Results: Between 2003 and 2011, the expenditure increased threefold. But, when these expenditures were analyzed; they expressed two sides to this question: On the one hand, they guaranteed 72% the population the constitutional right to access health care services. On the other hand, 28% of Brazilians are denied this right. Conclusion: The out-of-hospital mental health care expenditure is higher than hospitalization expenditures in Brazil but the advancement of psychiatric reform has been slow.

Keywords: mental health policy, funding, Brazil

---

* Corresponding author: Professor Maria LT Garcia, DSS/UFES, Programa de Pos-Graduacao em Politica Social, Pesquisadora CNPq, Antonio Honorio street, 41/502, Bento Ferreira. Vitoria/Espirito Santo, 29050-770, Brazil. E-mail: lucia-garcia@uol.com.br.

Introduction

"Financing is a critical factor in the realization of a viable mental health system. It is the mechanism by which plans and policies are translated into action through the allocation of resources. Without adequate financing, plans remain in the realm of rhetoric and good intentions. With financing, a resource base is created for operations and the delivery of services, for the development and deployment of a trained workforce, and for the required infrastructure and technology" (1).

World Health Organization (1) indicated that "... among the broad challenges faced by the financing of mental health care systems are: the diversity of resources among countries; the lack of financial data; the varying control and influence of mental health policy-makers and planners over mental health care financing; the varying levels of development of mental health systems between countries." Specifically, these concepts should be applied to understand the mental health system in Brazil. The Ministry of Health currently identifies that 3% of the population suffer from severe or persistent mental disorder where about 12% of the population needs some kind of mental health care, whether continuous or eventual (2), demonstrating an unmet need. As far as alcohol and psychoactive substances are concerned, more than 6% of the population has serious psychiatric disorders. In 2011, however, the Brazilian Ministry of Health spent 2.51% of its annual health budget on mental health (2). To fully understand the trend, this article analyzes reviewed a ten year pattern of federal funding for mental health services.

The primary profession serving mental health is social work making this debate fundamental understanding workforce issues as they relate to social work service provision. Data from Brazilian Institute of Geography and Statistics (3) shows that the number of social workers in health services in 2009 was 19.000 compared to the 2012 estimate by the Brazilian Federal Board of Social Work (4) of 120,000 registered social workers who were associated with health care, a significant increase in a three year period. This increase supports the perspective of a Psychiatric Reform (RP) within Brazil. Social workers contribute to the well-being and quality of the services provided within the mental health field and supports an individual's search for autonomy and social integration. Since there are a number of patients deprived from effective services then policy change is important in order to improve quality of life, not only for persons needing mental health care but in other areas as well.

This analysis encompasses pessimism of intellect and optimism of the will (as suggested by Gramsci). On the one hand, there is a struggle for advances in the field of mental health that contribute to psychiatric reform. On the other hand, there are the strains from multiple and contradictory interests that exist in an emerging country. This analysis required an objective assessment of the dynamics of Brazilian society within the context of an emerging world market. Our research made Bibliographical review and documental research on annual reports by the Brazilian Health Ministry's Mental Health Coordination (2001 to 2012).

Brazilian Mental Health Policy

After the creation of Brazilian Unified Health System (SUS) in the 1988 Federal Constitution, the implementation necessitated that the Brazilian Ministry of Health would be responsible for formulating and implementing mental health policies through National Mental Health Coordination, which happened in 1991 (5). This led to a new stage in public mental health policy construction. A "...theoretical-ideological uproar around the direction the Brazilian psychiatric reform was taking place and, as far as the healthcare system was concerned, the moment the laws regulating SUS were passed and implemented" (5, pp. 458), the Brazilian National Mental Health Coordination of the Health Ministry promoted changes contributing to psychiatric reform even before any Law of Psychiatric Reform was ever passed. The first change altered the funding to mental health by adopting Edict SNAS/MS 189/91, which changed SUS operating procedures. These proposed changes included diversifying therapeutic methods and techniques and restructuring outpatient and community services for people with mental disorders. In order to ensure thoroughness of health care to individuals with mental disorders and taking into account the need of matching mental health care procedures with the model proposed, the Ministry of Health passed the Groups and Procedures of the Hospital Information System Table (SIH-SUS) in mental health. This established a system to reduce prolonged hospitalizations for psychiatric patients while included new procedures, such as group care, performed by para-professionals with only college or high-school degrees; healthcare at Psychosocial Care Centers; therapeutic workshop care; and home visits by para-professionals with college degrees. This Edict meant healthcare facilities rendering mental health services for SUS would have to undergo supervision, control, and evaluation by federal, state and municipal technicians. Another change was the regulation of healthcare service operations (Edict SNAS/MS 224/92). In this, the Ministry of Health defined rules for SUS outpatient and inpatient services. This edict forbade the existence of restrictive spaces (cells); ensured the secrecy of letters to inpatients; and required the appropriate recording of diagnostic and therapeutic procedures adopted for patients.

The period between 1990 and 1996 marked the beginning of the discussion about mental health policies with the constitution of different work groups - formal partnerships with informal dialogues by various consultants. The goal was to speed up the process of psychiatric reform implementation in Brazil. In 1992, the Second Brazilian Conference on Mental Health (CNSM) was held. Most significant was the debates and hearings surrounding Bill no. 3657/89. This Bill provided more visibility for the interest groups involved – Psychiatric Reform Movement and Industry of Madness – as well as proposals by political action groups and their opponents. Another aspect that characterized this period was the work of Ministry of Health's Mental Health Coordination to organize health care aimed at de-hospitalization of mental health facilities through a process of evaluation and accreditation. The first edicts aimed at reorienting healthcare. Thus, even if the preferred psychiatric reform healthcare model had yet to be effectively constructed, the Brazilian Ministry of Health prepared the conditions to reach a consensus about the mental health policy (5). It is also worth noting that resistance to these proposals for change articulated by the Federation of Private Hospitals and the Brazilian Association of Psychiatry were strengthened during this period. These contradiction were in the form decreasing costs of psychiatric care at public psychiatric hospitals while reducing the public allocation of funding to the private sector "... to further enrich bourgeoisie and other conservative sectors that make up the basis of support for their political office" (6, pp.43).

Between 1990 and 1996, the process of systematic restructuring of the normative outline regulating psychiatric care in Brazil was begun. Edicts 189/91 and 224/92 regulated the services of Psychosocial Care Centers (CAPS), broadening the community care services (20). The challenges posed were to meet the actual needs projected with universal access and inverting the mental asylum model by deconstructing it with the creation of new services. The milestone of this situation was a meeting between the Brazilian National Coordination of Mental health and the Pan American Health Organization (PAHO) that composed a document establishing the mental health policy to be adopted in Brazil. Key elements of the policy were two-fold: a) overturn the poor quality and expensive health care at both financial and social levels; b) change the iatrogenic model by diversifying therapeutic resources and promoting decentralization of care that was believed to be the result "...of new political and cultural relations" (5, pp. 458). It departed from the premise that the "mental health" question should be solved locally, at municipal level. However, funding this network would still take place at this management (municipal) level.

Global funding for SUS mental health has increased over the past 11 years. However, that may be misleading since following the passage of Psychiatric Reform Law no. 10.216 in 2001 the funding slowed but not significantly enough. The law regulating mental health policy in Brazil emerged as an important gain to all those defending the psychiatric reform. Data from the World Health Organization (1) showed that 60% of member countries having mental health laws (covering 72% of all the world's population) were approved after the year 2000 with significant growth after 2005 (see Figure 1).

Following the passage of the Brazilian law there was a visible shift in the funding patterns as the money started to migrate from inpatient to outpatient hospital care – according to the change in model. This happened in such a way that by the end of 2006, the territorial and community element (CAPS, outpatient clinics, therapeutic homes, and living centers) were receiving more funding than hospital care for the first time. As a reference point, in 1997 the inpatient/outpatient ratio was 92% to 8% of the funds characterizing a dramatic shift in public psychiatry services that were built almost exclusively on Hospital Admission Orders (AIH).

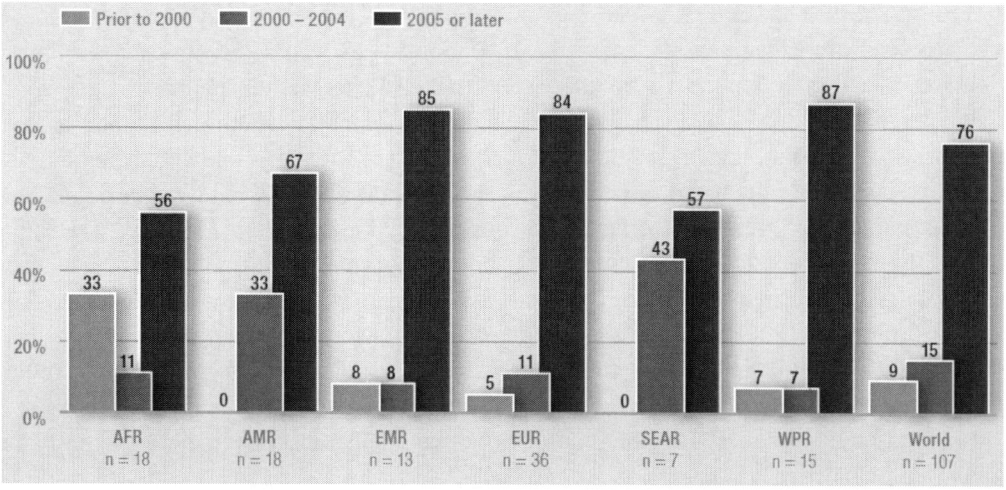

Figure 1. Countries with mental health laws (1).

Financing Services	2002	2003	2004	2005	2006	2007	2008	2009	2010	2011
Inpatients Services and Programs	465,98	452,93	465,51	453,68	427,32	439,90	458,06	482,83	534,25	522,07
Outpatients Services and Programs	153,31	226,00	287,35	406,13	541,99	760,47	871,18	1012,35	1.280,60	1.290,70

Figure 2. Brazilian mental health financing (in millions of reais – Brazilian Money) (2).

The mental health policy in Brazil parallels what has transpired in developed countries. Over the past 30 years, health systems in developed countries evolved from very centralized into a decentralized model where the responsibility for the implementation of policies and services transferred from central structures to local ones. This process affected the delivery of services in developing countries as the emphasis has been to reduce costs through efficiency and the creation of public-private contracts for the provision of services. The question arises as to whether decentralizing services is the best type of service for persons with mental health problems. Many times, people with mental problems have a chronic condition with strong likelihood for repeated or long periods requiring treatment. Instead of being treated by a mental health professional, then, in Brazil it is the police who are providing services during crisis episodes. The police are near the population resulting in the person in crisis being placed in custody, away from other, rather than being hospitalized and treated. There is the need to create more community-based emergency service units, such as Psychosocial Care Centers III with overnight beds, to address decentralized treatment modality. Currently, only 13 states of the Brazilian federation (7) have established such centers. There is some change happening as evidenced by the IV National Conference on Mental Health (held in Brasilia in 2010) where legislation was being proposed (for example, resolution 373 of 2009) to expand the number of CAPs in Brazilian states, especially CAPs III (open all day) and CPSsi (especially for child and adolescents). Between 2006 and 2010 the percentage of CAPs I and CAPs III grew on average 69%. However, the CAPs III deficit continues to be a challenge to mental health service delivery.

For the World Health Organization (8), mental health funding should take three key recommendations into account: a) resources for developing community services in face of partial closing of hospitals; b) investment in new services so as to facilitate transition from hospitals to community; and c) financial coverage of a given level of institutional care after community base services are established. In other words, building an adequate transition while funding the Pact for Health to make sure that the CAPs network and other community devices keep expanding (facing the challenge of access with quality). That is why consolidating mechanisms for the transition of the Compensation and Strategic Actions Fund (FAEC) is crucial to mental health policies. The Edict GM 2867/08 of 2008 modified CAPs funding procedures to come from resources that were reallocated through the financial municipal ceilings (9).

The Pact for Health management guidelines ensures incentives for expanding the network. The challenge is how to pay for it. Federal expenditures on health have steadily grown over the past few years but the proportion of the Expenditure on the Mental Health Program (GSM)/Public Health Action and Service (ASPS) has been stable (around 2% and

2.5%) (7). Although the World Health Organization recommends a 5% growth rate, the GSM/ASPS ratio in Brazil has been negligible. The Brazilian Ministry of Health would need to increase the GSM/ASPS by 100% just to be on par with the World Health Organization recommendation.

Between 2003 and 2006, the Brazilian Ministry of Health proposed that the Pact for Health would ensure maintenance and progressive enlargement of extra-hospital network funding or the resources allocated to the community should not be limited to financial and human resources transferred from the hospital. The report continues by identifying a need to increase funds to mental health services by at least 3% of the 2007-2009 health budgets increasing it to at least 4.5% by 2010. The report proposed transferring resources from other ministries to support inter-sectorial projects in the areas of culture, leisure, sport, jobs, social development that include mental health (10).

To create new areas for a shared management, the Brazilian Ministry of Health published the Pact for Health in 2006 (Edict no. 399 issued on February 22, 2006). The central idea of this Pact for Health was to implement institutional reforms in SUS — in the three management spheres (Union, states and Municipalities), replacing the directives proposed in NOB/96 and NOAS/2001 by the Commitment and Management Term. The goals of Pact for Health established a new funding agreement with new responsibilities, sanitation goals, and shared healthcare responsibilities in the three government management spheres (11). For healthcare managers, this was a reaffirmation for a commitment to SUS and its principles of strengthening of Primary Care and for more health care resources.

Mental health care funds after the Pact for Health in 2007-2009

Mental health advocates and other stakeholders in many countries are concerned about four areas: Access, quality, results, and efficiency (8). These translate into the following key questions: 1. Access - Are the people who need the services actually receiving them? 2. Quality - Are the services provided adequate and of high-quality? 3. Results – Are the outcomes of the people receiving services improving? 4. Efficiency - Are the services provided in an efficient manner? This study analyzed the funding provided to mental health actions and services to address these four questions. Data from the Brazilian Ministry of Health showed that expenditure on mental health was 1,494,000,000 BRL Reais (R) (around US$ 796,460,177.00) — R$482 million on inpatient care and R$1 billion, 12 million on outpatient care.

The Brazilian mental health policy proposes organizing a full care network made up of instruments to provide psychosocial care to people with mental disorders. This expenditure expresses two sides to this question: On one side, 67% of the population would be granted the constitutional right to access health care services leaving 33% of Brazilians without this right. Thus, not everyone who needs these services receives them (access). Although outpatient mental health care expenditures are higher than hospitalization expenditures, the number people served in outpatient services is far greater. Even though Brazilian psychiatric reform has slowed down, the services people received remained of a high quality (quality).

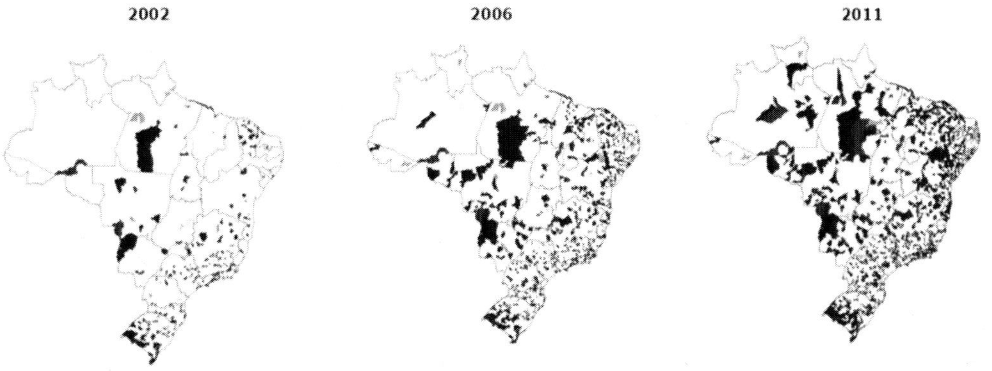

Figure 3. Coverage Caps by Brazilian municipalities (parameter 1 CAPS per 100,000 population) (2). Legend: color black – cities with mental health services; color white cities without services.

The Pact for Health introduced important changes in the forms of resource transfers from state to municipal level, grouping resources transferred into "Funding Blocks" defined as: a) Primary care block; b) Average and High Complexity Out and Inpatient Care Block; c) Health Surveillance Block; d) Pharmaceutical Care Block; e) Management Block. The new rules were regulated by Edict GM/MS no. 204, issued on January 29, 2007 (11). Mental health is placed in the "Management Block" (article 31), which defines: "... the component for implanting Health Actions and Services includes incentives currently designated: I – Implantation of Psychosocial Care Centers (CAPS); II – qualification of Psychosocial Care Centers (CAPS); III Implantation of Mental Health Therapeutic Homes; IV – Promotion of damage-reducing actions at CAPs ad" (11).

Taking the implantation of CAPs III as an example in our tripartite system, the federal government provides one third of the costs for this health care service while the state and municipal governments cover the balance of the costs. In the current scenario, only very politically engaged municipalities can manage to obtain financial support from their respective states, otherwise the municipality would have to cover two thirds of the service costs, since few state governments have contributed to direct maintenance of psychosocial care services. As a result, in May 2010, 46 Psychosocial Care Centers (CAPS) III had been implanted in 13 Brazilian states (59% of them in southwestern states).

See Figure 1 shows the gaps in mental health service coverage in some regions in Brazil (mainly North and Northeastern Regions).

The Brazilian National Health Plan (2012-2015) foresees the strengthening of the mental health care network, providing wide access to quality and diverse treatment for users of alcohol, crack, and other drug addicts, as well as family care services. The Plan aims at expanding the number of Psychosocial Care Centers (CAPS), as well as implanting sheltering units by increasing the number of psychiatric homes in general hospitals serving as urgent and emergency mental health care centers (2). This expansion is justified because of the 26 Brazilian states, only 18 have at least one 24hour CAPS (III or ADIII). On the other hand, 5 states do not have any CAPSi and one state does not have a CAPSad (thus denying them the universal right to health care).

Brazilians live with a structural political problem for funding SUS. In the current political and economic scenario, the Brazilian federal government there is structural obstacles to expand current outpatient mental health care services to effectively replace inpatient care. The current laws and financial resources generated by deactivating psychiatric beds should be allocated to the outpatient mental health services. However, the current structure identifies hospitalization funds as federal while the maintenance of therapeutic homes and CAPs is municipal. To complicate things further, psychiatric hospitals are mainly private while the patients in them are not necessarily residents of the municipalities in which the hospitals are based. Although according to the law the funds resulting from the deactivation of inpatient psychiatric bed should be reallocated to the municipality to which de deinstitutionalized patients are moved, there is no guarantee that the resources deriving from the decrease in mental health care beds will be forwarded to outpatient care services, especially when patients go to a municipality different from that in which they had been hospitalized (12).

Released shortly before the IV CNSM (Portuguese acronym for Brazilian Conference on Mental Health), the Mental Health bulletin states, "... the access to mental health care increased achieving 63% coverage" (7). The IV CNSM articles supporting the funding item highlighted the regulation of constitutional amendment no. 29; different funding modalities to services and co-management systems; overcoming of the procedural funding; regular resources to pharmaceutical care and quick and up-to-date communication and information mechanisms to support their findings.

The Pact for Health defined Mental Health as priority, allowing funding that took the per capita model into account for substitute services. This allowed not only regular health care procedures, but also community meetings, tours, cultural activities and activities apart from the general service. However, the funding question is far from the minimum predicted. In 2009, the expenditure on Mental Health in the health care budget was 2.38% (a little lower than in 2007 and 2008), and the percentage of the Expenditure on the Mental Health Program in relation to the Expenditure on Public Health Actions and Services was 2.57 (very far from the goal described in the management report of 2003-2006) (see Figure 4). Thus, mental disorders in Brazil are responsible for over 18% of the global overload of diseases in the country and rely on only 2.5% of the health budget (13).

The main discussion during the IV CNSM was the financial sustainability of mental health actions and services that created mechanisms guaranteeing mental health priority in the agreements at the three management levels of SUS. For example, in the 2008 management report of SAS, mental health is said to have had an agreement with 26 states, the main indications were coverage rate CAPs/100,000 inhabitants; and with 15 states, a complementary indication: Coverage rate of the "Back Home Program."

The challenge of ensuring that the resources from closing psychiatric hospital beds are invested in the mental health network still remains, as well as that of increasing the percentage invested and creating more effective mechanisms to monitor this process.

As far as mental health is concerned, there is also the funding of medication (essential and atypical) (14). Data from the 2010 Brazilian Ministry of Health (7) point to an increase in expenditures considered excessively high with payments for exceptional mental health medications (27.46% of total outpatient expenditure, expenses that are close to the federal funding to all CAPs network — a little over 33%). The current cost is disproportionate to the indication of usage in the high-cost medication program (patients with refractory schizophrenia diagnosis), which points to the need to re-evaluating the protocol and possibly broadening the indications and implanting clinical protocols of user control.

Column1	2002	2003	2004	2005	2006	2007	2008	2009	2010	2011
% Expenditure on the Mental Health Program into all expenditure on Public Health Actions and services	2,55	2,50	2,30	2,31	2,38	2,62	2,73	2,57	2,93	2,51

Figure 4. Percentage of the Expenditure on the Mental Health Program in relation to the Expenditure on Public Health Actions and Services (2).

In 2007, the Brazilian Ministry of Health spent 1 billion, 200 million on mental health (of which R$440 million were on hospital care and R$760 million on outpatient care (15). Of the outpatient expenditure, 33.19% are on CAPs; 38% on essential medication and 27.46% on exceptional medication. The mental health exceptional medication expenditure expresses two sides to this question: One is that the access to medication is essential to guarantee the constitutional right to health. The other is that it is now a reason for concern because of increase in expenditure (while the total expenditure on health increased by 9.6%, those on medication increased by 123.9% between 2002 and 2006) (16). The 2010 Budgetary Law of the Brazilian Government foresaw a decrease in resources in the Ministry of Health to acquire and distribute "exceptional" medications worth R$2,430,000,000.00 for a R$90,000,000.00 or a 3.47% decrease compared to the previous year budget. The 2010 Brazilian Board of Health Managers identifies the Ministry of Health's budget proposal for "exceptional" medications are insufficient.

Two guiding principles of psychotropic usage are: 1) medications rarely represent the whole response to patient's help need but represent a fragment of the response. The medications work as mediators to relieve the burden of some symptoms for the patient to allow patients to better relate with themselves, the people around them, and the health agents to whom the help requests were addressed. 2) The psychotropic medications neither reduce the symptom nor facilitate interpersonal relations in every case but should only be administered when it is effective to reducing discomfort — real or imaginary — and when it has beneficial results in relation to the risks inherent to treatment itself (17). On the other hand, anti-psychotic medications are also associated to different risks and several side effects. These effects can have an ever greater influence on the choice of the medication to long-term treatment compared to treatment during the acute phase (17).

CONCLUSION

Brazil's mental health financing could be summarized by Carvalho's sentence, "... the destination of funds shows the path of politics," (18). Considering the implementation of global health funding, social policy restrictions by each Brazilian state goes against the interests of SUS universal policy as it relates to public health funding. In other words, "Universal SUS goes against International Monetary Funds' (IMF) commands to cut costs and high primary surplus" (19). Current tax collection distribution is 60% to the Union, 24% to the states, and 16% to municipalities compared to 2007 health funding distribution that was 47% to the Union; 26% to states and 27% to municipalities. The difference between current health funding and 2007 funding excessively overtaxes municipalities and has exempted the federal government (constitutional amendment no. 29) through governmental actions that have eased the burden on the Union by more than 50% and overloaded the states by more than 20% and municipalities by more than 50% (18).

Specifically, outpatient mental health expenditures remain higher than inpatient care, partially resulting from medication expenditures that are not always prescribed adequately. This inversion of expenditures target the psychiatric reform movement and does not overcome the greatest obstacle to health and mental health policy today that being expenditures are lower than needs showing the underfunding of SUS. The underfinancing of health and mental health care demonstrates the centrality of economic policy to the detriment of social policy. This underfinancing disrespects the constitutional principle that health is a right to all and it is the Brazilian State's duty to provide access for every Brazilian citizen. This disrespect in shown by the coverage percentage of mental health policy: 72%. This uneven coverage in the Brazilian territory is more unfair to those living in the North and Northeastern Regions, which correspond to the poorest regions in Brazil.

The actions of the pharmaceutical industry are another aspect highlighted by the scenario of medicalization of "madness." These issues mean that Brazil continues have an inequity as it relates to universal health policy. There is much to do in the field of mental health. And this fight starts in the field of funding and passes through all the axes of health care policies.

All health care professionals, including social workers are affected by these policies. Social workers interact with those in greatest need for services at the intersection of the people and the organized social movements in the mental health field. Among these experiences are the social professionals and movements who fight for public health care for all.

This discussion shows that as mental health researcher and analyst "... my hope is immortal. I know we cannot change the beginning. But if we want, we can change the end" (21). Changing the end here will mean reinforcing the politics to defend the advances of a psychiatric reform (whose challenges increase every year) to ensure rights, increase resources to prevention, promotion, recovery and social reintegration in a fairer and less socially unequal country.

REFERENCES

[1] World Health Organization. Mental health atlas. Geneve: WHO, 2011.

[2] Brazil Ministry of Health. Saude Mental em dados 10. Brasilia, DF: Ministerio da Saude, 2012. URL: http://portal.saude.gov.br/portal/arquivos/pdf/mentaldados10.pdf.

[3] IBGE. Estatisticas da Saude: Assistencia Medico-Sanitaria 2009. Rio de Janeiro: IBGE, 2010. URL:http://www.ibge.gov.br/home/estatistica/populacao/condicaodevida/ams/2009/default.shtm.

[4] Brazilian Federal Board of Social. Assistente Social: um guia basico para conhecer um pouco mais sobre essa categoria profissional. URL: http://www.cfess.org.br/arquivos/deliberacao3comunica-material-midia-POSNACIONAL-final.pdf.

[5] Borges CF, Baptista TWF. O modelo assistencial em saude mental no Brasil: a trajetoria da construcao politica de 1990 a 2004. Caderno Saude Publica 2008; 24(2): 456-68.

[6] Bisneto JA. Servico Social e saude mental: uma analise institucional da pratica. Sao Paulo: Cortez, 2007.

[7] Brazil Ministry of Health. Saude Mental em dados 7. Brasilia, DF: Ministerio da Saude, 2010. URL: http://portal.saude.gov.br/portal/arquivos/pdf/smdados.pdf.

[8] World Health Organization. Mental health financing. Geneve: WHO, 2003.

[9] Brazil Ministry of Health. Saude Mental no SUS: As Novas Fronteiras da Reforma Psiquiatrica: Relatorio de gestao 2007-2010. Brasilia, 2011. URL: http://portal. saude.gov.br/ portal/ arquivos/ pdf/gestao2007_2010.pdf.

[10] Brazil Ministry of Health. Portaria GM/MS n. 204, de 29 de janeiro de 2007. Regulamenta o financiamento e a transferencia dos recursos federais para as acoes e os servicos de saude, na forma de blcos de financiamento, com o respectivo monitoramento e controle. Brasilia, DF: Ministerio da Saude, 2007. URL: http://dtr2001. saude.gov.br/sas/PORTARIAS/Port2007/GM/GM-204.htm.

[11] Santos L, Andrade LOM, editor. SUS: o espaco da gestao inovada e dos consensos interfederativos. Sao Paulo: Prisma Printer, 2007.

[12] Kilsztajn S, Lopes ES, Lima LZ, Rocha PAF, Carmo MSN. Leitos hospitalares e reforma psiqui?trica no Brasil. Cad. Saude Publica 2008; 24(10). URL: http://www.scielosp.org/scielo.php?script=sci_arttext&pid=S0102311X2008001000016&lng=en&nrm=iso.

[13] Mari JJ. Nao ha Saude sem Saude Mental. Psiquiatria Hoje J Assoc Brasileira Psiquiatria 2008; 5: 4-5.

[14] Aguiar MTA. Evolucao dos gastos federais com antipsicoticos atipicos no SUS: de 1999 a 2005. [Dissertation]. Sao Paulo: Universidade Catolica de Santos, 2008.

[15] Brazil Ministry of Health. Departamento de Informatica do SUS. 2008. Gastos em saude mental Brasilia, DF: Author, 2008. URL: http://w3.datasus.gov.br/datasus /datasus.php.

[16] Vieira FS. Gasto do Ministerio da Saude com medicamentos: tendencia dos programas de 2002 a 2007. Rev. Saude Publica 2009; 43(4). URL: http://www.scielo.br/ scielo.php?script=sci_arttext&pid=S0034-8910200900040 0014&lng=pt&nrm=iso.

[17] Falkai P, Wobrock T, Lieberman J, Glenthoj B, Gattaz WF, Möller HJ, et al. Diretrizes da Federacao Mundial das sociedades de psiquiatria biologica para o tratamento biologico da esquizofrenia: Parte 2: tratamento de longo prazo. Revista de Psiquiatria Clinica 2006; 33(2): 65-70.

[18] Carvalho G. O financiamento da reforma psiquiatrica no pos constitucional: avancos e entraves. 2010. Brazilian. URL: http://www.google.com.br/url?sa=t&rct=j&q=&esrc=s&frm=1& source=web&cd=2&ved=0CDEQFjAB&url=http%3A%2F%2Fwww.idisa.org.br%2Fimg%2FFile%2FGC_SAUDEMENTALeFINANCIAMENTO.ppt&ei=opeDUfCyLOfC0QGK4IGoBw&usg=AFQjCNHpKJSwir59LbCivwEoDYvJzGpdmg.

[19] Marques R M, Mendes A. Os dilemas do financiamento do SUS no interior daseguridade social. Economia e Sociedade 2005; 14(1): 159-75.

[20] Tenorio, F. A reforma psiquiatrica brasileira da decada de 1980 aos dias atuais: historias e conceitos. Historia Ciencia Saude-Manguinhos 2002; 9(1): 25-59.

[21] Lucinda E. Poema da Ética, 2012. URL: http://www.gustavussilverius.blogspot.com/2012/03/poema-da-etica-poem-of-ethics.html.

In: Public Health Yearbook 2016
Editor: Joav Merrick
ISBN: 978-1-53610-947-4

Chapter 14

NUESTRA CASA: AN ADVOCACY INITIATIVE TO REDUCE INEQUALITIES AND TUBERCULOSIS ALONG THE US-MEXICO BORDER

Eva M Moya[1,*], PhD, LMSW, Silvia M. Chávez-Baray[1], PhD, William W. Wood[2], PhD and Omar Martinez[3], JD, MPH, MS

[1]The University of Texas at El Paso College of Health Sciences Department of Social Work, El Paso, Texas, US

[2]University of Wisconsin-Milwaukee Department of Anthropology, Milwaukee, Wisconsin, US

[3]School of Social Work, College of Public Health, Temple University, Philadelphia, Pennsylvania, US

ABSTRACT

The US-Mexico border provides a rich learning environment for professional social workers and at the same time poses some challenges. This article explores some of the unique demographics and social and cultural characteristics in the border region. These characteristics have implications for social work teaching, research, policy and practice. The study of borders includes exploring social disparities and inequalities. Health risks and diseases travel fluidly between borders and kill indiscriminately. The US-Mexico border is at high-risk of elevated tuberculosis (TB) and HIV incidence due to socio-economic stress, rapid and dynamic population growth, mobility and migration, and the hybridization of cultures. Every minute, four people die from TB, and 15 more become infected worldwide. The number of deaths due to tuberculosis is unacceptable given that most cases of TB are preventable. Cross-border cooperation and collaboration among social workers, health professionals and public officials between communities and countries can reduce social injustices to move towards a healthier borderland, as demonstrated in the collaborative prevention of TB. Rather than limiting our work to

* Corresponding author: Eva M Moya, PhD, LMSW, Associate Dean College of Health Sciences and Assistant Professor, The University of Texas at El Paso College of Health Sciences Department of Social Work, 500 W University Ave, El Paso, Texas 79968, United States. E-mail: emmoya@utep.edu.

define social inequalities, we seek to further the conversation and suggest social action to address TB. This article contributes ideas and examples of experiences to encourage innovative, community-academic engaged inter- and multidisciplinary interventions like the Nuestra Casa (Our House) initiative. Nuestra Casa is an advocacy, communication and social mobilization strategy to address TB and HIV health disparities and inequalities in underserved communities, which we argue provides a useful model for combating TB and other inequalities plaguing the US-Mexico borderland.

Keywords: tuberculosis, health disparities, social work, U.S.-Mexico border

Introduction

The study of borders includes the study of social disparities. Borders create unique challenges and opportunities for social workers and public health professionals to address social inequalities and health disparities between groups. At borders, health risks and diseases travel and kill at will. These differences can affect how frequently a disease affects a group, how many people get sick, or how often the disease causes death. Healthy People 2020 defines a health disparity as "a particular type of health difference that is closely linked with social, economic, and/or environmental disadvantage. Health disparities adversely affect groups of people who have systematically experienced greater obstacles to health based on their racial or ethnic group; religion; socioeconomic status; gender; age; mental health; cognitive, sensory and physical disability; sexual orientation; gender identity; geographic location; or other characteristics historically linked to discrimination or exclusion" (1). From a health equity standpoint, we have the ability and responsibility to advocate for and provide culturally and linguistically appropriate services, and to promote policies that improve community health (2).

The US-Mexico border region is a distinct geographic, economic, cultural and social area that is affected by systematic social and economic injustice. This is evidenced by social and economic problems that are apparent throughout the region, including poverty, health disparities, social inequities, and low-wage assembly, service, seasonal, and agricultural employment. Endemic poverty co-exists with institutional racism, gender violence and structural violence (systematic oppressions). The area, while populated by resilient families and communities that have confronted governmental neglect and social isolation, is at the periphery of the American and Mexican economies (3).

The border spans almost 2,000 miles from the Pacific Ocean to the Gulf of Mexico and includes four US states, six Mexican states, 44 U.S. counties, and 80 Mexican municipalities. The border region, defined as the area within 62.5 miles of either side of the boundary, is home to approximately 13 million individuals and to 26 US federally recognized Native American tribes (4). Each country has a distinct system of policies and health care practices, each with a disproportionate share of health, environmental risks, and diseases. It is unlikely that any other binational border has such variability in health status, services, and utilization. Lower socioeconomic and educational levels, migration, immigration, and rapid industrial development accompanied by population growth from the implementation of the North American Free Trade Agreement in 1994 helps to explain some of the present complexity in this particular borderland (5). The policies, norms, and regulations of one side of the border are not applicable to the other. On the border, the developed and developing regions merge and mix to combine some of the best and worst of both worlds.

In some places, only a sign or a fence marks the border. In other places, the border is reinforced with barbed wire or tall steel fences (6). Although each nation operates under distinct legal and political systems as well as different health care and public health systems, the U.S.-Mexico border region is mutually dependent, sharing environmental, social, economic, cultural, and epidemiologic characteristics. Extensive family and cultural ties are shared by many of the people in the borderland. Health inequalities along the border especially affect indigenous and immigrant populations, who are vulnerable as a result of low socio-economic status, lack of health insurance, linguistic and cultural barriers, and limited access to healthcare and social services (5, 7). If the U.S.-Mexico border region were considered a state, the region would be comprised of the following characteristics: 1) rank last in access to health care; 2) second in death rates due to hepatitis; 3) third in deaths related to diabetes; 4) last in per capita income; 5) first in the number of school children living in poverty; and 6) first in the number of school children who are uninsured (8).

A SEMI-PERMEABLE MEMBRANE

The U.S.-Mexico border offers a stark context in cultural differences, social inequalities, and ever-present reminders of governmental power that limit individual opportunity by ascribing national identity. Although governed by different bodies, U.S. and Mexican border populations are highly connected through an integrated social and economic system. People on both sides of the border share similar cultures and are exposed to comparable environments. Population density and poverty in urban and rural areas near the border are high, and unincorporated communities—known as 'colonias'—often have inadequate housing, roads, sewage systems, drainage, and lack a potable water supply. Transborder trade; maquiladora (twin plants) industry; migration, mobility and energy trade; drug, arms and human trafficking; smuggling and other modalities of transnational organized crime are core economic activities in the border region (9).

The US-Mexico border is open to the movement of risk and disease but closed to the free movement of people, services, and cures. Since the US-Mexico border separates rich and poor countries with different types of healthcare systems, inequalities in access to health care are created and reinforced for those living between these two nations. The distribution of communicable diseases like TB is associated with other social disparities (e.g., wealthy versus poor, majority versus minority) in both access to medical care and treatment. In addition, considerable research in public health on the US-Mexico border has increased focus on individual behavior and social determinants (1, 5, 7).

The border region also attracts migrants from other areas of Mexico, Central and South America, Europe and Asia who seek opportunities and safety (8) and, in many cases, migration to the United States. These goals are not always achieved once they arrive to the region, thus creating populations that are displaced and vulnerable. According to the U.S. Customs and Border Protection, 57,525 unaccompanied children were apprehended at the southwest border between October 1, 2013 and June 30, 2014. More than three-quarters of unaccompanied minors come from mostly poor and violent cities in El Salvador, Guatemala and Honduras. Children from Mexico, once the largest group, now make up less than a quarter of the total - a small number from the 43 other countries (10). It is important to note that some right wing groups and conservative elected officials (federal and state government) have defended increased enforcement of deportation measures by pointing to fears of disease epidemics, including tuberculosis. However, tuberculosis does not appear to be a serious concern at the moment for this group. For instance, Carrie Williams, a spokeswoman for the Texas Department of State Health Services, said there have been only three cases of tuberculosis reported among the undocumented children who have come into Texas. This is not the case among adult immigrants, where recently 89 new cases of TB were reported. For every case of active TB, there are between 10-15 more individuals infected (11).

The large-scale movement of people, closeness of social interactions, large volume of trade, limitations of public health infrastructure, and environmental conditions are all factors that facilitate the transmission of infectious diseases among residents of the US-Mexico border region (12). Also intriguing are the so-called 'Hispanic or Latino health paradox' and the 'immigrant advantage,' referring to the contradictory finding that indicates that Latinos and immigrants in the U.S. tend to have significantly better health and mortality outcomes than the average population despite generally low socioeconomic status (13, 14). Findings from the Tomas Rivera Policy Institute (15) suggest that the Latino health paradox exists for mental health issues, asthma, maternal-child health, and high blood pressure. Results from this study indicate that Hispanic immigrants are healthier in terms of these four health outcomes when they first arrive in the United States; however, they become less healthy with greater amounts of acculturation.

El Paso, Texas - Ciudad Juarez Border Metropolis

El Paso County is intersected by the Franklin Mountain Range and encompasses a portion of the Chihuahuan Desert as well as several communities such as the City of El Paso. Combined, the population of El Paso County and its neighboring Ciudad Juarez in the state of Chihuahua, Mexico is approximately two million. El Paso is the fourth largest city in Texas, with a population of 800,647 (16). Over 80 percent of El Paso residents are Hispanic of Mexican-origin, with three quarters of the population speaking a language other than English at home. The median annual household income is $36,078. In El Paso, the unemployment rate in 2014 was 8.0 percent (17). The El Paso region experiences higher rates of unemployment, underemployment, and lower average wages than the rest of Texas. Texas, as a state, has the largest population of people who are uninsured, accounting for 28 percent of Texas's population or 6.1 million people (18). El Paso's uninsured rate is the highest in the state, with 30 percent being uninsured (19).

Ciudad Juarez is the largest city in the State of Chihuahua, Mexico, and the second most populated Mexican city on the US–Mexico border, after Tijuana in Baja California. Ciudad Juarez's population for 2010 was 1,332,131, and its metropolitan area is the eighth largest in Mexico. Approximately forty percent of the state of Chihuahua's population lives in Ciudad Juarez. More than 40 percent of the Juarez population lived in poverty in 2010 (20). Juarez borders with El Paso County in Texas, as well as Dona Ana County in New Mexico. In recent years, the national and international media have broadcast to the world examples of how violence, death, and organized crime have escalated in the border region and in particular in Juarez, naming the city as the most dangerous city in Mexico and among the most dangerous in the world (12).

The majority of people on either side of the border are permanent residents; some are 'borderlanders' (natives of the region that travel, live and work in both countries), others are bi-national, while others cross the border daily for work, school, business and to visit family members. Other individuals rarely cross the border, some have never crossed, and others are scared to cross. The public health consequences of these macro forces have been analyzed to some extent in conflict and transitional settings, but have not been considered in the context of Mexico's violent struggle against drug cartels and organized crime (21). While there is a great need for service provision, care is not provided to those that need it the most. Some of the reasons for this have to do with people's immigration status, border security and the enforcement of border laws, lack of linguistically appropriate services, and cultural understandings and misunderstandings (22).

THE CASE OF TUBERCULOSIS

In the United States, tuberculosis, HIV, viral hepatitis, and sexually transmitted infections (STI) are the most prevalent and most commonly reported infectious conditions. TB is described as a disease process resulting from the infection Mycobacterium tuberculosis. It is also understood as a social illness that causes great suffering, a disease of the "at-risk populations" and a sign of poverty and inequalities. TB is a medical and social condition that involves deep emotional experiences, narratives of illness, alienation from family members, isolation and stigmatization (23). TB remains a major global, social, and public health problem (24). Every minute, four people die from TB and 15 more become infected worldwide (25). In 2012, an estimated 8.6 million people developed TB and 1.3 million died from the disease, including 320,000 deaths among HIV-positive people (24). The number of deaths due to TB is unacceptable, especially given that most cases are preventable. While a myriad of communicable diseases exist in the U.S.-Mexico border region, TB, HIV and their co-morbidity are of upmost concern. TB and HIV account for substantial morbidity and mortality, with great social and financial costs to individuals, families, and societies. The US-Mexico border experiences a disproportionate burden of these conditions as compared to the rest of the countries and compared to other Western industrialized nations, with significant disparities observed across sub-groups and geographical regions (26).

There is recognition of the direct correlation between TB incidence and the prevalence of poverty (27). Although diseases like TB and HIV cross class lines and geographical locations, its highest toll has always been among immigrants, the foreign born, and the working class poor and their families. The patterns of diseases found in Hispanics, African Americans, Non-Hispanic Whites, Native Americans, Mexicans and foreign-born individuals along the border create unique challenges for social work and public health responses.

Poverty, increased violence, and family reunification are complex forces that move more poor people into the United States (from Mexico or any other underdeveloped countries like Honduras, El Salvador, Nicaragua, and Guatemala), and an increase in health risks and TB incidence is inevitable. The US-Mexico border is at high risk of elevated TB incidence and other health issues due to socioeconomic stress, rapid and dynamic population growth, mobility and migration, "cultural hybridization" and a young population (28). TB is a subtle and complex chronic infectious disease. The extent of the disease is likely to be underreported because of mobility and migration across the border as well as the long latency of the condition after infection occurs. The incidence of TB at the border far exceeds national incidence rates in both countries (see Figure 1).

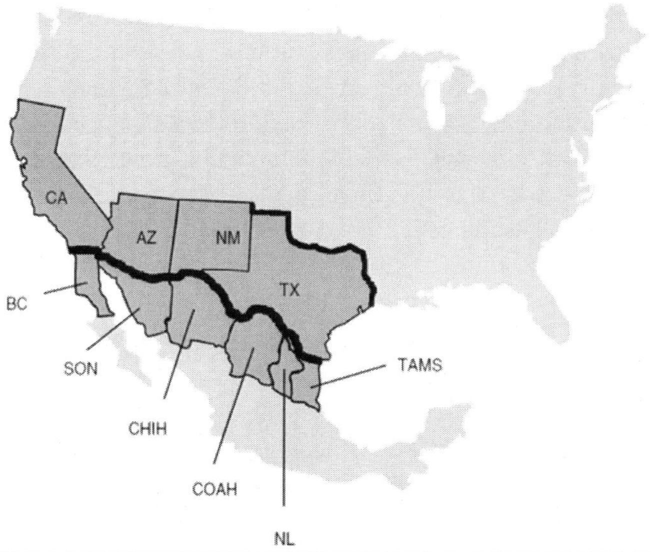

	2012 TB Cases	2012 TB Rate
Arizona (AZ)	211	3.2
California (CA)	2,191	5.8
New Mexico (NM)	40	2.4
Texas (TX)	1,233	4.7
U.S. Border States	3,675	6.1
U.S. Total	9,945	3.2
Baja California (BC)	1,853	54.8
Chihuahua (CHIH)	692	19.0
Coahuila (COAH)	614	21.2
Nuevo Leon (NL)	1,237	25.0
Sonora (SON)	855	30.0
Tamaulipas (TAMS)	1,109	32.0
Mexican border states	6,360	30.1
Mexican National	19,738	16.7

Figure 1.

[a] Border area is defined as the area extending 100 kilometers (62 miles) north-south of the U.S.-Mexico border. [b] Sources: Centers for Disease Control and Prevention. Reported Tuberculosis in the United States, 2013. U.S. Department of Health and Human Services, 2013. Preliminar 2013/Secretaria de Salud/Dirección General de Epidemiologia/Sistema Nacional de Vigilancia Epidemiológica. March 28, 2014.

There is little discussion among health policymakers, researchers, social workers, and health practitioners about how to address tuberculosis and migration as well as its connection to poverty and other social inequalities (29). As shown in Figure 1, in 2012, TB rates on each side of the border were two times their respective national averages, according to published (30) and unpublished sources (31).

Ongoing transmission, prolonged infection, delayed diagnosis, increased mobility, increased drug-resistance, limited access to health care, TB related stigma, increased mobility and migration make case management and completion of treatment difficult along the U.S.-Mexico border (5, 24, 32). TB presents unique characteristics that have their origin in the fact that society is divided into socioeconomic status-based groups or classes, and it is from these divisions that the resistance to the infection emerges. Mechanisms to reach out to educate and treat vulnerable populations for TB in both countries, including those that enter the US legally, need to be addressed and implemented.

In Mexico, every day there are 54 new TB cases, and every 6 hours a person dies from TB (31). TB continues to affect communities and individuals that are most vulnerable (e.g., the poor, underserved, malnourished, HIV positive, diabetic). Mexico's national TB rate for 2013 was 13.6 per 100,000 (31); this is over four times the rate in the United States of 3.2 per 100,000. Mexico's National TB prevalence rate for 2013 was 25.4 per 100,000; eight times higher than the United States rate of 3.2 per 100,000 (30).

Each of the six Mexican states that share a border with United States has higher TB rates compared to the national rate. Combined, they represent 29% of the total cases for Mexico in 2013, with the border municipalities of the states of Baja California, Nuevo Leon, and Tamaulipas having the largest concentration of TB cases (31). According to the Centers for Disease Control and Prevention (CDC), in the US in 2012, a total of 9,945 new TB cases were reported and the TB rate declined by 4.2% from 2006 to 3.2 cases per 100,000 (33). The national TB incidence rate in 2012 was the lowest since national reporting began in 1953. Despite this improvement, foreign-born persons and racial and ethnic minorities continue to bear a disproportionate burden of the disease in the US. TB rates among Mexican-origin individuals and other Hispanics, African Americans, Native Hawaiians and Other Pacific Islanders, and Asians were 5.3, 5.8, 12.3 and 18.9 times higher than among Non-Hispanic Whites respectively in 2012 (30).

We live in a society where risk and vulnerability have been globalized. At the same time and in seeming contradiction, the discourses of 'nation' (and assertions of 'national identity') are becoming more important in terms of globalization as an articulating device (34), which serves to distinguish 'insiders' from 'outsiders'. This helps to create risk categories (e.g., foreign-born, Mexican-origin) to justify enhanced surveillance while also serving to separate those who can manage the risk from those whose risk requires management under supervision (35). Risk management consequently represents a localized response to the globalized problems of TB, HIV and poverty. The risk of TB then becomes associated with particular social categories defined in terms of national identity, such as foreign-born, rather than the structural inequalities and processes that place people at risk. For example, TB is associated with poor quality and overcrowded housing, and minority ethnic groups are more likely to experience housing inequalities as well as reside in areas that experience disadvantage (36).

TB often coexists with other comorbidities like diabetes mellitus, substance abuse, and HIV that, if not treated, can produce fatal consequences. People who are HIV positive and infected with TB are 20 to 40 times more likely to develop active TB than people not infected with HIV in the same country (24). The focus on TB and HIV in the US-Mexico border is timely, given the evidence of increasing burdens and worsening health disparities for these conditions, the evolution in the understanding of the social and structural influences of disease epidemiology, and the implications of the global economic downturn. The global trends and impacts on health of TB, HIV and STIs remain among the most urgent public health challenges of our time (24). In a world characterized by globalization, policies concerning health security, communicable diseases, and healthcare are increasingly important. The advent of TB drug-resistance and the complexities of border population dynamics may cause a considerable threat to the population on either side (28). Health policies and health promotion actions tend to be unilateral in nature. Social workers, healthcare workers, and other professionals can help adapt and unify policies, actions, and interventions to address complex health disparities (37). We present a case study that describes the Nuestra Casa (Our House) Exhibit, an advocacy, communication and social mobilization strategy to increase the awareness of and social action for TB through public art as a medium for education and social engagement. This article describes the genesis and the evolution of this initiative.

NUESTRA CASA

Phase 1: Cross-border cooperation and innovation in TB awareness

The Nuestra Casa exhibition was several years in development and grew from a unique partnership between Project Concern International (PCI), the US Agency for International Development (USAID), the Alliance of Border Collaborative (ABC), Dr. Eva Moya (author and bi-national social worker) and Damien Schumman (South African-based photographer and artist). In 2008, Moya met Schumann at the 2008 International AIDS Conference in Mexico City, where the two developed the idea of working together to bring greater public awareness to the social and public health issues of TB and HIV. Schumann had gained notoriety in South Africa for the creation of "TB/HIV Shack" installations focused on public health and social justice issues. One of Schumann's Shack installations was on view in Mexico City, and there the two launched the idea of transforming the "The TB/HIV Shack" into the "Nuestra Casa" Initiative, focused on the issue of TB and HIV in the border region. In 2009, USAID awarded $20,000 to PCI to hire Schumann for the project and that same year the Nuestra Casa mobile exhibition began its tour in El Paso, Texas. The original house (see Photograph 1) was built by the artist with help from persons affected by TB in the El Paso and Ciudad Juarez border region.

The Nuestra Casa exhibition was an interactive experience where individuals entered a living space—a literal "mobile home for TB" (38). It was conceived as a movable house built out of discarded particleboard, wood, and other scrap materials easily found in Mexican communities and colonias. Nuestra Casa included a living room, kitchen, bathroom, a hallway or Corridor of Hope (Camino de la Esperanza), and a small patio at the main entrance. Photographs developed as part of the Border Voices and Images of TB Project that Professor Moya directed in 2008-2009 were included along with some of Schumann's photographic work.

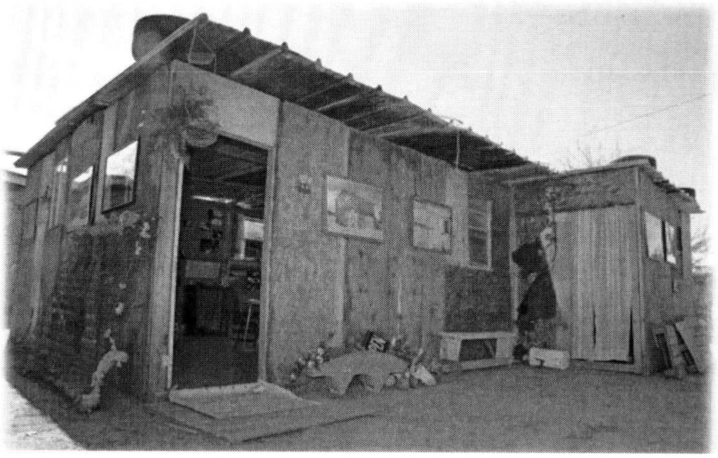

Source: Nuestra Casa Exhibit (2009). Courtesy of Damien Schumann.

Photograph 1. Nuestra Casa Exhibition.

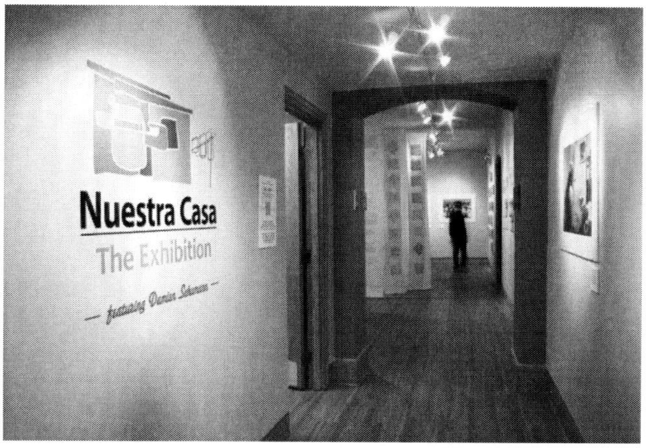

Photograph 2. Nuestra Casa returns to UTEP as an Initiative (2012). Courtesy of the University of Texas at El Paso Centennial Museum.

The creation of "trapitos" (small pieces of cloth that were made available for visitors to write their thoughts about TB, the lives of people living with and dying from TB, and their reactions to the exhibit) were central to the experience of visitors since the first exhibition in 2009. As Nuestra Casa presents the life stories of persons affected by TB and other health disparities, it is a lens into the socioeconomic and environmental realities that help to create health disparities but also the stories of resilience, empowerment, and hope of those living with (and dying from) TB.

As visitors went through the house, they were immersed in hundreds of photographs and stories showing the reality of TB. Visitors frequently asked questions, received health information and interacted with people affected by TB and HIV, social workers, students, health care workers, advocates and decision makers. After being on display on an outdoor pedestrian friendly patio on the university campus, the house tour was moved to Mexico in partnership with the National TB Program and the support of the State TB Programs in Quintana Roo, Oaxaca, Tamaulipas, and Tijuana, before ending at the CDC Museum in

Atlanta, Georgia in 2010. More than 1,500 trapitos were collected during the exhibit's tour in 2009 to 2010 and included comments such as the following:

> "I am now rethinking my career path so that I can do research to contribute to the efforts to combat TB. Also, I want to go abroad so that I can actively help out" - Atlanta, Georgia
>
> "It is so real that my lungs hurt" - Cancun, Mexico

While on tour in 2010, Nuestra Casa became an international phenomenon at the 40th UNION Conference on Lung Health and Tuberculosis in Cancun, Mexico. At the end of its 2010 tour and with cooperation from the CDC, Nuestra Casa opened the National TB Conference in Atlanta and remained on exhibit at the CDC Museum for four months. Nuestra Casa became an advocacy, communication and social mobilization model in Mexico and inspired local, state, national, and international TB programs to integrate perspectives of persons affected by TB (and comorbidities) in advocacy efforts.

Phase 2: Returning Nuestra Casa to the university: The initiative

Shortly after the tour ended at the CDC, coauthors Moya and Wood (then Director of UTEP's Centennial Museum) met to talk about how the exhibition's tour might be used as a catalyst to reengage the El Paso, Texas and Ciudad Juarez, Mexico communities to use advocacy, communication, and social mobilization (ACMS) efforts in TB prevention. They invited Schumann back to the university to reassemble the Nuestra Casa in a gallery of the Centennial Museum and to highlight the 1,500 trapitos. Having visitors to this second phase engage with the heartfelt messages on many of the trapitos was, they felt, a must.

In the fall of 2011, Moya brought together the project team for what would soon come to be called the Nuestra Casa Initiative (NCI) that included Wood; coauthor Dr. Silvia Chávez-Baray (Dept. of Social Work), Dr. Guillermina Nuñez (Anthropology), Dr. Arvind Singhal (Communications Department and Social Justice Initiative), Dr. Lucia Durá (Rhetoric Department), Azuri Gonzalez (Center for Civic Engagement), and Raquel Orduño (social work student and TB Advocate).

The NCI became an ACMS strategy to increase TB awareness, detection, and cure rates; improve collaboration among TB, HIV, and Diabetes Mellitus Programs to reduce risk of infection and increase information and co-morbidity detection; promote a person-centered approach in health services and in the community; mitigate the impacts of stigma and discrimination; honor community resilience and the narratives of affected persons; and promote social action.

Through a series of workshops led by university faculty, service learning students worked mostly in pairs with the trapitos from the locations the traveling exhibition had visited, coding the data, finding major themes, and identifying trapitos that most poignantly expressed a significant theme to be highlighted through a tendedero (clothsline) of trapitos in the installation at the Museum. In the final workshop, faculty took the students through a series of exercises where they shared their experiences with the NCI. As they shared with their classmates their "favorite trapitos," several of them were moved to tears as they explained just how profound the experience had been. The coding of the trapitos is posted online.

As faculty worked with students to code the trapitos and prepare them for installation, the Museum director worked with the artist, Museum staff and student interns to launch a web site and Facebook page, and to redesign the installation to include an art installation style display of Schumann's photo-narratives, web linked gallery content highlighting the 2009-10 tour, a computer kiosk to access online content (for those without handheld devises), a hands-on style trapito making station, and (of course) the tendederos of trapitos reconceptualized by Schumann as a forest that visitors would need to walk through as they approached Nuestra Casa.

In 2012, the project team launched the NCI at the UTEP Museum with the opening of a yearlong series of health and social programming developed by community advocates, faculty and students (see Photograph 2. The Museum's involvement in the NCI was conceived in terms of emerging ideas about how to make museums more "participatory" (39, 40) and "person-centered" in their educational goals and strategy while the wider initiative sought to advocate, engage, and mobilize communities of scholars, researchers, advocates, professionals, students, and persons affected by TB to work for a world free of TB and HIV. Multiple modalities of education and health promotion were utilized, including visual media, presentations, lectures, social work student-guided interactions, candlelight vigils and communications technology and social media.

The exhibition marked the first time in the Museum's history that an exhibit of this nature involving students, faculty, community advocates and staff had been developed and it proved to be a richly rewarding experience for all those involved. Over the course of 2012, nearly 25,000 people visited the Museum and attended supporting programming.

The NCI was especially successful in engaging social work students and persons affected by tuberculosis as they participated in the initiative. Five graduate social work students became museum docents for the exhibit and regularly provided guided tours for visitors from Ciudad Juarez and El Paso. Twenty students volunteered as part of service learning projects. A Digital Media student produced two YouTube documentaries on TB and the Nuestra Casa exhibit (they can be also found on the It is: https://www.facebook.com/NuestraCasaInitiative2011/), while others have conducted outreach as volunteers for the 2011-2012 Dia de los Niños-Dia de los Libros (Children's Day/Book Day), Binational Health Week, and community-wide events or through presentations in Ciudad Juarez and El Paso on TB and lung health. An NCI project dissemination guide (used by exhibit hosts to assist with assembly and dissemination), T-shirts and wristbands (For a world free of TB and HIV) were produced and disseminated.

In addition, Raquel Orduño, a person affected by TB, MSW graduate, activist and member of NCI, spoke about her experience in local, state, national and international forums. Her testimony reached hundreds of policy makers, advocates, and clinicians in the United States and Mexico, as well as officials during the 2013 World TB Day WHO Stop TB Partnership panel in Washington DC.

THE LEGACY AND CONTINUING IMPACTS OF THE NCI

The cross-border cooperation and innovation of the NCI was successful in terms of presentations, recognition, and publications. Nuestra Casa displayed at six principle venues:

1) the 40th and 42th International UNION Conferences on Lung Health and TB in Cancun, Mexico and Berlin, Germany respectively); 2) the 2010 National TB Conference (Atlanta, Georgia); 3) the 2011 National TB Conference in Mexico; 4) the 2012 International Social Work Conference in Stockholm; 5) the 2013 International Mental Health and Social Work Conference in Los Angeles; and 6) establishment of 20 academic, community and binational partnerships in the US-Mexico border supporting the 12-month display at the university.

Additionally, the exhibit was granted one of eight recognitions at the 2012 North American UNION Region Meeting and received notoriety at the 2011 Society for Applied Anthropology and the Western Social Science Association conferences. The exhibit was so successful that the Mexican Consulate in El Paso celebrated World TB Day 2012 by having the NCI team install several of Schumann's photo-narratives and trapitos, with an estimated viewership of 3,000. The 2012 World TB Day events were also launched at the university. At the event, the Pan American Health Organization released the 2012 TB and HIV/AIDS Comorbidity report for health care workers, which included an ACSM component highlighting the NCI. In 2013, NCI received the McGrath Community-University Engagement Regional award for innovation in interdisciplinary education and service.

Finally, this initiative has led to the publication of a book entitled *Social Justice in the US-Mexico Border* (Springer, 2012), authored by Moya in partnership with other scholars from the university. This publication features a chapter on TB and HIV, ACSM addressing challenges and opportunities for improving bi-national collaboration which include strategies like Nuestra Casa and the Border Voices and Images of TB (TB Photovoice Project). In 2013, the peer-reviewed article on the NCI was published in the journal *Reflections*, dedicated to scholarship on innovation in service learning. In 2014, the initiative was presented at the International Union Against Tuberculosis and Lung Disease Conference in Barcelona, Spain.

NCI fostered multi and interdisciplinary collaboration and capitalized upon the strengths of diverse professions and advocates to augment consciousness of tuberculosis. Faculty members used liberating structures and problem-based learning methods to work with students across disciplines. The participation of community members has also been critical to its success, as has re-conceptualizing museum gallery space as a public forum. The narratives of individuals affected by TB provide the human perspective necessary to contextualize the situation: namely, that all humans are vulnerable to the disease, and it is therefore imperative that policy be attentive to the challenges and needs of those affected.

The lessons learned that can be used to promote and strengthen macro social work practice and social mobilization efforts are as follows: 1) ACMS strategies are needed to effectively raise awareness, mobilize community members, leaders, and social workers; and to empower and engage persons affected by TB; to successfully prevent and care for those suffering from the diseases and its repercussions. 2) A person-centered approach to service delivery is required to improve detection, treatment, adherence, and cure, and to mitigate all forms of stigma related to TB. 3) NCI is a powerful ACMS intervention to increase social and political will to improve TB and HIV prevention and care and to mitigate stigma. 4) Macro social work interventions, community participation, as well as involvement of TB affected persons increased and is now fundamental for successful social mobilization. 5) Community-academic engagement partnerships and collaborative action in the United States and Mexico are essential.

The NCI also led to a formal "call to action" for increasing the visibility of persons affected by TB, their stories, lives, worries, concerns, vulnerabilities, and aspirations; promoting inclusion, parity, and the participation of persons affected by TB across all levels; and sustaining permanent lines of funding through efficient distribution mechanisms. The next steps of the NCI include: seeking to share our innovative findings with other communities, venues, and locations beyond the US-Mexico Border; launching ACMS strategies to increase collaboration and cooperation across the two countries; capitalizing on the use of viral technology to share the lessons learned and innovation online; and identifying publication and dissemination venues that value and may help us incorporate the visual elements of this initiative beyond the social work, health and education fields.

IMPLICATIONS FOR SOCIAL WORK

Implementing social determinant actions in health involves holistic understanding and interventions, identifying synergisms and antagonisms, and employing cost-effective strategies to achieve sustainable population coverage and scale (41).

The primary goal for local TB programs is to medically treat and eliminate TB in the jurisdiction that is being served. Social workers negotiate between multiple services and benefits within and across systems (42). Studies indicate that the rate of adherence to TB care continues to be low -approximately two thirds of all persons living with active TB and in treatment complete their medication regimen (24). TB interventions emphasize patient adherence with directly observed therapy (DOTS). Low adherence, stigma, TB comorbidities (i.e., HIV, diabetes, malnutrition, and substance abuse) significantly contribute to relapse rates, and may result in multidrug resistant TB. Social work, public health and medical literature point to factors associated with successful TB care: 1) medication regimen; 2) features of the health care system; and 3) features to the relationship between the person affected by TB, caregiver, and the health care provider (43, 44).

Based on the lessons learned and the evidence cited, social workers: 1) identify social and medical services and help find housing for homeless individuals affected by health disparities (like TB); 2) counsel individuals and families to deal with the emotional and financial ramifications of their diagnosis; 3) advocate for policies, programs and services grounded on person-centered care; 4) convene and participate in multi and interdisciplinary teams that work in collaboration to improve access to care and increase adherence to treatment; 5) engage in activities that involve navigation of services; and 6) identify resources for the client population.

Addressing the high rate of poverty, poor health indicators, and overall living conditions in the US-Mexico border and other low income communities requires social workers who possess the leadership skills and have the in-depth linguistic and cultural knowledge to overcome the barriers to the receipt of services people need. Social work programs residing in the U.S.-Mexico border have the exceptional challenges of preparing graduates and practitioners in the border region, and must thus distinguish their education offerings from programs in other areas of the world.

CONCLUSION

The border region does not fare well in terms of socioeconomic measures. The socioeconomic disadvantages are particularly marked among Hispanic border populations. Combined, the demographic and social determinants present a number of challenges to improving health at the border. Our experience with the NCI shows that "person-centered education model" about TB for the persons affected by TB, the family members and their social support network, health and human service professionals and the wider community is essential (45). The traditional medical model continues to emphasize adherence by individual persons, absent of a person-centered model, which fails to acknowledge or address social and structural determinants of health (46). Social workers offer an ecological perspective on person-centered care, incorporating cultural factors in a biopsychosocial assessment of the individual. Failing to adopt a holistic perspective that incorporates cultural factors, and focusing primarily on medical adherence, may lead to the perception that lack of adherence is due primarily to individual characteristics. Addressing health disparities requires structural interventions. Interventions must address TB screenings and treatment of persons infected while also preventing persons at risk from acquiring the disease. The social work profession stands in a position to provide a holistic framework.

Evidence from the international community demonstrates that political commitment to implementing health policies and structural interventions combined with existing knowledge, observational evidence, and evidence based innovative practices, may yield health improvements (47). By focusing attention on capacity building, leadership and governance, strategic partnerships, and effective health communication, person-centered approaches can help generate awareness, stimulate new dialogue and disseminate promising practices. Policy and systems change is essential for reducing health inequalities like TB and HIV, and creating communities of opportunity that support health equity. Local partnerships and cross sector collaborations is a key part of ensuring that every individual has access to high quality education, housing, transportation, jobs, safe places and health care (48). Finally, we hope that this article contributes to promoting an expanding field of research and social action which is highly needed in order to develop advocacy, communication and social mobilization strategies to understand the mix of social determinants of TB infection and care, the perspectives of persons affected by TB, and promising intervention strategies.

ACKNOWLEDGMENTS

Special thanks to the participants of this intervention and the organizations that contributed to the development, funding and the dissemination of the Nuestra Casa Initiative. We also want to thank Ethan C. Levine for proof-reading the article and Dr. Kathleen Curtis, Dean of the College of Health Sciences, the University of Texas at El Paso for her support.

References

[1] US Department of Health and Human Services. Health disparities. Healthy People 2020.Washington, DC: DHHS, 2014.

[2] Hernandez KE, Bejarano S, Reyes FJ, Chavez M, Mata H. Experience preferred: insights from our newest public health professionals on how internships/practicums promote career development. Health Promot Pract 2014; 15(1): 95-9.

[3] Moya EM, Lusk, M. Tuberculosis and stigma: Two case studies in El Paso, Texas, and Ciudad Juarez, Mexico. Professional Dev Int J Cont Soc Work Educ 2009; 12(3): 48-58.

[4] Robinson KL, Ernst KC, Johnson BL, Rosales C. Health status of southern Arizona border counties: a Healthy Border 2010 midterm review. Rev Panam Salud Publica 2010; 28(5): 344-52.

[5] Moya EM, Loza O, Lusk M. Border health: Inequities, social determinants and the case of tuberculosis and HIV. In: Lusk M, Staudt K, Moya E, eds. Social justice in the US-Mexico border region. New York: Springer, 2012.

[6] National Geographic. US-Mexico Border 2014. URL: http://education.nationalgeographic.com/education/media/tijuana-border-fence/?ar_a=1.

[7] United States-Mexico Border Health Commission. Annual Report. El Paso, TX: United States-Mexico Border Health Commission, 2010.

[8] National Rural Health Association. Addressing the health care needs in the US-Mexico Border region. Washington, DC: National Rural Health Association, 2010.

[9] Correa-Cabrera G. Security, migration, and the economy in the Texas- Tamaulipas border region: The 'real' effects of Mexico's drug war. Politics Policy 2013; 41(1): 65-82.

[10] Immigration Policy Center. Children in danger: A guide to the humanitarian challenge at the border. Washington, DC: American Immigration Council, 2014.

[11] Edelman G, Langford T. Some backlash in Texas to the housing of children crossing the border. New York Times 2014 Jul 19.

[12] Lusk M, Staudt K, Moya EM, eds. Social justice in the US-Mexico border region. New York: Springer, 2012.

[13] Acosta DA, Aguilar-Gaxiola S. Academic health centers and care of undocumented immigrants in the United States: Servant leaders or uncourageous followers? Acad Med 2014; 89(4): 540-3.

[14] Hayes-Bautista DE, Hsu P, Hayes-Bautista M, Iniguez D, Chamberlin CL, Rico C, et al. An anomaly within the Latino epidemiological paradox: the Latino adolescent male mortality peak. Arch Pediatr Adolesc Med 2002; 156(5): 480-4.

[15] Tamingco MT. Revisiting the Latino health paradox. Los Angeles, CA: Tomas Rivera Policy Center, 2007.

[16] United States Census Bureau. El Paso County, Texas. Washington, DC: United States Census Bureau, 2011.

[17] United States Department of Labor. Economy at a Glance: El Paxo, TX. Bureau of Labor Statistics, 2014.

[18] Texas Legislative Study Group. Texas on the Brink. Austin, TX: Legislative Study Group, 2013.

[19] City of El Paso. Department of Public Health. Community Health Assessment Draft Report. El Paso, TX: Department of Public Health, 2013.

[20] Instituto Nacional de Estadistica y Geografia. Poblacion total, municipio de Juarez, Chihuahua. Instituto Nacional de Estadistica y Geografia, 2010.

[21] Beletsky Llgc, Martinez G, Gaines T, Nguyen L, Lozada R, Rangel G, et al. Mexico's northern border conflict: collateral damage to health and human rights of vulnerable groups. Rev Panam Salud Publica 2012; 31(5): 403-10.

[22] Peralta F, Anderson SC, Roditti M. Working in the borderland: Implications for social work education. Professional Dev Int J Cont Soc Work Educ 2009; 12(3): 6-16.

[23] Castro A, Farmer P. Understanding and addressing AIDS-related Stigma: from anthropological theory to clinical practice in Haiti. Am J Public Health 2005; 95(1): 53-9.

[24] World Health Organization. Global tubercolosis report 2013. Geneva: World Health Organization, 2013.

[25] Chaisson RE, Harrington M. How research can help control tuberculosis. Int J Tuberc Lung Dis 2009; 13(5): 558-68.

[26] de Cosio FG, Diaz-Apodaca BA, Ruiz-Holguin R, Lara A, Castillo-Salgado C. United States-Mexico border diabetes prevalence survey: Lessons learned from implementation of the project. Rev Panam Salud Publica 2010; 28(3): 151-8.

[27] Centers for Disease Control and Prevention. CDC Health Disparities and Inequalities Report - United States, 2013. Atlanta, GA: Centers Disease Control Prevention, 2013.

[28] Fitchett JR, Vallecillo AJ, Espitia C. Tuberculosis transmission across the United States--Mexico border. Rev Panam Salud Publica 2011; 29(1): 57-60.

[29] Seung KJ, Omatayo DB, Keshavjee S, Furin JJ, Farmer PE, Satti H. Early Outcomes of MDR-TB treatment in a high HIV-prevalence setting in Southern Africa. PLoS One 2009; 4(9): 1-7.

[30] Iademarco MF. Availability of an assay for detecting mycobacterium tuberculosis, including rifampin-resistant strains, and considerations for its use, United States 2013. MMWR 2013; 62(41): 821-4.

[31] Bojorquez-Chapela I, Backer CE, Orejel I, Lopez A, Diaz-Quinonez A, Hernandez-Serrato MI, et al. Drug resistance in Mexico: results from the National Survey on Drug-Resistant Tuberculosis. IntJ Tuberc Lung Dis 2013; 17(4): 514-9.

[32] Lobato MN, Cegielski JP. Preventing and controlling tuberculosis along the U.S.-Mexican border: work group report. MMWR 2001; 50(RR-1): 1.

[33] Centers for Disease Control and Prevention. Reported tuberculosis in the United States 2012. Atlanta, GA: Centers Disease Control Prevention, 2013.

[34] Kolben K. Globalization and the future of labour law. Industr Labor Relat Rev 2008; 61(4): 580-2.

[35] Nadol P, Stinson KW, Coggin W, Naicker M, Wells CD, Miller B, et al. Electronic tuberculosis surveillance systems: A tool for managing today's TB programs. Int J Tuberc Lung Dis 2008; 12(3/1): S8.

[36] Acevedo-Garcia D. Residential segregation and the epidemiology of infectious diseases. Soc Sci Med 2000; 51(8): 1143-61.

[37] Horevitz E, Lawson J, Chow JCC. Examining cultural competence in health care: Implications for social workers. Health Soc Work 2013; 38(3): 135-45.

[38] Moya EM, Nunez G. Public art, service learning, and critical reflection: Nuestra Casa as a case study of tuberulosis awareness on the US-Mexico border. Reflections 2013; 13(1): 127-51.

[39] Simon N. The participatory museum: Museum 2.0; 2010.

[40] Anderson G, ed. Reinventing the museum: Historical and contemporary perspectives on the paradigm shift. Lanham, MD: Altamira, 2004.

[41] Dean HD, Williams KM, Fenton KA. From theory to action: Applying social determinants of health to public health practice. Public Health Rep 2013; 128(Suppl 3): 1-4.

[42] Graham JR, Shier ML. Profession and workplace expectations of social workers: Implications for social worker subjective well-being. J Soc Work Pract 2014; 28(1): 95-110.

[43] Craig GM, Booth H, Hall J, Story A, Hayward A, Goodburn A, et al. Establishing a new service role in tuberculosis care: the tuberculosis link worker. J Adv Nurs 2008; 61(4): 413-24.

[44] La Motte E. The nurse as a social worker. Public Health Nurs 2012; 29(2): 185-7.

[45] Cabrera DM, Morisky DE, Chin S. Development of a tuberculosis education booklet for Latino immigrant patients. Patient Educ Couns 2002; 46(2): 117-24.

[46] Hargreaves JR, Boccia D, Evans CA, Adato M, Petticrew M, Porter JDH. The social determinants of tuberculosis: From evidence to action. Am J Public Health 2011; 101(4): 654-62.

[47] Saldana R, Blas E. What can public health programs do to improve health equity? Public Health Rep 2013; 128(Suppl 3): 12-20.

[48] Schaff K, Desautels A, Flournoy R, Carson K, Drenick T, Fujii D, et al. Addressing the social determinants of health through the Alameda County, California, Place Matters Policy Initiative. Public Health Rep 2013; 128: 48-53.

In: Public Health Yearbook 2016
Editor: Joav Merrick

ISBN: 978-1-53610-947-4

Chapter 15

UNDERSTANDING SEXUAL MINORITY WOMEN AND OBESITY USING A SOCIAL JUSTICE LENS: A QUALITATIVE INTERPRETIVE META-SYNTHESIS (QIMS)

Tracey Marie Barnett**, PhD, LMSW,
Pamela H Bowers, PHD, MSW
and Amanda Bowers, BSN-RN, MSW
School of Social Work, The University of Arkansas at Little Rock, Little Rock, Arkansas, US and
Department of Social Work, Humboldt State University, Arcata, California, US

ABSTRACT

Obesity is a critical public health and social welfare issue affecting populations in the United States. One emerging area incorporates the interplay between obesity, sexual orientation, and identity. Sexual minority women (i.e., female identified lesbians, bisexuals, and transgender women) are disproportionately affected by the obesity epidemic, facing health disparities associated with outcomes such as high blood pressure, strokes, heart attacks, diabetes and more. Objective/Methods: Using a feminist social justice lens, the purpose of this qualitative interpretive meta-synthesis (QIMS) was to examine and understand the experiences of sexual minority women who struggle with obesity and obesity related diseases. Thus, Ethnography, Grounded Theory, and Phenomenology were among the frameworks identified in the nine included studies. Study group: The total sample consisted of 141 participants who self-identified as sexual minority women ages 18-71 years. Results: Four themes on weight attitudes and physical activity behaviors among sexual minority women emerged: Expectations, Culture, Interventions, and Health. Conclusions: As social workers and public health practitioners

* Correspondence: Tracey Marie Barnett, PhD, LMSW, The University of Arkansas at Little Rock, School of Social Work, 2801 South University Ave, Little Rock, AR 72204, United States. E-mail: tmbarnett@ualr.edu.

implement prevention practices for this population of women, culturally grounded lesbian, gay, bisexual and transgendered (i.e., LGBT specific) interventions are recommended. Furthermore, intervention and prevention efforts can be enhanced by practitioners who build cultural humility and gain knowledge and/or awareness of the health disparities experienced by sexual minority women as identified in these studies.

Keywords: sexual minority women, social justice, obesity, qualitative interpretive meta-synthesis, social inequalities, health disparities

INTRODUCTION

Obesity prevalence, prevention, and intervention is topping the priority lists for health practitioners in the United States and is considered a known risk factor for many preventable diseases such as heart disease, diabetes and some cancers (1,2). Obesity affects individuals in all age groups, socioeconomic levels, and ethnicities (3). According to the National Center for Health Statistics (3), obesity prevalence in the United States has increased 23% over the last 40 years. Given that 66% of the American population is overweight (3), obesity has been described as an epidemic. Among the US population, women have been associated with higher risk factors for obesity. This study explores the experiences of a sub-population of women: sexual minority women, who are disproportionately impacted by health inequalities: obesity and obesity related diseases. Our goal is to provide social workers and other helping professions a descriptive exploration of the health inequalities experienced by these women and provide recommendations addressing the related issues.

Literature review

One particularly disproportionate group affected by obesity and being overweight is sexual minority women, or those who identify as lesbian, bisexual and queer (LBQ). Specifically, sexual minority women have a greater likelihood of being overweight and obese than their heterosexual counterparts (4, 5). Moreover, several studies have found when comparing lesbians to heterosexual women, lesbians have consistently higher rates of being overweight and obese (5, 6, 10). Relatively little is known about sexual minority women who experience obesity-related health disparities, and researchers have documented the dearth of literature about health and health seeking behaviors of sexual minority women (7, 8).

When considering interventions for weight loss and healthy lifestyle improvements, researchers have recommended providers prescribe treatments for obesity to be inclusive of personal and individual characteristics including sexual orientation, race, age, and weight (9). Likewise, recommendations from the literature include a need for practitioners to have an increased awareness about the increased risk for obesity in sexual minority women (10). These recommendations highlight the gaps in our understanding of sexual minority women impacted by obesity health disparities. Thus, our research explores the issues of obesity experienced by sexual minority women from a qualitative perspective. In particular we use a feminist social justice lens to examine the compounded issues related to the intersections of privilege for this population of women. Furthermore, the theoretical perspective guiding our research comes from the social determinants of health as well as from a feminist social justice lens. To our knowledge, previous qualitative research on sexual minority women who experience obesity related health disparities has not been framed from a social justice perspective.

In 2008, the World Health Organization (WHO) launched the commission on the social determinants of health to support a movement that translates health knowledge into political action. In brief, the social determinants of health are defined as living conditions shaped by sociopolitical factors that contribute to the health of individuals and populations. In essence, factors related to the distribution of health include social position, education, occupation, income, gender, and ethnicity/race. While sexual orientation is not included within the social determinants of a health conceptual framework, sexual minorities experience significant and pervasive health disparities. For example, lesbian and bisexual women are less likely to seek cancer prevention services and have unequal access to care when compared to heterosexual women (11, 12). Not surprisingly, the literature has shown time and again that homophobia and heterosexism are at the forefront among barriers and access to health care (13, 14). Therefore, by incorporating a feminist social justice lens, we provide a context from which we focus towards developing interventions and treatment that empower individuals rather than place blame and/or subject them to further scrutiny, and to bring about a level of awareness of the issues facing this population of women.

Statement of purpose

The purpose of qualitative interpretive meta synthesis (QIMS) is to arrive at a new synergistic understanding of the social problem being explored. Aguirre and Bolton (15) explain the rigorous steps to data extraction and translation in the path toward collective understanding. A thorough explanation of QIMS is explained in the methods section. In this process, a research question must be identified. Using the social determinants of health model and a feminist social justice lens, our goal was to understand the experiences of sexual minority women (i.e., female identified bisexuals, lesbians, queer, and transgender women) and their experiences with obesity and obesity related issues. Thus, two questions guided the process: 1) What are the experiences of sexual minority women who struggle with obesity and other related health disparities? 2) What can we learn from these experiences to guide culturally inclusive social work practice for health inequalities?

METHODS

Synthesis of quantitative research via meta-analysis is well-established in social work; however only a few studies synthesizing qualitative research have been published (16). Grounded in social work values for practice and research and framed from the extensive applications in nursing, Qualitative Interpretive Meta-Synthesis (QIMS) was employed for this study. This method focuses on the "meanings of three words in 'interpretive meta-synthesis,' 'interpretive' meaning that we eschew aggregating findings quantitatively; 'meta' 'denoting a change of position or condition' and 'synthesis' being 'the combination of ideas to form a theory or system' (15, 17). Likewise, QIMS provides a means to synthesize a group of studies on a related topic into an enhanced understanding of the topic of study wherein the position of each individual study is changed from an individual pocket of knowledge of a phenomenon into a part of a web of knowledge about the topic where a synergy among the studies creates a new, deeper and broader understanding (15).

QIMS includes four components: instrumentation- role of the authors, sampling the literature, data extraction, and translation of data into a new synergistic understanding of the phenomenon being studied (15). QIMS is explained further in the following discussion of the steps in the method.

Instrumentation

For investigators to set aside their experiences as much as possible, the use of epoche (bracketing) is used as a way of examining a new phenomenon with a transcendental perspective (18). Moustakas (19) stated that seldom is this ever perfectly achieved. However, it is important for researchers to engage in this task when beginning a project before proceeding with the experiences of others (20). In qualitative research, the author(s) are the main instruments. Therefore, the following is a brief description of our credibility to conduct this study.

First author

As a heterosexual African American woman, the majority of women in my maternal and paternal family have all been diagnosed with at least one or more of the following cardiovascular disease risk factors: heart disease, heart failure, diabetes, high cholesterol, high blood pressure, and obesity. The idea of losing a curvaceous figure simply in the name of ideal heart health is not always appealing. Also, rejecting unhealthy, fried, lard-laden meals prepared by matriarchs at family gatherings is viewed as disrespectful. Today, poor cardiovascular health is too commonplace in the United States and my goal is to help create and improve effective prevention efforts to impede this epidemic yet preventable disease.

Second author

As a self-identified queer woman, I am keenly aware of the obesity related health disparities faced by women in my community and in my own family. I choose to bracket these experiences with the goal of refraining from overgeneralizing my own experiences to those faced by sexual minority women of color, those with disabilities, and other factors that may disenfranchise people in my community. I feel that my expertise in qualitative data analysis provides credibility that strengthens the rigor and trust-worthiness of our research.

Third author

As a sexual minority woman with extensive work experience as a Hartford Fellow in social work with older adult populations, and currently as a registered nurse in a large community emergency department, I have a unique perspective that incorporates a holistic approach centered in the care and empowerment of vulnerable populations. My self-identification as a lesbian coupled with my role as a health practitioner furthers my commitment to bring about a new awareness of health inequalities as they relate to sexual minorities. My diverse clinical and academic expertise enhances this research with a balance of field knowledge and practical application.

Sampling process

The studies included in this QIMS were identified using Google Scholar, Academic Search Complete, Health Source: Nursing/Academic Edition, EBSCO Host, Social Work Abstracts, Pro-Quest Dissertation and Theses Abstracts, PSYInfo, and One Search databases. The keywords used in varying combinations for the searches were those relating to the terms "obese," "lesbian," and "qualitative." These search terms were broadened using words such as obesity, overweight, fat, sexual minorities, bisexuals, transgendered, themes, focus groups, grounded theory, case study, phenomenology, narrative and ethnography. See Figure 1 for a summary of the retrieval and elimination process. To provide a comprehensive review, all years were included up to 2013. The initial search yielded approximately 200 articles with any of the words above either in the text or title. Sixty duplicates were removed, and then we scanned each article's title and abstract for inclusion criteria. A total of 100 studies were removed using a mixed methods approach, and/or included gay men and heterosexual men and women. After reviewing the 40 potentially relevant articles, only 22 met the inclusion criteria. After the first triangulation meeting with all authors and a closer look at the sample, 10 additional articles were removed from the sample due to these not being all inclusive of the specific criteria.

Table 1. Studies included in QIMS

Authors, Publication Year (Citation) and Discipline	Data Collection Strategy	N	Age, Race/Ethnicity	Location
Bowen et al., 2006 (26), Women and Health	Focus Groups	41 Sexual minority women	Ages: 22-71 Ethnicity: (33) White-not Hispanic, (3) White and Hispanic, (4) Asian or Pacific Islander; and (1) Bi/Multiracial	Seattle, WA
Huxley et al., 2013 (28), Health Psychology	Semi-structured interviews	15 Non-heterosexual women	Ages: 18–69 Ethnicity: white British or white Irish (13) and Jewish European (2)	Primarily urban areas of the United Kingdom
Jones & Malson 2011, (29), Psychology and Sexuality	Semi-structured interviews	5 Lesbians	Ages: 18 and 27 Ethnicity: White British	Britain

Table 1. (Continued)

Authors, Publication Year (Citation) and Discipline	Data Collection Strategy	N	Age, Race/Ethnicity	Location
Kelly 2007 (24), Health	Grounded theory	20 Lesbians	Ages: 32-57 Ethnicity: White (14), Hispanic American (2), Asian American (2), African (1) and Western Indian (1)	New Jersey, New York, and Canada
Maor 2012 (30), Lesbian Studies	In-depth interviews	3 Queer Lesbians	Ages: 22-40 Ethnicity: Jewish-Israeli	Israel
Millner 2004, (7) (Psychology)	Semi-structured interviews	11 Lesbians	Ages: 23-57 Ethnicity: European American (10) and Native and European American (1)	San Diego and Philadelphia
Roberts et al. 2009 (31), Clinical Nursing	Focus Groups	24 Lesbians	Ages: 22-60 Ethnicity: White (20) African American (3) and African American and Hispanic (1)	Massachusetts
Salkin 1997 (25) Applied Behavioral & Communication Science	Constructivist Methodology	8 Lesbian Women	Ages: 20-50 Ethnicity: Caucasian (7) and Biracial (1)	Oregon
Fogel et al., 2009, (32) Women and Health	Phenomenology & Grounded Theory	14 Lesbian Women	Ages: 33-68 Ethnicity: Caucasian (13) and African American (1)	Tennessee

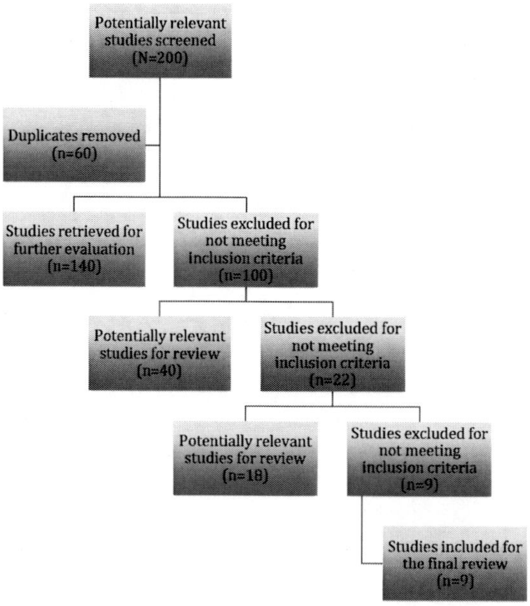

Figure 1. Quorum chart.

The final sample consisted of 9 articles which fit the following parameters: (1) experiences of sexual minority women who are obese (2) rigorous qualitative methodology (3) articles with representative quotes from key informants. While inclusion of only nine studies may appear to be small, other published studies using the same method (16, 21-22) only found four to five articles that met their inclusion criteria.

Data extraction

The first step involved extracting the themes, which were identified in the original studies (see Table 2). In order to maintain the integrity of each study, in Table 2 we used the exact language presented in the studies to represent the themes extracted. This was done to ensure that the data for our QIMS adhered to the authors' original interpretations.

Table 2. Themes extracted from original studies

Authors	Themes
Bowen et al.	-Healthy Eating and Physical Activity -Body Image -Health -Subgroup differences related to body -Intervention Ideas
Huxley et al.	-Normative Body Dissatisfaction -Mainstream Pressures -Critiquing Mainstream Pressures -Pressures within LGB communities -Are lesbian and bisexual women protected from body dissatisfaction
Jones and Malson	-Performing or Passing as a Straight Woman -Recovery as Self-And Social Acceptance
Kelly	-The Emergence of Body Silence -The Effect of Stigma -Body Silence -Lesbian Invisibility -Fear of Misinterpretation of Intent -Discomfort during intimacy -Questionable Feedback -Body Image and Sexual Identity
Maor	-Fat Acceptance -Political Marginality as a Value -Erotic Relations -The Natural and Neutral Body -Carving up Space -The Fantasy of Pure Resistance
Millner	-Strained Family of Origin Relationships -Impact of Coming out as Lesbians -Family of Origin Focus on Food and Weight -Ethnic and Cultural Identities -Genetic Component -Media -Body Image -Dieting -Weight Loss -Difficulty Maintaining Weight Loss -Development and Function of Binge Eating -Awareness of the problem -Binge Eating in Response to Feelings -Function of Binge Eating -Defining Recovery -Achieving Recovery -Recovery is an ongoing Process -Hindrances to Recovery -Preventing Relapse -Support -Supportive Romantic Relationships -Lack of Understanding

Table 2. (Continued)

Authors	Themes
Millner (continued)	-Lesbian Culture -Lesbian and Heterosexual Women -Protective Aspect of Lesbian Culture -Butch/Femme Identity -Fat Lesbians -Binge Eating Disorder Among Lesbians -Lack of Awareness in Lesbian Community -Other Mental Health Issues -Other Addictions -Exercise
Roberts et al.	-Generational differences -Acceptance of weight and body images -Effect of minority stress and depression on risk behaviors -Impact of stress and depression on healthy behaviors -Attitudes towards participation in weight reduction interventions -Lesbian Specific Interventions
Salkin	-Consistent Concern with Body Image -Similar Explanations for Body Image Concern -Lesbianism and Body Image Improvement -Unique Body Image Issues in the Lesbian Culture
Fogel	-Desire to improve health -History of weight loss attempts -Shame -Feelings-Being unaccepted related to sexual identity "not being able to be myself" -Searching for safety -The environment -The weight loss program -Community and social support -Safety and acceptance

Translation: Path to synergistic understanding

The next step which follows in the analysis is translation, which serves as a means to identify themes across the studies. Noblit and Hare state that translation "maintains the central metaphors and/or concept of each account in their relation to other key metaphors or concepts in that account. It also compares both the metaphors and concepts and their interactions in one account with the metaphors or concepts and their interactions in other accounts" (23).

To ensure accuracy of findings and representative of the sample, we used several methods of triangulation in addition to the triangulation essential in the original studies: a) studies were from different disciplines (i.e., triangulation of sources) and b) we triangulated with each other (i.e., triangulation of analysts). All extraction and translation of the data was first analyzed by the first author, followed by the second, and lastly third to ensure accuracy of the translations. A collection of themes emerged to create a new synergistic understanding of the phenomenon of sexual minority women and obesity.

Next, data synthesis followed theme extraction to the path of synergistic understanding of the phenomenon. This is a multi-phase process. Several meetings among the authors took place in order to generate an agreed upon translation. An integral part of this process involved keeping all authors aware of how their connection to the topic both provided an abundance of insight yet possibly introduced biases related to the topic. For this reason, we spent extended time discussing and processing during this QIMS. A synthesis of the studies emerged into a new, synergistic understanding of the experiences of sexual minority women who struggle with obesity and related cardiovascular disease risk factors.

RESULTS

Analysis of the nine studies identified four overarching themes that captured the experiences of sexual minority women who struggle with obesity and related health risk factors. Within the themes were dimensions and related categories for each dimension. Examples of each theme, dimension, and category are presented in Table 3. Following Table 3 is an extensive presentation of each theme.

Table 3. Themes, dimensions, categories, and example quotes

Themes	Dimensions	Categories	Example Quotes
Theme 1: Expectations	Self and Others: Image Expectations	Identity	''As soon as something got close to that [revealing sexual identity], you felt like you had to shut down, because you did not know the reaction of those people; you did not know how they would react.'' (32, p. 548).
		Body Image	"When I've dated women, I don't know, I just feel like, it's a lot more emotional than it is physical. So if I approach a woman, I'm much less likely to think, 'she won't like me because I am fat...'The level of superficiality isn't the same as it is if I'm interested in a man and approaching him." (26, p.88).
		Lesbianism	"Feminists and lesbians like to kid ourselves and think that we've escaped all those expectations, but the reality is that we haven't and we're still just as much a victim to it as anyone else and softening up or looking good for the camera or whatever you want to call it, is still just as important."(25, p.107).
		Consistent Concerns	''It is a very subtle kind of thing, like when you are in the other groups, you know, you just feel like, at any moment, you are going to get ambushed by, 'Oh, what does your husband think about your weight lost'? Tedious!''(32, p. 547).
	Self: Acceptance and Understanding	Acceptance	"I also think of fat as something truly positive. First of all, I find it physically attractive. As a concept, I find it attractive, it's nice, it really stems from the spirit of the community I hang out with..." (30, p.181).
		Lack of Understanding	"You're always going to get bullied for being a big girl, doesn't matter if you're gay, straight, bi, anything, you know. People see you as fat, they will call you fat. My weight has always been my, my one prime concern." (28, p.6).
	Self and Others: Social Expectations	Social Support	"I have gained a greater sense of myself, and being with other lesbians-that certainly is more affirming of who I am. And too, there is a greater acceptance, so there is a lot less punishment in coming to this group with all of us, because we just have this greater sense of acceptance of who we are as women already. (32, p.549).
		Mainstream Pressures	"If she could just 'look acceptable to a man,' he would want her, and she would not 'have to be a lesbian.'" (24, p.881).

Table 3. (Continued)

Themes	Dimensions	Categories	Example Quotes
Theme 2: Culture	Queer Culture	Being Protective of Culture	"I look at my niece, and I worry about her growing up where the ads show the stick figures. These are not real shapes."(26, p.87).
		Generational Differences	"Age is defining, you know now that I'm in my 40s…I think that older lesbians have different perspectives around weight and body changing and understanding that happens. I think when I look back on myself being younger and I wanted, you know, to be thin...but I knew that it was socially constructed, I got it even then." (31, p.1989).
		Intersections	"I was the little fat black girl. I think it was easier at the time to be black than fat. I seem to remember there were more black girls than fat ones. So when I was feeling bad about myself what did I do? Eat, my grandmother was a great cook." (24, p.877).
	Family Culture	Family of Origin Focus on Food and Weight	"They gave me a hard time about my weight because I was always heavier than them…they would say things to me like 'well, you should lose weight.'" (27, p.111).
		Generational	"My mother, my grandmother, we all have to deal with it. I don't think they feel different than I do" (31, p. 1989).
Theme 3: Interventions	Recovery and Support	Defining and Achieving Recovery	"…The support of my higher power…but I think just going to a (OA) meeting means you're asking for help. You're admitting that you have a disease, you're admitting that you're powerless over food and that you're there to get help…"(27, p.126).
		Process	"See for me the binging, I still have binging in my life. It hasn't stopped. I have more control over it and my hunch is that it's not going to stop. I have to be forever vigilant about it…being conscious about what I put in my body…I don't have it mastered by any stretch of the imagination, but you know I get closer to it every day." (27, p.127-128).
		Support	''I have gained a greater sense of myself, and being with other lesbians-that certainly is more affirming of who I am. And too, there is a greater acceptance, so there is a lot less punishment in coming to this group with all of us, because we just have this greater sense of acceptance of who we are as women already.''(9, p549).
		Barriers	"It's tougher to eat healthy than it is to eat crappy, and more expensive." (26, p.86).
	Interventions	Attitudes: Participation in Weight Reduction Interventions	"If you come to people with the information about nutrition, I mean I think it's true, if we each had nutritionists that could advise us on what they think is the best thing for us to eat, I think, that would be the ideal world." (26, p.89).
		Subgroup Differences Related to Body Intervention Ideas	"It's tough. The message is to be a real lesbian you have to like sports; you have to want to do these things, and I guess that makes me a fake lesbian."(26, p. 89).
		Sexual Minority Specific Interventions	"I think it gives you the opportunity to do lots of things like acknowledge the social pressures around body image and…you know, really try to tailor a message that's really positive about being healthful and fit…I've already said this but, tailoring it to, um....specific experiences of being in the lesbian community." (31, p.1990).

Themes	Dimensions	Categories	Example Quotes
Theme 4: Health	Health	Attitudes	"I want to be healthy and if I gain weight then I start feeling like I'm getting out of breath running for the bus...that concerns me, but in terms of the aesthetics I don't really, I don't really care." (28, p. 6).
		Definitions	"I think it's not about how I look; it's how I feel and how well it (body) works." (26, p.87).
	Weight	Difficulty Maintaining Weight Loss	"...First of all, I've never kept off any weight that I've lost, I've always put it back on right away..." (27, p. 120).
		Weight Loss	"It feels wonderful. I mean, people have noticed that the weight loss...I can put my seatbelt on in the car, I can close the door without having to keep on banging it shut about ten times...just socially it's a lot better..." (27, 119).
		Shame	"I would say there was a lot of shame based in going [to other groups]. Ah, I just always felt like there was something wrong with me...being fat is just something to be shameful about, and so I always felt a lot of shame." (32, p.547).
	Mental Health	Other Addictions and Obesity	"I think we probably do drink more and smoke more...it's the stress' but you know, I eat to comfort myself. I...reward myself, that sort of thing, you know..." (31, p.1990).
		Emotional Connection with Food	"I think I have an emotional connection with food. I've been a compulsive eater for a long time and struggled with weight loss, gain, loss, gain, loss, gain, loss, gain . . . a lot." (26, p. 86).
		Binge Eating	"It was an escape definitely when I binged, I didn't think about anything else except the food and that was, that was what I needed...I didn't want to think about all the other shit that was going on in my life, if I could just think about food that was, that was much easier to swallow." (27, p.123).

Theme 1: Expectations

The first theme was about expectations for the women including image expectations, social expectations, and acceptance and understanding of expectations. The image expectations dimension fell into four categories including identity (relating to sexual identity), image expectations (how themselves or others felt they should look), lesbianism (image expectations relating to lesbian culture), and concerns (ongoing from themselves and others).

Image expectations related to both being overweight as a woman, and being overweight as a lesbian. For example in (24) two women revealed:

> "My mother thought I became a lesbian because I was too fat to find a man." And, "My sister said but you are beautiful, you're thin . . . girlie . . . I don't get it...My mother just said, 'What a waste, many men have been interested in you.' I was really hurt. She didn't get it at all." (24).

The image expectations were different once the women self-identified as other than heterosexual (e.g., lesbianism):

> "I was less concerned about my weight when I came out and when I was around other lesbians. It's the same thing; it's more accepting about not having to fit into society's ad of what we should look like." (26)

Another woman remarked:

> "Well there's bound to be much greater empathy, isn't there? Because, because, you know, she's got the same sort of body as me, in terms of sort of gender and general overall things [. . .] I think there's more empathy, more, kind of, understanding about issues and problems and how you feel and so on in, in a way that I never experienced in all my, kind of, relationships with men . . ." (28)

Some of the women, for example, discussed how the expectations are different in their own community and it can be easier to feel less concerned with body image:

> "I feel much more forgiving about my size and weight with women than I ever did when I was heterosexual, and I don't know what that's about" (26). "I think it might be easier in being in the lesbian community because women are more accepting of the variety of sizes and shapes." (26)

Across the data were remarks from women who felt there were consistent concerns for passing as heterosexual or having to "out" themselves as a queer woman. For example, one woman said:

> "It is a very subtle kind of thing, like when you are in the other groups, you know, you just feel like, at any moment, you are going to get ambushed by, 'oh, what does your husband think about your weight loss.'? Tedious!" (32).

The concerns of having to worry about outing themselves if they were not comfortable created unnecessary stress. Another woman remarked:

"…I guess I told myself that's the, that's the right way to be, the right way to look, maybe I was trying to keep myself, looking straight maybe" (31).

Acceptance and understanding were about how the women internalized their status as obese. With regard to acceptance, one said, "I also think of fat as something truly positive. First of all, I find it physically attractive. As a concept, I find it attractive, it's nice, it really stems from the spirit of the community I hang out with…" (30). Another remarked, "my looks are a thermometer of my happiness…I think about it all the time" (25). While many of the women accepted the reality of obesity (whether positive or negative in their eyes), there was also a lack of understanding on the part of others. For example several women shared the sentiment that if they were overweight they would be bullied no matter what and people on the outside had no understanding for their experience, "you're always going to get bullied for being a big girl, doesn't matter if you're gay, straight, bi, anything, you know. People see you as fat, they will call you fat" (28). A certain level of shame was experienced with this lack of understanding from the outside:

> "As a feminist, I have so many problems with the ways that people think about weight loss, and the shame attached to, you know, being overweight" (32).

There were also mainstream pressures experienced by this population of women. One said:

> "A lot of the societal pressures about bodies and size and shape comes from…women wanting to look the way they think men want them to look, and if you're taking men even partially out of the equation then that becomes a whole lot less important" (28).

Another shared sentiment regarding to how others used men and certain heterosexual image expectations as a reference category to judge their size:

> "If she could just 'look acceptable to a man' he would want her and she would not have to be a lesbian" (24).

Unlike many of the aforementioned stressors for the women, social support was an important aspect of the expectations theme. In a lesbian-specific intervention one woman said

> "I have gained a greater sense of myself, and being with other lesbians-that certainly is more affirming of who I am. And too, there is a greater acceptance, so there is a lot less punishment in coming to this group with all of us, because we just have this greater sense of acceptance of who we are as women already." (32)

Likewise, there was an agreement that other sexual minority women are more accepting of each other's varying bodies; for example one woman said:

> "We're more apt to accept each other for who and what we are so if we gain a little weight, so what?" (31).

Theme 2: Culture

The second theme that emerged related to culture: queer and family cultural differences. Queer culture fell into categories including being protective of culture (concern with younger family members' future weight issues), generational differences (idea of weight changes over the lifespan), and intersections (coalescing ethnic minority status and weight). One protective aunt contemplates on her concerns regarding her niece's weight:

> "I look at my niece, and I worry about her growing up where the ads show the stick figures. These are not real shapes" (26).

Generational differences was a category within queer culture. One woman discusses a paradigm shift in terms of her weight.

> "Age is defining, you know now that I'm in my 40s…I think that older lesbians have different perspectives around weight and body changing and understanding that happens. I think when I look back on myself being younger and I wanted, you know, to be thin...but I knew that it was socially constructed, I got it even then." (31)

Lastly within queer culture, we hear from a woman who comments on the struggles she faced growing up as an obese ethnic minority child (intersections).

> "I was the little fat black girl. I think it was easier at the time to be black than fat. I seem to remember there were more black girls than fat ones. So when I was feeling bad about myself what did I do? Eat, my grandmother was a great cook." (24).

Family culture was the second dimension under the culture theme. Here, a female discusses unhelpful opinions from her family regarding her weight:

> "They gave me a hard time about my weight because I was always heavier than them…they would say things to me like 'well, you should lose weight." (27)

However, another female was able to find solace in her family as they all had similar weight issues as she (generational):

> "my mother, my grandmother, we all have to deal with it. I don't think they feel different than I do." (31)

Theme 3: Interventions

The third theme was about interventions, recovery, and support. We classified four categories under the dimension of recovery and support: defining and achieving recovery, process, support and barriers. One woman discusses how she depends on a higher being for support with her weight issues. She goes on to discuss a sense of freedom with knowing that she can give her issues of weight to this higher power and "he" will help her in addition to her overeaters anonymous group meetings (defining and achieving recovery):

> "…The support of my higher power…but I think just going to a (OA) meeting means you're asking for help. You're admitting that you have a disease, you're admitting that you're powerless over food and that you're there to get help…" (27)

Another woman comments on the progress that it will take and has taken for her to control her eating patterns. She realizes that change will not occur over night and that with everything in life, things will happen in its due season (process).

> "See for me the binging, I still have binging in my life. It hasn't stopped. I have more control over it and my hunch is that it's not going to stop. I have to be forever vigilant about it…being conscious about what I put in my body…I don't have it mastered by any stretch of the imagination, but you know I get closer to it every day." (27)

One woman spoke about why recovery from obesity was so important to her now of all times: Now it's very important because I have a four-year-old granddaughter, and I really think I can help in her upbringing a lot, and I definitely will be around a good long time for her (26). Another key informant discusses the acceptance and support she found in likeminded peers (support).

> "I have gained a greater sense of myself, and being with other lesbians-that certainly is more affirming of who I am. And too, there is a greater acceptance, so there is a lot less

punishment in coming to this group with all of us, because we just have this greater sense of acceptance of who we are as women already." (9)

However, another informant mentions that there are numerous barriers to weight loss and the huge discrepancy in prices of health and unhealthy foods (barriers). "It's tougher to eat healthy than it is to eat crappy, and more expensive" (26).

"For many of the women, setting unrealistic goals created a barrier for them: I think one of the things that I realized recently was I was making some lofty goals that would be pretty challenging to succeed in, in terms of my schedule. It was like, if I didn't exercise for an hour a day it didn't happen at all. So it was like all or nothing . . . and nothing happened more than all." (26)

Others struggled with information overload and a lack of education about weight loss:

"I think what my main obstacle has been is there is so much information, I don't get it" (26).

One person discussed feeling subpar or as a "fake lesbian" because she had no desire for anything recreational (sub group differences). She said:

"It's tough. The message is to be a real lesbian you have to like sports; you have to want to do these things, and I guess that makes me a fake lesbian" (26) (p. 89).

Interventions tailored specifically for lesbians was another dimension under this theme, specifically in terms of weight loss programs (attitudes toward participation in weight reduction interventions).

"If you come to people with the information about nutrition, I mean I think it's true, if we each had nutritionists that could advise us on what they think is the best thing for us to eat, I think, that would be the ideal orld." (26)

Part of participating in a weight reduction intervention was to have the right attitude, and for this woman it was about goal setting:

"I mean ultimately I have goals of being in better shape and just every day knocking away a little bit by what I'm eating, or treadmill till where it takes me to where I want to be physically." (26)

Lastly, being able to relate was a major theme that emerged. Women desired to lose weight under interventions that were aimed at their specific needs and experiences because they saw these as being most effective (sexual minority specific interventions).

"I think it gives you the opportunity to do lots of things like acknowledge the social pressures around body image and...you know, really try to tailor a message that's really positive about being healthful and fit...I've already said this but, tailoring it to, um....specific experiences of being in the lesbian community." (31)

On how an intervention could change to be more relevant for this population of women, one said:

"I think it gives you the opportunity to do lots of things like acknowledge the social pressures around body image and...you know, really try to tailor a message that's really positive about being healthful and fit .... I've already said this but, tailoring it to, um ...specific experiences of being in the lesbian community." (31)

Theme 4: Health

The last theme that appeared was health and within this were three dimensions: health (attitudes and definitions), weight (difficulty maintaining weight loss, weight loss, and shame) and mental health (other addictions and obesity, emotional connection with food, and binge eating). One woman describes her outlook in terms of weight was not for beauty purposes, but for overall health and wellbeing (attitudes).

"I want to be healthy and if I gain weight then I start feeling like I'm getting out of breath running for the bus...that concerns me, but in terms of the aesthetics I don't really, I don't really care." (28)

Another female agreed with similar statements (definitions): "I think it's not about how I look; it's how I feel and how well it (body) works" (26). The second dimension under the theme of health was weight, which included three categories: difficulty maintaining weight, weight loss and shame. Weight loss and weight gain are a part of life and this key informant discusses how her weight has always been an "up or down" issue (difficulty maintaining weight loss):

"... First of all, I've never kept off any weight that I've lost, I've always put it back on right away..." (27).

However another female seems to have maintained her weight loss (weight loss):

"It feels wonderful. I mean, people have noticed that the weight loss...I can put my seatbelt on in the car, I can close the door without having to keep on banging it shut about ten times...just socially it's a lot better ..." (27)

Next, a woman discusses her embarrassment with her weight (shame):

"I would say there was a lot of shame based in going [to other groups]. Ah, I just always felt like there was something wrong with me...being fat is just something to be shameful about, and so I always felt a lot of shame." (32)

The last dimension under the theme of health was mental health, which encompassed three categories: other addictions and obesity, emotional connection with food, and binge eating. Women stated that their level of stress was so high that substance use and overeating were often used as methods of rewards for dealing with numerous mental health issues (other addictions and obesity):

> "I think we probably do drink more and smoke more…it's the stress' but you know, I eat to comfort myself. I…reward myself, that sort of thing, you know …" (31)

Others stated they had an emotional connection to food which resulted in weight gain when they were sad or depressed and weight stabilization when they were happy (emotional connection to food).

> "I think I have an emotional connection with food. I've been a compulsive eater for a long time and struggled with weight loss, gain, loss, gain, loss, gain, loss, gain . . . a lot." (26)

Lastly, a female discusses how she enjoyed binge eating as it served as a method of escape from all of her problems (binge eating).

> "It was an escape definitely when I binged, I didn't think about anything else except the food and that was, that was what I needed…I didn't want to think about all the other shit that was going on in my life, if I could just think about food that was, that was much easier to swallow." (27)

Discussion

The utilization of a social justice framework throughout the analysis in this QIMS exploration highlights the context of health inequality faced by sexual minority women specifically as it relates to obesity. To the best of our knowledge, the identification of health inequalities for sexual minority women and obesity has not been previously discussed within the literature through a social justice lens. The field of social work just recently began to acknowledge the health inequalities and healthcare needs of the lesbian, gay, bisexual, transgender and queer population (33). Because social workers serve clients from diverse backgrounds who encounter numerous life threatening health related issues, physical health inequalities should be a top priority for the profession to help alleviate the prevailing issues (34). This emphasis provides a unique perspective that enhances our understanding of empowerment for this population, rather than exposing them to further social stigma.

The following four major themes were elicited in this study: Expectations, Culture, Interventions, and Health. The synthesis of data describes at least two perspectives seen previously in the literature: one, how sexual minority women experience obesity health disparities, which may be different from the experiences of heterosexual women (35); two, how sexual minority women experience some of the same experiences described in the literature by a general population of women (36). What this study adds to the literature, however, is that while very little is known about sexual minority women who experience obesity health disparities, they often have unique and separate experiences relating to obesity and the intersections of sexual orientation and race, among other things.

Health inequalities as it relates to sexual minority women who experience obesity were described within the studies. The dimension of mainstream pressures was unique to sexual minority women studied throughout this QIMS. The pressure to meet societal expectations regarding gender presentation was echoed in many of the aforementioned studies. Whether the participant self-identified as lesbian, bisexual, or queer, sexual minority women discussed the burden of conforming to mainstream gender norms (i.e., feminine, long hair etc.). The dichotomy between what men find attractive and what women find attractive was surpassed by the overarching societal pressure to be thin. Moreover, sexual minority women who experienced obesity frequently mentioned the increased stress, fear, and shame associated with stigmas surrounding both obesity and sexual minority status within mainstream society. This theme is important to highlight as it delineates key features of health inequalities faced by self-identified obese sexual minority women.

In the second theme of culture, key informants discussed a need for practitioners to have a greater understanding of the importance of culturally tailored prevention and intervention strategies specific to sexual minority women. For example, women in the lesbian-specific weight loss groups felt more comfortable as they did not fear being "outed" as a lesbian or bisexual, they could talk more freely, and most importantly could focus on improving their overall health. Culturally tailored interventions have the potential to ameliorate the health inequalities faced by these women in a group setting.

Through this QIMS, another key finding was focused on how the experience of being obese differs greatly depending on the current way the person identifies. Identifying more as a woman, more as a lesbian, more as a woman of color, or some combination of those, for example, created sub-group differences. Thus, some sexual minority women experience obesity with a focus more on the biological family dynamic and ethnic food practices, while others experience obesity with regard to their sexual orientation and did not feel pressure about their body shape/size. Additionally, because of the stress and stigma associated with being a sexual minority woman, binge eating was also one of the many manifestations of experiencing obesity. Several of the women also shared similarities with an emotional connection to food, as well as other addictions to alcohol, tobacco, and substance abuse. Regardless, it was clear that having a "healthful" attitude made a difference for this population of women. Social workers are in a unique position to empower and support these women to identify a healthful attitude and related attributes.

Limitations

While this QIMS provides a closer look into the lives of sexual minority women who experience obesity health disparities, some limitations are present. Although we systematically reviewed all known exploratory/qualitative articles on this topic, only nine studies fit our inclusion criteria. Thus, our sample, while larger than the original studies individually, was still constrained by missing variables. For example, there were very few women of color and transgender identified women. Additionally, some of the original authors noted limitations in their samples as the majority of their participants were Caucasian, able-bodied, and middle-class. The goal of this qualitative review was to reach a deeper understanding of the experiences of these women and assist practitioners. We did not aim to generalize our findings to the overall population of sexual minority women who experience obesity related health inequalities.

CONCLUSION

When crafting culturally grounded interventions for sexual minority women at risk for health disparities, numerous implications should be considered to ensure effectiveness. Practice implications for social workers include having awareness about sexual minority women who may be at a great risk for obesity and comorbid conditions. Therefore, access to cultural competency training for providers is paramount in reducing health inequalities for this population of women. The women in this QIMS frequently brought up issues of shame and fear when disclosing their sexual orientation to their health care providers. Providers are encouraged to avoid heteronormative assumptions in their service provision. Furthermore, public health efforts can be enhanced by practitioners who build cultural humility, and gain knowledge and/or awareness of the health disparities experienced by sexual minority women, as identified in these studies. Similarly, nurses, who serve as health educators, patient navigators and advocates, and hands on practitioners are in a unique position to help sexual minority women in obtaining access to culturally relevant prevention and intervention services.

Policy implications are formed based on the scarcity of information about sexual minority women and obesity. Social workers and other health practitioners need access to better data for health policy and research. As obesity has been linked to higher overall health care costs, national organizations should require lesbian, gay, bisexual and transgendered (LGBT) specific demographic data collection in their organizational policies to increase access to more representative samples. Similarly, calls for funding from national organizations such as the National Institutes of Health should include blocked funding specifically for this group to increase knowledge leading to policy change aimed at reducing health disparities.

Future research is needed to explore and identify population specific health essentials surrounding obesity and related diseases for sexual minority women. Small organizations may benefit from conducting needs assessments of their consumer base to further understand the specific treatment and interventions necessary for practice. In general, further research is needed to understand the unique needs, differences, and overall health of sexual minority women. Additionally, research investigating sexual minority women of color, transgender women, women with disabilities, and women from lower socio-economic statuses should be explored and included in future research.

REFERENCES

[1] American Cancer Society. Cancer facts and figures. Cancer Pract 2000;8: 105-8.

[2] Haslam D, James W. Obesity. Lancet 2005; 366(9492):1197-1209.

[3] CDC. Products - Health E Stats - Overweight prevalence among adults 2005-2006. URL: http://www.cdc.gov/nchs/data/hestat/overweight/overweight_adult.htm.

[4] Bowen D, Balsam K, Ender S. A review of obesity issues in sexual minority women. Obesity 2008;16(2):221-8.

[5] Case P, Bryn Austin S, Hunter D, Manson J, Malspeis S, Willett W, et al. Sexual orientation, health risk factors, and physical functioning in the Nurses' Health Study II. J Womens Health 2004; 13(9):1033-47.

[6] Valanis BG, Bowen DJ, Bassford T, Whitlock E, Charney P, Carter R. Sexual orientation and health: Comparisons in the women's health initiative sample. Arch Fam Med 2000; 843-53.

[7] Boehmer U, Bowen D. Examining factors linked to overweight and obesity in women of different sexual orientations. Prev Med 2009; 48(4):357-61.
[8] Diamant A, Wold C. Sexual orientation and variation in physical and mental health status among women. J Womens Health 2003; 12(1):41-9.
[9] Fogel S, Young L, Dietrich, M, Blakemore D. Weight loss and related behavior changes among lesbians. J Homosex 2013; 59(5):689-702.
[10] Struble CB, Lindley LL, Montgomery K, Hardin J, Burcin M. Overweight and obesity in lesbian and bisexual college women. J Am Coll Health 2010;59(1);51-6.
[11] Brandenberg DL., Matthews AK, Johnson TP, Hughes TL. Breast cancer risk and screening: a comparison of lesbians and heterosexual women. J Womens Health 2007;45(4):109-30.
[12] Buchmueller T, Carpenter C. Disparities in health insurance coverage, access, and outcomes for individuals in same-sex versus different-sex relationships, 2000--2007. Am J Public Health 2010;100(3):489.
[13] Coker T, Austin S, Schuster M. The health and health care of lesbian, gay, and bisexual adolescents. Rev Public Health 2010;31:457-77.
[14] Eliason M, Schope R. Original research: Does "don't ask don't tell" apply to health care? Lesbian, gay, and bisexual people's disclosure to health care providers. J Gay Lesbian Med Assoc 2001; 5(4):125-34.
[15] Aguirre R, Bolton K. A qualitative interpretive meta-synthesis in social work research: Uncharted territory. J Soc Work. 2013 2014;14(3):279-84.
[16] Smith M, Aguirre R. Reproductive attitudes and behaviors in people with sickle cell disorders: A qualitative interpretive meta-synthesis. Health Soc Work 2012;51(9):757-79.
[17] Meta. Oxford Dictionaries Online. URL: http:// oxforddictionaries.com/definition/meta.
[18] Husserl E. The crisis of European sciences and transcendental phenomenology. Evanston, IL: Northwestern University Press, 1970.
[19] Moustakas C. Phenomenological research methods. Thousand Oaks, CA: Sage, 1994.
[20] Creswell J, Creswell J. Qualitative inquiry and research design. Thousand Oaks: Sage, 2007.
[21] Frank L, Aguirre R. Suicide within United States jails: A qualitative interpretive metasynthesis. J Sociol Soc Welfare 2013;40(3):31-52.
[22] Aguirre RTP, Bolton K. Why do they do it? A qualitative interpretive meta-synthesis of volunteer motivation in high-stress volunteer situations. Soc Work Res 2013;37:1-12, doi: 0.1093/swr/svt035.
[23] Noblit G, Hare R. Meta-ethnography: Synthesizing qualitative studies. Newbury Park, CA: Sage, 1998.
[24] Kelly L. Lesbian body image perceptions: The context of body silence. Qual Health Res 2007;17:873-83.
[25] Salkin NB. A qualitative study of body image and lesbian self-identity. Dissertation. Ann Arbor, MI: University Oregon, 1997.
[26] Bowen DJ, Balsam KF, Diergaarde B, Russo M, Escamilla GM. Healthy eating, exercise, and weight: Impressions of sexual minority women. J Womens Health 2006;44(1):79-93.
[27] Millner RE. The experiences of lesbians who have a history of binge eating disorder: A qualitative investigation. Dissertation. Ann Arbor, MI: Alliant International University, 2004.
[28] Huxley C, Clarke V, Halliwell, E. A qualitative exploration of whether lesbian and bisexual women are 'protected' from sociocultural pressure to be thin. J Health Psychol 2013; 18(11):1478-92.
[29] Jones R, Malson H. A critical exploration of lesbian perspectives on eating disorders. Psycho Sex 2013;4(1):62-74.
[30] Maor M. The body that does not diminish itself: Fat acceptance in Israel's lesbian queer communities. J Lesbian Stud 2012;16(2):177-98.
[31] Roberts SJ, Stuart-Shor EM, Oppenheimer RA. Lesbians' attitudes and beliefs regarding overweight ad weight reduction. J Clin Nurs 2010; 19:1986-94.
[32] Fogel S, Young L, McPherson B. The experience of group weight loss efforts among lesbians. J Womens Health 2009;49(6-7):540-54.
[33] Wheeler DP, Dodd S. LGBTQ capacity building in health care systems: a social work imperative. Health Soc Work 2011;36:307-9.

[34] Dowler E, Spencer N. Challenging health inequalities: From Acheson to 'choosing health'. Bristol, UK: Policy Press, 2007.

[35] Beren SE, Hayden HA, Wilfley DE, Grilo, CM. The influence of sexual orientation on body dissatisfaction in adult men and women. Int J Eat Disord 1996;20(2):135-41.

[36] Dworkin AH. Nor in man's image: Lesbians and the cultural oppression of body image. Women Ther 1988;8:27-39.

In: Public Health Yearbook 2016
Editor: Joav Merrick
ISBN: 978-1-53610-947-4

Chapter 16

RISK AND PROTECTIVE FACTORS RELATED TO THE WELLNESS OF AMERICAN INDIAN AND ALASKA NATIVE YOUTH: A SYSTEMATIC REVIEW

Catherine E Burnette*, PhD and Charles R Figley, PhD
School of Social Work, Tulane University,
New Orleans, Louisiana, US

ABSTRACT

In comparison with the general population, research indicates a need for greater health equity among American Indian and Alaska Natives (AI/AN). AI/ANs have demonstrated remarkable resilience in response to centuries of historical oppression, yet growing evidence documents mental health disparities. Consequently, some AI/AN youth, defined as 18 years or younger, experience elevated rates of suicide, substance use disorders, conduct and oppositional defiant disorders, attention deficit-hyperactivity disorders, and posttraumatic stress disorders. In this article we systematically review the growing body of research examining the culturally specific risk and protective factors related to AI/AN youth wellness. This review includes published, peer-reviewed qualitative and quantitative research on AI/AN youth between the years 1988 to 2013. Organizing risk and protective factors within a ecosystemic resilience framework, the following broad risk and protective factors are critically reviewed: societal factors (historical oppression and discrimination), cultural factors (ethnic identity, spirituality, and connectedness), community factors (community environment, school environment, peer influence, and social support), family factors (family support, family income, parental mental health, family trauma and stressful life events), and individual factors. The review includes a discussion of the risk and protective factors accounting for AI/AN youth mental health disparities, implications for correcting disparities, and importance of incorporating familial and community level interventions for AI/AN youth.

* Correspondence: Catherine E Burnette, School of Social Work, Tulane University, 6823 St Charles Ave, Bldg 9, Rm 208, New Orleans, LA 70118, United States. E-mail: cburnet3@tulane.edu.

Keywords: American Indian, Alaska Native, disparities, mental health, protective factors, risk factors, substance abuse, systematic review, wellness

INTRODUCTION

A goal of the United States Affordable Health Care Act is to move the nation a step closer toward health equity, a priority of the Healthy People 2020 initiative (1, 2). If health equity, or reaching and maintaining the highest health for all people, is a desired outcome, then understanding the current inequalities is of utmost importance (2). American and Alaska Natives (AI/AN) inequities experience some of the most widely documented health disparities in the United States (3, 4). This is due, in part, to the disconnect between the paradigms employed in mainstream social work practice and research and the worldviews more salient among AI/AN populations (5, 6). For example, rather than separating mental health from physical health, many AI/AN populations value the strong connection between physical, mental, emotional and spiritual health (7, 8); emotional health is viewed from a perspective of wellness (7, 8). We argue that the AI/AN nations deserve medical and mental health services that complement their cultural heritage that have sustained them for many centuries. We define wellness as the balance between the intertwined mind, body, soul, and spirit, (7). Researchers recommend this holistic and strengths-based perspective about health (7, 8). Therefore, this systematic review focuses on wellness, which we view as resilience in the form of prosocial emotional and academic outcomes, as well as mental health disparities.

With a trust responsibility, based on treaty agreements with sovereign tribes requiring the United States federal government to provide for the healthcare of AI/AN populations in exchange for 400 million acres of land (9), a critical barrier to health equity among AI/AN populations exists. Great heterogeneity exists across AI/AN populations, and research consistently finds significant differences in prevalence of mental health disparities across these populations (3, 4, 10-12). Despite this variability, psychiatric distress in the form of mental health disorders tends to be disproportionately high across populations (3).

AI/ANs represent over five million people and 1.7% of the U.S. population (13). With rapidly changing demographics, AI/ANs increased by almost twice the rate of the general U.S. population between the years 2000 and 2010. In total, 78% of AI/ANs live off of reservation land (13). Yet, this percentage differs among people who identify as either multiethnic or solely AI/AN, with more AI/AN's living off of reservation land in the former than the latter (13). On average, these populations are more likely to live in poverty, experience violent victimization and traumatic loss, domestic violence, and educational inequities than non-AI/AN populations (4). AI/AN youth between the ages of 12 and 19 are more likely than non-AI/AN youth to experience serious violent crime and be affected by a sudden traumatic death (4). Rates of witnessing intimate partner violence and experiencing child maltreatment are also elevated (4). Given the disproportionately high rates that AI/AN youth experience inequity in income and education, as well as traumatic stressors, it is not surprising that many also experience mental health disparities (4).

RESILIENCE AMONG AI/AN YOUTH

Although the research available on AI/AN youth is relatively small, studies document elevated rates for substance use disorders, conduct and oppositional defiant disorders, attention deficit-hyperactivity disorders, and posttraumatic stress disorders (PTSD) (3, 4). Moreover, the suicide rate for AI/AN youth ranges from three to six times higher than non-AI/AN peers (4). Indeed suicide is the 2nd leading cause of death for AI/ANs ages 15-34 years (14).

With these concerning statistics, the fact that the majority of AI/AN youth are healthy and not experiencing mental health disparities can often be overlooked (12). Despite the undoubted resilience of AI/AN populations after centuries of historical trauma, loss, and oppression, current research tends to focus on risk factors (15). Given the over-focus on problems, resilience, or positive adaptation in response to adversity is especially relevant (11, 16, 17). Adversity is typically characterized by challenging life experiences, such as experiencing discrimination or trauma (17). These challenging life experiences can be thought of as risk factors, which increase the probability of negative outcomes, such as mental health disparities (11, 12, 18). Protective factors, in contrast, are associated with positive life outcomes and bolster individual and family resilience.

The ecosystemic perspective emerged within social work literature (17). According to this perspective, rather than being a static "trait" or concept, resilience is a multi-determined and constantly changing result of people's interaction within the ecosystemic context (17). An ecosystemic resilience framework highlights the interconnections and interactions among individuals, families, communities, and societies (17). Thus, researchers, not only examine characteristics and patterns within a given system, but they also examine how multiple systems interact. A focus is the continual adaptation and interaction between individuals and families with their environments (17). Therefore, a risk factor in one context may be protective in other contexts (17). Resilient individuals and families are often able to withstand and recover from adversity with greater skills and capacity than before experiencing the challenge (11, 12, 18).

CULTURALLY SPECIFIC RISK AND PROTECTIVE FACTORS

Distinct tribes have varying historical contexts, languages, cultural practices, values, and social structures. Despite this variability, there is an absence of localized understanding of culturally specific risk and protective factors relating to AI/AN populations youth (19-21); this absence persists, even with a research emphasizing the variability of resilience across contexts the need for its greater understanding (19-21). Although overlap between AI/AN and non AI/AN risk and protective factors exist, such as social support, self-esteem, family support, school factors, community safety, parental education and mental health, and exposure to traumatic events (15, 16, 22-27), culturally distinct factors are also significant for AI/AN youth, such as historical loss, spirituality, extended family, ethnic identity, and connectedness (25-31).

A major societal risk factor health inequity is historical trauma and oppression (32). Indeed, any examination of mental health disparities incorporate the ubiquitous effects of the disproportionate rates of historical and contemporary traumas continually experienced by AI/AN populations (4, 10). Intergenerational trauma and historical trauma are concepts used to indicate the trauma inflicted on groups sharing an ethnic or national background (33-35). Campbell and Evans-Campbell (34) emphasize the pervasive effects of historical trauma on AI/AN youth, families, and communities. The historical loss and oppression incurred by AI/AN peoples throughout colonization, including widespread disease, warfare, starvation, cultural genocide, forced relocation and boarding school participation, discrimination, and poverty, are linked to mental health disparities among AI/AN youth (8, 8, 24, 26, 31, 34, 36, 37). Burnette (38) has extended the concept of historical trauma to incorporate historical oppression, to not only encompasses the pervasive and continued effects of chronic, internalized, insidious, and intergenerational experiences of subjugation, but to also include daily experiences of oppression, such as discrimination and poverty. Although the relationship of historical oppression and health inequities is commonly proposed in research, empirical support for this relationship is in its preliminary stages (39).

Because it influences how people approach, appraise, and respond to adversity, the influence of culture is thought to be an essential component for research on resilience (20, 21, 40, 41). Culture encompasses the beliefs, values, rituals, and norms of social groups, which are affected by historical and social factors (42). Identification with one's culture is thought to have a buffering effect against mental health problems (16, 43-45), yet complexities related to its measurement and understanding have created the need for more research (46). Relatedly, spirituality and connectedness have been found to be particularly important for AI/AN youth (47-51). Finally, community, and especially extended family, are thought to be particular instrumental to AI/AN youth (4, 7, 12, 15, 19, 41, 44, 52, 53). AI/AN extended families can include blood relations, as well as clan, tribe, and adopted family relationships (54). Likewise, resilience research tends to examine individual resilience including stress management, sleeping success, and other variables. Very few studies have focused on the risk and protective factors at the family, community, cultural, or societal levels (19, 20); this is a severe limitation, given the primacy of family and community to AI/AN youth (12).

With the absence of systematic reviews examining the risk and protective from an ecosystemic resilience framework, this review fulfills several purposes. First, although connections among risk and protective factors related to AI/AN and non-AI/AN populations exist, AI/AN sovereignty and heterogeneity make culturally distinct factors important to uncover. This review examines AI/AN youth distinctly. Second, this review examines the existing empirical evidence validating culturally specific risk and protective factors, such as historical oppression, spirituality, and ethnic identity. Third, the majority of existing research examines isolated risk and protective factors in relationship to an outcome. However, many risk and protective factors relate to multiple outcomes. Therefore, a holistic, ecosystemic examination is needed to understand the context of mental health disparities and the wellness of AI/AN youth across multiple levels (17).

This holistic examination of risk and protective factors can identify gaps in current research and inform social work interventions, which can be developed based on relevant factors. Therefore, this review fills the gap in understanding about the context of mental health and substance use disparities that could not be understood through individual component studies. This systematic review examines the following question: What are the risk and protective factors related to AI/AN wellness across societal, cultural, community, familial, and individual levels?

METHODS

This review includes peer-reviewed quantitative and qualitative research articles on the wellness of AI/AN youth published between the 25 year span of 1988 to 2013. These years were chosen because research on mental health equity and inequity is relatively new; articles published within this period encompass all relevant research that could be located by this review. To offset the tendency of research to focus on problems and deficits (19), the inclusion criteria were empirical research articles relating to AI/AN youth wellness as measured by resilience and pro-social outcomes and mental health a disparities experienced by AI/AN youth, such as suicide, PTSD, attention-deficit disorder, conduct disorder, and substance use disorders. Only empirically-based research articles with samples incorporating AI/AN youth were included; articles with solely adult samples were excluded.

Initial decisions about articles that were included were made based on articles' full reports by the first author and were reviewed by the second author to assess reliability. An example of an article that was included was an article with a sample of 221 AI/AN youth to investigate risk and protective factors related to alcohol and drug use (43), whereas a study investigating the relationship between intimate partner violence and alcohol, drug, and mental health disparities among AI/AN adult women was excluded (55).

A multitude of social science and health related databases were used to search for relevant articles, including Google Scholar, Social Work Abstracts, SocINDEX with Full Text, Social Sciences Full Text, PsychARTICLES, PsychINFO, The Educational Resource Information center (ERIC), Academic Search Complete, Family Studies Abstracts, MEDLINE, Race Relations Abstracts, and Health Source: Nursing/Academic Edition. Search terms included the following:

- "American Indian," OR "Alaska Native," OR "Native American,"
- AND "Mental Health," OR "Substance Abuse,"
- AND "Risk Factor," OR "Protective Factor," OR "Resilience," OR "Resiliency,"
- AND "Youth," OR "Adolescent."

Based on inclusion criteria, 51 empirical studies are included in this systematic review. Among this research, 47 articles used quantitative research methods, whereas four articles employed qualitative methods. With exception of these qualitative inquiries, the vast majority of research examined isolated independent variables in relationship to dependent variables, such as mental health or substance use outcomes. Articles described ages of samples either by grade or age, with other research identifying "adolescents" or "middle schooler." The age inclusion criterion for this article was that the research article included participants ages 18 or younger. Research articles that did not include participants 18 or younger were excluded from this review article. The majority of articles described grades between six and twelve and ages ranging from 10 to 18. Three articles included ages that ranged from 15 into the mid-50's and described their samples as adolescents and young adults (56-58).

Regarding geographic context, 58% of reviewed articles sampled reservation AI/AN populations, 20% of samples were urban, 14% had samples from both urban and reservation based populations, and 8% did not specify whether the AI/AN population was reservation or urban based (See Figure 1).

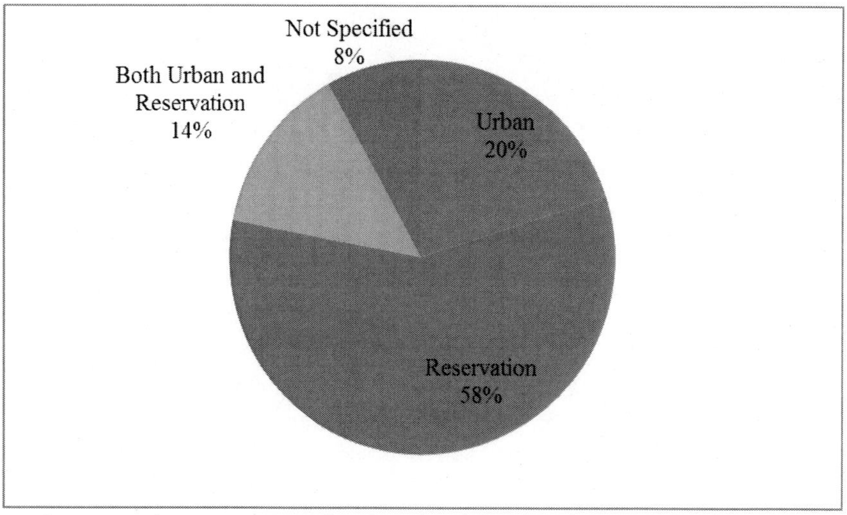

Note. Figure 1 portrays the percentages of reviewed articles that drew samples from reservation based populations, urban based populations, both urban and reservation based populations, as well as articles that did not specify geographic locale.

Figure 1. Percentages of Reservation and Urban Based AI/AN Samples.

Figure 2 portrays the percentages of samples drawn from differing geographic regions with 7% of articles not specifying geographic region, and approximately 20% of articles sampling multiple regions.

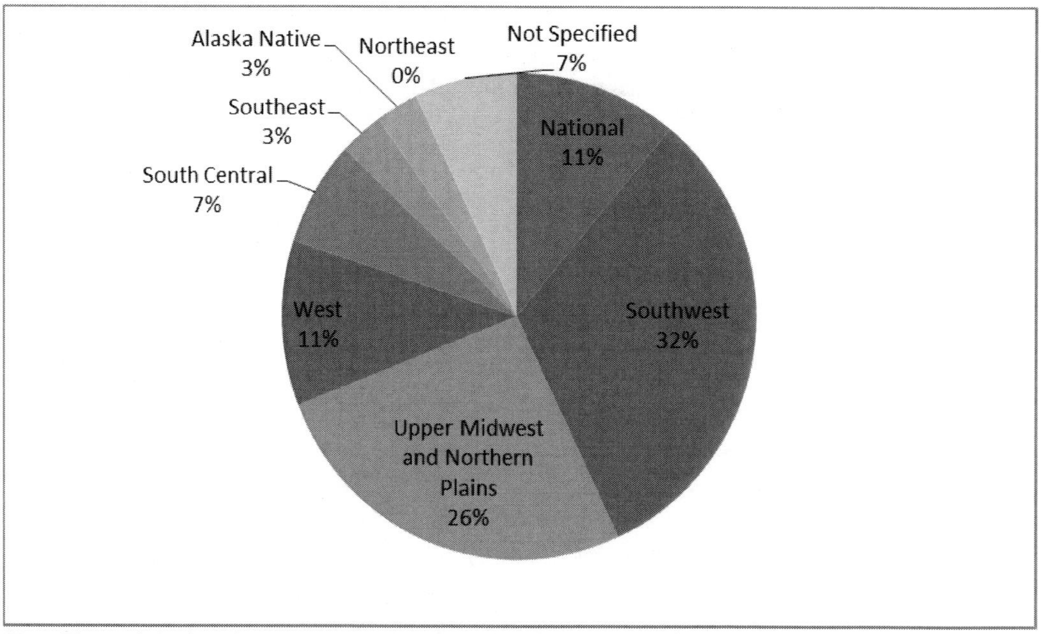

Note. Figure 2 depicts the percentage of samples in this systematic review that originated from National U.S. Samples, as well as those from the Southwest, Upper Midwest and Northern Plains, West, South Central Southeast, Alaska Native, Northeast, Not specified.

Figure 2. Percentages of Samples by Geographic Region of the United States.

Three articles who sampled multiple tribes included those from Canada and the upper Midwestern United States. These articles were retained in the review. The majority, 32% of articles had samples from the southwestern United States, with 26% of samples being drawn from each the Northern Plains and Upper Midwest. National samples and samples from the West compromised 11% of samples, and 7% came from either the south central United States. The remaining samples came from Alaska Natives or the Southeast, with these compromising only 3% of the total. No identified samples were included from the Northeast. Thus, there was a significant deficit of tribes sampled from these regions, with only 2 articles attending to each the Southeast and Alaska Natives and none from the Northeast.

RESULTS

Using an ecosystemic framework, overarching risk and protective factors for AI/AN youth mental health and substance use disparities and resilience are organized by societal, community, familial, and individual levels. Figure 3 presents the overarching factors organized within this framework.

Among the total number of risk and protective factors reported to be relevant within studies, 7% were at the societal level, 16% were at the cultural level, 23% were at the community level, 41% were at the family level, and 13% were at the individual level (See Figure 4). Taken as a whole, 59% of factors had to do with relationships. Because risk and protective factors can vary by context and situation (17), the details of these factors are delineated within each subheading.

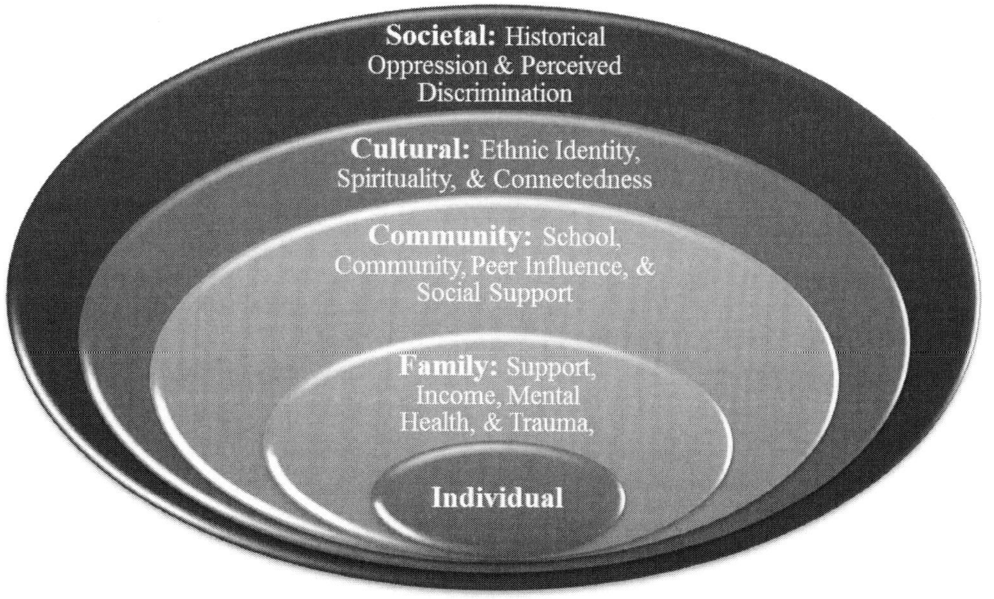
Societal: Historical Oppression & Perceived Discrimination
Cultural: Ethnic Identity, Spirituality, & Connectedness
Community: School, Community, Peer Influence, & Social Support
Family: Support, Income, Mental Health, & Trauma,
Individual

Note. Figure 3 portrays risk and protective factors arranged across an ecosystemic framework at the societal, cultural, community, familial, and individual levels.

Figure 3. Risk and Protective Factors for AI/AN Youth within an Ecosystemic Framework.

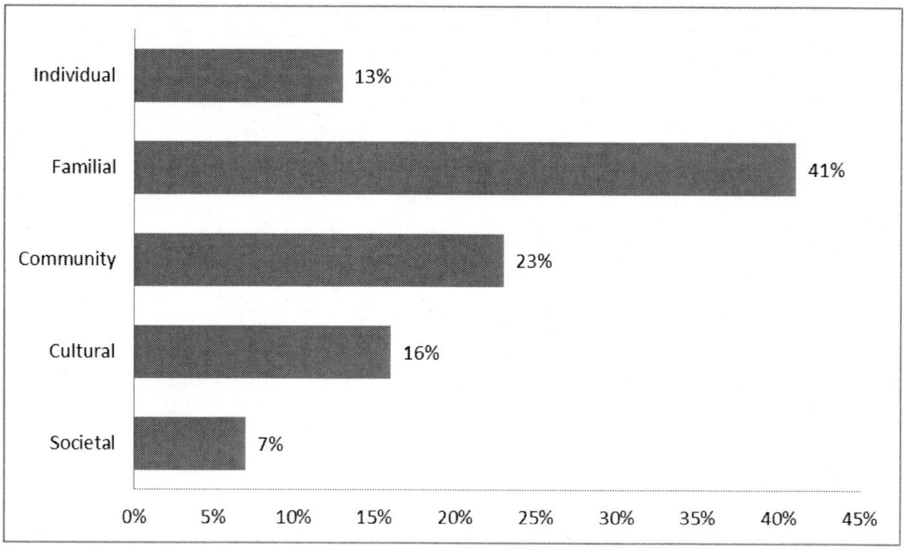

Note. Along with identified factors, 59% of factors had a relationship aspect. The factors with the most research supporting their relevancy were both within the family level and included family support, as well as family trauma and stressful life events. The second and third most supported risk factors were within the community level and included peer influence and school environment.

Figure 4. Percentages of Factors with Empirical Support across Ecosystemic Levels.

SOCIETAL FACTORS

Historical oppression. Perceived historical loss, including loss of language, land, traditional spirituality, culture, and respect for elders, has been associated with emotional and behavioral consequences among AI/AN youth (59). For instance, AI/AN youth reported experiencing daily thoughts of historical loss, which were positively associated with depressive symptoms (59). Furthermore, using a focus group study with elders, parents, youth workers and youth, across three tribal communities, loss of language and culture were identified as major risk factors for delinquent behaviors among adolescents in the Southwest (12).

Perceived discrimination. A form of historical oppression, perceived discrimination, is a well-established risk factor for mental distress across populations (60-65), and this finding extends to AI/AN groups. For example, perceived discrimination was an identified risk factor substance abuse and externalizing behaviors among AI/AN youth (24, 26). Likewise, perceived discrimination significantly contributed to internalizing symptoms (66) and suicidality among AI/AN youth (53, 67). Finally, perceived discrimination predicted AI/AN's depressive symptoms, even when controlling for other factors (31). Therefore, the effects of historical oppression and perceived discrimination and AI/AN youth's mental health are increasingly substantiated in research.

In summary, although the vast majority of research includes societal factors, such as historical oppression, in the explanation of challenges experienced by AI/AN populations, additional empirical research supporting this explanation is needed. Difficulty in measuring historical effects undoubtedly present research challenges, yet studies have begun to substantiate societal factors relating to AI/AN disparities (12, 59). For instance, historical loss was associated with depressive symptoms and delinquent behaviors among AI/AN youth (59). More research is needed to disentangle the relationship between historical oppression and mental health disparities. Contextual information on the experiences of oppression, such as relocation, discrimination, poverty, and boarding schools, and their effects on AI/AN populations will add necessary information to further knowledge development in this substantive area. Finally, perceived discrimination is a well-established risk factor across populations (60-65), and this finding extended to AI/AN youth, as it is related to substance use, externalizing behaviors, internalizing symptoms, depressive symptoms, and suicidality (24, 26, 31, 53, 67). The focus now shifts to cultural factors that have buffered risk factors and bolstered resilience among AI/AN youth.

CULTURAL FACTORS

Ethnic identity

Enculturation, or the degree that individuals learn about, identify with, and are embedded in their ethnic culture, is reported as protective against substance abuse and mental distress (68). Among AI/AN youth living on or near reservation communities in the Upper Midwest, increased levels of enculturation were predictive of decreased suicidal behavior (69). Similarly, enculturation has been predictive of prosocial outcomes, such as academic achievement and substance non-use (16, 26). Finally, using the National American Indian Adolescent Health Survey, involvement in traditional activities was found to be protective against suicidal attempts and ideation for males (30).

Other research has found mixed results for enculturation as a protective factor (10). For example, ethnic pride was associated with fewer alcohol symptoms; however, engagement in generic pow wows was not protective in this context, as it they were associated with a social group engaged in informal drinking (27). Contrarily, other researchers identified tribal language, engagement in ceremonies and pow wows to be protective against adolescent delinquent behaviors (12). However, ethnic identity was not predictive of alcohol involvement directly or indirectly in other research (22, 70, 71). Although ethnic identity did not directly affect mental health and substance abuse outcomes among AI/AN adolescents in another study, it was positively associated with social support, which was protective against negative outcomes (43); therefore, enculturation may indirectly affect mental health and substance use disparities (43).

Finally, biculturalism, or identifying and navigating effectively in more than one culture without comprising either, has been protective for self-esteem, mental health, and substance abuse among AI/AN populations (25, 72-75). Indeed, modest support was reported for bicultural skills in preventing substance abuse AI/AN adolescents residing on two reservations in the Northwest (74).

Spirituality

Related to enculturation, engagement in traditional spiritual practices and religious activities, more broadly, have been found to be protective for AI/AN youth. Religious affiliation and spirituality have been identified as protective against adolescent alcohol abuse/dependence (27, 28). In one study, Christian beliefs and belonging to the Native American Church were associated with lower levels of substance abuse (49). Because they were associated with anti-drug attitudes, norms, and behaviors, traditional spiritual beliefs are thought to serve protective functions for AI/AN populations (49). However, in contrast to commitment to Christianity or beliefs in cultural spirituality, commitment to cultural spirituality was associated with a reduction in suicide attempts among AI/AN populations (57). Therefore, although spirituality and religious involvement may have a protective effect, this effect is dependent on complex factors such as belief systems, commitment beliefs, measurement issues, and the social context.

Connectedness

Connectedness emerged as protective across multiple dimensions and domains of AI/AN wellness. Hill's research uncovered connectedness, or interrelatedness to community, family, nature, the Creator, land, environment, and ancestors, as a protective factor for adult AI/AN populations against suicide (47). Extreme alienation from family and community, in contrast, was a reported risk factor for suicide attempts among AI/AN adolescents (76). Likewise, relationship loss and feeling unsupported were risk factors for impaired AI/AN youth resilience, whereas connectedness fostered youth resilience (41, 77, 78). Finally, feeling cared for and connected to others was protective against depression and negative health outcomes (15).

Thus, existing research indicates enculturation, spirituality, and biculturalism are protective in certain contexts. Ethnic identity emerged as a powerful protective factor (16, 26, 30, 69). That said, other research reports were mixed (22, 27, 70, 71). This is not surprising when considering the complexity of measurement of social variables and heterogeneity across AI/AN populations (43). Spirituality was another empirically supportive protective factor (27, 28, 49). Like ethnic identity, however, it depended on the content and context of research investigations (57).

Lending support to the notion that any one factor can serve as a risk factor or protective factor, depending on the context, all factors, including spirituality must be assessed holistically within the social environment. There is some evidence that connectedness was a culturally-specific protective factor associated with suicide risk, level of resilience, level of depression, among other health outcomes (41, 76-78). Finally, modest support was found for biculturalism being protective against substance (74), yet more research is needed to provide additional evidence. More investigation about factors that may account for variability is warranted. Risk and protective factors at the community level are now examined.

COMMUNITY FACTORS

Community environment

AI/AN adolescents are situated within broader environments. Community and school environments may serve as either protective or risk functions, depending on their quality. For example, community support was found to be protective in fostering adolescent prosocial behaviors (26). However, gang involvement and gun availability were risk factors for suicide attempts (23). Moreover, neighborhood safety, particularly the presence of crime and drug sale, predicted depressive symptoms and substance abuse among AI/AN adolescents (79). Not only were unsafe communities risk factor, a positive association was reported between neighborhood poverty and lifetime alcohol use, but not illicit drug use (80).

School environment

Connectedness extended to the domain of school, and school belonging was protective against substance abuse (29). Likewise, school connectedness was protective against violent perpetration among AI/AN urban youth (81) and negative emotional health outcomes (52). School safety emerged as a key issue, and an unsafe school environment to be a risk factor for substance abuse, whereas school attachment was a protective factor (82). Furthermore, a negative school environment was risk factor for substance abuse (27).

Parallel to these findings, school bonding was protective against substance abuse among AI/AN students (83). Moreover, positive feelings about school were protective against suicidality, hopelessness (30), suicide attempts (71), and substance abuse (24). Educational prevention efforts, such as anti-drug use campaigns were reported to be protective against AI/AN drug use (84). A non-parental adult role model was protective against alcohol use (28). Finally, school mentors and role models were found to be protective, whereas a lack of teacher support was a risk for AI/AN adolescent delinquent behavior (12).

Peer influence

Parallel to school environment, peer influence was highly predictive of AI/AN mental health and substance use outcomes. Specifically, peer alcohol use and peer deviance were risk factors, whereas peer support was protective against substance abuse and mental health problems (22, 23, 27, 80, 83, 85-87). First, peer encouragement of alcohol use was a risk factor for substance abuse (87). Second, peer alcohol use predicted substance abuse (22), a finding paralleled in more recent research (83). Third, peer deviance, defined as those engaging in substance abuse or who have non-negative attitudes about missing school, stealing things, picking a fight, or attacking with the intent of harm, is an additional risk factor for AI/AN adolescent substance abuse (27, 80, 83, 86, 88).

Among protective factors, discussing problems with friends, in contrast, was protective and associated with decreased levels of suicidality (23). Having prosocial peers was also protective against suicide attempts (84, 89), whereas a friend attempting suicide was a risk factor for suicide ideation (90). Finally, peer support was found to be protective against substance use and risk behavior among AI/AN adolescents (43).

Social support

Social support is protective within the general population, a finding also evident among AI/AN populations. Social support was protective against suicide attempts among AI/AN (71, 90). Furthermore, caring adults, neighbors, and tribal leaders were protective against suicidality, suicide attempts, and hopelessness for AI/AN adolescents (30, 89). Finally, adult warmth and social support is negatively associated with depressive symptoms (31, 43). Social support from peers, adults, and community members is integral, and the focus shifts now to the centrality of family for AI/AN resilience.

To summarize, among many AI/AN populations, community is especially instrumental in facilitating or impairing the resilience of their youth. It is not surprising that empirical research parallels this finding (23, 26, 79, 80). Although community support fostered prosocial behaviors and resilience (26), a lack of neighborhood safety, manifested through the presence of gangs, firearms, crime, drugs, and poverty, was a risk for depressive symptoms, substance abuse, and suicide attempts (23, 79). The school environment and peer influence were the third and fourth most frequently supported factors relating to AI/AN wellness. A positive school environment along with school connectedness and bonding were protective against negative emotional health outcomes, violent perpetration, substance abuse, suicidal thoughts and actions (29, 30, 52, 81, 83). Unsafe schools and a lack of school bonding, in contrast, were associated with substance abuse (27, 82). Education-based prevention programs were linked with less drug use (84), and school role models were protective against delinquent behaviors and substance use (12, 28).

Peers influence could be protective or a risk; peer deviance, suicide attempts, and substance use were risk factors for substance use, suicide attempts, risky behaviors, and mental health problems, whereas discussing problems with friends, peers support, were protective factors (22, 23, 27, 43, 80, 83, 85-90). Parallel to the general population, social support was found to be protective against suicide attempts and depressive symptoms (31, 43, 71, 90). Peer influence clearly plays an integral role in AI/AN adolescent functioning, and bolstering individual resilience may warrant community and school based efforts.

FAMILIAL FACTORS

Family support. Family is especially instrumental to the wellness of AI/AN adolescents and youth, and the following research provides its empirical support. Family satisfaction was protective against suicide (67), and family support, caring, parental warmth and communication protect against substance use and risky behavior (28, 80, 91, 92). First, family communication was reported as protective against AI/AN adolescent substance abuse (28). Second, family support was found to be protective against depression (15). Discussing problems with family, as well as family connectedness were protective against suicide attempts (23). Family could have a differential effect based on gender and ethnic background.

A caring family, family attention, and parental expectations were protective against suicidality and hopeless for AI/AN adolescent girls, whereas, a caring family was protective for adolescent boys (30).

Parental warmth emerged as a protective factor in four studies (26, 31). First, maternal warmth was protective for academic success and abstaining from substance abuse (26). Second, parental warmth was protective against depressive symptoms (31). Third, parental warmth was associated with positive feelings about school, which protected against AI/AN adolescent problem drinking (24). Fourth, family caring explained 15% of the variance in emotional health outcomes among AI/AN adolescents (52). Similarly, parental attachment was protective against substance abuse (80). Coercive parent, such as yelling, and caretaker rejection, in contrast, was predictive of suicidality (53). Therefore, the quality of family relationships had measurable direct and indirect effects on behaviors related to AI/AN mental health and substance use disparities.

Positive family relationships (27) and family sanctions against drugs and alcohol were protective against substance abuse (22, 84, 93). Importantly, family sanctions against drug use had direct and indirect influence on AI/AN adolescent drug use, which differed from the Anglo sample (93). Parental disapproval of substance abuse was similarly protective (88). In a focus group study, sibling and cousin influence were found to be particularly important in the substance abuse decision-making among AI/AN youth (54). Moreover, family members could either serve as a protective or protective function against or risk function on substance abuse decisions, depending on family members' attitudes toward substance abuse (54).

Family income

Family income could also be a risk or protective factor for AI/AN mental health and substance use outcomes. For instance, in a quasi-experimental and longitudinal study, family income supplements were protective against mental health disorders (94). Family financial strain, in contrast, was a risk factor for both mental health problems and substance abuse (27, 31, 58). Parental education, which could affect family income, was protective against substance abuse among AI/AN adolescents (80, 95).

Parental mental health

Parental mental health and substance use behaviors were also relevant to AI/AN wellness. For example, parental substance abuse was identified as a risk factor for lifetime substance abuse of participants (24). Parental substance abuse was also associated with substance abuse and mental health problems, including suicidality, in other research (27, 58, 67). Having a parent with major depression also placed AI/AN adolescents at greater risk for substance abuse (24). Finally, having a family member attempt or complete suicide tended to be a risk for AI/AN adolescent mental health disorders and suicidality (67, 76, 85). Clearly, family affected AI/AN mental health and substance related outcomes based on factors, including the quality of communication, parental caring and warmth, parental expectations, norms against substance use, family income, and parental wellness.

Family trauma and stressful life events

Parallel to the influence of family, the impact of experiencing trauma and stressful life events are well-documented risk factors. Stressful life events, family violence, and experiencing trauma and abuse are well documented risk factors for mental health and substance use problems, and often, family is the context for which this trauma occurs (96). Stressful life events and adverse childhood experiences, such as having a loved one attempt suicide, having family member with substance abuse problems, experiencing abuse, unemployment, experiencing a breakup, experiencing a death/loss of a loved one, the serious injury of a family member, and being gossiped about, have been associated with mental health and substance abuse problems among AI/AN adolescents (43, 69, 70, 87, 91, 97-99).

Family violence is another major risk factor for AI/AN youth. Witnessing family violence and trauma are risk factors for substance abuse among AI/AN adolescents (56, 95, 99). Paternal violence problems were associates for youth and adolescent mental health problems (58). Experiencing violent victimization in childhood was a risk for both substance abuse and suicide attempts among AI/AN adolescents (89, 100), and perpetrating violence was a risk factor for suicide attempts among male AI/AN adolescents (101). Parallel to non-AI/AN samples, experiencing childhood physical and sexual abuse was also an overwhelming risk factor for negative outcomes including suicide attempts, substance abuse, and mental health disorders (23, 27, 52, 56, 58, 76, 82, 100).

Therefore, the relationship between family and AI/AN wellness was ubiquitous along multiple dimensions, and families, encompassing 41% of the reported risk or protective factors related to wellness, are particularly instrumental to many AI/AN communities (102). Family satisfaction, caring, warmth, support, and positive communication, were protective against depression, suicide attempts, risky behaviors, substance abuse, whereas, coercive parenting predicted suicidality (15, 24, 26, 28, 30, 52, 53, 67, 80, 91, 92). Families could also deter substance abuse by imposing sanctions or expressing their disapproval of substance use, and parents, siblings, and cousins could also increase the likelihood of substance abuse depending on their own attitudes and orientations (22, 54, 84, 88, 93). Family income and education were protective against mental health disorders; whereas financial strain could heighten the risk of substance abuse and mental health challenges (27, 31, 58, 80, 94). Family influence seemed to supersede non-family influence, and is thus an important factor for continued investigation (54). Parental mental health and substance abuse challenges were associated with substance abuse, suicidality, and mental health problems (24, 27, 58, 67, 76, 85).

Stressful life events, adverse child experiences, and family violence are all associated risk factors for substance abuse and mental health problems. Similar to non-AI/AN samples, experiencing childhood physical and sexual abuse was an ubiquitous risk factor for negative outcomes including suicide attempts, substance abuse, and mental health disorders across the life course (97, 103-105).With extended family being especially relevant to many AI/ANs (75), more information about the effects of siblings, grandparents, as well as aunts, uncles, and cousins is needed. Furthermore, contextual factors about the family environment need to be delineated, and this may be best achieved through ethnographic and qualitative inquiry (17). Finally, we shift focus to research examining risk and protective factors at the individual level.

INDIVIDUAL FACTORS

Individual lever risk factors also played a role in AI/AN mental health and substance abuse outcomes. Self-esteem and subjective wellness fostered prosocial outcomes, such as substance non-use, and was protective against suicide ideation among AI/AN adolescents (16, 23, 90). Low self-worth, in contrast, was a risk factor for substance abuse (76, 86). Moreover, embodying an internal locus of control was protective against suicide ideation (90). Similarly, positive perceptions about oneself and one's family were protective against mental health problems (70). Pride in one's body was also protective for emotional health (52). Embodying an academic orientation was found to be protective against AI/AN adolescent substance abuse and suicide (98). Negative views about substance use were protective against abuse (88). Associated positive affect, in contrast, was protective against violent perpetration for AI/AN youth, whereas, risk factors included substance abuse and suicidal thoughts (81, 101).

Risk factors interacted and tended exacerbate each other. Impulsivity was a risk factor for substance abuse (80). Further, substance abuse, feeling depressed, feeling life had no purpose, anxiety, antisocial behavior, and depression were risk factors for suicide attempts among AI/AN adolescents (53, 67, 71, 82, 89, 90). Finally, Substance abuse, angry feelings, delinquent behavior, and sexual activity to be risk factors for depression and health compromising behaviors, including substance abuse (15, 23, 66, 76, 85, 95, 106, 107). Therefore, mental health and substance use outcomes were simultaneously risk factors for subsequent negative outcomes; the interactions between these factors must be considered holistically.

In closing, individual factors are the well-studied among youth in the general population, and many of these are also relevant to AI/AN populations. Within this review, impulsivity, delinquent behavior, mental health problems, substance abuse, were simultaneously risk factors and negative outcomes related to each other (15, 23, 53, 67, 71, 76, 82, 85, 89, 90, 106, 107). Self-esteem, subjective wellness, an internal locus of control, positive self and family perceptions, pride in one's body, an academic orientation, and positive affect were protective factors for mental health and substance use disparities (16, 23, 52, 70, 76, 81, 86, 88, 90, 101).

DISCUSSION

This systematic review examined risk and protective factors across the societal, cultural, community, familial, and individual levels across several outcomes. Results reveal considerable overlap of risk factors across mental health outcomes. Depression and suicide, for example, share similar risk factors as substance abuse. These overlapping risk factors compound the potential for mental health service disparities related to AI/AN wellness.

Despite overlap, much of the research found significant variability in risk factors based on specific demographic information, namely gender, geographic region, and urban versus reservation dwelling populations. First, variability was consistently found by gender (22, 24, 30, 37, 52, 58, 69, 70, 76, 78, 100, 106). For instance, family sanctions against alcohol use was protective for females but not for males (22). Likewise, the risk factor of child sexual abuse was more prevalent among females (100). Clearly, gender is an important construct in the examination of risk and protective factors.

Second, although the majority of AI/AN populations reside in urban areas, almost 60% of research focused on reservation dwelling samples (13). Despite this imbalance, some research conducted research across regions and with both urban and reservation-based populations. Third, regional differences and variability among samples was consistently reported (10). Despite this variability, there was an absence of research with AI/AN populations residing in Alaska, the Southeast, and the Northeast. With variability across AI/AN populations, more research is needed from these regions.

With the majority of risk and protective factors being present at the family, community, and cultural levels, these are particularly important areas for intervention development. Moreover, additional research is needed to empirically delineate the relationship of historical oppression to AI/AN wellness to further delineate this societal factor. Research examining wellness holistically is needed to synthesize the many overlaps across factors and outcomes.

However, rather than examining resilience holistically, which is recommended for work with AI/AN populations (17, 19), the majority of research tends to use quantitative methods to examine distinct risk and protective factors in isolation and relate them to specific mental health disparities. Despite the undoubted benefit of identifying the effects of specific variables related to mental health disparities, there is first a need to establish a comprehensive understanding of how risk and protective factors are culturally defined and situated within localized contexts. Toward this aim, qualitative research (16), and in particular, ethnographic research is recommended for the study of human resilience (17). As Waller elaborated (17), important protective factors, that may not be readily apparent to researchers, are illuminated with a holistic understanding of how people appraise experiences of adversity. Without this comprehensive understanding, important mechanisms that promote or prevent resilience may be missed (20, 21).

Implications for treatment

The identified culturally specific risk and protective factors are not only important for future research to delineate in more complexity, they can inform social work interventions development. Indeed, the incorporation of family, spirituality, and community are recommended for suicide prevention and intervention development (108). Concepts, such as "mental health" are socially constructed, however, AI/AN constructions typically involve a holistic understanding of wellness, which includes body, mind, and spiritual dimensions and the balance between these dimensions (7, 8). Indeed, risk and protective factors, such as spirituality and connectedness consistently predicted mental and substance abuse outcomes for AI/AN youth. Rather than addressing risk and protective factors separately, this systematic review indicates that the balance and reciprocal interaction between factors across ecosystemic levels are important foci in developing interventions to address health inequities related to mental health and substance abuse. Bolstering protective factors and reducing risk factors within an culturally congruent ecosystemic framework is a promising approach for mitigating health disparities experienced by AI/AN youth.

In reviewing the research, a paucity of evidenced-based prevention and interventions for AI/AN youth were uncovered (109). Current available interventions for AI/AN youth span along a continuum between culturally-based and culturally relevant programs to evidenced-based programs, typically developed with non-AI/AN populations (109). Research has identified barriers to effective social work interventions in the form of underfunded health care systems, disregard for AI/AN traditional practices, and the uncritical use of evidence-based practices (EBP) (4, 37). Many interventions are used from existing EBPs, which are assumed to be culturally appropriate and superficially adapted for AI/AN populations (109). The challenge with EBPs is that traditional healing tends to be excluded from these practices, and these practices haven't included AI/AN samples (37, 110). Moreover, some AI/ANs have felt that the reliance on EBP has led to the imposition of Euro-American worldviews, which is thought to be a continued form of colonization (111). Within these interventions, lies a reported failure to integrate adequate cultural sensitivity (110, 112). Some scholars state that these interventions are internally flawed and culturally irrelevant to AI/AN youth (109). Indeed, some AI/ANs have been found to be uncomfortable with the dominance of Euro-American approaches to substance abuse treatments (111).

Culturally-based and culturally relevant prevention and interventions programs, in contrast, emerge from AI/AN worldviews, but largely lack and empirical basis (109). Indeed, one study found no manualized interventions to address the need of AI/AN youth in a culturally appropriate manner (113). Recent research documents that many AI/AN populations prefer traditional healing (111, 113, 114), and there is a growing body of work that delineates traditionally informed intervention and prevention efforts (44, 108-115). However, with the heterogeneity across AI/AN populations, preferences are variable and context specific; individuals and families preferences vary along a continuum of traditionally-based to more conventional treatments. Thus context-specific and individualized treatment options are needed. Clearly, more culturally relevant and culturally specific prevention and interventions are needed. Integrating culturally definitions of wellness and mental health and culturally relevant interventions are recommended (8).

EBTs, then, are recommended to be integrated within culturally specific and culturally relevant AI/AN social work interventions rather than the reverse, which is most commonly the case (111). Whitbeck (116) proposed a promising multi-stage model for developing evidenced based culturally specific intervention and assessment models for AI/AN populations. First, familiarity with key risk and protective factors are gained, such as those synthesized in this review (116). Second, familiarity with culturally specific research is followed by a cultural partnership with cultural experts (116). Finally, culturally specific measures and interventions are developed in partnership with AI/AN communities (116).

In closing, culturally specific risk and protective have been identified across ecosystemic levels, including the societal, cultural, community, familial, and individual levels. With family, community, and culture being especially salient to many AI/AN communities, prevention and treatment interventions should be situated within the historical context and reflect the their prominence. These factors are largely represented in the personal connections among community members. Given that almost 60% of factors identified in this review were relationship oriented, interventions that highlight the relational context are recommended. Culturally relevant, sensitive, and specific interventions, developed by and with AI/AN communities are needed to build upon identified protective factors. It is the responsibility of those aware of these factors to work cooperatively to build a system of care for the AI/AN communities, families, and individuals that ameliorate risks, and work toward uncovering and applying additional factors that bolster wellness.

REFERENCES

[1] Andrulis DP, Siddiqui NJ, Purtle JP, Duchon L. Patient Protection and Affordable Care Act of 2010: Advancing health equity for racially and ethnically diverse populations. Washington, DC: Joint Center for Political and Economic Studies, 2010.
[2] US Department of Health and Human Services, Office of Disease Prevention and Health Promotion. Healthy people 2020. URL: http://www.cdc.gov/nchs/healthy_people/hp2020.htm.
[3] Gone JP, Trimble JE. American Indian and Alaska Native mental health: Diverse perspectives on enduring disparities. Annu Rev Clin Pychol 2012;8:131-60.
[4] Sarche M, Spicer P. Poverty and health disparities for American Indian and Alaska Native children. Ann NY Acad Sci 2008;1136(1):126-36.
[5] Burnette CE, Sanders S, Butcher HK, Rand JT. A researcher's toolkit for balancing rigor with cultural sensitivity: An application with indigenous communities. Ethics Soc Welfare 2014; doi: 10.1080/17496535.2014.885987.
[6] Getty GA. The journey between Western and Indigenous research paradigms. J Transcult Nurs 2010;21(1):5-14.
[7] University of Maryland Center for School Mental Health. Promoting wellness in American Indian youth. Baltimore, MD: University Maryland Center School Mental Health, 2011.
[8] West A, Williams E, Suzukovich E, Strangeman K, Novins D. A Mental health needs assessment of urban American Indian youth and families. Am J Commun Psychol 2012 06;49(3):441-53.
[9] US Commission on Civil Rights. Native American health care disparities briefing: Executive summary. Washington, DC: US Commission Civil Rights, 2004.
[10] Alcantara C, Gone JP. Reviewing suicide in Native American communities: Situating risk and protective factors within a transactional–ecological framework. Death Stud 2007;31(5):457-77.
[11] Lane DC, Simmons J. American Indian youth substance abuse: Community-driven interventions. Mount Sinai J Med 2011;78(3):362-72.
[12] Mmari KN, Blum RW, Teufel-Shone N. What increases risk and protection for delinquent behaviors among American Indian youth? Findings from three tribal communities. Youth Society 2010;41(3):382-413.
[13] United States Census. The American Indian and Alaska Native population: 2010. URL: http://www.census.gov/prod/cen2010/briefs/c2010br-10.pdf.
[14] Centers for Disease Control. Suicide: Facts at a glance, 2012. Atlanta, GA: CDC, 2012.
[15] Barney DD. Risk and protective factors for depression and health outcomes in American Indian and Alaska Native adolescents. Wicazo Sa Rev 2001;16(1):135-50.
[16] Stumblingbear-Riddle G, Romans JS. Resilience among urban American Indian adolescents: Exploration into the role of culture, self-esteem, subjective well-being, and social support. Am Indian and Alsk Native Ment Health Res 2012;19(2):1-19.
[17] Waller MA. Resilience in ecosystemic context: Evolution of the concept. Am J Orthopsychiatry 2001;71(3):290-7.
[18] Greene RR. Risk and resilience theory: A social work perspective. In: Greene RR, ed. Human behavior theory & social work practice, 3rd ed. Piscataway, NJ: Aldine Transaction, 2009:315-434.
[19] McMahon TR, Kenyon DB, Carter JS. My culture, my family, my school, me: Identifying strengths and challenges in the lives and communities of American Indian youth. J Child Fam Stud 2013;22:694-706.
[20] Ungar M. Resilience across cultures. Br J Soc Work 2008;38:218-35.
[21] Walters KL, Simoni JM. Reconceptualizing Native women's health: An "Indigenous" stress-coping model. Am J Public Health 2002;92(4):524-24.
[22] Bates SC, Beauvais F, Trimble JE. American Indian adolescent alcohol involvement and ethnic identification. Subst Use Misuse 1997;32(14):2013-31.
[23] Borowsky IW, Resnick MD, Ireland M, Blum RW. Suicide attempts among American Indian and Alaska Native youth: risk and protective factors. Arch Pediatr Adolesc Med 1999;153(6):573.

[24] Cheadle JE, Whitbeck LB. Alcohol use trajectories and problem drinking over the course of adolescence: A study of North American indigenous youth and their caretakers. J Health Soc Behav 2011;52(2):228-45.
[25] Herman-Stahl M, Spencer DL, Duncan JE. The implications of cultural orientation for substance use among American Indians. Am Indian Alsk Native Ment Health Res 2003;11(1):46-66.
[26] LaFromboise TD, Hoyt DR, Oliver L, Whitbeck LB. Family, community, and school influences on resilience among American Indian adolescents in the upper Midwest. J Commun Psychol 2006;34(2):193-209.
[27] Yu M, Stiffman AR. Culture and environment as predictors of alcohol abuse/dependence symptoms in American Indian youths. Addict Behav 2007;32(10):2253-9.
[28] Beebe LA, Vesely SK, Oman RF, Tolma E, Aspy CB, Rodine S. Protective assets for non-use of alcohol, tobacco and other drugs among urban American Indian youth in Oklahoma. Matern Child Health J 2008;12(1):82-90.
[29] Napoli M, Marsiglia FF, Kulis S. Sense of belonging in school as a protective factor against drug abuse among Native American urban adolescents. J Soc Work Pract Addict 2003;3(2):25-41.
[30] Pharris MD, Resnick MD, Blum RW. Protecting against hopelessness and suicidality in sexually abused American Indian adolescents. J Adolesc Health 1997;21(6):400-6.
[31] Whitbeck LB, Walls ML, Johnson KD, Morrisseau AD, McDougall CM. Depressed affect and historical loss among North American indigenous adolescents. Am Indian Alsk Native Ment Health Res 2009;16(3):16.
[32] King M, Smith A, Gracey M. Indigenous health part 2: The underlying causes of the health gap. Lancet 2009;374(9683):76-85.
[33] Brave Heart MYH. Oyate Ptayela: Rebuilding the Lakota Nation through addressing historical trauma among Lakota parents. J Hum Behav Soc Environ 1999;1(1-2):109-26.
[34] Campbell CD, Evans-Campbell T. Historical trauma and Native American child development and mental health: An overview. In: Sarche MC, Spicer P, Farrell P, Fitzgerald HE, eds. American Indian children and mental health: Development, context, prevention and treatment. Santa Barbara, CA: Praeger, 2011:1-26.
[35] Duran E, Duran B, Brave Heart MYH, Yellow Horse-Davis S. Healing the American Indian soul wound. In: Danieli Y, ed. International handbook of multigenerational legacies of trauma. New York: Plenum, 1998:341-54.
[36] Gary FA. Perspectives on suicide prevention among American Indian and Alaska Native children and adolescents: A call for help. Online J Issues Nurs 2005;10(2):6.
[37] Goodkind JR, Ross-Toledo K, John S, Hall JL, Ross L, Freeland L, et al. Rebuilding trust: a community, multiagency, state, and university partnership to improve behavioral health care for American Indian Youth, their families, and communities. J Community Psychol 2011;39(4):452-77.
[38] Burnette CE. From the ground up: Indigenous women's after violence experiences with the formal service system in the United States. Br J Soc Work 2014; doi: 10.1093/bjsw/bcu013.
[39] Burnette CE. Unraveling the web of intimate partner violence (IPV) with women from one Southeastern tribe: A critical ethnography. Dissertation. Iowa City, IA: University Iowa, 2013.
[40] McCubbin H, Thompson EA, Thompson AI, Fromer JE. Stress, coping and health in families sense of coherence and resiliency. Thousand Oaks, CA: Sage, 1998.
[41] Wexler L, Moses J, Hopper K, Joule L, Garoutte J. Central role of relatedness in Alaska Native youth resilience: Preliminary themes from one site of the circumpolar indigenous pathways to adulthood (CIPA) study. Am J Commun Psychol 2013;52(3-4):393-405.
[42] Cruz MR, Sonn CC. (De)colonizing culture in community psychology: Reflections from Critical Social Science. Am J Commun Psychol 2011;47:203-14.
[43] Baldwin JA, Brown BG, Wayment HA, Nez RA, Brelsford KM. Culture and context: Buffering the relationship between stressful life events and risky behaviors in American Indian youth. Subst Use Misuse 2011;46(11):1380-94.
[44] Garrett MT, Torres-Rivera E, Brubaker M, Agahe Portman TA, Brotherton D, West-Olatunji C, et al. Crying for a vision: The Native American Sweat Lodge Ceremony as therapeutic intervention. J Couns Dev 2011;89(3):318-25.

[45] Pridemore WA. Review of the literature on risk and protective factors of offending among Native Americans. J Ethn Crim Justice 2004;2(4):45-63.
[46] Markstrom CA, Whitesell N, Galliher RV. Ethnic identity and mental health among American Indian and Alaska Native Adolescents. In: Spicer P, Farrell P, Sarche MC, Fitzgerald HE, eds. American Indian children and mental health: Development, context, prevention, and treatment. Santa Barbara, CA: Praeger, 2011:101-32.
[47] Hill DL. Relationship between sense of belonging as connectedness and suicide in American Indians. Arch Psychiatr Nurs 2009;23(1):65-74.
[48] Kulis S, Napoli M, Marsiglia FF. Ethnic pride, biculturalism, and drug use norms of urban American Indian adolescents. Soc Work Res 2002;26(2):101.
[49] Kulis S, Hodge DR, Ayers SL, Brown EF, Marsiglia FF. Spirituality and religion: Intertwined protective factors for substance use among urban American Indian youth. Am J Drug Alcohol Abuse 2012;38(5):444-9.
[50] Mohatt NV, Fok CCT, Burket R, Henry D, Allen J. Assessment of awareness of connectedness as a culturally-based protective factor for Alaska Native youth. Cult Diversity Ethn Minority Psychol 2011;17(4):444.
[51] Yeh CJ, Hunter CD, Madan-bahel A, Chiang L, Arora AK. Indigenous and interdependent perspectives of healing: Implications for counseling and research. J Couns Dev 2004;82(4):410-9.
[52] Cummins JC, Ireland M, Resnick MD, Blum RW. Correlates of physical and emotional health among Native American adolescents. J Adolesc Health 1999;24(1):38-44.
[53] Walls ML, Chapple CL, Johnson KD. Strain, emotion, and suicide among American Indian youth. Deviant Behav 2007;28(3):219-246.
[54] Waller MA, Okamoto SK, Miles BW, Hurdle DE. Resiliency factors related to substance use/resistance: Perceptions of Native adolescents of the Southwest. J Sociol Soc Welfare 2003;30(4):79-94.
[55] Oetzel J, Duran B. Intimate partner violence in American Indian and/or Alaska Native communities: A social ecological framework of determinants and interventions. Am Indian Alsk Native Ment Health Res 2004;11(3):49-68.
[56] Boyd-Ball AJ, Manson SM, Noonan C, Beals J. Traumatic events and alcohol use disorders among American Indian adolescents and young adults. J Trauma Stress 2006;19(6):937-47.
[57] Garroutte EM, Goldberg J, Beals J, Herrell R, Manson SM. Spirituality and attempted suicide among American Indians. Soc Sci Med 2003;56(7):1571-1579.
[58] Libby AM, Orton HD, Novins DK, Beals J, Manson SM. Childhood physical and sexual abuse and subsequent depressive and anxiety disorders for two American Indian tribes. Psychol Med 2005;35(3):329-40.
[59] Whitbeck LB, Adams GW, Hoyt DR, Chen X. Conceptualizing and measuring historical trauma among American Indian people. Am J Commun Psychol 2004;33(3/4):119-30.
[60] Dawson BA. Discrimination, stress, and acculturation among Dominican immigrant women. Hispanic J Behav Sci 2009;31(1):96-111.
[61] Kessler RC, Mickelson KD, Williams DR. The prevalence, distribution, and mental health correlates of perceived discrimination in the United States. J Health Soc Behav 1999;40(3):208-30.
[62] Landry LJ, Mercurio AE. Discrimination and women's mental health: The mediating role of control. Sex Roles 2009;61:192-203.
[63] Padela AI, Heisler M. The association of perceived abuse and discrimination after September 11, 2001, with psychological distress, level of happiness, and health status among Arab Americans. Res Pract 2010;100(2):284-91.
[64] Rospenda KM, Richman JA, Shannon CA. Prevalence and mental health correlates of harassment and discrimination in the workplace: Results from a national study. J Interpers Violence 2009;24:814-43.
[65] Seaton EK, Yip T. School and neighborhood contexts, perceptions of racial discrimination, and psychological well-being among African American adolescents. J Youth Adolesc 2009;38:153-63.
[66] Whitbeck LB, Hoyt DR, McMorris BJ, Chen X, Stubben JD. Perceived discrimination and early substance abuse among American Indian children. J Health Soc Behav 2001;42(4):405-24.

[67] Freedenthal S, Stiffman AR. Suicidal behavior in urban American Indian adolescents: A comparison with reservation youth in a southwestern state. Suicide Life Threat Behav 2004;34(2):160-71.

[68] Whitbeck LB, Xiaojin C, Hoyt DR, Adams GW. Discrimination, historical loss, and enculturation: Culturally specific risk and resiliency factors for alcohol abuse among American Indians. J Stud Alcohol 2004;65(4):409-18.

[69] Yoder KA, Whitbeck LB, Hoyt DR, LaFromboise T. Suicidal ideation among American Indian youths. Arch Suicide Res 2006;10(2):177-190.

[70] Fisher PA, Storck M, Bacon JG. In the eye of the beholder: Risk and Protective Factors in Rural American Indian and Caucasian Adolescents. Am J Orthopsychiatry 1999;69(3):294-304.

[71] Howard-Pitney B, LaFromboise TD, Basil M, September B, Johnson M. Psychological and social indicators of suicide ideation and suicide attempts in Zuni adolescents. J Consult Clin Psychol 1992;60(3):473.

[72] LaFromboise T, Coleman HLK, Gerton J. Psychological impact of biculturalism: Evidence and theory. Psychol Bull 1993;114(3):395-412.

[73] Oetting ER, Beauvais F. Orthogonal cultural identification theory: The cultural identification of minority adolescents. Subst Use Misuse 1991;25(S5-S6):655-85.

[74] Schinke SP, Orlandi MA, Botvin GJ, Gilchrist LD, Trimble JE, Locklear VS. Preventing substance abuse among American-Indian adolescents: A bicultural competence skills approach. J Couns Psychol 1988;35(1):87.

[75] Weaver HN. Social work with American Indian youth using the orthogonal model of cultural identification. J Contemp Hum Serv 1996;77(2):98-107.

[76] Grossman DC, Milligan BC, Deyo RA. Risk factors for suicide attempts among Navajo adolescents. Am J Public Health 1991;81(7):870-4.

[77] Wexler L, Jernigan K, Mazzotti J, Baldwin E, Griffin M, Joule L, et al. Lived challenges and getting through them: Alaska Native youth narratives as a way to understand resilience. Health Promot Pract 2014;15(1):10-7.

[78] Zitzow D, Desjarlait F. A study of suicide attempts comparing adolescents to adults on a northern plains American Indian reservation. Am Indian Alsk Native Ment Health Res 1994;4:35-69.

[79] Nails AM, Mullis RL, Mullis AK. American Indian youths' perceptions of their environment and their reports of depressive symptoms and alcohol/marijuana use. Adolescence 2009;44(176):965-78.

[80] HeavyRunner-Rioux AR, Hollist DR. Community, family, and peer influences on alcohol, marijuana, and illicit drug use among a sample of Native American youth: An analysis of predictive factors. J Ethn Subst Abuse 2010;9(4):260-83.

[81] Bearinger LH, Pettingell S, Resnick MD, Skay CL, Potthoff SJ, Eichhorn J. Violence perpetration among urban American Indian youth: Can protection offset risk? Arch Pediatr Adolesc Med 2005;159(3):270.

[82] Mackin J, Perkins T, Furrer C. The power of protection: a population-based comparison of Native and non-Native youth suicide attempters. Am Indian Alsk Native Ment Health Res 2012;19(2):20-54.

[83] Dickens DD, Dieterich SE, Henry KL, Beauvais F. School bonding as a moderator of the effect of peer influences on alcohol use among American Indian adolescents. J Stud Alcohol Drugs 2012;73(4):597.

[84] Tragesser SL, Beauvais F, Burnside M, Jumper-Thurman P. Differences in illicit drug-use rates among Oklahoma and Non-Oklahoma Indian youth. Subst Use Misuse 2010;45(13):2323-39.

[85] Manson SM, Beals J, Dick RW, Duclos C. Risk factors for suicide among Indian adolescents at a boarding school. Public Health Rep 1989;104(6):609.

[86] Radin SM, Neighbors C, Walker PS, Walker RD, Marlatt GA, Larimer M. The changing influences of self-worth and peer deviance on drinking problems in urban American Indian adolescents. Psychol Addict Behav 2006;20(2):161.

[87] Spicer P, Novins DK, Mitchell CM, Beals J. Aboriginal social organization, contemporary experience and American Indian adolescent alcohol use. J Stud Alcohol Drugs 2003;64(4):450.

[88] Chen H, Balan S, Price R. Association of contextual factors with drug use and binge drinking among white, Native American, and mixed-race adolescents in the general population. J Youth Adolesc 2012;41(11):1426-41.

[89] Chino M, Fullerton-Gleason L. Understanding suicide attempts among American Indian adolescents in New Mexico: modifiable factors related to risk and resiliency. Ethn Dis 2005;16(2):435-42.

[90] Novins DK, Beals J, Roberts RE, Manson SM. Factors associated with suicide ideation among American Indian adolescents: Does culture matter? Suicide Life Threat Behav 1999;29(4):332-46.

[91] Dick RW, Manson SM, Beals J. Alcohol use among male and female Native American adolescents: Patterns and correlates of student drinking in a boarding school. J Stud Alcohol Drugs 1993;54(2):172.

[92] Marsiglia FF, Nieri T, Stiffman AR. HIV/AIDS protective factors among urban American Indian youths. J Health Care Poor Underserved 2006;17(4):745.

[93] Swaim RC, Oetfing ER, Thurman PJ, Beauvais F, Edwards RW. American Indian adolescent drug use and socialization characteristics. A cross - cultural comparison. J Cross-Cultural Psychol 1993;24(1):53-70.

[94] Costello EJ, Erkanli A, Copeland W, Angold A. Association of family income supplements in adolescence with development of psychiatric and substance use disorders in adulthood among an American Indian population. JAMA 2010;303(19): 1954-60.

[95] O'Connell JM, Novins DK, Beals J, Whitesell N, Libby AM, Orton HD, et al. Childhood characteristics associated with stage of substance use of American Indians: Family background, traumatic experiences, and childhood behaviors. Addict Behav 2007;32(12):3142-52.

[96] Figley CCR, Kiser LLJ. Helping traumatized families, 2nd ed. New York: Routledge, 2013.

[97] Koss MP, Yuan NP, Dightman D, Prince RJ, Polacca M, Sanderson B, et al. Adverse childhood exposures and alcohol dependence among seven Native American tribes. Am J Prev Med 2003;25(3):238-44.

[98] LeMaster PL, Connell CM, Mitchell CM, Manson SM. Tobacco use among American Indian adolescents: Protective and risk factors. J Adolesc Health 2002;30(6):426-32.

[99] Whitesell NR, Beals J, Mitchell CM, Manson SM, Turner RJ, AI-SUPERPFP TEAM. Childhood exposure to adversity and risk of substance-use disorder in two American Indian populations: The meditational role of early substance use initiation. J Stud Alcohol Drugs 2009;70(6):971-81.

[100] Clark DB, Lesnick L, Hegedus AM. Traumas and other adverse life events in adolescents with alcohol abuse and dependence. J Am Acad Child Adolesc Psychiatry 1997;36(12):1744-51.

[101] Pettingell SL, Bearinger LH, Skay CL, Resnick MD, Potthoff SJ, Eichhorn J. Protecting urban American Indian young people from suicide. Am J Health Behav 2008;32(5):465-76.

[102] Weaver HN, White BJ. The Native American family circle: Roots of resiliency. J Fam Soc Work 1997;2(1):67-79.

[103] Bohn DK. Lifetime physical and sexual abuse, substance abuse, depression, and suicide attempts among Native American women. Issues Ment Health Nurs 2003;24(3):333-52.

[104] Kunitz SJ, Levy JE, McCloskey J, Gabriel KR. Alcohol dependence and domestic violence as sequelae of abuse and conduct disorder in childhood. Child Abuse Negl 1998;22(11):1079-91.

[105] Robin RW, Chester B, Rasmussen JK, Jaranson JM, Goldman D. Prevalence, characteristics, and impact of childhood sexual abuse in a Southwestern American Indian tribe. Child Abuse Negl 1997;21(8):769-87.

[106] Gilder DA, Ehlers CL. Depression symptoms associated with cannabis dependence in an adolescent American Indian community sample. Am J Addict 2012;21(6): 536-43.

[107] May PA, Van Winkle NW, Williams MB, McFeeley PJ, DeBruyn LM, Serna P. Alcohol and suicide death among American Indians of New Mexico: 1980–1998. Suicide Life Threat Behav 2002;32(3):240-55.

[108] Goldston DB, Molock SD, Whitbeck LB, Murakami JL, Zayas LH, Hall GCN. Cultural considerations in adolescent suicide prevention and psychosocial treatment. Am Psychol 2008;63(1):14-31.

[109] Yellow Horse S, Brave Heart MYH. Native American children: A review of the literature. URL: http://dshs.wa.gov/pdf/dbhr/MH/resourceguide/Nativebestpract.pdf.

[110] Echo-Hawk H. Indigenous communities and evidence building. J Psychoactive Drugs 2011;43(4):269-75.

[111] Novins DK, Aarons GA, Conti SG, Dahlke D, Daw R, Fickenscher A, et al. Use of the evidence base in substance abuse treatment programs for American Indians and Alaska Natives: pursuing quality in the crucible of practice and policy. Implement Sci 2011;6(1):63-74.

[112] BigFoot DS, Funderburk BW. Honoring children, making relatives: The cultural translation of parent-child interaction therapy for American Indian and Alaska Native families. J Psychoactive Drugs 2011;43(4):309-18.
[113] Novins DK, Boyd ML, Brotherton DT, Fickenscher A, Moore L, Spicer P. Walking on: Celebrating the journeys of Native American adolescents with substance use problems on the winding road to healing. J Psychoactive Drugs 2012;44(2):153-9.
[114] Hartmann WE, Gone JP. Incorporating traditional healing into an urban American Indian health organization: A case study of community member perspectives. J Couns Psychol 2012;59(4):542-54.
[115] Novins DK, King M, Stone LS. Developing a plan for measuring outcomes in model systems of care for American Indian and Alaska Native children and youth. Am Indian AlskNative Ment Health Res 2004;11(2):88-98.
[116] Whitbeck LB. Some guiding assumptions and a theoretical model for developing culturally specific preventions with Native American people. J Commun Psychol 2006;34(2):183-92.

In: Public Health Yearbook 2016
Editor: Joav Merrick

ISBN: 978-1-53610-947-4

Chapter 17

ASIAN AMERICAN HEALTH INEQUITIES: AN EXPLORATION OF CULTURAL AND LANGUAGE INCONGRUITY AND DISCRIMINATION IN ACCESSING AND UTILIZING THE HEALTHCARE SYSTEM

Suzie S Weng*, PhD, MSW and Warren T Wolfe, III, MSW
Department of Sociology, Anthropology, and Social Work, University of North Florida, Jacksonville, Florida, and Community Health Department, Rockingham Memorial Hospital, Harrisonburg, Virginia, US

ABSTRACT

Asian Americans face health inequalities due to many barriers that exist in accessing and utilizing services. As one of the fastest growing racial groups, Asian Americans have not been subjected to the same level of inquiry on this topic. Historical trends identifying Asian Americans as a model minority have also served to discount challenges encountered by this group, including access to health care, level of care used, and quality of care. This article will explore impediments to healthcare access and utilization with a focus on cultural and language incongruity that contribute to discrimination and mistreatment encountered by Asian Americans within the healthcare system. With the majority of Asian Americans being immigrants and the older adult group growing at a faster rate than the overall Asian-American population, cultural and linguistic factors are particularly important, especially among more recent immigrants. Using the socio-cultural framework for health service disparities, we argue that there is not one particular factor that contributes to Asian American health inequalities but rather it is the combination of the multiple levels of social structures in the context of cultural and language incongruity and discrimination. The article concludes with implications for social work at the macro, mezzo, and micro levels.

* Corresponding author: Suzie S Weng, PhD, MSW, Assistant Professor, University of North Florida, Department of Sociology, Anthropology, and Social Work, 1 UNF Drive, Jacksonville, Florida 32224, United States. E-mail: s.weng@unf.edu.

Keywords: access to services, barriers to services, service use, health challenges, marginalization, healthcare access, immigrants, refugees, older adults

INTRODUCTION

Alegria and colleagues (1) state that, "race and ethnicity do play a role in health and health care" (p. 363) and argue that inequalities are compounded by the healthcare system, accessibility to the system, suitability of treatments and providers, and the way care is provided. Health inequalities are defined as systematic differences in health access, quality, and/or outcomes due to unequal positions in society based on social categories such as race. Outright expressions of discrimination experienced by members of nondominant racial and ethnic groups may have been reduced in the last few decades as societal attitudes towards overt expressions of discrimination have shifted to become less acceptable. More subtle forms, however, are still the reality for many. The World Health Organization's Commission on Social Determinants of Health (2) concluded that health inequities are influenced by inequities in people's daily circumstances; which are influenced by inequities in social structures that consist of power, money, and resources. In general, disadvantaged status groups have poorer physical and emotional health (3). Compared to European Americans, nondominant groups have less access to care and when they do, it is often inferior (4). Nondominant racial groups also receive fewer medical procedures and poorer quality of care (5).

Asian Americans have generally been characterized as the model minority who are perceived to be wealthy and healthy; however, this does not account for variability within the numerous subgroups that of which the racial group is comprised. Many of the underlying beliefs for the myth were based on the perception that Asian Americans had fewer challenges and issues to address as compared to other groups, which served as a reason to dissuade more in-depth research into health inequities and inequality encountered by this group. The overgeneralization has also masked inequities of subgroups within the Asian-American population and contributed to a neglect of major health concerns, lack of resources, and the barriers they face (6). An examination of health inequalities is important to comprehend the causes in order to reduce them.

The many barriers Asian Americans encounter in the health and human services system have been explored and identified and can be categorized as linguistic, cultural, economic, systemic, structural, governmental, and informational (7). This article highlights linguistic and cultural incongruities between Asian Americans and mainstream society in general and the healthcare system in particular that lead to health inequalities among Asian Americans and how the incongruities influence discrimination at multiple levels of social structures that contribute to poorer physical health outcomes. In addition to overcoming barriers to healthcare access and utilization, one of the primary challenges to achieving parity in health outcomes relates to quality of care. Compared to other racial groups, Asian Americans have reported higher dissatisfaction with heath care (8). Greater levels of satisfaction with service were found to be related to higher English proficiency and trust in Western health care and no experience of discrimination or disrespect in healthcare settings (9).

The socio-cultural framework for health service disparities (SCF-HSD) is used in this article as a tool to conceptualize the interactions occurring at the societal, organizational, and individual levels that may result in health inequalities (1). SCF-HSD focuses on how all levels of social structures, combined with culture, influence treatment and community systems. A key idea inherent in this framework is the idea of cumulative disadvantage, whereupon initial weaknesses or challenges are magnified over time that result in health inequities and illness. The framework is particularly relevant for social work in its conceptualization of domains at the macro, mezzo, and micro levels. In applying the framework to this paper, we argue that there is not one particular factor that contributes to Asian American health inequalities but rather it is the accumulation of the multiple levels of social structures in the context of discrimination influenced by cultural and language incongruity.

ASIAN AMERICANS AND HEALTH

Asian Americans comprise about 5.5% of the total United States population with 61.6% being foreign born immigrants or refugees (4). While Asian Americans age 65 and older made up 3.3% of the older adult population in 2007, they are projected to account for 7.8% by 2050 (10). Many older adults are immigrants with over 30% of Chinese, Filipino, and Korean and over 40% of Vietnamese and Indians having immigrated after age 60 (11). Great heterogeneity exists within the Asian-American population with more than 60 different subgroups speaking over 100 different languages (12).

American-born and immigrant Asian Americans vary significantly in terms of experiences. Immigrants experience dramatic changes in their social environment that may affect their health. Immigrants' migration may also result in adaptation stress to the new country that could lead to negative health outcomes. Individuals who immigrate to the United States as refugees have different experiences from those who come voluntarily. In a study of Cambodian refugees, the majority reported exposure to trauma and violence pre-migration including starvation (99%), forced labor (96%), murder of family or friend (90%), and torture (54%) (13). While socioeconomic status (SES) is not strongly associated with subjective health for Asian Americans (14), immigrants tend to have lower SES than their United States born counterparts. Immigrants are disproportionately represented in low-wage and lower-skilled jobs. They are more likely to be unemployed and work in jobs that are a mismatch to their abilities and skills that may lead to negative health outcomes. These jobs often are characterized by insecure employment, long working hours, lack of paid leave, and dangerous working conditions, all of which may contribute to negative health conditions. A study found 25% of patients sought delayed care due to their need to prioritize basic needs such as food and shelter (15). Other patients who delayed help seeking may have done so due to inability to take time off work. Finally, immigrants face more acculturative stress in terms of language ability in seeking employment (16).

Health variations exist between Asian Americans and European Americans as well as among Asian-American subgroups. In general, Asian Americans are similar to European Americans in terms of disability, mortality, and morbidity (17). Asian Americans are more likely to suffer from stomach cancer and liver cancer as well as mental health problems (18). Asian Americans are less likely to have health-related information and lower self-rated health (19). While Asian Americans as a group have a smoking rate of 18%; Laotians have 92%; Vietnamese, 65%; and Cambodians, 71% (20). Hawaiians have worse birth outcomes than other subgroups (21). Pacific Islander women have lower rates of prenatal care (22). Pacific Islanders reported higher rates of mortality, stroke, cancer, cardiovascular disease, body-mass index, hypertension, diabetes, arthritis, asthma, smoking, and alcohol intake but are also more physically active (23). Hmong Americans in California experience higher incidences of cervical cancer (6). Asian Indian Americans were found to have higher incidences for liver cancer for both genders and stomach, esophageal, and cervical cancer among female California cancer registrants (24). Pacific Islanders and Filipino Americans have higher levels of type 2 diabetes (25). Native Hawaiians have double the rate of coronary artery disease (20). New immigrants in general are healthier than American-born Asian Americans but this advantage decreases with more time in the United States (26). Refugees however, on average are in poorer health (26).

IMPEDIMENTS TO HEALTH CARE ACCESS AND UTILIZATION

The SCF-HSD posits that cumulative disadvantages in multiple social structures are magnified over time. Immigrants, particularly those who are older, face numerous barriers that block them from integrating into American society. When accessing and using health services in particular, immigrants have been found to face more barriers (16). Immigrants may not possess the basic literacy or cultural skills to access, navigate, and function within the mainstream healthcare system. They may experience discrimination within the healthcare system because of their race, country of origin, language spoken, or accent when speaking English. These disadvantages and challenges are compounded over time and the SCF-HSD predicts that they will result in health inequalities. While culture, language, and discrimination are often factors that are concurrently relevant, this section examines each factor separately to distinguish the differences and explores the literature of each factor as it relates to health inequalities.

CULTURE

One's culture and their general beliefs about health and health care can contribute to health inequalities. In general, the belief that fate is in control of one's destiny is relevant for Asian Americans. Health and illness beliefs are traditionally influenced by Confucianism, Taoism, Buddhism, and Hinduism that take a holistic view of health emphasizing a balance between the mind, body, and environment. There are also different health beliefs within subgroups. For example, Laotians view health as a result of spiritual causes and seek care from healers (6). In a study of Hmong-American women and their cervical cancer screening, participants faced barriers that included fear and embarrassment; which the researchers attribute to the women's shyness about their bodies and the belief that women's bodies should be kept private (6). Koreans believe health is related to lifestyle and living situation (27). Finally, in Japanese culture, disease is not spoken about whereas Korean culture spreads the word about disease (28, 29).

Asian Americans, particularly those who are immigrants and/or older adults may be heavily influenced by their native culture when interacting with the United States healthcare system. For one, symptom presentation may differ from what healthcare providers are trained to expect. There may also be differences in recognizing what is a problem or an illness. Asian-American patients may view illnesses influenced by their native culture as well as a historical perspective of their health in the past. Other notable impediments may be expectations as they relate to treatment and when it should be pursued (30).

Previous studies have consistently found immigrants adhere to their traditional lifestyles post migration (29). Asian Americans may prefer traditional means of treatment that are culturally dictated. Yi and colleagues (28) note Western medical professionals have different approaches to health from Koreans and suggest some Korean Americans may seek other sources of care. For example, Korean Americans were found to prefer home remedies in addressing health concerns (31). For some, there may be skepticism and mistrust of Western medicine. For others, there may be a desire to complement Western medicine with culturally-based healthcare remedies such as traditional Chinese medicine. When both traditional Eastern medicine or remedies and Western medicine are used, it can cause miscommunication in healthcare settings as there may be different attributions of causality for illness and approaches to addressing the illness.

Ethnic communities as well as their social cohesiveness and network interconnectedness can be a factor in health inequalities. Immigrants, particularly those who recently migrated, become part of ethnic communities because these communities provide a safe place for adjustment to the new country. Community members are critical links to healthcare services by way of knowledge of the system, referrals to healthcare professionals, and encouragement of service utilization and retention. When community members experience or have knowledge of others experiencing poor provider behavior or discrimination, that knowledge may extend back to the community. Repeated negative contact can lead to community mistrust that can then lead to service underutilization and health inequalities. Asian Americans who live in ethnic enclaves such as Chinatowns are segregated from the mainstream and are more likely to depend on medical care within the enclaves. The availability of healthcare facilities in minority and poverty communities is limited, however. According to Williams and Jackson (32), segregated minority communities are less likely to have pharmacies adequately stocked, less likely to be referred to specialty care, and more likely to have lower-quality physicians.

Inequalities experienced by immigrants may also be related to provider factors. When treating Asian Americans, healthcare professionals may be uncertain about the patients' beliefs and backgrounds and how they may manifest in the communication of symptoms and treatment. At times, healthcare professionals may stereotype based on their own assumptions about the racial or ethnic group. They may assume the needs and requests based on their stereotype of the patient's ethnic group. Negative stereotypes can bias interaction as well as care delivery (33).

LANGUAGE

Another significant impediment to having equal outcomes for health is related to the degree to which one is fluent in English with those who are proficient typically having better communication and connectedness to healthcare systems. Speaking fair or poor English have been found to associate with mental health and physical health outcomes (14). English proficiency is also related to access to health information and services as well as experience with the healthcare system (28). Immigrants are particularly affected by linguistic barriers as it relates to health inequality. Compared to the total United States population of 9%, 44% of Hmong Americans speak English "less than very well" (34). Among Korean Americans, 75% reported speaking only Korean at home and 47% having limited English proficiency (31). Korean Americans were found to prefer Korean-speaking doctors (31) but among all physicians in the United States, only 9% represent nondominant racial and ethnic backgrounds with most providers speak only English (35).

Asian American immigrants and older adults have low literacy skills that may affect their engagement with the healthcare system and health outcomes. Studies have suggested among Chinese Americans who are more acculturated that there is a greater tendency to be able to connect with the healthcare system and report greater ease in communicating with their physicians when compared to first generation immigrants who may be less acculturated and have language barriers (36). Yi and colleagues (28) found a lack of English proficiency and ethnic-specific resources as barriers for Korean Americans to receive health information. A review of the literature found lack of knowledge about health risks related to Asian Americans who engaged in risky health behavior (37). Compared to individuals with high literacy levels, those with low literacy skills are 1.3 to 3 times more likely to have adverse health outcomes (38).

Provider and patient language barriers can lead to inequalities in service delivery and health outcomes. Language incongruity may be in the form of health professionals and patients not listening or understanding what the other is saying. One study found 27% of Asian Americans reported their doctor did not listen to what they had to say, they did not understand what their doctor said, and they did not ask the doctor any questions during their visit (39). Limited English proficiency can compromise the quality of care if healthcare professionals are not able to address patient concerns. Language discordance can also result in poorer health outcomes and patient satisfaction (40). When patients and healthcare providers differ based on culture, language, and assumptions, it may lead to an increase in misdiagnosis and/or a mismatch of services to needs. Inappropriate diagnosis or services then in turn may result in greater disease burden and differential health outcomes (1). Patients who have difficulties communicating with healthcare providers have been found to have a higher charge for testing and longer stay in the emergency room (41). Patients have attributed unfair treatment to race or language spoken when in treatment (42). Finally, language incongruity may also lead to poor adherence to treatment and impede patient-physician communication in instances requiring more regular interaction, such as in the managing of chronic illness; which can be manifested in a number of manners such as missing or not scheduling appointments.

Federal guidelines urge health care providers to have trained interpreters on staff as well as offer linguistically and culturally adapted health information. These guidelines have been met with concern and resistance because of the additional costs required and the lack of bilingual staff available (43). Non-dominant ethnic and racial communities tend to have a disproportionally low supply of multilingual service providers (44). When providers fail to meet the diverse workforce suggested by the federal government, it may lead to greater inequalities for patients with limited English proficiency. According to Derose and Baker (44), providers who are not bilingual in ethnic communities can impact service inequality. Even in situations where an interpreter is present, there is a chance that their services are not fully utilized by medical staff who may perceive greater time pressures and be unreceptive to cultural anecdotes about different meanings of words or disregard patient narratives.

Having lower English proficiency is associated with more likelihood of not having insurance (6, 31). Compared to Asian Americans born in the United States, immigrants are more likely to be uninsured (16). Within the Asian American population, 31% of Korean Americans were uninsured compared to Filipino Americans who had the most coverage with 14% uninsured; which fails to achieve parity with 12% uninsured among European Americans (45). For Asian Americans in general and immigrants specifically, lack of health insurance has been found to be a significant barrier to healthcare utilization (16). This was also confirmed by Jang and colleagues (9) among older female Korean Americans. Having health insurance has been linked to service satisfaction. For example, older Korean Americans who had health insurance were more likely to be satisfied with service (9). But for some immigrants with insurance, there will be difficulty in interpreting the coverage and benefits. Once in the physician's office, limited English proficient immigrants will also have difficulty in completing all the required forms.

DISCRIMINATION

For Asian Americans, their culture in how it manifests in health beliefs and practices, their language and accent, and simply being Asian American all contribute to their potential discrimination in American society in general and the healthcare system in particular. The SCF-HSD posits that the interaction of individual instances of discrimination, influenced by culture and language, at multiple levels of society can magnify over time to result in health inequalities. Among Asian Americans, discrimination has also been found to be linked to lower satisfaction with life, self-esteem, sense of community, and social connectedness (46). Evidence suggests experience of discrimination is underestimated at the individual level (47). This may be particularly true for Asian Americans who do not want to lose face and bring shame to the family (7). Of those that are reported, Gee and colleagues (48), found 56% of Asian Americans reported experiencing discrimination due to their nationality, race, or skin color. Other domains in which Asian Americans experience discrimination are based on their language spoken and accent when speaking English. Studies have also found discrimination of Asian Americans due to the perception that they are a perpetual foreigner who is untrustworthy (49).

Discrimination is a negative experience across subgroups. A study found after resettlement in the United States, 70% of Cambodian Americans were exposed to violence (13). In comparisons among subgroups, Filipino Americans were found to report more discrimination than Chinese Americans while Vietnamese Americans reported less than the other two subgroups (50). The main reasons for the discrimination of Filipino Americans were race, ancestry, or skin color (48). Asian Americans who have lived longer in the United States have been found to experience more racial discrimination (51). Among Chinese Americans, studies have found immigrants to report higher rates of racial discrimination compared to those born in the United States (52). This may be because immigrants do not understand dominant cultural rules, do not speak English well, or are sensitive to discrimination because of lack of prior experience (52). Increasingly, Asian Americans are facing anti-Asian violence in the form of intimidation, threats, robbery, and vandalism. South Asian Americans are particularly vulnerable to discrimination because of the terrorist attacks on September 11, 2001.

According to Williams and Mohammed (53), "because racism is deeply embedded in the culture and institutions of society, discrimination can persist in institutional structures and policies even in the context of marked declines in individual level racial prejudice and discrimination" (p. 21). Jang and colleagues (9) agreed that access to healthcare among Korean Americans, particularly newer immigrants, is influenced by structural barriers. Racial discrimination can impact health through societal structures that influence employment, education, housing, and health care access, and quality of health care by ethnicity (53). Multiple studies have found discrimination in many societal systems such as labor markets, housing, education, and criminal justice (54). Historically, Asian Americans have been denied housing, citizenship, and the right to vote. While much progress has been made in eliminating the formal sanctions against Asian Americans, many still experience discrimination in terms of employment, education, home buying, and economic opportunities.

Evidence suggests racism to be a determinant of health and a driver of ethnic inequalities (53). According to the World Health Organization (56), racism may be a significant risk factor for poor health conditions among racial and ethnic minorities. In a review of empirical research, Williams and Mohammed (53) determined a pattern of racial inequalities in a wide range of contexts and for a broad array of health outcomes that suggest various ways racism can affect health. Paradies's (55) literature review noted 62% of the studies found an association between racism and physical health outcome for oppressed racial groups.

In a national study of the healthcare system, non-dominant racial and ethnic group members have reported high incidences of being treated unequally or with disrespect by medical providers (42). According to Bloche (57), uncertainty and stereotyping are the core of the problems, because they result in incomplete information for healthcare professions to administer efficacious intervention. Evidence suggests negative stereotypes can lead to unconscious discrimination that can be translated into biases in the delivery of care (33). Experiences of unfair treatment or disrespect may be a barrier to healthcare utilization and decrease service satisfaction. According to Blanchard and Lurie (42), patients who reported being treated with disrespect are less likely to receive good care for a chronic condition, follow the doctor's advice, or return for physical exams. Among Korean Americans, those who were more likely to be satisfied with their medical service were less likely to have experienced disrespect or discrimination (9). Discrimination can come in the form of lack of culturally responsive practices that then translate into mistrust of healthcare professionals (45). Distrust in Western medical care has been found to influence healthcare use and may impact service satisfaction (42). Asian Americans have been reported as having greater mistrust of health professionals and being less likely to utilize available care (58).

Numerous studies have associated the impact of discrimination on health. In general, these studies indicate a negative effect on health outcomes, risk factors, and service utilization across racial groups (53, 55). Hate crime may be a form of discrimination in which physical harm is the result. More subtle chronic discrimination can be just as important for health. Research has shown that discrimination is associated with negative effects on physical health, lower physical functioning, less deep sleep, high blood pressure, respiratory problems, higher rates of disease, somatic complaints, lower self-rated health, increases in mortality risk, chronic conditions, hypertension, incidences of breast cancer, and obesity (53, 55, 59). Unhealthy health behaviors such as smoking, overeating, alcohol abuse, and substance abuse has also been linked to discrimination (53). Unhealthy behaviors may be due to a decrease in an individual's self-control because of the energy needed and stress involved in dealing with discrimination. Other types of health behaviors connected to discrimination involve nonparticipation in promotion of good health including diabetes management, cancer screening, and condom use (60). Finally, not seeking preventative services has been linked to discrimination (61).

Numerous studies have linked discrimination, illness, and poorer overall health among Asian Americans (46, 48, 52, 59, 62). Positive correlations were found between discrimination and cardiovascular conditions, respiratory illness, pain, chronic conditions, obesity, headaches, and diabetes (59). In a national study of Asian Americans, everyday discrimination was found to be connected to chronic conditions as well as indicators of pain, respiratory illnesses, and heart disease (48). Discrimination of older adults can increase health effects given the health vulnerabilities of the population. Language discrimination was also found to be significantly associated with health conditions, with the relationship stronger for immigrants who have lived in the United States 10 years or more. The relationship between health and discrimination has also been researched with some larger subgroups specifically. Discrimination was significantly associated with cardiovascular conditions for Filipino, Vietnamese, and Chinese Americans (48). Chronic health conditions were associated with episodic and chronic discrimination in a study of Filipino Americans (62). The authors also found a relationship between chronic and acute racial discrimination and substance use. In a study of Korean Americans, Jang and colleagues (9) found an increase in discrimination with a decrease in care satisfaction.

Evidence is mixed, however, on the relationship between length of residency in the United States and discrimination of Asian Americans. Comparing native born and immigrants, age at immigration has a great influence on health inequality (63). For one, immigrants do not have the same opportunities and resources or the social networks that shape life trajectories and health that native born Asian Americans do (63). Thus, longer residence in the United States allows immigrants to better accumulate health resources such as access to healthcare services and insurance as well as more likely to obtain health information and knowledge that may lead to better health (63). Longer residency has also been linked to a decrease in discrimination in healthcare settings (51). The decrease may be because with time, individuals are able to identify healthcare providers who are sensitive to their issues and who they can trust. Increased time in the United States also has its disadvantages in terms of health. Longer residence is connected to negative health problems and behaviors with unhealthy behaviors and lifestyles, developmental hurdles, stress accumulation in the host country, and discrimination (59, 63). The increase in discrimination prevalence may be due to increased exposure, recognition, and reporting. Longer residence is also associated with more likelihood to develop a disability, activity limitation, higher body mass index, and chronic disease morbidity (26).

In a review of the literature on racism and health by Williams and associates (64), most of the studies focused on mental health and the studies largely reported a positive association between discrimination and mental distress. In another review, self-reported racism was reported to be significantly associated with mental health outcomes in 72% of the studies among oppressed racial groups (55). Both in cross-sectional and longitudinal studies, researchers have consistently found evidence to support the association of discrimination and a variety of negative mental health outcomes (53). The association between discrimination and mental health outcomes for Asian Americans has been documented. Studies have found discrimination to associate with depressive symptoms, mental disorders, psychological distress, and anxiety (48, 50).

Among the many negative mental health outcomes associated with discrimination, stress is most explored in the literature. In general, discrimination can be a direct stressor or as a mediator to poorer physical health (53). Experience of discrimination, particularly recurring instances, can be stressful as a pathway to illness and increased risk of physical health conditions. Psychosocial stress can result in physiological responses that lead to a wide range of negative health consequences as well as morbidity and mortality (53). Researchers have suggested stressors can impact the immune, cardiovascular, and somatic systems (48). Chronic stressors can also cause wear and tear on the body that may impact premature illness and mortality and faster progression of disease. Psychosocial stress can lead to negative health outcomes through risk behaviors such as smoking and alcohol consumption (53). Chronic stressors may overwhelm people's ability to cope, which can then lead to increases in injury, disease, and psychological problems. Cumulative stressors may also erode protective resources that can increase an individual's vulnerability to physical illness (48). Finally, psychosocial stress can influence individuals' fewer interactions with healthcare systems.

DISCUSSION

When there is language discordance, patients have been found to be less likely to continue services (65). Culture and language incongruity as well as experiences of discrimination may also lead to no follow-ups, noncompliance with doctors' advice, and lower utilization of preventative care and screening procedures. All these factors may eventually result in Asian Americans withdrawing from formalized healthcare systems thus contributing to health inequalities as predicted by the SCF-HSD. Disengagement from formalized healthcare systems may result in poorer outcomes as it relates to preventing illnesses or managing ongoing health conditions that require careful monitoring. Failure to confront such issues may in turn lead to individuals presenting to the healthcare system at later dates with more advanced or complex illnesses that consequently are associated with a worsened prognosis. Goggins and Wong (66) attribute the poor survival rates for Asian-Indian and Pakistani-American females with breast cancer to later diagnosis of the disease. Research supports this concern as Asian-American women had one of the lowest rates of screening for routine care including pap smears, mammograms, and breast cancer screening (30).

Heath inequalities are preventable differences. In applying the SCF-HSD, a system-wide comprehensive approach at the macro, mezzo, and micro levels by social workers is required to address health inequality for Asian Americans. Interventions at a single level or for a single issue may still fail to reduce inequalities because the problems are multilevel as posited by the SCF-HSD. For example, Fang and Baker (6) found it is not sufficient for Hmong-American women to overcome barriers of cervical cancer screening with only the availability of health insurance. This section provides a macro, mezzo, and micro discussion of social work implications on Asian American health inequalities and concludes with implications for research.

Among a review of health inequalities theories, McCartney and associates (67) argue structural theory offers the best explanation. In support of structural theory, research has shown a reduction in health inequalities when structural inequalities have diminished through an example of a community's health improvement when they were provided with more resources (68). Access to community resources is related to power imbalances. Thus, a shifting of power and the structural imbalances in society must be a focus. Immigrant and older adult populations are vulnerable and lack the social, political, and organizational power needed to advocate for policies that will improve their health and well-being. Accordingly, social workers must take an active role promoting health policies for the benefit of the vulnerable populations in which they serve because healthcare policies greatly shape healthcare systems. Health social workers must address programmatic and policy changes at the federal, state, and local levels. Specifically related to the Asian-American population, Title VI of the Civil Rights Act of 1964 promotes language access for limited English proficiency individuals when using healthcare services but only a limited number of states have implemented a comprehensive approach (69). Lack of insurance or underinsurance may have contributed to lack of access for Asian Americans. Therefore, expansion of insurance coverage for immigrants may reduce access inequalities (16). For minority youth, healthcare policies such as State Children's Health Insurance Programs are critical in reducing access barriers (1).

Cultural theories of health inequality can also provide some insight as to how health inequalities are generated at the macro level (67). In caring for the health of groups like Asian Americans and how their health concerns are influenced by their cultural backgrounds, culturally responsive services have been suggested in the literature as a strategy to address health inequalities (70). At the systemic level, cultural responsiveness involves multilingual services and literature specific to the target populations. Greater diversity of individuals who are bicultural and bilingual within the healthcare workforce is necessary. Policymakers and practitioners must develop strategies to overcome cultural and service use barriers as well as be committed to ensuring the availability of culturally appropriate health services.

Fang and Baker (6) suggest health literacy as a strategy to reduce health inequities because early diagnosis and education are vital to improving understanding of many health problems. It is important for service providers to implement an outreach campaign to help Asian-American families to become more aware and knowledgeable about health issues so that they can recognize symptoms and find out about the availability of existing resources and services. Education can also focus on reducing the stigma of seeking services. Use of community radio, television, newspapers, newsletters, and magazines are common outlets. Development of brochures in common subgroup languages can be used. Health social workers should involve Asian-American subgroups in the campaigns to ensure cultural appropriateness of the information.

Community members should also be involved in outreach and education because it is common among Asian Americans to share information about health and find treatments by relying on social networks. Individuals with strong cultural ties depend heavily on the ethnic community for health information. Korean Americans tend to rely on Korean-specific health information (27). Studies have found that Korean Americans who do not have the necessary health information due to language or cultural barriers assign more weight on other Korean Americans' experiences (28, 29).

At the mezzo level, a more comprehensive approach by healthcare organizations can be used to address the causes of racial and ethnic inequalities along the continuum of care. Because health inequalities and inequity are national issues that affect numerous vulnerable populations, all healthcare organizations should be required to have a plan for elimination and report their progress. To address cultural appropriateness at the organizational level, diversity in leadership as well as staff and providers, including those of Asian backgrounds, should be promoted. Leaders of different backgrounds may contribute to creating policies, procedures, and settings that are more sensitive to Asian Americans. Betancourt and colleagues (70) found organizations that are invested in cultural responsiveness committed to diversity, equity, and quality.

Ethnic centers can be used to create a sense of support as well as places for Asian Americans to learn how to better integrate into dominant society. Interaction with others of similar backgrounds can help immigrants and older Asian Americans build support networks that are important for their overall wellbeing (7). Social support has been identified as a potential moderator between perceived discrimination and health. When individuals experience discrimination, they can turn to their social support to talk about feelings and challenge the validity of events, thereby reducing self-doubt and rebuild self-worth. Having social support following experience of discrimination has been linked to lower depressive symptoms (71). In times of illness, a support system can provide resources such as health care, medicine, and food. Ethnic centers may increase one's ethnic identity, which can be a moderator between perceived discrimination and health. Group identity has been found to be a significant effect on coping with discrimination (72). According to Mossakowski (50), higher levels of identity are associated with lower depressive symptoms. Finally, because language proficiency greatly affects healthcare access and service use, English can be taught at the ethnic centers. Information about the healthcare system and insurance can also be shared.

Current interventions for health inequalities are focused on the healthcare system and the patient but they also need to consider healthcare provider attitudes and biases. Communication between healthcare providers and patients is associated with health outcomes, patient satisfaction, and adherence to medical instructions (40). At the micro level, being culturally responsive in matters of health is not limited to healthcare providers but crucial for social workers as well. Client presentations of symptoms and beliefs about health may be very different from ways with which social workers are familiar. Clients may share their distrust of Western medical care or experiences of discrimination with social workers. In being culturally responsive, social workers must recognize the diversity within the Asian-American population and be respectful of the uniqueness of subgroups as well as individuals. Health social workers must be aware of their own assumptions about populations who are different from themselves in order to avoid stereotyping. To avoid being ignorant of the Asian-American population as a whole and the subgroup clients may represent, practitioners can learn about the populations prior to working with them to have a starting point and modify their ideas about the client with additional interaction.

Aratani and Cooper (69) suggested developing multilingual, multicultural, non-stigmatizing strategies in settings frequented by diverse cultural groups. Health social workers can utilize several strategies in providing Asian friendly services. To overcome the language barrier, familial interpreters should be avoided as many are children who should not be held responsible for nor be expected to understand health concerns of the family (7). Social workers in medical settings should advocate for interpretation by nonfamilial members that are more appropriate and effective. One way is through the use of bilingual and bicultural service professionals that will be helpful in the delivery of services. To address cultural beliefs related to health, practitioners could use cultural brokers who understand both western and eastern cultures (73). For immigrants and older Asian Americans, lack of transportation is a barrier to services (7). Therefore, providing transportation to and from services will increase access and service use. Another strategy to overcome transportation barriers is through the use of mobile medical units.

In general, data collection by healthcare providers should be consistent across all racial and ethnic groups for comparison purposes, including patient data related to race, ethnicity, and language. Additionally, research on Asian-American population and their health as it relates to characteristics, prevalence, utilization, and outcome must continue and expand, including data on distinct ethnic groups because of the heterogeneity within the racial group. The first step in adequate data collection is by the federal health programs and hospitals. The data will allow healthcare organizations to identify where inequalities exist and determine what the mechanisms were, and monitor the impact of inequalities interventions. Collection of adequate data is crucial to comprehending health inequality and inequity that can facilitate the breakdown of barriers and development of culturally responsive services to improve health service access, use, and quality for Asian Americans.

ACKNOWLEDGMENT

We would like to thank Jacqueline Robinson for her contributions to this paper.

REFERENCES

[1] Alegria M, Pescosolido BA, Williams S, Canino G. Culture, race/ethnicity and disparities: Fleshing out the socio-cultural framework for health services disparities. In: Pescosolido BA, Martin JK, McLeod JD, Rogers A, eds. Handbook of the sociology of health, illness, and healing. A blueprint for the 21st Century. New York: Springer, 2011: 363-82.

[2] World Health Organization Commission on Social Determinants of Health. Closing the gap in a generation: health equity through action on the social determinants of health. Accessed 2012 August 30. URL: http://whqlibdoc.who.int/publications/2008/9789241563703_eng.pdf.

[3] Alwin DF, Wray LA. A life-span developmental perspective on social status and health. J Gerontol Soc Sci 2005; 60: S7-S14.

[4] U.S. Department of Health and Human Services. Agency for Healthcare Research and Quality. Accessed 2010 May 15. URL: http://www.ahrq.gov/qual/nhdrO9/nhdrO9.pdf.

[5] Smedley BD, Stith AY, Nelson AR. Unequal treatment: Confronting racial and ethnic disparities in health care. Washington, DC: National Academies Press, 2003.

[6] Fang D, Baker J. Barriers and facilitators of cervical cancer screening among women of Hmong origin. J Health Care Poor Underserved 2013; 24(1): 540-55.
[7] Weng SS. Dimensions of informal support network development in an Asian American community in the new south: A grounded theory. Saarbrücken, Germany: Scholar's Press, 2013.
[8] Meredith LS, Siu AL. Variation and quality of self-report health data: Asians and Pacific Islanders compared with other ethnic groups. Med Care 1995; 33: 1120–31.
[9] Jang Y, Kim G, Chiriboga D. Health, healthcare utilization, and satisfaction with service: Barriers and facilitators for Older Korean Americans. Am Geriatr Soc 2005; 53: 1613-7.
[10] US Department of Health and Human Services. A statistical profile of Asian older Americans aged 65 and older. Accessed 2009 July 2. URL: http://www.aoa.gov/AoAroot/Aging_Statistics/minority_aging/Facts-on-API-Elderly2008-plain_format.aspx.
[11] Mui AC, Shibusawa T. Asian American elders in the twenty-first century: Key indicators of well-being. New York: Columbia University Press, 2008.
[12] Institute of Medicine. Unequal treatment: Confronting racial and ethnic disparities in health care. Washington, DC: IOM, 2002.
[13] Marshall GN, Schell TL, Elliott MN, Berthold SM, Chun CA. Mental health of Cambodian refugees 2 decades after resettlement in the United States. JAMA 2005; 294: 571–9.
[14] John D, de Castro A, Martin D, Duran B, Takeuchi D. Does an immigrant health paradox exist among Asian Americans? Associations of nativity and occupational class with self-rated health and mental disorders. Soc Sci Med 2012; 75: 2085-98.
[15] Diamant AL, Hays RD, Morales LS, Ford W, Calmes D, Asch S, et al. Delays and unmet need for health care among adult primary care patients in a restructured urban public health system. Am J Public Health 2004; 94: 783–9.
[16] Carrasquillo O, Carrasquillo A, Shea S. Health insurance coverage of immigrants living in the United States: Differences by citizenship status and country of origin. Am J Public Health 2000; 90: 917-23.
[17] Grant BF, Hasin DS, Stinson FS, Dawson DA, Ruan WJ, Goldstein RB, et al. Prevalence, correlates, co-morbidity, and comparative disability of DSM-IV generalized anxiety disorder in the USA: Results from the National Epidemiologic Survey on alcohol and related conditions. Psychol Med 2005; 35(12): 1747-59.
[18] Miller BA, Chu KC, Hankey BF, Ries LAG. Cancer incidence and mortality patterns among specific Asian and Pacific Islander population in the U.S. Cancer Causes Control 2008; 19: 227-56.
[19] Sorkin D, Tan AL, Hays RD, Mangione CM, Ngo-Metzger Q. Self-reported health status of Vietnamese and non-Hispanic white older adults in California. J Am Geriatr Soc 2008; 56: 1543-8.
[20] Office of Minority and Multicultural Health. The health of minorities in New Jersey, Part III. Trenton, NJ: Office Minority Multicultural Health, 2000.
[21] Singh G, Yu S. Pregnancy outcomes among Asian Americans. Am Pacif Islander J Health 1993; 1: 63–78.
[22] Le LTK, Kiely JL, Schoendorf KC. Birthweight outcomes among Asian American and Pacific islander subgroups in the United States. Int J Epidemiol 1996; 25: 973–9.
[23] Bitton A, Zaslavsky A, Ayanian J. Health risks, chronic diseases, and access to care among US Pacific Islanders. J Gen Intern Med 2010; 25: 435-40.
[24] Jain RV, Mills PL, Parikh-Patel A. Cancer incidence in the south Asian population of California 1988–2000. J Carcinog 2005; 4: 21.
[25] Grandinetti A, Kaholokula JK, Theriault AG, Mor JM, Chang HK, Waslien C. Prevalence of diabetes and glucose intolerance in an ethnically diverse rural community of Hawaii. Ethn Dis 2007; 17(2): 250–5.
[26] Frisbie WP, Cho Y, Hummer RA. Immigration and the health of Asian and Pacific Islander adults in the United States. Am J Epidemiol 2001; 153: 372–80.
[27] Pourat N, Lubben J, Wallace S, Moon A. Predictors of use of traditional Korean healers among elderly Koreans in Los Angeles. Gerontologist 1999; 39: 711–9.
[28] Yi Y, Stvilia B, Mon L. Cultural influences on seeking quality health information: An exploratory study of the Korean community. Libr Inf Sci Res 2012; 34: 45-51.

[29] Kakai H, Maskarinec G, Shumay D, Tatsumura Y, Tasaki K. Ethnic differences in choices of health information by cancer patients using complementary and alternative medicine: An exploratory study with correspondence analysis. Soc Sci Med 2003; 56: 851–62.
[30] Sohn L, Harada ND. Knowledge and use of preventive health practices among Korean women in Los Angeles county. Prev Med 2005; 41: 167-78.
[31] Asian Pacific Islander American Health Forum. Health brief: Koreans in the United States. San Francisco CA: Asian Pacific Islander Health Forum, 2006.
[32] Williams DR, Jackson PB. Social sources of racial disparities in health. Health Aff 2005; 24: 325–34.
[33] van Ryn M. Research on the provider contribution to race/ethnicity disparities in medical care. Med Care 2002; 40: I140–51.
[34] Pfeifer ME, Lee S. Hmong population, demographic, socioeconomic, and educational trends in the 2000 Census. Hmong 2000 Census Publication: data and analysis. Washington, DC: Hmong National Development, Hmong Cultural and Resource Center, 2004.
[35] Fiscell K, Franks P. Impact of patient socioeconomic status on physician profiles: a comparison of census derived and individual measures. Med Care 2001; 39: 8–14.
[36] Chun K, Chesla C, Kwan C. "So we adapt step by step": Acculturation experiences affecting diabetes management and perceived health for Chinese American immigrants. Soc Sci Med 2011; 72: 256-64.
[37] Esperat M, Inouye J, Gonzalez E, Owen D, Feng D. Health disparities among Asian Americans and Pacific Islanders. Ann Rev Nurs Res 2004; 22: 135-59.
[38] Dewalt D, Berkman N, Sheridan S, Lohr KN, Pignone M. Literacy and health outcomes: A systematic review. J Gen Intern Med 2004; 19: 1228–39.
[39] Collins KS, Hughes DL, Doty MM, Ives B, Edwards J, Tenney K. Diverse communities, common concerns: Assessing health care quality for minority Americans. New York: Commonwealth Fund, 2001.
[40] Stewar M, et al. Evidence on Patient-Doctor Communication. Cancer Prev Control 1999; 1: 25–30.
[41] Hampers L, Cha S, Gutglass D, Binns H, Krug S. Language barriers and resource utilization in a pediatric emergency department. Pediatrics 1999; 103: 1253–6.
[42] Blanchard J, Lurie N. R-E-S-P-E-C-T. Patient reports of disrespect in the healthcare setting and its impact on care. J Fam Pract 2004; 53: 721.
[43] Flores G, Laws MB, Mayo SJ, Zuckerman B, Abreu M, Medina L, et al. Errors in medical interpretation and their potential clinical consequences in pediatric encounters. Pediatrics 2003; 111: 6–14.
[44] Derose KP, Baker DW. Limited English proficiency and Latinos' use of physician services. Med Care Res Rev 2000; 57: 76–91.
[45] Lee S, Martinez G, Ma G, Hsu C, Robinson E, Bawa J. Barriers to health care access in 13 Asian American communities. Am J Health Behav 2010; 34: 21-30.
[46] Yoo HC, Lee RM. Ethnic identity and approach-type coping as moderators of the racial discrimination/well-being relation in Asian Americans. J Couns Psychol 2005; 52: 497–506.
[47] Mellor D, Bynon G, Mallor J, Cleary F, Hamilton A, Watson L. The perception of racism in ambiguous scenarios. J Ethn Migr Stud 2001; 27: 473-488.
[48] Gee GC, Spencer M, Chen J, Takeuchi D. A nationwide study of discrimination and chronic health conditions among Asian Americans. Am J Public Health 2007; 97: 1275–82.
[49] Sue DW, Bucceri J, Lin AI, Nadal KL, Torino GC. Racial microaggressions and the Asian American experience. Cultural Diversity and Ethnic Minority Psychology 2007; 13: 72–81.
[50] Mossakowski KN. Coping with perceived discrimination: Does ethnic identity protect mental health? Journal of Health and Social Behavior 2003; 44: 318–31.
[51] Goto SG, Gee GC, Takeuchi DT. Strangers still? The experience of discrimination among Chinese Americans. J Commun Psychol 2002; 32: 211–24.
[52] Ying YW, Lee PA, Tsai JL. Cultural orientation and racial discrimination: predictors of coherence in Chinese American young adults. J Commun Psychol 2000; 30: 427–42.
[53] Williams DR, Mohammed SA. Discrimination and racial disparities in health: evidence and needed research. J Behav Med 2009; 32: 20-47.

[54] Blank RM, Dabady M, Citro CF. Measuring racial discrimination. Washington, DC: National Research Council, 2004.
[55] Paradies Y. A systematic review of empirical research on self-reported racism and health. Int J Epidemiol 2006; 35: 888-901.
[56] World Health Organization. The world health report 2001 – Mental health: New understanding, new hope. Geneva: WHO, 2001.
[57] Bloche MG. Race and discretion in American medicine. Yale J Health Policy Law Ethics 2001; 1: 95-131.
[58] Quach T, Nuru-jeter A, Morris P, Allen L, Shema SJ, Winters JK, et al. Experiences and perceptions of medical discrimination among a multiethnic sample of breast cancer patients in the Greater San Francisco Bay Area, California. Am J Public Health 2012; 102: 1027-34.
[59] Yoo HC, Gee GC, Takeuchi D. Discrimination and health among Asian American immigrants: Disentangling racial from language discrimination. Soc Sci Med 2009; 68: 726–32.
[60] Ryan AM, Gee GC, Griffith D. The effects of perceived discrimination on diabetes management. J Health Care Poor Underserved 2008; 19: 149-63.
[61] Trivedi AN, Ayanian JZ. Perceived discrimination and use of preventive health services. J Gen Intern Med 2006; 21: 553–8.
[62] Gee GC, Chen J, Spencer M, See S, Kuester O, Tran D, et al. Social support as a buffer for perceived unfair treatment among Filipino Americans: Differences between San Francisco and Honolulu. Am J Public Health 2006; 96: 677–84.
[63] Lee S, Ma GX, Juon H, Martinez G, Hsu CE, Bawa J. Assessing the needs and guiding the future: Findings from the health needs assessment in 13 Asian American communities of Maryland in the United States. J Immigr Minor Health 2011; 13: 395-401.
[64] Williams D, Neighbors H, Jackson J. Racial/ethnic discrimination and health: Findings from community studies. Am J Public Health 2003; 93: 200-208.
[65] Manson AMD. Language concordance as a determinant of patient compliance and emergency room use in patients with asthma. Med Care 1988; 26: 1119–1128.
[66] Goggins W, Wong G. Cancer among Asian Indians/Pakistanis living in the United States: Low incidence and generally above average survival. Cancer Causes Control 2009; 20: 635-43.
[67] McCartney G, Collins C, Mackenzie M. What (or who) causes health inequalities: Theories, evidence, and implications? Health policy 2013; 113: 221-7.
[68] Krieger N, Rehkopf DH, Chen JT, Waterman PD, Marcelli E, Kennedy M. The fall and rise of US inequities in premature mortality: 1960–2002. PLoS Med 2008; 5(2): e46.
[69] Aratani Y, Cooper J. Racial and ethnic disparities in the continuation of community-based children's mental health services. J Behav Health Serv Res 2012; 39: 116-29.
[70] Betancourt J, Green J, Carrillo J, Park E. Cultural competence and health care disparities. Key Perspect Trends 2005; 24: 499-505.
[71] Noh S, Kaspar V. Perceived discrimination and depression: Moderating effects of coping, acculturation, and ethnic support. Am J Public Health 2003; 93: 232–8.
[72] Noh S, Beiser M, Kaspar V, Hou F, Rummens J. Perceived racial discrimination, depression, and coping: A study of Southeast Asian refugees in Canada. J Health Soc Behav 1999; 40: 192–207.
[73] Robinson J, Weng SS. Cultural broker. In: Cousins LH, Golson JG, eds. Encyclopedia of human services and diversity. Thousand Oaks, CA: Sage, 2014.

In: Public Health Yearbook 2016
Editor: Joav Merrick

ISBN: 978-1-53610-947-4

Chapter 18

KEEP THEM SO YOU CAN TEACH THEM: ALTERNATIVES TO EXCLUSIONARY DISCIPLINE

Kevin F McNeill, MSW, MPA, MA, Bruce D Friedman*, PhD and Camila Chavez, BA
Department of Business and Public Administration and Department of Social Work, California State University, Bakersfield and Dolores Huerta Foundation, Bakersfield, California, US

ABSTRACT

Exclusionary discipline (expulsion and suspension) practices to reduce undesired behaviors have been the mainstay disciplinary practice in schools. The problem is that exclusionary discipline creates a negative school climate that has negative consequences to all students, especially those receiving them, and also creates a value conflict with educational doctrine. Further, minority students are disproportionately the recipients of these exclusionary discipline practices. A comprehensive literature review revealed two possible alternatives: Restorative Justice (RJ) and Positive Behavior Interventions and Supports (PBIS). Each alternative was contrasted with the current exclusionary discipline approach. Potential outcomes as well as approaches to cultural responsive practices that address the disproportionality of high numbers of students of color were addressed. Outcomes suggest that implementation of either intervention would improve the educational climate and enhance student educational outcomes. Additionally, Peer Mediation (PM), a student-driven approach, compliments aspects of both RJ and PBIS, and may be beneficial as an ancillary to either. Preliminary results suggest substantial health benefits are associated with both PBIS and RJ. Further, replacing the punitive model with either intervention has consistently resulted in dramatic decreases in suspensions (50-80% decrease within approximately one month to a school year), and effectively addresses minority expulsion and suspension disproportionality issues. Differences in how these approaches target undesired behavior suggest that the

* Correspondence: Professor Bruce D Friedman, PhD, ACSW, CSWM, LCSW, Director, Department of Social Work, California State University Bakersfield, 25 DDH-9001 Stockdale Highway, Bakersfield, CA 93311-1022, United States. E-mail: bfriedman@csub.edu.

application of selected portions of each may be particularly effective, and is worth serious consideration.

Keywords: exclusionary discipline, suspension, expulsion, PBIS, restorative justice

INTRODUCTION

In Kern County, California, there is more than a 30% chance (1) that a student will be suspended prior to graduation. The likelihood of suspension also means that there is the potential for multiple suspensions and even expulsion since each suspension places the student academically further behind. For example, during the 2011-2012 school year, the Kern (California) Union High School District (KUHSD) averaged thirty-one suspensions per one hundred students – a rate three times the state average (1), and seven times the last recorded national average in 2006. That same year, the KUHSD expelled 2,578 students (about 7% of the approximately 37,000 student body) (2). In fact, the KUHSD has consistently led the state in suspensions and expulsions since at least 2006 (3).

These numbers are not unique to Kern County however, and approaches to discipline such as these have been utilized within public education in the United States for at least the past half a century. Beginning in the 1950s, approaches focusing on groups dynamics (4), or utilizing the concepts of Democracy and the idea of teachers correcting students' mistaken goals (5), were popularized. These approaches yielded in the 1970s to the more structured strategies of assertive discipline proposed by Canter and Canter (6), which flourished for the next two decades. Then, Curwin and Mendler (7) introduced the notion of categorizing discipline programs according to their intended focus: with obedience models focusing on rules and consequences, and responsibility models aimed at the acquisition of skills to make independent and responsible choices. Despite their differences, however, they all shared one feature: exclusionary discipline practices. Further, exclusionary discipline (i.e., suspension and expulsion) continues to be a mainstay of public education, and its use has actually increased dramatically in recent years.

However, there is a large body of research documenting both the ineffectiveness of exclusionary discipline in reducing undesired behaviors, and its association to additional negative consequences for the students receiving it, as briefly detailed below. Perhaps even more surprising is the virtual absence of any studies supporting the efficacy of its use.

Exclusionary discipline is used inappropriately

For over two decades, researchers have maintained that exclusionary practices have a place, but should only be used for the most dangerous and destructive behaviors displayed by students (8). These recommendations are not reflected in the contemporary use of suspensions and expulsions, however. In fact, Ryan, Peterson, Tetreault, and van derHagen (9) found that exclusion was frequently being used more for students leaving an assigned area and class disruptions, than for violent behaviors. "Zero Tolerance" policies were instituted in the mid-1990s in response to perceived increases in school violence and may partially account for increased implementations of suspensions and expulsions (10). Still, the use of exclusionary discipline practices for relatively minor offenses persists despite research indicating that they are ineffective, administered in a biased way, and may interfere with some student's normal development (11).

Research supporting the past use of exclusionary school-wide programs is limited. Assertive discipline used during the 1970s and 1980s, (6) was the most popular school-wide discipline approach yet subsequent studies concluded that the "evidence" for its use was either misleading, reported selectively, or altogether absent, and found no evidence of its efficacy. (12).

Exclusionary discipline is administered in a biased way

In addition, exclusionary discipline is dis-proportionally overrepresented by African American (or other students of color) students (12), students with disabilities (13), and children living below the poverty line (14), without any evidence that these groups misbehave at higher rates (15). Racial/ethnic minority students, especially, are not only more likely to receive exclusionary discipline, they are more likely to receive it for less severe actions (16).

Since the 1970s, suspension/expulsion rates have increased for all groups. Yet, while White students are 66% more likely to receive exclusionary discipline than they were 30 years ago, African American, and Latino students are 150%, and 133% more likely, respectively (17). Students with disabilities, as a group, are twice as likely to be suspended, as compared to the overall population, and students with behavioral disorders and learning disabilities are up to three times more likely (11). Achilles, McLaughlin, & Crononger. (15) found that students with attention deficit hyperactivity disorder (ADHD), who are typically served under the other health impaired (OHI) disability category, were more likely to have been suspended or expelled than students with diagnosed learning disabilities who are most likely in a special education program and protected as a result of the disability.

In terms of gender, boys are more likely to be suspended and expelled than girls (11, 14, 17). Finally, high suspension rates have also been associated with teacher perceptions of low student competence, low parental school involvement, and students' perceptions that teachers were uninterested in them (18, 19).

Exclusionary discipline is not effective

In an era of accountability, federal legislation has called for schools to use only those interventions that are research-based and proven effective. The problem is so extensive that the state Governor has signed legislation that will essentially forbid the use of exclusionary discipline, unless documentation is presented showing how other, less severe, measures have been tried and failed. Schools and school administrators assert that the use of exclusionary discipline is supported by research showing it to be effective in lowering rates of disruptive behavior or improving overall school safety. However, no such evidence exists to support these assertions that school climate is improved. To the contrary, the research consistently concludes that exclusionary discipline is linked to increases in negative outcomes for students (20) suggesting that suspensions reinforce rather than extinguish inappropriate behavior (21).

Exclusionary discipline is associated with negative impacts for students

In the long term, school suspension has been found to be a moderate-to-strong predictor of school dropout (22). This suggests that exclusionary practices have contributed to students gradually disengaging from academics and social interactions thus increasing the probability for academic failure and dropping out (23-26). About 35- 45% of students who are suspended become repeat offenders (27, 28) and suspensions are associated with increased involvement in the juvenile justice system (29). This process begins in elementary schools with the likelihood of later suspensions in middle school (30) with the likelihood that students who have been suspended three times are more will drop out of school altogether (26, 30). McCrystal, Percy, and Higgins (31) found that adults who received school exclusions reported higher levels of drug use and antisocial behavior.

Table 1 provides a summary of these and other research findings. As this table reveals, exclusionary discipline is an ineffective disciplinary strategy while being associated with many negative outcomes for students. This study explored viable alternatives.

Table 1. Selected Summary of Findings and Conclusions Made Regarding Exclusionary Discipline

Exclusionary Discipline is Administered in a Biased Way:
• Children living below the poverty line are disproportionally exposed to exclusionary practices (27, 32-34).
• Students with physical disabilities are twice as likely to be suspended compared to students without physical disabilities (14)
• Students with behavioral disorders and learning disabilities are disproportionately suspended at rates two to three times higher than for students without disabilities (11).
• Since the 1970s, rates have increased 150% for African Americans, and 133% for Latinos, but only 66% for Whites (16)
Exclusionary Discipline is Administered Inappropriately:
• Should be used only for "the most dangerous and destructive behaviors displayed by students." However, less than 1% meet this criteria (9-10)
• Over 85% for non-violent offenses (9)
Exclusionary Discipline Does Not Serve its Intended Purpose: • Does not reduce negative behaviors (20) • Does not improve school climate (21) **Exclusionary Discipline is Associated With Additional Negative Outcomes:** • Suspension may encourage inappropriate behavior (21). • Students who have been suspended are three times more likely to drop out (22) • Eight times more likely to get involved in the juvenile justice system (26) • May be used "cleanse" the school of "troublemakers" (27). **Exclusionary Discipline is Conceptually Flawed** • Does not consider student's motivation for their behavior (36) • Has no mechanism for changing student's behavior (37) • Presumes that complex student behavior problems can be addressed using simple and general approaches (36).

METHODS

A full text, keyword search of the Academic Search Premier database was used to identify alternative behavior models. Searches were also made in the LexisNexis Academic Search, as well as the Social Sciences Full Text and Social Services Abstracts databases, because of their particular relevance to Public Administration and Social Work, respectively. Additionally, a search was conducted of the Internet using the Google search engine.

Specific entry of the search terms were Suspension OR Expulsion OR Exclusionary Discipline AND Student OR Education OR School. This yielded over 180,000 articles published between 1961 and the present. Additional searches restricting keyword location to "author supplied key words," reduced the number to 9,320. The titles and abstracts of these articles were then screened for relevancy. Costs and time constraints were also factors considered. Ultimately, approximately 200 articles were chosen for review.

RESULTS

Removing a student from school, for whatever reason, is counterintuitive since it punishes a student by removing him or her from the learning environment. Additionally, research identifies that such suspensions are not a deterrent to future misbehavior. From a public viewpoint, it is better to keep students in schools. Therefore, it is important to provide alternatives models that enhance the school climate and keep students in schools. This study identified and explored two alternative behavior models - Restorative Justice (RJ), a reactive approach, and Positive Behavior Intervention and Support (PBIS), a proactive approach, both show promise for schools. Additionally, Peer Mediation, a student driven approach, was revealed to have potential as a complement to either or both RJ and PBIS, and is also summarized briefly. Table 2 presents a comparison among these models on several relevant aspects.

Restorative justice (a reactive approach)

Restorative justice is a process for repairing harm that has been done. Unlike more typical responses, which focus on punishing the offender, restorative justice emphasizes restoring a sense of well-being not only to those who were harmed, but to the individual who committed the harm and to the surrounding community members. Originating out of the indigenous cultures of New Zealand, Canada, Australia, and the American Indian and Alaskan Native (AI/AN) cultures in the United States (38). The philosophy of restorative justice focuses on when an individual does harm, there is an effect not only the victim but also on the community and the person who caused the harm. The restorative process works to repair that harm by giving the person who caused the harm an opportunity to make peace with both the victim and the encompassing community. Justice is achieved when an offender repairs the harm he or she committed against both the other person and/or the school community.

Restorative practices can change the culture of a school and greatly improve school climate. Research shows that schools who implement restorative justice programs see a lowered reliance on detention and suspension; a decline in disciplinary problems, truancy, and dropout rates; and an improvement in school climate and student attitudes (38). Although there are different RJ models (Victim-Offender Mediation, Family Group Conferencing, and Circles), each all them generally involve the same three phases.

Table 2. Comparing the Alternative Approaches to Each Other and Against the Punitive Model

	PBIS	Restorative Justice (VOM)	Peer Mediation	Punitive Model
Main Purpose	To Provide and Encourage an Environment Supportive of Positive Behaviors	To Repair Damaged Relationships	Conflict Resolution; Development of Mediation Skills	Retribution; To Punish the offender
Underlying Principal	Positive Reinforcement – Desired behaviors can be developed by rewarding them.	Victim impact, as well as perpetrator motivation and environmental consequences, are important considerations to achieve healing.	The development of good communication skills aids in negotiation and conflict resolution.	Punishment- Exposure to an unpleasant event (punishment) will result in a decrease of the undesirable behavior that precipitated the event. undesired behavior
Primary Outcomes Sought	Increase in Positive Behaviors	Return "balance" to immediate parties and surrounding area	Reduce or eliminate negative impact of conflict	Decrease in Undesired Behavior
Are Actual Outcomes Consistent with Primary Outcomes	YES – Schools have reported significant decreases in office referrals, and up to 80% fewer suspensions	YES - For Victim and Offender; reduction of suspensions 30-50%; 95% of those involved in process reported process was beneficial	*In General* YES - Difficult to measure direct impact accurately, but schools have reported up to 50% decreases in suspensions after implementation.	NO – This model has never been associated with a later decrease in undesirable behaviors
Potential Weaknesses?	PBIS requires a Multi-Year Commitment. Implementation is incremental (one level per year in most cases. Could take up to two years for students most in need of intervention. Extensive planning is also required before implementation, as well as regular follow-up.	The VOM component of RJ is not consistent with many Western viewpoints, so participants may be reluctant to volunteer. Potential for different solutions may undermine support	Peer mediation requires strong student and administrative support to have appreciable positive impact. Requires ongoing training of new peer mediators (to replace graduates)	Seeks only to alter behavior; does not address underlying causes or consider motivations for initial behavior. Removing students may create or worsen existing education-related problems.
Research Support?	YES	YES	YES	NO

The first phase involves an agreement by the affected parties to participate, and an assessment to determine if the matter is a good candidate for RJ. The second phase is the meeting itself (or, series of meetings) where under the guidance of a mediated facilitation, the victim, offender, and other affected parties work together to find a mutually acceptable resolution to the harm caused. Phase three occurs after the meeting, when the mediator conducts follow-up with both the offender and the victim to ensure that the person who caused the harm is held accountable to the agreement made by the parties (39).

This process empowers victims by giving them a voice and allowing them to hear why they were harmed by the individual. Those who caused the harm hear the consequences of their actions and how the victims were affected, which encourages them to develop empathy for the victims. In many cases, the restitution agreement is less important to victims than the opportunity to share their feelings face to face with those who caused the harm. Having direct involvement with the restitution process and plan gives the victim greater satisfaction with the outcome (40). Also, the individual who caused the harm is now far more aware of the effect of his or her behavior the victim and the larger community. The participants gain skills in conflict resolution and are made aware of their collective responsibility to any conditions that may have existed that contributed to the offender's behavior.

These practices are now being acknowledged for their transformative powers in addressing school climate and behavioral issues. These practices contribute to students' social and emotional development by teaching them valuable skills in building and repairing relationships with their classmates, teachers, family, and community. Restorative practices also keep students in school, learning, rather than removing them for suspension or expulsion

A proactive approach

Positive Behavioral Interventions and Supports (PBIS), also known as School Wide Positive Behavioral Support (SWPBS), is a universal, school-wide prevention strategy for improving behavior and school climate. PBIS uses a three-tiered public health model to create primary (school-wide), secondary (targeted) and tertiary (individual) systems of support. At the school-wide level, schools create three to five clear behavioral expectations and rules that all students and teachers know. Responses to inappropriate behavior are clearly defined, such as a teacher response – like a warning, time out, and privilege loss or parent contact – versus sending a student to the principal's office or suspension or expulsion (41).Teachers and school leaders implement a rewards system to encourage students to exhibit positive behavior and be leaders for their peers. Students receive points or token rewards for positive behavior and are recognized periodically for their success. Students who do not improve their behavior under this universal level of support receive more targeted interventions at the 2nd and 3rd level. For example, at the secondary level, students may participate in group therapy sessions or role-playing exercises. At the individual (tertiary) level, students can have an individualized behavioral functional analysis and/or receive individualized therapy (42).

The initial goals of PBIS are focused on the development and maintenance of an optimal environment for good education and positive relationships, such as increasing positive and civil social behavior, encouraging increased family engagement in schools, and improving school climate for students and staff. Long-term outcomes sought include: enduring positive changes in behavior; reduction in the need for serious disciplinary measures such as suspension and expulsion; and improvements of outcomes for all students, including those with challenging behavior and educational disabilities (43).

Positive Behavioral Interventions and Supports aims to improve school culture and climate and improve student behavior so that teachers can teach and children can learn. The principles and practices of PBIS can also be used at home and in community settings such as youth athletic teams and youth clubs (44).

Schools that have implemented PBIS have successfully reduced office referral, raised academic achievement, and improved school climate by setting clear behavioral expectations, rewarding appropriate behavior, utilizing progressive discipline, and providing individualized interventions for students with chronic behavior problems.

Peer mediation (a supplemental, student-driven approach)

While probably not appropriate as a primary intervention, peer mediation does have aspects which complement and support both PBIS and RJ. Further, the empowerment it provides to students, as well as its "student-led" focus, could be advantageous in bolstering, securing, and maintaining student support. The potential for increased positive outcomes suggest that its use warrants consideration, and we have included a brief summary of some of its key aspects.

Peer mediation is a form of conflict resolution based on integrative negotiation and mediation. Within a dispute, the sides communicate with the goal of finding a mutually satisfying solution to their disagreement while a neutral third party facilitates the resolution process (45). The salient feature of peer mediation as opposed to traditional discipline measures and other forms of conflict resolution is that, outside of the initial training and ongoing support services for students, the mediation process is entirely carried out by students and for students.

In accordance with the principles of conflict resolution, peer mediation programs start with the assumption that conflict is a natural part of life that should neither be avoided nor allowed to escalate into verbal or physical violence. Equally important is the idea that children and adolescents need a venue in which they are allowed to practically apply the conflict resolution skills they are taught. Peer mediation is intended to prevent the escalation of conflict (46). Initially mediators work in teams, observing designated school areas and responding to signs of antagonism between students as they arise. They will approach the disputants, ask if they need help, and take them aside for mediation, if the disputants agree.

Typically, the mediator generates options by encouraging both parties to brainstorm how they might resolve the problem. The mediator writes down all the solutions, marking the ones that are mutually agreed upon. The mediator then writes a contract using the solutions to which both parties agree and then sign. After a period of time the former disputants will report back to the mediator whether the contract is being upheld by both parties.

Although it is difficult to accurately determine the success of peer mediation programs, one meta-analytic review reported a 93 percent success rate, with 88 percent of the participants satisfied with the agreements (47). Students do learn and retain the knowledge of conflict resolution techniques, and those who participate in mediation, either as mediators or as disputants, benefit from the experience. One of the reasons for the success of peer mediation is the fact that it is student run. Peer mediators build a culture of positive peer pressure where the student body can begin to establish independence from adult guidance

(48). When given the opportunity, they are capable of using their own judgment to creatively solve disputes, and often their solutions are less punitive than those of adults.

Discussion

A positive school environment is healthy for the learning experience. However, current exclusionary disciplinary practices challenges that premise by removing the student from the school, decreasing instructional time (49), and contribute to the high incidence of drop-out and other types of early departure among minority students (22). Studies have revealed that only 40 percent of students disciplined more than 10 times graduate from high school, yet they are eight times more likely to be incarcerated (16). Additionally, not completing high school can have lifelong effects on employment and earning potential as well (50).

A child might miss school for many reasons, including health problems or other excused absences, unexcused absences (truancy), and exclusionary punishments (suspensions and expulsions). Regular school attendance is a predictor of academic success, and research shows that suspensions and expulsions can exacerbate student academic problems, amplify the achievement gap between low-income children and their higher income peers, and contribute to student involvement in the juvenile justice system (10).

Current approaches to discipline focus on the student, with a determination made about whether the behavior is "good" or "bad" dependent on the perceived severity of current and past actions, and the student is disciplined accordingly. Unfortunately, when the subject is discipline, the focus is overwhelmingly "bad." To avoid stigmatizing the student by a behavior incident, approaches to discipline need to be aligned to the behavior and not the student. PBIS does this by encouraging desired behaviors through reward while Restorative Justice accomplishes this through an understanding of the effects of those behaviors and subsequent provisions to repair damage and restore balance. Peer Mediation supports both of these approaches by instilling skills likely to facilitate good behavior outcomes.

A PBIS Model utilizes a system-wide tiered framework focused on the expectation, shaping, and support of agreed upon behavioral expectations. Using this framework, behaviors having positive results within the context are displayed and rewarded, with the expectation that this will reinforce and encourage desired behaviors in the future. Proactive in focus, PBIS aims primarily to prevent the occurrence of problem behaviors all together, while also having mechanisms to reduce the incidence and minimize the severity of current problem behaviors.

A Restorative Justice (RJ) framework employs a responsive regulatory approach that identifies social engagement as the key element for repairing bonds that have been broken. Using this framework, behaviors having negative results are considered in the context of understanding what happened, listening to the needs of those who have been most affected, and responding to the harm done (51). Reparations considered as part of the healing process also include a consideration of disruptions believed to have occurred to the larger community. In contrast to more traditional approaches, justice is marked by a return to homeostasis and well-being for the community as well the offender and victim.

Each intervention presented is also supported by a body of research attesting to its potential for improving important educational outcomes for students. Research also suggests that replacing the punitive model with either proposal could reasonably be expected to be followed by a dramatic decrease in suspensions rather quickly (50-80% decrease within approximately one month to a school year). There are some key differences between these models, however, and they do not promote these positive outcomes in the same way, as shown in Figure 1.

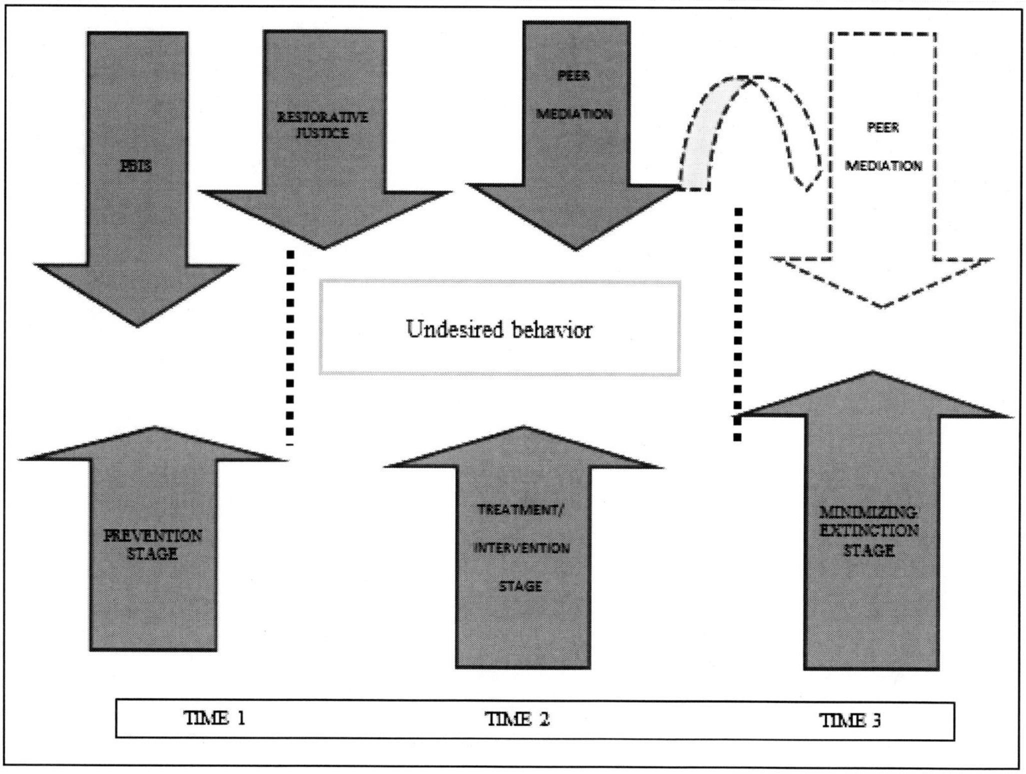

Figure 1. How PBIS, RJ, and PM target undesired behaviors.

The objective is to have an optimal school environment for learning. Each views problem behaviors (defined however they may be) as disruptive, and seeks to minimize or eliminate them. For PBIS, the best way to do that is to prevent them. A focus on the prevention of negative behaviors is admirable, but it does so at the cost of addressing those currently occurring. Additionally, full implementation can take years, when results are desired in weeks or months at most.

With Restorative Justice, this goal is best derived by bringing the affected parties together to negotiate, possibly educate, to arrive at a mutual understanding, as well as appropriate, but usually very specific, solutions. Although much benefit can be had by targeting problem behaviors, this focus may do little to address the potential origins of that behavior. No behavior, good or bad, just happens. Rather, a person exhibits a behavior in response to earlier experiences. Very few behaviors occur in isolation, so simply treating the behavior, without a consideration of why it occurred (except in that particular situation) may do little in reducing its future occurrence. By allowing the directly affecting parties discretion regarding appropriate sanctions may also raise concerns among administrators seeking equitable accountability.

Peer mediation focuses on the successful acquisition and refinement of social skills, although positive outcomes are often also a beneficial outcome of its use. Even so, switching the focus away from the behavior, and more toward the use of skills to handle the behavior could lead to resolutions that are more social and less punitive - similar to restorative justice

As shown in Figure 1, undesired behaviors can be mitigated in three primary ways: intervening before they occur to prevent them (prevention stage); intervening as they occur to treat them (treatment state); or by developing skills to minimize their impact, effectively extinguishing them (minimize/extinguish stage). It follows, then, that an intervention intended to address behavior would, ideally, have mechanisms targeting undesired behaviors at each level.

Each of the proposed interventions has the capability of independently changing a school climate – that is, PBIS, Restorative Justice, and Peer Mediation have all been used as the sole intervention, and each has successfully achieved desired goals. However, differences in how they achieve these goals suggest that each may be targeting a specific stage. For example, the PBIS approach of determining desired behaviors a priori, then seeking to manifest them through shaping and reward, gives this approach important advantages over the others at the prevention stage, Restorative Justice focuses on repairing the "harm done" rather on "harmer/harmed" sets it apart as the preferred approach at the treatment stage, while the conflict negotiation skills developed through Peer Mediation are applicable across many situations and are the best candidate to mitigate the impact of future, often unknown or undefined, negative behaviors (see Figure 1). However, it may be possible to combine aspects of these approaches, in a way that emphasizes the particular strengths of each, to arrive at a strategy worth consideration

By design, a PBIS Model is introduced incrementally (typically, one level per year, so that it takes up to three years for full implementation). Similarly, with Peer Mediation, the necessary training of student mediators prevents school-wide introduction immediately, although the lag time for this intervention is much shorter (one to three months). However, if there are mediators trained in Restorative Justice techniques already present in the community, it is possible to implement this model immediately.

This sets the stage for the following scenario: A school could simultaneously introduce Restorative Justice, and also begin Level I (School Wide) of PBIS. Since Restorative Justice seems better suited to address current manifesting problem behaviors, and PBIS better suited to focus on the prevention of those behaviors, there should be little or no chance of conflict between them. In fact, the potential exists for the two to be an especially potent combination, addressing behaviors at two keys areas. At the same time, selection and training of Peer Mediators could commence from among students who either volunteered or were otherwise identified as potential candidates. At the completion of their training, these students would make up a third aspect of this approach.

There could be two disciplinary tracts: 1) "traditional" (punitive), for major violations, actual (not perceived) threats to school safety; and chronic offenders (only after evidence that less punitive measures have consistently failed); and 2) "Alternative" (non-exclusionary) – for all others, as well as violent 1st offenders that may require an off-site location for additional protections, providing all students and/or parents agree to the process and all parties agree to be bound by terms of resolution(s). As an added incentive, a probationary component could form part of the "alternative" tract, with all record of the incident purged from the offending student's file upon successful completion. Should the same or similar behaviors be repeated, then the student would risk more punitive sanctions. Another potential advantage of this strategy is that it allows the impact of several interventions to be assessed at the same time.

Certainly, addressing undesired behaviors at multiple levels would certainly be advantageous, but limitations in funding and other resources available may not allow for such a comprehensive approach. During the process of introducing these approaches, it may become evident that one is clearly superior for a particular environment. Having mechanisms in place from multiple approaches not only allows for greater flexibility in approaching discipline, but also facilitates easier transitions when favoring one approach over another.

If adopted, and after beneficial outcomes have begun to manifest, it is possible that this approach could be adapted to facilitate better outcomes in most or all social encounters involving students. Depending on the situation, focusing on one approach over another may result in more positive outcomes overall. For example, student-student conflicts may be best served by an approach favoring restorative justice. This approach seeks redress for a specific transgression, and allows for specific, sometimes uniquely appropriate resolutions. Giving the participants greater control and latitude in resolving their dispute may also result in more commitment on the part of each. Providing a forum for perpetrators to explain reasons and motivations for committing the act, and for victims to explain the impact and other experiences resulting from it, may also have powerful benefits.

Parents seeking to improve or change their child's behavior, on the other hand, may find PBIS-type strategies are a better option. Prior to implementing PBIS, schools first make determinations and reach consensus about what actually constitutes "good" versus "not good" behavior. Parents (as well as many other entities, for that matter) can follow the same process in seeking desired behaviors from children.

Often, the most pertinent issue in negotiations between school officials and students is not the behavior that necessitated the meeting, but the actual (and perceived) difference in status between them. Students, especially, may feel that their views are not important, or that their position was not given adequate consideration in resolving a matter. The use of peer mediators, however, may help to level this perceived power imbalance, resulting in greater support for administrative decisions, higher levels of student satisfaction (regardless of outcome), and increased compliance overall to school policies.

The United States government maintains that any interventions adopted in schools should be "evidence-based" – in this case, that means that school policies regarding discipline should be based on research showing it is effective. Yet, absent in the literature are any studies lending support to the notion that the use of suspensions and expulsions relates to a subsequent reduction is student misbehavior. There is no evidence to suggest that exclusionary discipline works. There are, however, an abundance of studies attesting to its negative impacts. What is perhaps even more astonishing is the realization that, despite all this, the use of suspensions and expulsions to address student misbehavior has actually increased substantially in recent years. We can reasonably conclude that teachers, school administrators, and legislative policy makers have access to this body of research, and are aware that suspensions/expulsions lack both efficacy and support.

Therefore, current policies regarding student discipline must change. The dogmatic reliance on exclusionary discipline is archaic and contrary to the intent of education.

Although research has not revealed a "single-best" disciplinary system, it is clear that current approaches favoring harsher discipline do not reduce targeted negative behaviors, and cannot be justified by existing research. Moreover, the observed disparities suggest the possibility of unlawful discrimination. Non-exclusionary models such as PBIS and Restorative Justice are gaining support as a matter of sound general education strategy; and are worthy of serious consideration. Further, the dynamics and intended goals of peer mediation meld well with both PBIS and RJ – its potential as a viable ancillary supportive strategy should similarly be investigated.

Implications for social work practice

Teachers are trained to teach information, not control the classroom. There are multiple factors that can affect the classroom environment, and many are social conditions that are exacerbated by income inequalities. Social workers are trained to address the effects of income inequalities on the human condition, be it at the macro, mezzo, or micro levels. This suggests the need for a comprehensive relationship between social work and education to address what is happening in schools today as the social conditions are affecting the students to a point where it is difficult for a teacher to just be able to teach.

On a local level, Kern County High Schools continue to rely on suspension and expulsion as the primary means of "correcting" undesired student behavior despite abundant research documenting its lack of effectiveness. This is not unlike placing a "Band-Aid" over a wound and expecting that whatever caused the injury will magically also correct itself. This approach is superficial and short-sighted, and does nothing to address underlying causes.

Researchers in the behavioral sciences have explored many of the variables thought to impact learning and behavior in education (the individual, the peer group, the family, the "educational system" as a whole, etc.). However, most have done so by examining them as distinct entities, without much consideration regarding how one might impact another. Regarding school discipline, these approaches do not adequately account for the potential interplay among variables involved in education which may occur. Perspectives in social work, as well as the social workers who employ them, can be particularly useful in addressing these gaps.

For example, the person in environment (or PIE) perspective stipulates that behavior cannot be understood adequately without a consideration of the various aspects of that individual's environment – family, peer group, school, among others. In contrast to approaches aimed solely on changing a student's behavior, or maintaining a calm learning environment, a consideration of environmental influences provides a more comprehensive basis for determining the etiology of a student's behavior, as well as mitigating factors and/or strengths that may be used in addressing issues. In contrast to approaches considering the student and the environment, PIE (as well as systems theories like them) seeks to explain behavior from the perspective of the student within the environment.

It is important to note that students (like all people) are hardwired to learn – the ability to gain knowledge from our environment and social experiences is a core aspect of who we are as a species, and it is how we survive. Perhaps the reason exclusionary discipline is so ineffective at changing behavior is because it removes the student from the very environment where behavior change is expected. As social workers, it is incumbent on us to address this, and seek alternatives allowing the student to both focus on behavior change (where necessary) and remain in school.

ACKNOWLEDGMENTS

We wish to acknowledge and thank R. Steven Daniels, Ph.D., and Roberto Reyes, M.S. for their thoughtful comments and helpful suggestions on earlier drafts of this manuscript. Additionally, the authors gratefully acknowledge the staff at the Dolores Huerta Foundation – especially Lori DeLeon, Erika Brooks and, of course, Dolores Huerta – for their abundant provision of much needed encouragement and support.

REFERENCES

[1] US Department of Education. National and state projections, 2006 Accessed 2013 Mar 01. URL: http://ocrdata.ed.gov/Projections_2006.aspx.

[2] California Department of Education. Dataquest, 2011. Accessed 2013 Feb 11. URL: http://data1.cde.ca.gov/dataquest/Expulsion/ExpReports/StateExp.aspx?cYear=2010-11&cChoice=ExpData1&Pageno=1.

[3] California Department of Education. Dataquest, 2012. Accessed 2013 Feb 11. URL: http://data1.cde.ca.gov/dataquest/page2.asp?level=District&subject=Expulsion&submit1=Submit.

[4] Redl F, Wattenberg W. Mental hygiene in teaching; New York: Harcourt Brace World, 1951.

[5] Dreikurs, R. Character education and spiritual values in an anxious age. Boston, MA: Beacon Press, 1952.

[6] Canter L, Canter, M. Assertive discipline: A take-charge approach for today's educator. Seal Beach, CA: Lee Canter,1976.

[7] Curwin RL, Mendler AN. We repeat, let the buyer beware: A response to Canter. Educ Leadership 1989;46(6): 83.

[8] Farmer GL. Disciplinary practices and perceptions of school safety. J Soc Serv Res 1999;26(1):1–38.

[9] Ryan JB, Peterson R, Tetreault G, van der Hagen E. Reducing seclusion timeout and restraint procedures with at-risk youth. J At-Risk Issues 2007;13(1):7–12.

[10] Sundius J. Farneth M. Putting kids out of school: What's causing high suspension rates and why they are dangerous to students, schools, and communities? 2008. Accessed 2015 Feb 01. URL: http://www.acy.org/upimages/ OSI_Suspensions.pdf

[11] Skiba RJ. Special education and school discipline: A precarious balance. Behav Disord 2002;27:81–97.

[12] Render GF, Nell J, Padilla M, Krank HM. What research really shows about assertive discipline. Educ Leadership1989;46(6):72–5.

[13] Fenning P, Rose J. Overrepresentation of African American students in exclusionary discipline: The role of school policy. Urban Educ 2007;42: 536–59.

[14] Fiore TA, Reynolds KS. Analysis of discipline issues in special education research. Triangle Park, NC: Research Triangle Institute, 1996.

[15] Ruck MD, Wortley S. Racial and ethnic minority high school students' perceptions of school disciplinary practices: A look at some Canadian findings. J Youth Adolesc 2002;11:185-95.

[16] Fight Crime. Classmates not cellmates: Effective school discipline cuts crime and improves student success. Accessed 2015 Feb 01. URL: http://fightcrime.s3.amazonaws.com/wp-content/uploads/CA-School-Discipline-Report.pdf.

[17] Hayden C. Primary-age children excluded from school: A multiagency focus for concern. Child Soc 1994;8:257–73.

[18] Christle C, Nelson CM, Jolivette K. School characteristics related to the use of suspension. Educ Treat Child 2004;27:509–26.

[19] Morrison GM, D'Incau B. The web of zero-tolerance: Characteristics of students who are recommended for expulsion from school. Educ Treat Child 1997;20:316–35.

[20] American Psychological Association Zero Tolerance Task Force. Are zero tolerance policies effective in the schools? An evidentiary review and recommendations. Am Psychologist 2008;63:852-62.

[21] Tobin T, Sugai G, Colvin G. Patterns in middle school discipline records. J Emot Behav Disord 1996;4(2):82-94.

[22] Balfanz R. High poverty secondary schools and the juvenile justice system. In: Wald J, Losen DJ, eds. Deconstructing the school to prison pipeline. San Francisco, CA: Jossey-Bass, 2003:77-8.

[23] Bakken R, Kortering L. The constitutional and statutory obligation of schools to prevent students with disabilities from dropping out. Remedial Spec Educ 1999;29:360–6.

[24] Bock SJ, Tapscott KT, Savner JL. Suspension and expulsion: Effective management for students? Intervent Sch Clinic 1998;34:50–3.

[25] DeRidder LM. How suspension and expulsion contribute to dropping out. Educ Digest 1991;56(6): 44–7.

[26] Ekstrom RB, Goertz ME, Pollack JM, Rock DA. Who drops out of school and why? Findings from a national study. Teachers Coll Record 1986;87: 357–73.

[27] Bowditch C. Getting a hand on troublemakers: High school disciplinary procedures and the production of dropouts. Soc Problems 1993;40: 493–507.

[28] Costenbader VK, Markson S. School suspension: A survey of current policies and practices. NASSP Bull 1994;78:103–07.

[29] Fabelo T, Thompson MD, Plotkin M, Carmichael D, Marchbanks MP III, Booth EA. Breaking schools' rules: A statewide study of how school discipline relates to students' success and juvenile justice involvement. New York: Council State Governments Justice Center, 2011.

[30] Raffaele Mendez LM. Predictors of suspension and negative school outcomes: A longitudinal investigation. In: Wald J, Losen DJ, eds. New directions for youth development. Deconstructing the school-to-prison pipeline. San Francisco, CA: Jossey-Bass, 2003:17-34.

[31] McCrystal P, Percy A, Higgins K. Exclusion and marginalization in adolescence: The experience of school exclusion on drug use and antisocial behavior. J Youth Stud 2007;10:35–54.

[32] Achilles GM, McLaughlin MJ, Croninger RG. Sociocultural correlates of disciplinary exclusion among students with emotional, behavioral, and learning disabilities in the SEELS national dataset. J Emot Behav Disord 2007;15:33–45.

[33] Casella R. Punishing dangerousness through preventive detention: Illustrating the institutional link between school and prison. Wald J, Losen DJ, eds. New directions for youth development. Deconstructing the school-to-prison pipeline. San Francisco, CA: Jossey-Bass, 2003:55-70.

[34] Christle CC, Nelson M, Jolivette K. School characteristics related to the use of suspension. Educ Treat Child 2004;27:509-26.

[35] Sprague J, Walker H, Golly A, White K, Myers DR, Shanon T. Translating research into effective practice: The effects of a universal staff and student intervention on indicators of discipline and school safety. Educ Treat Child 2001;24:495–511.

[36] Maag JW. Behavior management: From theoretical implications to practical applications, 2nd ed. Belmont, CA: Wadsworth/Thomson Learning, 2004.

[37] McNeill KF. Recommendations for decreasing minority suspension/expulsion rates in Kern County high schools. Dissertation. Bakersfield, CA: California State University, 2013. URL: http://www.csub.edu/library/thesis/mcneill_k_pa_sp13.pdf).

[38] Graves D, Mirsky L. American Psychological Association report challenges school zero tolerance policies and recommends restorative justice. Restorative Practices E-Forum, 2007. URL: http://www.safersanerschools.org

[39] Bazemore G, Umbreit M. A comparison of four restorative justice conferencing models. Juv Justice Bull 2001; Febr:1–18.

[40] Umbreit M, Greenwood J. Guidelines for victim-sensitive victim-offender mediation: Restorative justice through dialogue. Minneapolis, MN: Center Restorative Justice Peacemaking, 2000.

[41] Horner RH, Sugai G, Smolkowski K, Eber L, Nakasato J, Todd AW. A randomized, wait-list controlled effectiveness trial assessing school-wide positive behavior support in elementary schools. J Pos Behav Intervent 2009;11:133–44.

[42] OSEP Technical Assistance Center on Positive Behavioral Interventions and Supports, Effective Schoolwide Interventions, 2009. Is school-wide positive behavior support an evidence-based practice? URL: http://www.pbis.org/research/ default.asp.
[43] Horner RH, Sugai G. School-wide positive behavior support: An alternative approach to discipline in schools. In: Bambara L, Kern L, eds. Positive behavior support. New York: Guilford, 2005:359-90.
[44] Lewis TJ, Jones SEL, Horner RH. School-wide positive behavior supports and students with emotional /behavioral disorders: Implications for prevention, identification, and intervention. Exceptionality 2010;18: 82–93.
[45] Cohen R. Students resolving conflict: Peer mediation in schools. Culver City, CA: Good Year Books, 2005.
[46] Schrumpf F, Crawford DK, Bodine RJ. Peer mediation: Conflict resolution in schools: Program guide. Chmpaign, IL: Research Press, 1997.
[47] Burrell NA, Zirbel CS, Allen M. Evaluating peer mediation outcomes in educational settings: A meta-analytic review. Conflict Resolut Quart 2003; 21:7–26. doi: 10.1002/crq.46.
[48] Sellman E. Peer mediation, school culture and sustainability. Pastoral Care Educ 2002;20:7–11. doi: 10.1111/1468-0122.00223.
[49] Centers for Disease Control and Prevention. Health risk behaviors among adolescents who do and do not attend school. United States, 1992. MMWR 1994;43(08):129-32.
[50] Heilbrunn JZ. Pieces of the truancy jigsaw: A literature review, 2007. National Center for School Engagement. URL: http://www.schoolengagement.org/Truancyprev entionRegistry/Admin/Resources/ Resources/PiecesoftheTruancyJigsawALiteratureReview.pdf.
[51] Zehr H. The little book of restorative justice. Intercourse, PA: Good, 2002.

In: Public Health Yearbook 2016
Editor: Joav Merrick
ISBN: 978-1-53610-947-4

Chapter 19

BANDAGE IT OR WRITE IT: EXPERIENCES WITH HEALTH INEQUALITIES OF HOSPITAL SOCIAL WORKERS IN TURKEY

Gonca Polat**, PhD, Lana Sue Ka'opua, PhD, MSW, Arzu I Coban, PhD and Seda Attepe, PhD

Ankara University, Faculty of Health Sciences,
Department of Social Work, Ankara, Turkey;
Myron B Thompson School of Social Work and the Cancer Research
Center of Hawaii, University of Hawaii, Honolulu, Hawaii, US;
Department of Social Work, Faculty of Health Sciences,
Baskent University, Ankara, Turkey

ABSTRACT

In the last decade Turkey has attempted to tackle health inequalities through a transformation of its health services. Objective: This paper describes the challenges of health care transformation and its reflection on health inequalities as experienced by hospital social workers in Ankara. Methods: Using a semi-structured schedule of questions, we conducted 24 in-depth interviews with social workers from nine hospitals. Interviews were transcribed verbatim and content analysis was performed to detect the impact of transformation efforts on the social work profession and the persons who they serve. Results: Findings indicate that respondents viewed disparities as persistent and emphasized continuing difficulties in health services access experienced by socioeconomically disadvantaged consumers from both urban and rural areas. Further, access was compromised by discrimination in the health care system, as experienced by persons living with HIV and other stigmatized conditions. Respondents indicated that interventions for tackling health inequalities fell into two major categories: 1) "bandage it" [the wound] or providing short-term solutions such as temporary housing and emergency financial assistance and 2) "write it" or filing reports to government agencies

* Correspondence: Gonca Polat, PhD, Ankara University Faculty of Health Sciences, Department of Social Work, Şükriye Mah. Plevne Cad. Aktaş Kavşağı No:5 Altındağ/Ankara, Türkiye. E-mail: goncapolat@ankara.edu.tr.

on patterns of patient discrimination. Discussion and Conclusion: Social workers' response to health inequalities was necessary but at the same time was perceived as ineffective to address the social determinants of health inequalities. Indicated is the need for professional advocacy to leverage a more central role for social workers in development of health care transformation policies and programs which might offer the hopeful prospect of health and well-being for all.

Keywords: content analysis, health inequalities, health care transformation, social work, Turkey

INTRODUCTION

The World Health Organization (WHO) defines health inequalities as differences in health status or in the distribution of health determinants between different groups (1). Certain models were developed in order to present the dynamics of health inequalities such as psychosocial theories, political economy of health (2) and eco-social model (3). Additionally, the Commission on Social Determinants of Health (CSDH) initiated by WHO proposed a model of social determinants of health which contains three groups of variables that effect health directly or indirectly. These are socio-economic and political context; structural determinants for individual socioeconomic position (e.g., education, income, gender, occupation, social class race/ethnicity) and intermediary determinants which point out the "underlying social stratification and, in turn, determine differences in exposure and vulnerability to health-compromising conditions" (2). As can be inferred from this model, health inequalities are closely linked with social inequalities (4) and thus, health inequalities of a country reflect the overall inequalities occurring in its socioeconomic system.

HEALTH INEQUALITIES IN TURKEY

Turkey is an upper-middle income country with Gross National Product of $789.3 Billion, as reported by the World Bank (5). The population is 75,627,384 million in the year 2012, with a population increase rate of 12% (6). As a developing nation, Turkey experienced multiple challenges associated with income and other socioeconomic disparities (7). After the economic crises of 2001, health inequalities intensified. Despite relative progress in the economy over the last 10 years, Turkey ranked 29 of 30 among countries with high rates of unequal income distribution. Within Turkey, income disparities were exacerbated by cross-regional differences (7-8) especially between eastern and western part of the country.

A closer look at inequalities burdening specific segments of the population, presents a less than optimistic picture. In comparison to other nations, Turkey experiences inequalities in child-youth and elder poverty, as well as among those who work but do not earn a living wage (9-10). For example, 29 percent of those who work fall at or below poverty line (11). The poverty of those who are disabled is not fully known due to lack of data (12).

Health inequalities in Turkey need to be considered within a historical framework. This historical view will reflect both improvements and persistent problems among the indicators of health inequalities such as data on life expectancy, infant and child mortality and health expenditures. In the 1940s, the life expectancy was 30 years for men and 33 years for women (13). However in 2012, life expectancy for women increased to 77 years, compared with 72 for men (14). Infant and child mortality is another important indicator of health inequalities. High rates of infant mortality point out lack of effective maternal and child health services and it can also be seen as a result of poverty. Turkey had a significant problem of infant and child mortality, despite its increasing economic level. In the past years, while adult mortality rates were not considerably different from similar-income countries, the life expectancy from birth were lower due to high infant and child mortality rates. In 1960's the infant mortality rate was 163%, in 1980s 121% and in 1990s 66% (13). After 2000s, with high awareness of the policy makers, it started to decrease. In 2011, Turkey succeeded in decreasing the infant mortality rate to7.7% (6). With this success, Turkey is considered as one of the few countries to accomplish the Millennium Developmental Goals on infant mortality, as set forth by United Nations Children's Fund (UNICEF) (13). In the same year, the mortality rate for children <5 years was 11.3% and maternal mortality rate was 21.2% (6).

Finally, the expenditures in health is the another indicator of the health of a particular society. Like other expenditures such as education, social services, health expenditures are lower in Turkey when compared to other OECD Countries. Total health spending accounts for 6.1% of Gross Domestic Product (GDP) in Turkey, more than three points below the average of 9.5% across OECD countries (14).

The literature on health equity and social determinants is based largely upon data collected in high-income countries. Such literature may not be directly relevant to Turkey and other middle to low income countries. Health inequalities in middle and low income countries need to be more explicitly observed. Turkish case is remarkable with the recent transformation in health policy and its consequences for health inequalities in the Country.

HEALTH CARE TRANSFORMATION IN TURKEY

Reform efforts in health care are observed beginning from 1990's in different regions of the world. According to Hurst (16), "most of the health care systems in the industrialized world cope with a common reality: they operate in a state of continuous change, striving to adjust to the economic, political, and social demands of the moment." Technological improvements in the health care sector and more awareness in health problems increased access to health care services. This in turn, raised problems in financing of health services. During the reform process, countries review their own health policy objectives, their health care institutions (16), and the finance and service provision system in health care (17). For example, in Europe reform efforts mainly included four reform themes such as roles of state and the market; decentralization of administrative and policy authority; patient rights and empowerment and role of public health (18). In the US, health care reform sought to achieve the Triple Aims of better health (improved population health with a focus on preventive health), better care (improved patient experience and quality of care), and lower costs per capita (decreasing cost by focusing on the "super utilizers" or populations with the highest risks and utilization patterns) (19-20).

Since the 1980s, the Republic of Turkey has undertaken several reform efforts aimed the structure or organization of health services delivery and ways of financing health care services. While the 1961 Constitution saw the State as the main body responsible for ensuring the right to health care and social security; the 1982 Constitution had a different perspective for health care, seeing the responsibility of health as residing with individuals, as well as the State. The 1982 Constitution functioned to reduce the responsibility of the State to one of monitoring the public and private health care institutions. Another important aspect in 1982 Constitution was articulation of General Health Insurance and Contributions for the first time. This paradigm shift in health policy was also included in Seventh (1996-2000) and Eighth (2001-2005) Development Plans (21-22).

In 2003, with the awareness of growing problems in access, quality and standardization of health services, the Government planned and implemented the "Transformation in Health." It is also possible to claim that this transformation cannot be considered apart from the international trends, including the World Health Organization's policy of Health for All in the 21st Century, as well as the Accession Partnership document prepared by the EU (23).

The main components of the transformation included the re-organization of health services especially in the primary level health care (family practitioners), General Health Insurance system (a worker and premium payment-based, mostly individualized insurance system), promoting the privatization of health insurance system and a performance based, for-profit system of management at health care institutions (21, 24-25). In terms of insurance system, the program included a transition from a system of multiple insurance schemes that cover only about two-thirds of the population to a single-payer system aiming to achieve universal coverage (26).

With the transformation, one goal as stated by the Government was, "accessible, high quality health care services spread across the Country" (27). Thus, the transformation was a step to reduce the observed inequalities in accessible and high quality health services.

The research on the results of transformation is still far from giving a clear picture of the consequences. Some research indicated positive outcomes of increased access to treatment and medication (28-29); while other research reported negative outcomes on service quality and health care workers' rights (25 p16, 30-32). An empirical analysis of transformation indicated that while the general population sees positive results, efforts have not adequately addressed health inequities (22).

SOCIAL WORK AND HEALTH CARE

As a part of the health care system, social workers in hospitals and clinics were able to directly observe the effects of transformation on real people. That is, by being on the front line, social workers were able to observe the need for reforms, as well as results of reform efforts. Taking a role in service provision, they carry the reform from rhetoric to practice. Social workers are also affected by the reform processes. How social workers function in the hospital settings or in other areas of practices are determined by the content of the reforms and transformations in the health care policies (19).

Within the health care system, the problems of persistent health inequalities are the central focus for social workers. Health inequalities are considered a critical area of human rights practice and thus directly related to the responsibility of social workers to promote social and economic justice for all people, with an emphasis on addressing persistent poverty (33-37). Activities aim to reduce health inequalities contain both policy level and practice level efforts in which social workers take an active role. Social Work's response to health inequalities should not be, as stated by Backwith and Mantle (38) "behaviorally or individually oriented," rather, a public health approach should be employed. Because, "(t)he systematic occurrence of health inequalities is a product of the social determinants of health: they are generated by structural inequalities which are best addressed at a collective, rather than individual, level" (38).

Social workers have direct and indirect impact on reducing health inequalities. Bywaters emphasized their direct roles in providing the resources necessary for supporting health and helping people to manage illness as well as their indirect roles in enabling service users to access health care services or health services to reach disadvantaged populations more effectively and efficiently. Also, social workers have an impact on actions taken to address the social determinants of health (36). Therefore, the perspective of social workers working in hospital settings should include micro to macro levels of intervention.

The efforts to tackle health inequalities were generally grouped in two directions as downstream and upstream interventions. Downstream interventions were described as the interventions which aim to tackle the effects of inequalities characterized by a range of measures of death or ill-health (39). In other words, these interventions mainly target a change in the results or causes of ill-health mostly at individual level. Therefore social workers may take an active role in raising awareness for individual's own health, promote healthy life style, or to meet the individual with the health service so that the results of ill-health would be overcome. The action social workers take in order to increase the access of health services for the general population is another example of these downstream interventions.

Upstream interventions, however, aim to tackle the underlying causes of inequality: the structural and social determinants of health which include poverty, discrimination, unemployment, educational achievement and poor housing (39). These interventions may take place inside or outside of the hospital setting and targets to reduce general inequalities in the society as well as the ill-health.

Objectives

Through in-depth interviews, we sought to obtain a description of the challenges of health care reform from the perspective of hospital social workers in Ankara, Turkey. Of particular interest were challenges social workers experienced in assisting and advocating for persons who are exposed to health inequalities.

METHODS

Through in-depth interviews with hospital social workers we aimed to obtain a rich description of two phenomena namely, the ways in which health inequalities are experienced by persons presenting in hospitals and clinics of Ankara, Turkey and the ways in which social workers intervene in cases involving health inequalities.

Participants

The final sample was comprised of 24 social workers. Participants were employed in a variety of departments and service units associated with State and university medical centers located in Ankara. We used a convenience sample with participants drawn from the capital city of Ankara where is located in the central Turkey and receives many patients from all regions of Turkey.

In the year 2011, the total number of hospitals in Ankara was 73; 35 of them were under the Ministry of Health (public hospital), 9 of them were University hospitals and 29 were Private hospitals (40).

The participants were determined according to purposeful sampling strategy, based on the hospital types. It is believed that social workers' experiences and perceptions are closely related to the roles and tasks they undertake in different hospital types. We sought to recruit practitioners from all types of hospitals including University/research, general and specialty care hospitals. The hospitals in the sample reflected all hospital types in Ankara. The first type of hospitals as University and specialty (e.g., Veterans hospital) hospitals, are accepted as tertiary level of health care institutions where education and research is the aim behind the services given to general population or certain groups such as veterans or drug and alcohol addicted patients. General hospitals are accepted as secondary care institutions which are more accessible for general public.

We received the informed consent of all participants. We conducted in-depth interviews with 24 social workers at total. 18 social workers were female while 6 of them were male. Their ages ranged from 28 to 48 with a mean age of 38. Additional participant characteristics are displayed in Table 1.

Procedures

The researchers determined the hospitals from which to elicit social workers' participation. During this process, we sought to include all possible types of hospitals. Upon determining the facilities, researchers made telephone contacts with social workers. Social workers were informed about the research content and asked whether they would like to participate or not. The main aims of the research, privacy of the personal and research data, the length of possible interviews were explained during the telephone calls. Two of the social workers declined participation due to time constraints. Social workers agreed to participate were given an appointment at a time and place convenient to them. Without exception, social workers chose to meet in their office or in a quiet place close to the site of their employment

Interviews were conducted by six researchers; three of the authors and three post graduate students. All interviewers had successfully completed a doctoral level qualitative research course, had experiences in qualitative data collection, and received pre-interview training and ongoing supervision from the principal investigator. The consent of the social workers for participating the research was taken individually. Consent for digital recording was specifically sought.

Table 1. Descriptive characteristics of participants

Sample Characteristic	N	%
Gender		
Female	18	75
Male	6	25
Total	24	100
Age		
Minimum	26	
Maximum	48	
Mean	38,04	
Std Deviation	6,708	
Health Social Work Experience		
Minimum	3 years	
Maximum	32 years	
Mean	11.7	
Std Deviation	7.086	
Hospital Types		
State	11	45.9
University-affiliated	8	33.3
Specialized (tertiary) state facility	3	12.5
Veterans	2	8.3

After obtaining consent, the interviews were conducted using a semi-structured interview guide (see appendix 2). Interviews lasted between 60-90 minutes.

Digitally-recorded and noted interviews were transcribed verbatim by the interviewers as soon as the interview has been conducted. Data analysis was performed manually, using Word Processor (Microsoft Office Word 2010). Researchers followed the undermentioned stages in the analysis process: Stage 1.Researcher completed the interview, filled out the observation form; Stage 2. Researcher transcribed the digitally recorded interview; Stage 3. Researcher reviewed his/her own transcribed material and made open-coding (line-by-line coding); Stage 4. Second researcher read all the transcribed material and the initial codes given by the interviewers. Using a deductive approach to data analysis, the researcher determined the themes in accordance with the interview guide; Stage 5. The themes determined were constantly compared for each interview script in terms of similarities and differences; Stage 6. Coding system of headings and categories were developed; Stage 7. Two experienced researchers in the team reviewed the system of headings and categories and Stage 8. The findings were written according to the determined themes and categories. The narratives were used for presenting the results.

Measures: Semi-structured interview

The topics in the interview guide were grouped in three headings: 1) the demographic information and the roles undertaken at the hospital, 2) discussion of the concept of health inequalities 3). How do they challenge and how they function about health inequalities?

RESULTS

In the background of the conceptualizations of health inequalities, we realized the discussion on the health care transformation in Turkey. This transformation seemed to be reflected on social work practice in health. While participants define health inequalities, they somehow made reference to health care transformation. All of the participants stressed these transformations at the core of health inequalities. Some of them saw transformation as having negative effect on health inequalities, 8 participants importantly stressed its positive outcome in increasing the access to health care. However all of them also pointed out the contradictory results in quality of health services. The negative reflections of the health care transformation according to the participants can be summarized as:

- The negative effect of performance-based system on medical examination and treatment period;
- Increased rate of privatization and limitation of access to good quality health care services for the poor;
- Contributing costs and the changing perception of health services as a purchasable right.

Besides the transformation, we observed a changing pattern in social workers' roles and responsibilities in the hospitals. The client profile changes according to the hospital type they work. For example, participants working at the social service units encounter primarily, "economically deprived, unable to pay the treatment costs, aged, homeless patients." Patients coming from other cities and have difficulties in accommodation during treatment often referred to social service units.

> When we look at the client profile…I can say that patients from all over the country come here. (…) poverty and lack of education is very common among patients. (Participant No:2, University Hospital Social Worker)

> Patients who are unaccompanied, aged, disabled, homeless, uninsured patients...these days, patients from other cities, refugees… (Participant No: 20, State Hospital Social Worker).

Participants explain their roles at the hospital and generally stress two basic functions. The first area of functioning is termed as "routine work" (e.g., providing socio-economic support for the patients who could not afford cost of treatment, providing accommodation and/or travel allowance, placement of homeless and unaccompanied patients to social service agencies). In this framework several routine channels already are established with certain agencies and standard documents are being used.

> I am responsible for meeting all kind of needs of patients. Financial support, recreational activities, accommodation support, etc. (Participant No:6, State Hospital Social Worker).

> We sometimes help patients out of town and arrange accommodation to them but this kind of intervention is a short term one. We use the resources of municipalities. Other than that, we make placements to social service agencies. Preparing documents of the patients and arrange the health reports of them, make assessment of the client, referral... (Participant No:5, State Hospital Social Worker).

This routine work is often described as "administrative," "involving non-social work tasks," "routine tasks," "paper work," "compulsory work."

Social workers' second function is stressed as "real social work" and includes assessment-based interventions involving emotional and informational support, as well as some tangible assistance. Participants describe the role dichotomy of "non-social work" and "real social work" in terms both explicit and implied. A few participants express different perspective and complain that their work centered on referral work, which they do not consider "social work":

> Some of our colleagues don't think that their work is related with financial support! I think this is some kind of arrogance. Essentially, patients with green card have multiple problems. They are mistreated, have language difficulties, don't know anybody, maybe come to Ankara for the first time in their life... 'eee,' what do I do? I don't make a financial assessment only, I tell them their rights...For example I say, "You can apply to this place for a job if he is unemployed or apply that place for support for rent. Well then, isn't that social work? (Participant No: 3, University Hospital Social Worker).

Health inequalities: "The fact of my country!"

The following definition (41) of health inequality was read to participants at the beginning of this section of interviews:

> "Health inequality can defined as any health differences between social groups, which are avoidable and preventable and thus, unjust and unacceptable. This inequality can be observed in two areas; the health state and the access and use of health care services"

Participants were asked to express their perspective on this definition. Most of them view health inequalities as an important problem in the Turkish context. One of the participants explains this inequality "as the fact of the country," with socioeconomic determinants reflected in health inequalities as well as in other areas such as education:

> In many fields we experience this inequality. In terms of the conditions, opportunities, access to services, it brings to my mind the fact of my country! The economic conditions of the people, social conditions, the environment they live...all of

> them are important indicators of how healthy they are. If you have money, if you are well-educated, if you are able to make yourself understood and have your rights, then you can access to and use the health care services properly. But if you are one of the "people of my country"[an average citizen in this Country] then you will take what has given to you…will not ask for more. (Participant No:17, Specialized State Hospital Social Worker).

Problem in access to health care services is the mostly stated characteristic about health inequalities. All of the participants stress the importance of access to services as the key to equity in health care:

There should be equality. Access to an important surgery should be available to everyone. Then we have equality.

> Equality should be here; for an important surgery, this hospital (a tertiary level, university hospital) should be accessible…accessible for everyone… then we can talk about equality. (Participant No:3, University Hospital Social Worker).

Geographical differences are stressed by participants as an obstacle of equality in health care services. Here, these differences are related to service access;

> For example, dialysis patients may need to migrate from their hometown because of lack of services there. Unlike inhabitants of metropolitan areas, people form rural areas and small towns do not have access to dialysis and other services. This is a kind of inequality. (Participant No:15, Specialized State Hospital Social Worker).

Problems of special populations in utilization of health care services: Uninsured patients, green card owners and asylum seekers are also stated as other important components of health inequality conceptualization of social workers. While participants were explaining health inequality, they usually referred to certain population groups and their disadvantage in access and utilization of health care. Among these groups, uninsured patients and asylum seekers are the mostly mentioned;

> [Health] "Equality" is based on personal income I think…if you have no income, then there is no social security. Not everyone can or should be equal in income but should be a part of the social security system… (Participant No: 3, University Hospital Social Worker).

> Foreign patients (asylum seekers) are subjected to serious discrimination. The same is true for green card owners…for example this group may be uninsured and cannot access emergency care services… the administration doesn't want to accept the uninsured patients to ER unless there is certain risk of death! (Participant No:24, University Hospital Social Worker).

Discrimination based on certain characteristics of the patients (HIV, Addicted, and/or other Socially Stigmatized Statuses) is the last sub-theme in participants' conceptualization of health inequalities. When participants' direct contact with the polyclinics increases, they are more likely to be aware of and to mention the disadvantages which certain client groups experience.

> I remember a case... An HIV patient from X(city) had to go into dialysis. The state hospital in that city refused to have this patient in dialysis. However, they didn't have the right to refuse care! They said that other patients would be infected. However dialysis machines are really hygienic and are controlled and cleaned in that manner. If they don't do this routine cleaning, then not only HIV but any kind of microbe could be transmitted. This case somehow reached us...The governorship arranged accommodation for the patient. And he continued his treatment here in Ankara. Besides we had contacts for him to receive disability payment. It was a good work for advocacy. (Participant No:1, University Hospital Social Worker).

> The polyclinics are not designed for disabled patients. For example it is difficult for visually impaired patients to reach the hospital (Participant No: 18, State Hospital Social Worker).

> We work with drug addicts, who are already discriminated in the society. They are also discriminated by the health care service itself. (...) Thus, this is a group who experience problems during receiving services. A further step is that, sometimes the function of addiction treatment facilities is also being questioned. Sometimes some ideas are coming up such as, should we treat these patients or not...so...they are really disadvantaged in that manner (Participant No: 22, State Hospital Social Worker).

Social worker conflict: Bandage it or write it!

Many of the participants review their tasks in the hospital within the framework of health inequalities and conclude that they are the professionals who tackle these inequalities. One participant reviews his/her job definition in the frame of health inequalities.

> We, in fact, as social workers, are working directly with patients who experience health inequalities... so to speak, it is very difficult for an uninsured patient to access health services. The costs are really hard to cover. We work in order to cover them. We try to close the gap between insured, well-educated, non-poor patients and poor, uninsured, homeless, unaccompanied patients (Participant No: 20, State Hospital Social Worker).

Bandage the wound or write it!: Participants usually employ two methods for tackling health inequalities. First, they describe functioning as broker to meet the economic needs of patients. Mostly mentioned resources that social workers use are financial assistance from Governorship, some NGOs, Social Assistance and Solidarity Foundations and local administrations (Municipalities). However, because of the limitations of resources in the community, this method doesn't always end in equity.

> This morning a patient came for example. Since he doesn't have social insurance, nothing was done for him. Well, we, as the unit (social service unit) don't have such a fund for him to cover the expenses. Moreover, there is not an NGO that we can refer the patient. Nobody tries to cover the treatment payment for him... (Participant No:21, State Hospital Social Worker).

Correspondence with the health bureaucracy is another way that participants tackled health inequalities. Correspondence sometimes addresses legal gaps in a client's care or client's rights that had been violated. Participants mention that such interventions are disadvantaged by long waiting periods and at times, bring no positive results at all.

> For example one of our veterans needed a prosthesis in K4 level [an advanced level of dysfunction]. But when SSA [Social Security Agency] didn't pay for this prosthesis and the medical firm then get this prosthesis back from the patient. At this point, the patient asks why he cannot have the appropriate prosthesis for his disability, but take the cheaper, inappropriate one that the SSA covers. We wrote report for that to Ministry of Family and Social Policy, the report is sent to competent authorities but well...its going to be processed…or not…what will happen next. How many years pass… (laugh)…we experience such situations…but we write it [correspondence], anyway... (Participant No:9, Veterans Hospital Social Worker).

Among the Units participants work, Patient Rights Units (PRU) have a special position because of its structure enabling health inequalities to be more visible. The regulation on patient rights in Turkey required establishment of PRU at hospitals and social workers took a leader role in these units and most hospital social workers started to work under that structure. Participants mostly observe the problems of patient-doctor relationship as the main reason for application to PRU. Health inequalities or other kind of inequalities are not mentioned by participants in these units.

> In fact we expect the patients who experience violations in rights to come. However most of the complaints are nonsense. (...) it is like, the problem about access to services are solved, so that the expectations rose. The positive changes in health care system changed the complaints/applications. It is all about catharsis! They express their aggression! The target of this aggression is the doctor! (Participant No: 4, State Hospital Social Worker).

This shift in the problems of patients is associated by the participants with the "new" health care system which usually face patients with doctors.

How to Tackle? If I could, I surely would!: Participants indicate the inadequacy, indeed the futility of interventions used for addressing health inequalities. They advocate systems interventions rather than individually-focused ones.

> How can we tackle this? With policy, only...there is only one thing we can do at this point, which is to refer patient to resources… suppose the 200 TL for an examination. The governorship pays this amount without problem. But suppose the patient has to have an operation…who will pay it? (Participant No: 14, State Hospital Social Worker).

> We have to think within the policy context...We shouldn't focus on small scaled problems (Participant No:4, State Hospital Social Worker).

> The greatest resource for eliminating health inequalities is the power held in the hands of legislators (Participant No:16, Specialized State Hospital Social Worker).

However, this "power in the hands of legislators" is seen as far from the social worker's area of action:

Not only in health, but I don't believe that any inequalities in that country could be removed. There is no such thing…so I believe that neither social workers nor other professionals can do anything about that! The only solution is a political solution (Participant No: 15, Specialized State Hospital Social Worker).

Our people like the things that "come from the big guns." They accept it, like it, do it, see it as a rule...that's why, it will be better if it comes this way (Participant No: 16, Specialized State Hospital Social Worker).

On the other hand, one participant emphasizes the essential role of social worker in observing the individual differences that are not reflected to the policy and legislations and so that, from this point, social workers can have important contributions for the system to become more flexible at the individual level.

In Turkey's system, it is like two times two makes four. There is legislation but it doesn't take the individual differences into account. The health system should be individualized, I think…the system doesn't see the individual differences but you work with the patients face-to-face…you see the problems s/he encounters because of the system...But the system ignores this individuality. So you still have to struggle yourself, even for one client (Participant No: 8, Veterans Hospital Social Worker).

Advocacy is viewed as critical intervention in addressing policy changes. One participant reports his/her doubts about the efficacy of advocacy work:

This inequality is very related to advocacy. But social workers here may not be able to do what social workers in developed countries do. Do the structures, the organizations give us enough space for advocacy? The issue is about Professional competency. To what extent does my advocacy serve the client's needs? I say that it is not enough...The decision I take, the report I write…they are not restrictive, not functional…Of course advocacy is the central issue when talking about inequalities. But how functional we are? How is the legal infrastructure? (Participant No: 22, State Hospital Social Worker)

DISCUSSION

In this research we aimed to understand how the health inequalities within the context of current health transformations in Turkey is observed and experienced by hospital social workers in Turkey and how they tackle these health inequalities. In the lived experiences, social workers have a critical role in observing the positive and negative effects of transformations in the front-line and respond to these inequalities for a more just society.

The experiences of social workers can be understood within a general perspective of their roles at the hospitals. Several limitations are stated by social workers, which are also closely related to their action against health inequalities. The dichotomy of social work roles is an important challenge for analyzing and responding to health inequalities. Social workers make a distinction between financial interventions and psychosocial interventions. This dichotomy is an obstacle for a holistic view to client's needs and interventions in order to meet them.

Financial assessment and interventions are the dominant roles of social workers at hospitals. But it is mostly in the form of brokering with resources that are limited. This finding closely parallels with other research with hospital social workers in Ankara (42, 43). When taken into consideration with a health inequalities perspective, this work has a critical role. However, with a radical perspective (44), social workers' function in meeting the financial needs of patients at micro level, it can be regarded as a remedial function of social work and thus needs to be critically examined. As Solar and Irwin (2) stated, the concept of power becomes important when dealing with inequalities. And it is arguable that such power can be gained by the disadvantaged groups through such a limited economical support.

Conceptualization of health inequalities of social workers are in parallel with the current literature. Inequalities are conceptualized in relation to the widespread incapability experienced by the disadvantaged population in Turkey (45). When describing health inequalities, study participants explicitly emphasize four points, including: problems with access to health care services, geographical differences, poverty and discrimination.

Access to health care is an important dimension of health equity, however is taken into consideration with the discussion in the literature on quality of services (30, 46). Social workers see an improvement in access to health care services with the current transformations, however are worried about the quality of service. Their concern is also supported by the Turkish literature evaluating the transformation (46).

With regard to their experiences while tackling health inequalities, social workers are eager to see health inequalities at the hearth of their work, even if it is a new framework for them to see the problems from the lens of health inequalities. Most social workers couldn't respond as they heard the term "health inequality" for the first time, however after discussion of the definition; they easily connected the concept with their everyday practice arena. Social workers' experiences against health inequalities include two important components. The first component is temporary, rather than permanent solutions, such as responding the urgent need of client in order to take the necessary support for receiving services. Some examples to these temporary solutions are mostly related with the financial support such as referring the client to an economical resource or helping client to manage treatment costs, paying the hospital bills, etc. These temporary actions are important in tackling with health inequalities that they can be regarded as the response of social work to the disadvantaged clients in the short term. However, as stated in the literature (33, 35), tackling poverty and income distribution is one of the main steps in reducing inequalities in health. Social workers are reluctant to make macro level changes and effect both economic and health policies. There can be many explanations for this reluctance. First of all, macro level roles of social workers are usually not actively taken in Turkey and national social work policy in the field of health is still absent (43). Although the social work education in Turkey is for a long time adapted a generalist view, micro-mezzo and macro levels of roles are not undertaken by social workers as an integrative manner. This point of view is seen in the narratives that social workers feel powerless and "out of charge" when they state that tackling health inequalities needs a policy-level action. We think that this feeling of powerlessness is related to the general ineffectiveness of social workers in the rapid changes in policies including their professional status. Cilga (47) stressed this process as the "exclusion of social work as a science and profession" in Turkey. Loss of Professional rights, deprofessionalization process and lack of evidence-informed political decisions dominant in the country is expected to affect the social workers working in the field of health.

Social workers' position in tackling health inequalities show that they are most likely to respond health inequalities using upstream interventions as described in the study of Fish and Karban (39), however it is far from structural interventions. Social workers mostly perform upstream interventions at individual level in order to increase the availability of health services and utilization of treatment for their clients who are directly referred to them.

When the data on tackling health inequalities is analyzed in terms of the health care service delivery, it is possible to infer that health care system itself is in the risk of becoming the source of inequalities in health as it is claimed in CSDH. (35) The ineffectiveness of social workers in tackling health inequalities may be regarded as an example of this mechanism.

However, a positive and encouraging finding is social workers' awareness of legal gaps in the health care system and their use of this gap for the benefit of disadvantaged client. Even social workers state that individual level solutions are not effective for a widespread struggle; these individual solutions are important contributions for the everyday practice against health inequalities.

Despite these findings, this study should be considered with its methodological limitations. First of all, the qualitative nature of the study makes it impossible to generalize findings to social workers in Ankara and in Turkey. Another limitation of the study is that the authors were not able to employ a method for inter-coder reliability during the analysis of the data, due to resource and time constraints. Lastly, social approval bias is another limitation. It is possible that social workers in the field may feel uncomfortable in entering theoretical discussions or talking about their roles with investigators who were university academics.

Nonetheless, we believe that this research is still an important contribution to the discussion of health inequalities in Turkey and in other countries experiencing similar transformations in health. It is also important to discuss the position of social work as it is practiced at the heart of health care system. As Whitehead (48) stated, health care system itself is an important component of health inequalities and to overcome obstacles in the system, awareness-raising is a must, in order to explain the true extent of the problem and increase understanding of the effects of diverse policies on health, especially that of vulnerable groups. Social workers are the most powerful team members in the hospitals that have direct interaction with these disadvantaged groups and therefore the voice of social workers in the current state of inequalities should be heard.

Limitations notwithstanding, the study included participants from diverse healthcare settings. Thematic analysis of interview content from this diverse sample of social workers indicates concordance on challenges to achieving health equality for all.

CONCLUSION

Results describe the challenges social workers encounter when addressing health inequalities. Most of the challenges are related to development of a comprehensive approach for tackling health inequalities. The study also provides important considerations for health social workers in other developing countries, where health care transformations are taking place, by outlining critical areas that social workers should take into account during their daily practice. We summarize our major findings and possible implications for social work in Appendix Table 2. The positioning of social work in overall policy processes in Turkey is reflected in the problems in health care specifically. Lack of integrated roles at hospitals (dichotomy of roles), ineffective political stance, and lack of adequate professional authority may be overcome with a more powerful professional stance. This may include more powerful advocacy work and lobbying among the agents of health care system.

APPENDIX 1. MAJOR THEMES AND IMPLICATIONS FOR SOCIAL WORK PRACTICE

	Themes	Recommendations	Social work implications
Health Inequalities	Widespread inequalities in the country	-integrating the work against all kinds of inequalities	-taking active role for tackling with HI and other inequalities with other professionals
	Disadvantaged groups -Geographical differences - Asylum seekers -Uninsured patients -Certain groups (HIV; Drug addicts)	-Additional regulations for disadvantaged groups to support them during access to services and service utilization.	- Using empowerment approach and function as advocator - Lobbying for service planning in order to improve human rights for disadvantaged groups
Social Work Function	Two faces of social workers: A Dichotomy on the roles	- Reevaluate the role of hospital social workers - standardized Professional responsibilities including all of the social worker's tasks.	-Awareness of the holistic view gained through the education -Supporting the socio-economical assessment with psychosocial interventions -Improving the physical standards of the workplace
Tackling Health Inequalities	Common feeling of desperation	- Getting more powerful and being able to be heard	-Sharing the "good practices" -being organized effectively as hospital social workers
	Seeking individual solutions to increase access to services	-Standardization of pathways to individual solutions	-transfer this experiences to a macro level work
	Paperwork based struggle	-using paperwork (correspondence) for a more structured and systematic means of struggle	- using other ways of struggle such as lobbying, awareness-raising, brokering, fund-raising while using reports at the macro level.

Appendix 2. Interview Guide

Semi-Structured Interview Guide

- **Introduction of self**
  - Socio-demographical characteristics (age, gender, educational background, marital status, children)
  - Professional background (work experiences and duration of current work/position, past work experiences)

- **Professional roles and activities**
  - How would you describe the unit that you are currently working? What is the client profile?
  - Can you describe your roles and responsibilities in general at your hospital/department/service?
  - How do you feel about your function/ effectiveness in the hospital? What more could you do, instead of your current tasks?
- **Conceptualizing Health Inequalities**

Read the following definition aloud to him/her (in Turkish)
"*Health inequality can defined as any health differences between social groups, which are avoidable and preventable and thus, unjust and unacceptable. This inequality can be observed in two areas; the health state and the access and use of health care services*"

  - What does it mean to him/her? What does he/she understand?
  - What comes to his/her mind first, when talking about health inequalities? What are examples of health inequalities as they affect patients and families? What are his/her experiences as a social worker?
- **Tackling Health Inequalities**
  - Which specific activities and roles you undertake in order to tackle with health inequalities (consider this for specific cases, either)
  - A case example that she/he remembers (in these, what were your goals? plan of action? what were you able to do? what might you like to have done? how do you assess/evaluate the effectiveness of the intervention?)
  - What barriers did you encounter in intervening? (Patient-related? hospital systems-related? policy-related? social worker related?)
  - What resources did she/he used during this work? (Patient-related? hospital systems-related? policy-related? social worker related?)
  - How can health inequalities be reduced? What strategies can be effective? How social workers can contribute to this process?
  - How does he/she observe the current transformation of health system in relation with the health inequalities?

ACKNOWLEDGMENTS

A previous version of this paper was presented at the 3rd ENSACT Joint European Conference in Istanbul, Turkey, 19 April, 2013. Dr. Ka'opua's work on this project was supported in part by an award from the National Institute on Minority Health and Health Disparities to the University of Hawai'i (U54MD007584). The content is solely the responsibility of the authors and does not necessarily represent the official views of the National Institutes of Health. Authors would like to thank to Gizem Celik, Emre Ozcan and Melike Tunc for their contribution during the data collection process.

REFERENCES

[1] World Health Organization. Health impact assessment. Accessed 2014 Feb 21. URL: http://www.who.int/hia/ about/glos/en/index1.html.

[2] Solar O, Irwin A. A conceptual framework for action on the social determinants of health. Social Determinants of Health Discussion Paper 2 (Policy and Practice). Geneva: World Health Organization, 2010.

[3] Krieger N. Theories for social epidemiology for the 21st century: an ecosocial perspective. Int J Epidemiol 2001;30(4):668-77.

[4] Krasnik A, Rasmussen NK. Reducing social inequalities in health: evidence, policy, and practice. Scand J Public Health. 2002;30(59):1-5.

[5] World Bank. Turkey. Accessed 2013 Oct 13]. URL: http://data.worldbank.org/country/turkey.

[6] Turkiye Istatistik Kurumu (TUIK). [Address-based population registration system 2012]. Accessed 2013 Oct 13]. URL: http://www.tuik.gov.tr/PreHaberBulten leri.do?id=13425 Turkish.

[7] World Bank. Turkey-joint poverty assessment report (Report No. 29619-TU). Ankara: Human Development Sector Unit, Europe and Central Asia Region, 2005.

[8] Candas A, Bugra A, Yilmaz V, Gunseli S, Yakut Cakar B. [Inequalities in Turkey: An overview of persistent inequalities]. Istanbul: Bogazici Universitesi Sosyal Politika Forumu, 2010. [Turkish].

[9] United Nations Children's Fund. Preventing child poverty. Ankara: UNICEF Turkey, 2006.

[10] Organization for Economic Co-operation and Development (OECD). Doing better for children 2009. Accessed 2013 Nov 11. URL: http://www.keepeek.com/ Digital-Asset-Management/oecd/social-issues-migra tion-health/doing-better-for-children_9789264059344-en#page1.

[11] Turkiye Istatistik Kurumu (TUIK). [2008 Poverty work results] Ankara: Turkiye Istatistik Kurumu (TUIK), 2009. [Turkish]

[12] Turkiye Cocuk Vakfi. [Quantitative child warning report on world children's day]. Accessed 2013 Feb 6. URL: http://www.cocukvakfi.org.tr/resource/pdf/Rapor lar/4yenibinyilin_dunya_cocuklari_raporu.pdf.

[13] Koc I, Eryurt MA, Adali T, Seckiner P. [Demografic transformation of Turkey: Fertillity, family planning, mother child health and change in under-five mortality 168-2008]. Ankara: Hacettepe University, 2010. [Turkish].

[14] OECD. Better Life Index. Accessed 2013 July 31. URL: http://www.oecdbetterlifeindex.org.

[15] Blas E, Kurup AS. Introduction and methods of work. In: Blas E, Kurup AS, eds. Equity, social determinants and public health programmes. Geneva: World Health Organization, 2010:3-11.

[16] Hurst JW. Reforming health care in seven European nations. Health Aff 1991;10(3):7-21.

[17] Hayran O. [Globalisation and health]. Yeni Turkiye 2001;7(40):1110-6. [Turkish].

[18] Saltman RB, Figueras J. Analyzing the evidence on European health care. Health Aff 1998;17(2):85-108.

[19] Reisch M. The Challenges of health care reform for hospital social work in the United States. Soc Work Health Care 2012;51(10):873-93.

[20] Reardon C. The health care reform puzzle - How does social work fit? Soc Work Today 2011;11 (1):18-21.

[21] Elbek O, Adas EB. [Transformation in health: a critical evaluation]. Turkiye Psikkyatri Dernegi Bult 2009;12 (1):33-44. [Turkish].

[22] Celikay F, Gumus E. [Empirical analysis of transformation in health] Accessed 2013 Oct 20. URL: http://mpra.ub.uni-muenchen.de/42363/.

[23] Kisa A, Younis MZ, Kisa S. A comparative analysis of the European Union's and Turkey's health status: how health-care services might affect turkey's accession to the EU. Public Health Rep 2007;122(5):693–701.

[24] Aksakoglu G, Kilic B, Ucku R. [The model/system of family medicine is not suitable for Turkey]. Top Hek 2003;18(4):251-61. [Turkish].

[25] Turk Tabipleri Birligi (TTB). [General health insurance], 2nd ed. Ankara: TTB Yay, 2005. [Turkish].

[26] Yildirim HH, Yildirim T. Health care financing reform in Turkey: context and salient features. J Eur Soc Policy 2011;21(2):178-93.

[27] Saglik Bakanligi. [Development report Turkey health transformation programme]. Ankara: Saglik Bakanligi, 2008. [Turkish].

[28] Bostan S, Kilic T, Acuner T. [The changing effect of health transformation program on hospitals: hospital managers views]. TISK Akademi 2012;7(14):109-23 [Turkish].

[29] Kocak O, Tiryaki D. [The Importance of health Policies in the welfare state mentality and the evaluation of changing health policies: A survey from Yalova]. Istanbul Ticaret Univ Sos Bil Dergisi 2011;10(19):55-88. [Turkish].

[30] Soyer A. ["Transformation in health" and public health workers]. Turk Tabipleri Birligi Mesleki Sag Guv Der 2011;(42):12-4. [Turkish].

[31] Ozdemir O, Ocaktan E, Akdur R. [The assesment of primary health care services in Turkey and european countries due to health reform in Turkey]. Ankara Univ Tip Fak Mecmuasi 2003; 56(4):207–16. [Turkish].

[32] Hatun S. [While medical schools are being dragged into crises]. Accessed 2011 Apr 3: URL: http://www.radikal.com.tr/radikal2/tip_fakulteleri_krize_suruklenirken-1045106. [Turkish].

[33] Marmot M. Social determinants of health inequalities. Lancet 2005; 365(9464):1099-1104.

[34] Whitehead M, Dahlgren G. Concepts and principles for tackling social inequities in health: Levelling up Part 1. (Studies on social and economic determinants of population health, No. 2). University of Liverpool: WHO Collaborating Centre for Policy Research on Social Determinants of Health, 2007.

[35] Commission on Social Determinants of Health. Closing the gap in a generation: health equity through action on the social determinants of health. Final report of the commission on social determinants of health. Geneva: World Health Organization, 2008.

[36] Bywaters P. Tackling inequalities in health: a global challenge for social work. Br J Soc Work 2009;39 (2):353-367.

[37] IFSW Policy Statement on Health [Internet]. International Fedaration of Social Workers, 2011. Accessed 2013 Apr 2. URL: http://www.ifsw.org/p3800 0081.html.

[38] Backwith D, Mantle G. Inequalities in health and community-oriented social work: Lessons from Cuba? Int Soc Work 2009;52(4):499-511.

[39] Fish J, Karban K. Health inequalities at the heart of the social work curriculum. Soc Work Educ Int J 2013;33(1):15-30.

[40] Turkiye Istatistik Kurumu (TUIK). [Distribution of hospitals and beds by provinces, 2012. Accessed 2013 Oct 13. URL: http://www.tuik.gov.tr/PreTablo.do?alt_ id=1095.

[41] Belek I. [Class inequalities in health and socio-economical status: a longitudinal research in Antalya].1th ed. Ankara: Turk Tabipleri Birligi (TTB, 2004. [Turkish].

[42] Aydemir I, Duyan V. [Patients problems faced by social workers who are working at Ministry of Health and services they address for these problems]. Sag Top 2005;15(1):82-9. [Turkish]

[43] Ozbesler C, Coban AI. [Social work practice in the hospital setting: The case of Ankara].Top Sos Hiz 2010;21(2):31–46. [Turkish].

[44] Payne M. Modern social work theory, 3rd ed. New York: Palgrave Macmillan, 2005.

[45] Sen A. Why health equity. Health Econ 2002;11(8):659–66.

[46] Aka A. [Projections of Neoliberal transformation on health: basic healthy actors perception of these outlines]. Top Sos Hiz 2012;23(1):167-86. [Turkish].
[47] Cilga I. [The dynamics of social exclusion, exclusion of the science, the profession, and the foresights]. Top Sos Hiz 2009;20(2):7–26. [Turkish].
[48] Whitehead M. The concepts and principles of equity and health. Copenhagen: WHO Regional Office Europe, 1990.

In: Public Health Yearbook 2016
Editor: Joav Merrick

ISBN: 978-1-53610-947-4

Chapter 20

MEXICAN ADOLESCENTS' INTENTIONS TO USE DRUGS: GENDER DIFFERENCES IN THE PROTECTIVE EFFECTS OF RELIGIOSITY

Marcos J Martinez*, PhD, Flavio F Marsiglia, PhD, Stephanie L Ayers, PhD and Bertha L Nuño-Gutiérrez, PhD

College of Public Health and Social Work, Florida International University, Miami, Florida, US; Southwest Interdisciplinary Research Center, Arizona State University, Phoenix, Arizona, US; and Centro de Estudios e Investigaciones en Comportamiento, Universidad de Guadalajara, Guadalajara, Mexico

ABSTRACT

Cultural and social norms contribute to gender differences in substance use and health outcomes. Religiosity is an important facet of Mexican culture that reinforces familial and societal gender norms and behaviors, which may result in aspects of religiosity having differential protective effects on intentions to use substances for male and female youth. Applying an ecodevelopmental perspective, this article examines gender differences in religiosity and its subsequent impact on intentions to use substances in a cross-sectional sample of Mexican adolescents (N = 390; M = 13.01) from Jalisco, Mexico. A bi-national team of researchers from universities in Mexico and in the US conducted this study in accordance with the Institutional Review Board at both universities and followed policies for protecting human subjects. Using OLS regression, a significant relationship between gender and internal (β = .23, p < .05) and external religiosity (β = .31, p < .05) was found. This association was stronger for males. Internal religiosity was protective for females against intentions to use alcohol (β = -.23, p < .001) and cigarettes (β = -.18, p < .01), while external religiosity was protective for males against intentions to use alcohol (β = -.11, p < .01). Despite rapidly changing cultural

* Correspondence: Marcos J Martinez, PhD, College of Public Health and Social Work, Florida International University 11200, SW 8th St., AHC5 565 Miami, Florida 33199, United States. E-mail: marcmart@fiu.edu; marsiglia@asu.edu.

norms, most girls in the sample appear to be adhering to more traditional conceptions of gender roles that could be reinforced at least in part by internal religiosity. Boys, on the other hand, appear to be benefiting more from external religiosity and organized religion's sponsored environments and networks. Given the role of the family in the transmission of culture to youth, social work implications from this study suggest the need to approach substance use prevention with Mexican youth, and perhaps with Mexican heritage youth in the US, from a gendered and culturally informed perspective that recognizes the protective facets of religiosity for boys and girls.

Keywords: religiosity, Latino adolescents, substance use

Introduction

Over the past decade, substance use rates among Mexican adolescents have continued to increase (1-3). Mexican adolescents have reported increases in alcohol and tobacco use as well as earlier ages of initiation (4, 5), with males drinking alcohol and smoking tobacco earlier than their female counterparts (6-8). While gender differences in substance use among Mexican adolescents have been found (9), those differences have narrowed over time with females reporting increased rates of substance use (3). This rise is of critical concern given the association of early substance use with deleterious long-term health and social outcomes including the development of drug dependency (10, 11), academic failure, unintended accidents, risky sexual behavior, and criminal activity (5, 12-14).

Given these negative outcomes associated with substance use, it is critical to understand the factors that protect Mexican adolescents from engaging in substance use. Religiosity has been identified as an important socio-cultural protective factor for Mexican adolescents against substance use (5, 15, 16). Despite its noted importance, few studies have examined if religiosity operates differently for males and females and its subsequent impact on substance use. Religiosity may reinforce traditional masculine and feminine norms, and in turn, may contribute to an exaggeration of gender differences. Therefore, a polarized approach that does not recognize the gender differences among youth may lead to lack of access or underutilization of health services and prevention programs (17). From an ecodevelopmental perspective, this article investigates if religiosity operates differently among Mexican adolescent boys and girls in relation to intentions to use alcohol and cigarettes. The overall hypothesis guiding the study is that religiosity will be protective for both boys and girls, and girls will benefit the most from the protective effects of religiosity against intentions to use alcohol and cigarettes.

Ecodevelopmental theory

The Ecodevelopmental Theory focuses on the interrelationships between adolescents' multiple social contexts and how those environments have a different influence on both adolescents' development and risk behaviors (18-20). Specifically, this theoretical approach considers the relationships between the micro, meso, exo, and macro social contexts as a multidimensional process that impacts adolescent development and behavior.

The micro system, the most proximal system to adolescents, is the context that youth are directly involved with the most (e.g., parent-adolescent relationship, parental monitoring, and parent discipline) (18, 19). The meso system, the next most proximal system, examines processes that influence youth indirectly, such as degree of parental involvement in their child's schooling. Exo system factors are those that do not directly influence youth (parents receiving emotional support from their social network) and macro factors are the larger structural (e.g., economy) and cultural processes (e.g., religiosity) that influence the interpersonal relationships between families and youth (19, 20). Although exo and macro factors are not directly related to a youth's risky behaviors, they require important consideration when researching the etiology of adolescent substance use and in the structuring of sustainable and culturally relevant prevention programming (21).

Culture, a macro factor, is thought to operate through familial processes (22, 23), as families play a critical role in not only child rearing and behavior socialization but also in transferring cultural values (24, 25). Culture can be defined as a group's distinct worldviews, beliefs, practices, and attitudes that are shared by the members (21, 26) and understanding the role that culture has in influencing adolescents' multiple contexts is essential since it is thought to "permeate all aspects" of an individual's social ecology (18).

Religiosity is an important aspect of Mexican and the broader Latino cultures and can act as a source of strength and information to guide youth in how to behave and interact with family members, peers, and elders (27). Religiosity appears to have positive and constructive influences in the lives of youth (28) and plays a critical role in identity formation as youth transition from childhood into adolescence (24, 29). This transition is particularly important since youth begin to examine their religious values and beliefs as they start searching for purpose in their lives during this developmental period (24, 29-31). It is believed that the significance that is ascribed to religious beliefs in Mexican culture may be a protective buffer against substances use.

Religiosity as a protective factor

Religiosity may be protective for Mexican and Latino youth because it promotes normative and prosocial behavioral expectations (28). Religious institutions provide a setting where youth can share their spiritual values and beliefs while simultaneously exploring their emerging self-identities in a venue that functions as a supportive and culturally specific community (32). In this community setting, adolescents can interact with adult role models in the church (32-34). These adults may reinforce ideas about normative behavior that can discourage youth from engaging in taboo, harmful, anti-social, damaging, and risky acts which may be detrimental to their physical, mental, and social health.

Being integrated at an early age into cultural and religious networks can provide youth with even greater protection as they enter adolescence (32, 35, 36). For example, Jang and colleagues (33) found that children who grew up in religiously conservative households, as well as children that had parents who felt religious service and attendance were important, had lower rates of substance use in late adolescence and early adulthood compared to children who did not grow up in religious households. Similarly, Flanzer's study of substance abuse in the Jewish community found low rates of substance abuse among Jewish adolescents; it was suggested that the low rates of adolescent substance abuse was a result of the strong religious values held within the Jewish community, which led to a stronger sense of connection among members (37, 38). With Mexican youth in particular, it is difficult to separate religiosity from other aspects of Mexican culture. On both sides of the Mexico-US border, many of the main Mexican holidays and festivities celebrated by families and communities (e.g., baptisms, weddings, quince eras, Christmas, Towns' patron saint days, the feast of Our Lady of Guadalupe, etc.) have a connection to the Roman Catholic tradition even among those who are not actively involved in organized religion (39, 40).

Two aspects of religiosity, internal and external, are often viewed as protective mechanisms. Internal religiosity, sometimes called intrinsic religiosity, constitutes the importance that one places on their faith/religion and is generally considered to be one's commitment to their faith (5, 41, 42). External religiosity, also called extrinsic religiosity, refers to an individual's outward participation in religious activities such as attending church (5, 41, 42). A Mexico-based study with adolescents reported that youth with strong internal and external religiosity were less likely to drink alcohol compared to their peers with low internal and external religiosity (5). Another study investigating the relationship between religiosity and psychological adjustment among adolescents found that youth reporting higher internal religiosity had significantly higher self-esteem and lower depression compared to individuals who were not religious (43).

Despite its protective nature, religiosity is not uniformly and consistently protective. For example, Mexican adolescents who exhibited strong external religiosity but weak internal religiosity were found to be at greater risk for alcohol and cigarette use, while youth who were not internally or externally religious were less likely to smoke cigarettes (5). This difference may be due to the differing religious salience among males and females. Females, in a multiethnic US-based sample, reporting significantly higher internal religiosity when compared to males (43). As well, a large meta-analysis of more than 70 studies found that women consistently reported higher scores on internal religiosity measures than men (44), indicating that internal religiosity has greater salience for females. Although studies have not found any statistically significant gender differences in external religiosity, they have suggested that this difference may be fully mediated through strict adherence to traditional societal and culturally-based gender roles (43, 44).

Religion, gender roles, and culture

Traditional cultural norms encourage and promote differential or polarized gender norms that give boys and girls different messages about how they are "supposed" to behave both at home and in their broader social environments (45) and are often endorsed and accepted by both Mexican men and women (46, 47). The traditional Mexican gender roles have generally been known as "machismo" and "marianismo" (48). Introduced by the Spanish when they came to the Americas, machismo endorses the supremacy of men (patriarchy), men as the primary leaders and breadwinners and views women as caretakers of the home, disciplinarians to the children, and managers of household finances (49, 51). Machismo (24, 39) has been described as a form of exaggerated masculinity that is expressed in an aggressive manner most often seen through dominance over women and culturally sanctioned sexual promiscuity.

Not all dimensions of machismo are negative. One dimension known in the literature as "caballerismo" has been associated with positive traits such as being "dignified, protector, responsible, nurturing, spiritual, faithful, respectful, friendly, caring, sensitive, trustful" (39). Lastly, social class, occupational and educational statuses, as well as place of residence and religious beliefs appear to explain the great variation in contemporary Mexican men's perceptions about masculinity, machismo and caballerismo (52).

On the contrary, behavioral and societal expectations for women are rooted in the concept of marianismo. Marianismo is related to a broader interpretation of the Roman Catholic archetype of the Virgin Mary image, or specifically in Mexico, the Virgin of Guadalupe (48). The Virgin Mary has been historically presented as a symbol of female purity in Mexican society (40), however adherence to this traditional gender ideal varies greatly within Mexico based on social class, rural versus urban, and other factors (52, 53). Nonetheless, the Marian image is important as it links together identities in social, religious, and political contexts; the concept of marianismo emphasizes the traditional role of women in the household and society where needs of family members are placed over her individual needs (54). As a result of socialization processes, it is speculated that adolescent girls may alter and suppress their self-expression in order to maintain important social relationships (55). Although the oppressive dimensions of the marianismo archetype for women and men have been well documented, the Marian image itself has also been identified as an empowering representation of both faith and culture that highlights the important roles that Mexican women identify with such as mother, healer, leader, and consoler (48).

Religious institutions are one way to reinforce and promote traditional gender roles (33, 56). Dating back to the times of the Spanish Conquest in the late 1490s, the imposition of Catholicism on the indigenous populations (57, 58) solidified the gender norms which have, to varying degrees, survived to the present day among some communities in Mexico. Organized religion has historically been perceived as playing a powerful institutional role in shaping gender-differentiated normative and behavioral patterns: popular beliefs and practices originally connected to organized religion reinforce the primary facets of machismo and marianismo (53). For example, the modern day Roman Catholic Church hierarchy provides an example of gender-based roles as men traditionally hold the dominant and most prestigious positions of pope, bishops and priests whereas women act in subordinate and supportive roles (48, 59).

Gender norms and risk behaviors

Socially prescribed traditional gender roles often set a double standard for male and female youth regarding certain risk behaviors such as substance use and sexual activity. Machismo and marianismo may result in parents becoming increasingly protective of female adolescents yet being lenient towards male adolescents regarding their social behavior. For example, alcohol use in certain contexts is socially acceptable for men but not for women (60, 61). Women are discouraged from, and stigmatized for, consuming any type of drug or alcohol.60 Furthermore, for women who do consume alcohol are, drinking to intoxication is perceived negatively and is usually controlled and monitored by men (9, 47).

Thus, as a result of this behavioral double standard, males and females may act, process, and respond to social situations in a different manner. For example, studies examining strategies concerning refusal strategies for drug offers have noted differences among male and female youth (63, 64). It has previously been found that differences in refusing drugs was directly aligned with the behavioral and gender social norms that are held within traditional Mexican culture (63-65). The specific demarcation of gender roles and expectations may impact not only communication patterns and relationships between boys and girls but substance use behavior as well (40, 64).

Current study

The primary aim of the current study is to first determine if there are gender differences in internal and external religiosity, and second, examine how these processes operate on substance use intentions. It is hypothesized there will be gender differences in religiosity identification. Females will report significantly higher internal religiosity, while males will report greater external religiosity. Second, it is hypothesized that these gender differences in religiosity identification will provide differing protective effects against substance use intentions; internal religiosity will provide increased protection for females and external religiosity will be more protective for males.

METHODS

This study utilized a cross-sectional sample consisting of adolescents (mean age of 13 years; 54.8% female), from Guadalajara, Jalisco, Mexico (N = 390), who participated in Mantente REAL, the Spanish language version of keepin' it REAL. keepin' it REAL is a SAMHSA model drug abuse prevention model that teaches drug resistance strategies to assist in deflecting drug offers [Refuse, Explain, Avoid, Leave] (68). Two universities, one from the U.S. and one from Mexico, collaborated in this study and chose Jalisco as an ideal setting to pilot test Mantente REAL. Jalisco was chosen because of 1) its large Guadalajara metropolitan area and 2) the existing bi-national research collaboration between researchers from Jalisco and the US. Two urban secondary schools (approximately middle school grades in the US) were recruited and accepted to participate. Ten classrooms (5 classrooms at each school) participated in the pilot study.

Survey administration

This study was conducted in accordance with the Institutional Review Board at both universities and followed policies for protecting human subjects. Participants were notified that the survey was part of a university sponsored research study and were made aware that participation was voluntary and their answers in the survey were confidential. Written student assent was obtained and parents were informed before the study began that their child would be participating in Mantente REAL. Parents were told that if they did not want their child to participate in the program or had questions about it, to contact the school where the child attended or the researchers conducting the study. Assenting students completed the questionnaires in Spanish. There was no personally identifying information on participants.

A one-hour, classroom based survey questionnaire gathered information on demographic characteristics, substance use, substance use norms and attitudes, and intentions to use substances. Although the original survey questionnaire was developed in English, back translation procedures (67) were used to translate the survey into Spanish. Once survey questionnaires were complete, the Mexican-based research team entered the data into Excel and shared the data set with the US-based team for analysis and joint manuscript development. This article only reports findings based on the baseline (pretest) surveys from both schools.

Measures

Intentions to Use Substances. The most commonly used substances by Mexican youth are alcohol and tobacco and are the focus of this study (7, 8). Due to the overall low substance use rates among participants, intentions to use alcohol and intentions to use cigarettes were the main outcome variables for this study. Previous research has found substance use intentions to be directly correlated with actual substance use (69, 70). Students were asked about their intentions to use alcohol or cigarettes using the following questions: "If you had the chance this weekend, would you use alcohol?; Would you smoke cigarettes?" Likert type responses for both intentions to use alcohol and intentions to use cigarettes ranged from [1] = 'Definitely No' to [4] = 'Definitely Yes.'

Internal and External Religiosity. Internal religiosity was measured by asking youth: "How important is your religion to you?" Likert style responses ranged from [0] 'Not important' to [4] 'Very important'. External religiosity was measured by asking youth: "How often do you attend church?" Responses ranged from [0] 'Never' to [5] 'Each week.' Previous research has used these single item measures for internal and external religiosity (5). Gender was coded as [0] female and [1] male.

Control variables included parental monitoring, parent education level, substance use offers, grades, and living arrangement. Students were asked how often their parents monitored their behavior and response categories ranged from [1] 'Never' to [4] 'Always'. Living arrangement measured if the youth lived at home with both parents and was a dichotomous variable: [1] 'yes' and [0] 'No.' Average grades were coded as [1] 'D's & F's' to [4] 'A's'. For substance use offers, participants were asked the frequency that they had been offered substances in the last 12 months, with responses ranging from [0] 'Never' to [5] 'More than 10 times.'

Analysis strategy

The analysis for this study was based on pre-test questionnaires and was conducted using the statistical software package, IBM SPSS Statistics for Windows, Version 21.69 Due to the small variance in religious affiliation (94% Roman Catholic), the analytic sample was limited only to youth who identified as Roman Catholic, which put the final sample just under 400 participants (N = 390). Descriptive statistics were gathered to review the characteristics and distribution of the sample. Then, ordinary least squares regression was used to examine (a) the relationship between gender and religiosity and (b) the relationship between external/internal religiosity and substance use intentions.

RESULTS

Descriptive statistics for this study are presented in Table 1. The sample consisted of more females (55%) than males (45%). The mean age was 13.01 years (SD = .44) but ranged from 12 to 15 years of age. Average grades were between C's and B's (M = 2.90, SD = .41). Seventy nine percent of students lived in a two-parent household (M = .79, SD = .41). Over the past 12 months, 78% of students had never been offered substances while 21% had been offered substances at least once (M = .33, SD = .76). Youth in the sample had low intentions to use alcohol (M = 1.71, SD = .88) and intentions to use cigarettes (M = 1.51, SD = .77). More than eighty percent of youth reported that their parents monitor their behavior regularly (M = 3.12, SD = .74). On the measure of internal religiosity, most students felt that their religion was important or very important (M = 3.25, SD = .84) to them. Regarding external religiosity, a large majority of students reported attending church every week (M = 3.44, SD = 1.46).

Results for the OLS regression models examining gender differences and religiosity are presented in Table 2. Gender was significantly associated with internal religiosity ($\beta = .23$, $p < .05$) and external religiosity ($\beta = .31$, $p < .05$): males reported significantly higher levels of both internal and external religiosity. Parental monitoring ($\beta = .12$, $p < .05$) and parent education level ($\beta = -.07$, $p < .01$) were significantly associated with internal religiosity; however, no other control variables were significantly associated with external religiosity. As a result of the statistical significance between gender and both internal and external religiosity, separate models that include male participants only and models including female participants only were regressed on intentions to use alcohol and intentions to use cigarettes.

Table 3 reports the results for the gender specific OLS regression models with intentions to use substances (alcohol and cigarettes) as the main outcome variables.

Table 1. Descriptive Statistics for Variables in the Analysis

Variables		Range		
	Mean (SD)	Min	Max	N
Dependent Variables				
Internal Religiosity (Females)	3.19(.85)	1	4	229
Internal Religiosity (Males)	3.36(.83)	1	4	189
External Religiosity (Females)	3.40(1.44)	1	5	229
External Religiosity (Males)	3.53(1.50)	1	5	188
Use Intentions-Alcohol (Females)	1.77(.90)	1	4	226
Use Intentions-Alcohol (Males)	1.67(.84)	1	4	190
Use Intentions-Cigarettes (Females)	1.52(.76)	1	4	228
Use Intentions-Cigarettes (Males)	1.55(.79)	1	4	190
Independent Variables				
Gender	.45(.50)	0	1	390
Parental Monitoring	3.12(.74)	1	4	384
Parent Education Level	6.38(1.67)	2	8	388
Substance Use Offers	.32(.76)	0	5	385
Grades	2.90(.83)	1	4	389
Living Arrangement	.79(.41)	0	1	381

Table 2. OLS Regression Results for Internal and External Religiosity

	Internal Religiosity ($N = 371$)		External Religiosity ($N = 370$)	
	B	SE	B	SE
Gender (1=Males)	.23*	.09	.31*	.16
Parental Monitoring	.12*	.06	.18	.11
Parent Education Level	-.07**	.03	-.05	.05
Substance Use Offers	-.03	.06	.06	.10
Grades	.01	.05	.19	.10
Living Arrangement	.13	.10	.34	.19
R^2	.05		.04	

*p < .05; **p < .01; ***p < .001.

Table 3. OLS Regression Results for Male Alcohol and Cigarette Use Intentions

	Male Alcohol Use Intentions ($N = 174$) B(SE)	Male Cigarettes Use Intentions ($N = 173$) B(SE)
Independent Variables		
Internal Religiosity	.05(.08)	.03(.07)
External Religiosity	-.11(.04)**	-.07(.04)
Parental Monitoring	-.14(.08)	-.09(.08)
Parent Education Level	-.02(.04)	-.05(.03)
Substance Use Offers	.35(.09)***	.27(.08)***
Grades	-.07(.07)	-.18(.07)**
Living Arrangement	.10(.15)	.07(.14)
R^2	.16	.15

*p < .05; **p < .01; ***p < .001.

For females, internal religiosity was significantly associated with lower intentions to use alcohol
($\beta = -.23$, $p < .001$) and lower intentions to use cigarettes ($\beta = -.18$, $p < .01$), while external religiosity was significantly associated with higher cigarettes use intentions ($\beta = .08$, $p < .05$). Parental monitoring was significantly associated with intentions to use alcohol ($\beta = -.37$, $p < .001$) and intentions to use cigarettes ($\beta = -.26$, $p < .001$). Substance use offers were significantly associated with intentions to use alcohol ($\beta = .28$, $p < .001$) and intentions to use cigarettes ($\beta = .29$, $p < .001$).

Male only models. External religiosity was significantly associated with lower intentions to use alcohol ($\beta = -.11$, $p < .01$) for males but was not significantly associated with intentions to use cigarettes ($\beta = -.07$, $p > .05$). Substance use offers was significantly associated with intentions to use alcohol ($\beta = .35$, $p < .001$) and intentions to use cigarettes ($\beta = .29$, $p < .001$). Internal religiosity was not significantly associated with intentions to use alcohol ($\beta = .05$, $p > .05$) or intentions to use cigarettes ($\beta = .03$, $p > .05$). Having higher grades was negatively associated with intentions to use cigarettes ($\beta = -.18$, $p < .01$).

Table 4. OLS Regression Results for Female Alcohol and Cigarette Use Intentions

	Female Alcohol Use Intentions ($N = 213$)	Female Cigarette Use Intentions ($N = 215$)
	B(SE)	B(SE)
Independent Variables		
Internal Religiosity	-.23(.07)***	-.18(.06)**
External Religiosity	.05(.04)	.08(.03)*
Parental Monitoring	-.37(.08)***	-.26(.07)***
Parent Education Level	-.03(.04)	-.02(.03)
Substance Use Offers	.28(.07)***	.29(.06)***
Grades	-.04(.07)	.07(.06)
Living Arrangement	.02(.14)	-.15(.11)
R^2	.23	.24

*p < .05; **p < .01; ***p < .001.

DISCUSSION

This article explored the relationship between external and internal religiosity and substance use intentions among a sample of Mexican youth from Jalisco, Mexico. Similar to previous studies (5, 15, 16), this study found that religiosity was protective for youth against intentions to use substances, albeit in different ways. Thus, the study's findings confirmed the stated hypothesis. To the best of the research team's knowledge, this study is one of the few studies to examine gender differences in the salience of internal and external religiosity and how these processes operate differently for Mexican male and female youth on intentions to use substances. From an ecodevelopmental perspective, this is a particularly significant area of study given the important role of religiosity in Mexican culture (24, 25). Religiosity may act as a proxy and as an enforcer of familial and societal gender expectations regarding adolescents' pro-social behavior (e.g., abstaining or delaying drug use) (27) and understanding this dynamic process can provide insight into substance use treatment and prevention efforts that target Mexican and Mexican American youth on both sides of the Mexican-US border.

The initial research question motivating the study asked if there were gender differences among Mexican adolescents in internal and external religiosity identification. It was hypothesized that gender differences would exist in religiosity identification due to culturally prescribed gender socialization: specifically, females would exhibit higher internal religiosity and males would exhibit higher external religiosity. This hypothesis was partially supported in the model that accounted for both males and females: there were significant gender differences in religiosity but surprisingly males were found to overall have greater internal and external religiosity compared to females.

The second research question asked if internal and external religiosity operate differently for males and females on intentions to use alcohol and cigarettes. It was hypothesized that internal religiosity would be more protective for females while external religiosity would be more protective for males. This hypothesis was supported: findings indicated that internal religiosity was protective for females against intentions to use alcohol and cigarettes while external religiosity was found to be protective for male youth against intentions to use alcohol.

Internal religiosity may be more salient for females since they are socialized to maintain positive relationships with those around them and are given the message that they are mainly responsible for the household. The concept of marianismo, within a religious context, reinforces these behavioral and social expectations and the pressures to conform to traditional gender roles (43) and may result in girls being more reserved, reflective and spending more time at home (57). For example, girls may be more reserved in or avoid certain social situations such as parties in order not to upset their interpersonal relationships in addition to maintaining a "pure" image (48). Conversely, since the Marian image can represent, in a positive manner, the important roles of women in society (e.g., mother, leader, consoler), girls that have greater internal religiosity may be empowered to not engage in taboo behavior such as substance use in order to fulfill these important culturally prescribed and enforced roles.

In this sense, the State Survey on Values for residents of Jalisco (72) found the most important thing for adolescent boys and girls currently and over time was family, work, and religion. An analysis comparing Jalisco to the rest of the country found that ninety percent of Jalisco residents were Catholic. Women also reported that religion was more important to them and also attended mass more often than men. Women may be searching for a sense of belonging that is more spiritual and internal, and church attendance may be a way to obtain that.

On the contrary, external religiosity was protective for males against intentions to use alcohol. Since males are not as scrutinized to the degree that females are regarding drinking and smoking, participating in religious' sponsored activities (external religiosity) may provide male's access to networks where alcohol, tobacco and other drug use may not be expected, which may also explain why external religiosity was protective for males. Culturally, males are socialized to be the breadwinner and the socially perceived head of the household and are given more freedom with their behavior as well as who they are allowed to socialize with, which may result in males being more exposed to risky situation outside of the home (62, 64). Previous studies have found that involvement in religious social networks at an early age can be protective for youth as they mature (32, 35-38). Religion may provide a forum where boys can receive positive guidance from adult role models in the church that reinforce messages of pro social behavior (32-34). For example, adult role models in the church may provide males with positive direction and accountability that may keep them from engaging in substance use.

Organized religion and a broader sense of religiosity are important components of Mexican culture that espouse gendered messages regarding behavioral expectations. These cultural traits may help explain the consistent gender differences that were found in the way internal and external religiosity operated for male and female youth on intentions to use alcohol and cigarettes. Although previous studies have found behavioral and gender social norms in Mexican culture to be related to differences in male and female youths' refusal of drug offers (63-65), this study contributes an important finding to the literature, specifically that religiosity within Mexican culture influences youths' intentions to use alcohol and cigarettes in differential ways for boys and girls.

Findings from this study suggest that religiosity operates in a different way for males and females as a result of cultural and gendered processes. Given that cultural norms are vital in shaping this developmental process, from an ecodevelopmental perspective, it is also important to consider the role of the family in transmitting these gendered social expectations. The family is considered to be the main socialization agent for youth, are the main transmitter of culture, and they play an important role in conveying values and beliefs that are rooted in culture (22, 23, 45, 46). The family, therefore, may be most important unit of prevention since it is a direct conduit for youth regarding normative behavior and what it means to be male or female in society.

Further, religiosity and religious iconography and organized religious rituals and activities may be working in different ways as protective factors for boys and girls in a very rapidly changing Mexican cultural landscape. Church sponsored social activities appear to have been traditionally more protective for boys due to their documented higher risk levels. These findings need to be interpreted in tandem with the rapidly raising rates of female alcohol, tobacco and other drug use in Mexico. These findings also highlight the opportunity as well as the emerging need to better address young women's prevention needs in Mexico and the US and reassess older ideas of Latinas' femininity, risk and health within and outside the realms of organized religion.

Limitations

The use of one-item measures to assess internal and external religiosity do not capture the multifaceted construct of religiosity. While the concepts of internal and external religiosity are important, other facets and nuances of religiosity are unable to be examined in this study and are needed in order to further the understanding of how religiosity operates for boys and girls on substance use behavior. Further, the use of substance use intentions as the main outcome is limited in assessing actual substance use. The use of substance use intentions was a result of how young the current sample is as well as the low rate of actual reported substance use.

Given the cross sectional nature of this study we cannot infer causality or generalize these findings beyond Mexican or Mexican heritage youth. The generalizability of this study is limited to Mexican youth residing in predominately urban area and may not apply to Mexican adolescents living in rural areas or to Mexican youth in the US. While these findings could have great implications for Mexican-heritage youth in the U.S. due to powerful processes such as globalization and circular migration, the differing socio-cultural contexts of these two countries (Mexico and US) as well as the integration of mainstream American norms by Mexican heritage youth through acculturation remains unclear. Findings from this study highlight the need to approach drug use prevention research as a gendered phenomenon in Mexico and to some degree within recent Mexican heritage immigrants and other Latino communities in the US.

CONCLUSION

Religiosity appears to be protective for male and female youth in different ways and traditional Mexican and other Latino cultural norms may help explain these differences.

Social work implications from this study indicate the need to have a culturally and gender informed perspective when working with Mexican and other Latino families and communities. Building effective partnerships with organized religion with the goal of effectively reaching out to both young Mexican men and women on both sides of the border can be highly beneficial from a prevention science point of view. Approaching substance use prevention as a gendered phenomenon might help reinforce effective substance use prevention interventions for both girls and boys and might also help the design and evaluation of culturally relevant and responsive services that are addressing the rapidly changing norms of Mexican youth in Mexico and other Latino youth.

ACKNOWLEDGMENTS

Research assistance for data analysis and manuscript development was supported by training funds from the National Institute on Minority Health and Health Disparities of the National Institutes of Health (NIMHD/NIH), award P20 MD002316-07 (F.F. Marsiglia, P.I.). The content is solely the responsibility of the authors and does not necessarily represent the official views of the National Institute on Minority Health Disparities or the National Institutes of Health.

REFERENCES

[1] World Health Organization. Global status report on alcohol and health. Geneva: WHO, 2011.

[2] Instituto Nacional de Salud Publica. Encuesta Nacional de Adicciones, 2008. Mexico: Instituto Nacional de Salud Publica INSP, 2009.

[3] Benjet C, Borges G, Medina-Mora ME, Fleiz C, Blanco J, Zambrano J, et al. Prevalence and socio-demographic correlates of drug use among adolescents: Results from the Mexican Adolescent Mental Health Survey. Addiction 2007;102:1261-8.

[4] Villareal J, Medina-Mora ME, Amador N, Bermudez P, Hernandez H, Fleiz C, et al. [Drug, alcohol, and tobacco use among students in Mexico D.F.]. Mexico: INP-SEP, 2004.

[5] Marsiglia FF, Ayers SL, Hoffman S. Religiosity and adolescent substance use in central Mexico: Exploring the influence of internal and external religiosity on cigarette and alcohol use. Am J Commun Psychol 2012;49:87-97.

[6] Herrera-Vazquez M, Wagner F, Velasco-Mondragon E, Borges G, Lazcano-Ponce E. Onset of alcohol and tobacco use and transition to other drug use among students from Morelos, Mexico. Salud Publica Mexico 2004;46(2):1-9.

[7] Instituto Nacional de Salud Publica. Encuesta Nacional de Adicciones, 2011. Mexico: Instituto Nacional de Salud Publica, 2012.

[8] Instituto Nacional de Salud Publica. Encuesta Nacional de Adicciones, 2012. Mexico: Instituto Nacional de Salud Publica, 2013.

[9] Kulis S, Marsiglia FF, Lingard EC, Nieri T, Nagoshi J. Gender identity and substance use among students in two high schools in Monterrey, Mexico. Drug Alc Depend 2008;95(3):258-68.

[10] Robins LN, Przybeck TR. Age of onset of drug use as a factor in drug and other disorders. Washington, DC: National Institute Drug Abuse Monograph 56, DHHS Publication No ADM 87-1335, 1987:178-92).

[11] Volkow ND, Li T. Drug addiction: The neurobiology of behaviour gone awry. Nat Rev Neurosci 2004;5:963-70.

[12] Latimer W, Floyd LJ, KariisT, Novotna G, Exnerova P, O'Brien M. Peer and sibling substance use: Predictors of substance use among adolescents in Mexico. Rev Panam Salud Publica 2004;15(4):225-32.
[13] Medina-Mora ME, Cravioto P, Villatoro J, Fleiz C, Galvan-Castillo F, Tapia-Conyer R. Drug use among adolescents: Results from the National Survey on Addictions, 1998. Salud Publica Mexico 2003;45:S16-S25.
[14] Miller MA, Alberts JK, Hecht ML, Trost M, Krizek RL. Adolescent relationships and drug use. Mahwah, NJ: Erlbaum, 2000.
[15] Johnson BR, Jang SJ, Li SD, Larson DB. The "invisible institution" and black youth crime: The church as an agency of local social control. J Youth Adolesc 2000;29:479-98.
[16] Nonnemaker JM, McNeely CA, Blum RW. Public and private domains of religiosity and adolescent health risk behaviors: Evidence from the national longitudinal study of adolescent health. Soc Sci Med 2003;57:2049-54.
[17] Sen G, Ostlin P, George A. Unequal, unfair, ineffective and inefficient gender inequity in health: Why it exists and how we can change it. World Health Organization 2007. Accessed 2014 Mar 10. URL: http://cdrwww.who.int.ezproxy1.lib.asu.edu/social_determinants/resources/csdh_media/wgekn_final_report_07.pdf.
[18] Coatsworth JD, Pantin H, Szapocznik J. Familias Unidas: A family centered ecodevelopmental intervention to reduce risk for problem behavior among Hispanic adolescents. Clin Child Fam Psychol Rev 2002;5:113-32.
[19] Pantin H, Schwartz SJ, Sullivan S, Coatsworth JD, Szapocznik J. Preventing substance abuse in Hispanic immigrant adolescents: An eco-developmental, parent-centered approach. Hisp J Behav Sci 2003b;25(4):469-500.
[20] Bacio GA, Estrada Y, Huang S, Martinez M, Sardinas K, Prado G. Ecodevelopmental predictors of early initiation of alcohol, smoking, and drug use among Hispanic adolescents. J School Psychol;53:195-208.
[21] Szapocznik J, Coatsworth JD. An ecodevelopmental framework for organizing the influences on drug abuse: A developmental model of risk and protection. In Glantz M, Hurtel CR, eds. Drug Abuse: Origins and Interventions. Washington, DC: American Psychological Association, 1999:331-6.
[22] Prado G, Huang S, Schwartz SJ, Maldonado-Molina MM, Bandiera FC, De la Rosa M, Pantin H. What accounts for difference in substance use among U.S.-born and immigrant Hispanic adolescents? Results from a longitudinal prospective cohort study. J Adolesc Health 2008;45:118-25.
[23] Martinez MJ, Huang S, Estrada Y, Sutton M. The relationship between acculturation, ecodevelopment, and substance use among Hispanic adolescents. J Early Adolescence 2016;1-27.
[24] Koss-Chioino JD, Vargas LA. Working with Latino youth: Culture, development, and context. San Francisco, CA: Jossey-Bass, 1999.
[25] Szapocznik J, Prado G, Burlew AK, Williams RA, Santisteban DA. Drug abuse* in African American and Hispanic adolescents: Culture, development, and behavior. Annu Rev Clin Psychol 2007;3:77-105.
[26] Marsiglia FF, Kulis S. Culturally grounded social work: Diversity, oppression, and change. Chicago, IL: Lyceum, 2008.
[27] Marsiglia FF, Kulis S, Nieri T, Parsai M. God Forbid! Substance Use Among Religious and Nonreligious Youth. Am J Orthopsyhiatry 2005;75:585-98.
[28] Smith C. Theorizing religious effects among American adolescents. J Sci Relig 2003;42(1):17-30.
[29] Erickson E. Identity: Youth and crisis. New York: Norton; 1968.
[30] Marcia JE. Development and validation of ego identity status. J Pers Soc Psychol 1966;5:551-8.
[31] Miller L, Davies M, Greenwald S. Religiosity and substance use and abuse among adolescents in the national comorbidity survey. J Am Acad Child Adolesc Psychol 2000;39:1190-7.
[32] Hodge DR, Marsiglia FF, Nieri T. Religion and substance use among youths of Mexican heritage: A social capital perspective. Soc Work Res 2011;35:137-46.
[33] Jang SJ, Bader CD, Johnson BR. The cumulative advantage of religiosity in preventing drug use. J Drug Issues 2008;38:771-98.

[34] Jang SJ, Johnson BR. The effects of childhood exposure to drug users and religion on drug use in adolescence and young adulthood. Youth Soc 2011;43:1220-45.
[35] Hodge DR, Cardenas P, Montoya H. Substance use: Religious participation as protective factors among rural youths. Soc Work Res 2001;25:153-61.
[36] Bartkowski JP, Xu X. Religiosity and teen drug use reconsidered: A social capital perspective. Am J Prev Med 2007;32:S182-94.
[37] Flanzer, JP. Alcohol use among Jewish adolescents: A 1977 sample. Curr Alcohol 1979;6:257-68.
[38] Friedman, BD. Building a spiritual based model to address substance abuse. Soc Thought 2000;19:23-8.
[39] Castro RG. Chicano folklore: A guide to the folktales, traditions, rituals, and religious practices of Mexican-Americans. Oxford: Oxford University Press, 2001.
[40] Stephen L. Sexualities and Genders in Zapotec Oaxaca. Lat Am Perspect 2002;29(2):41-59.
[41] Fiala WE, Bjorck JP, Gorsuch R. The religious support scale: Construction, validation, and cross validation. Am J Commun Psychol 2002;30:761-786.
[42] Nasim A, Utsey SO, Cornoa R, Belgrave, FZ. Religiosity, refusal efficacy, and substance use among African American adolescent and young adults. J Ethn Subst Abuse 2006;5(3):29-49.
[43] Milevsky A, Levitt M. Intrinsic and extrinsic religiosity in preadolescence and adolescence: Effect on psychological adjustment. Ment Health Relig Cult 2004;7:307-21.
[44] Donahue MJ. Intrinsic and extrinsic religiousness: Review and meta-analysis. J Pers Soc Psychol 1985;48:400-9.
[45] Castro FG, Coe K. Traditions and alcohol use: A mixed-methods analysis. Cultur Divers Ethnic Minor Psychol 2007;13:269-84.
[46] Castro FG, Stein JA, Bentler PM. Ethnic pride, traditional family values, and acculturation in early cigarette and alcohol use among Latino adolescents. J Prim Prev 2009;30:265-92.
[47] Medina-Mora ME, Rojas Guiot E. Mjuer, probeza, y addiciones. Perinatol Reprod Hum 2003;17:230-44.
[48] Pena M, Frehill LM. Latina religious practice: Analyzing cultural dimensions in measures of religiosity. J Sci Study Relig 1998;37:620-35.
[49] Alvarez L, Ruiz P. Substance abuse in the Mexican-American population. In Straussner LA, ed. Ethnocultural factors in substance abuse treatment. New York: Guliford, 2001:111-36.
[50] Medina C. Towards an understanding of Puerto Rican ethnicity and substance abuse. In Straussner LA, ed. Ethnocultural factors in substance abuse treatment. New York: Guliford, 2001:137-63.
[51] Rothe E, Ruiz P. Substance abuse among Cuban Americans. In Straussner LA, ed. Ethnocultural factors in substance abuse treatment New York: Guliford, 2001:97-110.
[52] Velez-Ibanez CG. Border Visions: Mexican cultures of the southwest United States. Tucson, AZ: University Arizona Press, 1996.
[53] Hunt LL. Religion, gender, and the Hispanic experience in the United States: Catholic/Protestant differences in religious involvement, social status, and gender role attitudes. Rev Relig Res 2001;43(2):139-60.
[54] Perea A, Slater D. Power distance and collectivist/individualist strategies in alcohol warnings: Effects by gender and ethnicity. J Health Commun 1999;4:295-310.
[55] Spira MK, Grossman SF, Wolff-Bensdorf J. Voice and identity in a bicultural/bilingual environment. Child Adolesc Social Work J 2002;19:115-38.
[56] Smith C, Denton ML, Faris R, Regnerus M. Mapping American adolescent religious participation. J Sci Study Relig 2002; 41: 597-612.
[57] Rodriguez, J. Our lady of Guadalupe: Faith and empowerment among Mexican-American women. Austin, TX: University Texas Press, 2010.
[58] Basham R. Machismo. Frontiers: J Women Studies 1976; 1(2): 126-143.
[59] McGuire, MB. Gendered spirituality and quasi-religious ritual. In Greil A, Robbins T, eds. Between Sacred and Secular: Research on Theory and Quasi-Religion. Greenwich, CT: JAI Press, 1994.
[60] Kulis S, Marsiglia FF, Hurdle. Gender identity, ethnicity, acculturation and drug use: Exploring differences among adolescents in the Southwest. J Commun Psychol 2003;31:1-22.

[61] Wycoff CS. The Garcia family: Using a structural systems approach with an alcohol-dependent family. Fam J Alex Va 2000;8(1):47-57.

[62] Felix-Ortiz M, Villatoro-Velazquez JA, Medina-Mora ME, Newcomb MD. Adolescent drug use in Mexico and among Mexican American adolescents in the United States: Environmental influences and individual characteristics. Cultur Divers Ethnic Minor Psychol 2001;7:27-46.

[63] Hecht ML, Trost M, Bator R, MacKinnon D. Ethnicity and gender similarities and differences in drug resistance. J Appl Commun Res 1997;25:75-97.

[64] Kulis S, Marsiglia FF, Hecht ML. Gender labels and gender identity as predictors of drug use among ethnically diverse middle school students. Youth Soc 2002;33:442-75.

[65] Kulis S, Marsiglia FF, Castillo J, Becerra D, Nieri T. Drug resistance strategies and substance use among adolescents in Monterrey, Mexico. J Prim Prev 2008;29:167-92.

[66] Deutsch FM, Zalenski CM, Clark, ME. Is there a double standard of aging? J Appl Psychol 1986;16:771-5.

[67] Robler H. The meaning of culturally sensitive research. Am J Psychiatry 1989;146:296-303.

[68] Marsiglia FF, Hecht ML. Keepin'it REAL: An evidence-based program. Santa Cruz: ETR Associates, 2005.

[69] Andrews JA, Tildesley E, Hops H, Duncan SC, Severson HH. Elementary school age children's future intentions and use of substances. J Clin Adolesc Psychol 2003;32:556-67.

[70] Maddahian E, Newcomb MD, Bentler PM. Adolescent drug use and intention to use drugs: Concurrent and longitudinal analyses of four ethnic groups. Addict Behav 1998;13:191-5.

[71] IBM Corporation. IBM SPSS statistics for windows, version 21.0. Armonk: IBM Corporation, 2012.

[72] Cortés-Guardado MA, Shibya-Soto CS. Los valores de los jaliscienses. Encuesta Estatal de Valores. Mexico: Universidad de Guadalajara, 1999.

In: Public Health Yearbook 2016
Editor: Joav Merrick
ISBN: 978-1-53610-947-4

Chapter 21

PERCEPTIONS AND ATTITUDES ABOUT CHILDHOOD OBESITY AMONG ADULTS IN THE LOWER RIO GRANDE VALLEY

George S Eyambe, PhD, Bruce D Friedman*, PhD and Esmeralda Rawlings, MSW

Clinical Laboratory Sciences, University of Texas Pan American, Edinburg, Texas, US;
Department of Social Work, California State University, Bakersfield, California, US;
and Doctors Hospital McAllen, McAllen, Texas, US

ABSTRACT

Childhood obesity is a health and social problem in the United States. Childhood obesity leads to increased problems of diabetes, heart disease, and other health factors as the children become adults, thus increasing the costs of health care. Is this a universal problem or one that may have specific geographic or cultural considerations was explored. A mixed methods study of low income individuals in the Lower Rio Grande region of the United States was done. The qualitative data identified a number of factors relating to obesity as both cultural and socio-economic problems that cut across multiple intervention strategies. Meaning that it is an individual problem with the need for some mezzo and macro interventions. The study recommends four intervention strategies including: three generational intergenerational educational programs since grandparents are very engaged in the upbringing of the children in this Mexican-American population; the increase of intergenerational exercise opportunities since things are better supported if parents and grandparents are engaged in the process; a multiple disciplinary approach that shares the burden between physicians who do not have adequate time to address the issues and other health professions; and finally, increasing the number of safe recreational areas within communities, especially in the low income areas of a community where there are minimal safe recreational areas. The study identified that the problems of obesity are multifaceted needing additional research. Cultural factors

* Corresponding author: Professor Bruce D Friedman, PhD, ACSW, CSWM, LCSW, Director, Department of Social Work, California State University Bakersfield, 25 DDH-9001 Stockdale Highway, Bakersfield, CA 93311-1022, United States. E-mail: bfriedman@csub.edu.

contributed to the problem meaning solutions should incorporate the cultural values of the population when developing interventions.

Keywords: childhood, obesity, public health, health, intervention

Introduction

Obesity and childhood obesity in particular have been receiving more and more attention as a social problem in the United States. The issues of obesity are not just factors of being overweight, but that there are complications to other health problems as a result of being obese. These complications are in the form of increased issues of diabetes, heart disease, and other complications (1). Some speculate that it is a simple fix in addressing the obesity problem of reducing ones calorie intake while burning more calories. However, it is not that easy. There are a number of contributing factors associated with changes in the types of foods that people are eating, the advent of technology as it has related to lifestyle changes, and culture. The problem has been ever increasing over the past three decades with the trend being that all regions in the United States have been getting heavier leading to a public health crisis (1, 2).

Although the problem is a national health problem, there are racial and ethnic differences in the problem (2). Several studies have reported that non-Hispanic Blacks and Mexican Americans had higher prevalence of obesity problems than other groups with over a 10-percentage point differential (2). With the South Texas area having a higher percentage of Mexican Americans than many other parts of the country, it was important to understand the factors that contribute to the obesity problem in this region. Specific CDC county data by state also shows that Hidalgo and Starr Counties, Texas have some of the highest values of both obesity and diabetes in Texas with values of 9.7% of the Hidalgo population having diabetes problems and 34.2% with obesity problems and the Starr county data represents 8.9% and 34.2% respectively (3). This area of south Texas is along the Mexico-Texas border and is classified as the lower Rio Grande. When looking at other factors, this area also reflects higher levels of persons with less than a high school education (49.5% compared to 24.3%) and higher levels of poverty (34% compared to 16.3%) than other parts of Texas (4).

Causes of obesity

The causes of obesity are very complex and multifactoral (5, 6). It cannot be simply described as the need to reduce food intake in combination with increasing exercise as there are multiple factors associated with the problem of obesity. On the one hand, Mayer's (7) glucostatic theory states that glucose (sugar) is an inhibitor to food intake and that alone will not cause obesity but lead to a positive energy balance. Wang and Beydoun (2) show that there are numerous factors including gender, socioeconomic, racial/ethnic, and geographic issues that contribute to obesity. Thus, a complex strategy needs to be developed in order to arrive at solutions to address this national epidemic.

Caprio et al. (3) look at the racial and ethnic factors as relating to a social construct. Even though there may be some commonalities between racial and ethnic groups, it is not possible to generalize across them. Thus, it is important to incorporate other factors that may be contributing to the obesity epidemic in various areas. Caprio et al. (3) look at race/ethnicity as one factor but combine it with factors of socioeconomic status, biology and culture not only as causal factors associated with obesity but also as addressing some of the prevention and treatment modalities as well. However, Hunt et al. (8) warn that it is important to be careful not to look at ethnic factors as a form of stereotyping when taking them into consideration as part of health disparities.

Poston and Foreyt (9) identify that there are major environmental factors that contribute to obesity. These may come in the form of lifestyle factors that may lead individuals to lifestyles that are not compatible to the person's evolutionary makeup. They argue that environment rather than genetic factors are the true cause of obesity.

Childhood obesity

To this point, there has been a discussion of obesity in general but the question is whether there are inherent factors that may lead to the increase in childhood obesity. For if some of these factors can be addressed early enough then maybe there would not be so many obese adults. Yet, over the past thirty years, there has been an increase in the number of obese individuals in the United States and there has been an increasingly alarming number of obese children. Such factors as both parents being obese, the number of hours watching television, maternal smoking during pregnancy, reduced sleeping patterns, and percent weight gain in the first year were all factors that contributed to obese children (10, 13). Since the problem is continuing to increase, it is evident that previous interventions have been unsuccessful in addressing these factors. Reilly et al. (10), suggest the need for early intervention but a true understanding of the issues associated with childhood obesity still persists.

Epstein et al. (11) demonstrated that there is a familial relationship associated with obesity. In their study, when a family incorporated lifestyle changes, such as eating more fruit, then there was an ability to reduce the level of obesity in that family. However, they also mentioned that the behavior needs to be sustained or else the family will resort back to prior behaviors.

Childhood obesity continues to be a leading public health concern (9) particularly among minority and low income children (12). The Pediatric Nutrition Surveillance System (PedNSS) is the only nationally compiled obesity data obtained at the state and local levels. The data showed that obesity trends among low-income, preschool-aged children increased steadily between 1998 and 2008 (13). A total prevention method will need to be incorporated to address this problem.

There was no available data on the PedNSS for Texas in 1998 but between 2003 and 2008, Texas showed an increase in prevalence percentage of obesity in children between ages 2 and 4 years from 14.4 to 16.2 (14). With the high percentage of low-income and minority children in the Lower Rio Grande Valley region of Texas, the research team decided it was important to find out from the community those factors that they believe contributed to childhood obesity in the area and if there was a perception as to whether the obesity was different here than the rest of the United States. This led to the development of a mixed methods research project that would identify key stakeholders to ascertain the cause and extent of childhood obesity in the Lower Rio Grande Valley region of Texas. In addition, by identifying key informants, then it would be possible to understand from those who are closest to the situation what the factors are and enable the development of appropriate intervention strategies for the region. Flanagan's (16) Critical Incident technique was used in the development of focus groups that were used with the key informants to arrive at the qualitative data.

METHODS

With the purpose of the study to not only identify factors that contribute to childhood obesity, but to also develop some intervention strategies, it was felt that the University needed to engage community-based organizations and primary healthcare practitioners in the Lower Rio Grande Valley. To move in this direction, a mixed method research approach was introduced. To identify baseline data on perceptions as to whether obesity was a problem and whether it differentiated from the rest of the United States, a survey was developed, piloted for validity and reliability, and distributed to physicians and other health professionals, dieticians, and health educators. The second phase of the project was to conduct focus groups to provide a more in-depth understanding of the obesity problem in the Lower Rio Grande Valley in order to develop an intervention strategy. The focus group data was analyzed following Flanagan's Critical Incident Technique with the use of N-VIVO 9 (QSR Intl., Melbourne, Australia) research software to categorize the qualitative data.

FINDINGS

The Rio Grande Valley is one of the poorest areas in the United States with a Hispanic population of over 90%. It is also one of the areas of the country with high rates of juvenile diabetes and high rates of acanthosis nigricans. These are all elements that relate to childhood obesity. So the question posed was, what factors lead to childhood obesity in the Rio Grande Valley? In addition, is childhood obesity different in the Rio Grande Valley than the rest of the United States?

These questions led to a process of engaging a variety of community professionals, lay health educators, and parents with obese children living in Hidalgo, Cameron, Starr, and Willacy counties in Texas, all along the lower Rio Grande River. The community professionals consisted of physicians (family and pediatricians), school dieticians, nurse practitioners, and health educators. Because there is a high percentage of community members where Spanish is either the first or the only language in the home, we included a number of lay health professionals called promotoras - laypersons trained to work within the colonias (undeveloped housing complexes) in the Rio Grande Valley, as part of the stake holders engaged in the project. The third group consisted of parents, mostly those living in colonias, with overweight children undergoing therapy.

Table 1. Weight Perception Survey Summary Statistics

Category	Problem in US	Problem in LRGV	Perceived Difference between LRGV & US	Comparison between LRGV and US	Contributing factors	Diet	Rated Obesity in LRGV
Dietician (n = 14)	Yes = 14	Yes = 14	Yes = 8 No = 6	Above = 10 Same = 3 Below = 1	Stress = 2 Lack of Education = 12 Culture = 12 Lack Exercise = 13 Low Self Esteem = 2 Lack Leisure Activity = 4	Carb = 13 Snacks = 13 Soft Drinks = 12 Fast Food = 11 Meats = 9 Dairy = 2	Above = 10 Same = 3 Below = 1
Physician (n = 22)	Yes = 22	Yes = 22	Yes = 18 No = 4	Above = 20 Same = 2	Stress = 3 Lack of Education = 21 Culture = 17 Lack Exercise = 20 Low Self Esteem = 7 Lack Leisure Activity = 10 Other = 10	Carb = 22 Fruit = 1 Snacks = 20 Soft Drinks = 19 Fast Food = 22 Meats = 16 Dairy = 11	Above = 21 Same = 1
Physician Assistant (n = 15)	Yes = 15	Yes = 15	Yes = 11 No = 4	Above = 11 Same = 3	Stress = 5 Lack of Education = 12 Culture = 12 Lack Exercise = 14 Low Self Esteem = 8 Lack Leisure Activity = 8	Carb = 15 Fruit = 2 Snacks = 14 Soft Drinks = 15 Fast Food = 13 Meats = 14 Dairy = 5	Above = 12 Same = 2 Below = 1
Community Member (n = 60)	Yes = 56 No = 4	Yes = 57 No = 3	Yes = 25 No = 35*	Above = 25 Same = 28 Below = 6	Stress = 10 Lack of Education = 28 Culture = 17 Lack Exercise = 25 Low Self Esteem = 18 Lack Leisure Activity = 13 Other = 4	Carb = 32 Fruit = 24** Snacks = 23 Soft Drinks = 21 Fast Food = 30 Meats = 35 Dairy = 16	Above = 23 Same = 29 Below = 9

Significance *<.05; ** <.01.

This study was supported by a grant from the National Institues of Child Health and Human Development, National Institutes of Health.

The quantitative data appears in Table 1 and represents a comparison between the stakeholders. All groups felt that there was an obesity problem in the United States yet when the community members were compared to the professionals, there was a significant difference in perception as to whether the problem was different in the Lower Rio Grande Valley compared to the United States with the professionals feeling that the problem was greater whereas the community members did not (F = 11.747 significant to the .01 level). It was also interesting to note that the perception of diet showed some significant differences when the professionals were compared with the community members. The professionals did not see hardly any fruits and vegetables as part of the diet, yet over half of the community members mentioned that fruit and vegetables were part of their diet (F value of 28.271 significant at the .01 level). Other than that there were no significant differences between the professionals and the community members.

This still led to a number of questions as to how to make sense of the problem of obesity in the Lower Rio Grande Valley. To address these questions, thirteen focus groups were conducted to solicit participants' attitudes and perceptions about childhood obesity in both the United States and the Rio Grande Valley and some ideas for solutions to address the problem. The focus groups followed a semi-structured set of questions (Table 1) to elicit open discussion about the attitudes and perceptions. Each person in the focus group was perceived to be an expert of his/her knowledge and experience in order to help the research team gather information that will help to develop a planned intervention for the Lower Rio Grande Valley region to address the issues about childhood obesity.

The focus groups were recorded. Since the primary language for many of the promotoras and community members was Spanish, the focus groups were translated into English and transcribed into an N-Vivo data file for analysis. The responses from the participants identified 33 different variables relating to what the participants felt were contributing factors to childhood obesity in the Rio Grande Valley. Some of these variables are interrelated and linked together. Seven overriding variables seem to encompass the problems. First were lifestyle factors that have changed over the years. Second were cultural factors associated with being in the Rio Grande Valley. Third were genetic issues that may be unique to the area. Fourth were climatic factors in the Rio Grande Valley that keep people in-doors during the summer. That also relates to the fifth factor of a lack of safe recreational places in the area. Most of the people interviewed either worked with the poor or were poor, there were mixed perceptions about the sixth factor of socio-economic issues. These seemed to cut across between the professionals and the non-professionals with the non-professionals feeling that socio-economic status was a contributing factor. The basic overriding issue goes back to the basic premise of calories in versus calories out. Thus, lifestyle and marketing with a variety of other psychological factors are contributors to the seventh factor of portion sizes. A brief discussion of each of these factors is given below.

Lifestyle factors

All groups felt that one of the biggest contributors to childhood obesity in the United States is changes in lifestyle. Some of these factors relate to the need to have two working parents. One participant stated, "When you are a working parent you don't have time to go and play with kids, also because you are tired you tell them to watch TV so you can keep them busy while you do things. That is not healthy either if that is all they do." A number of participants struggling with balancing work and family time including no time to prepare dinner for the children repeated that sentiment. They stated that it was easier to get fast food or eat out than to cook and that created somewhat of a sedentary lifestyle, as relayed by another participant, "now our days the whole world is getting bigger and bigger for the same reason that parents don't have time, and pick up food on the way home. A lot of us had our moms that stayed home all day and they were making tortillas all day and they cook and stuff."

Although lifestyle factors and working parents is a national phenomenon, the participants felt that when combined with culture, lack of recreation, and climatic factors, that these factors were exacerbated here in the Rio Grande Valley. A number of participants stated, "The heat is what's keeping the kids inside, they don't want to be outside because it is too hot." and, "there is a lack of recreational activities for the children, we don't have theaters, there is really nothing here to do, and we are too far away from anything." Thus, the combination of climate and lack of recreational activities, keeps the children in the home watching television or playing video games. The Hispanic culture of our region is used to eating more traditional foods like tacos, tortillas, and tamales; however, the parents said that their children prefer to eat the food that is served in the schools. A number of parents voiced this sentiment, "Many times you can't give your children what you want because they will not eat it. They are so used to eating the food from school that when they get home they don't want to eat the food we make because they want food like school, pizza, and hamburger and so on."

Cultural factors

Cultural factors were another reason used to differentiate the differences between obesity in the Rio Grande Valley and the rest of the United States. Many of the participants reported that food is a central component to the Mexican-American culture. People use food for all types of celebrations. The food that is used is not healthy foods but the "three Ts" or tacos, tortillas, and tamales, usually made with Manteca (lard). Some participants reported that when asked to use vegetable oil, the participants reported that the older generation would say that they could not because it just would not taste good.

Another factor associated with culture is the relationship of chubby children associated with being healthy. One participant stated that the value of her parents was "gordito es bonito," or fat is beautiful. That idea is attributed to children who are under two years of age. Some of the physicians participating in the focus groups stated that this idea could be problematic since as children develop there are certain fat pockets that develop during certain periods. Once those pockets develop, they exist for life. Thus, there are factors associated with chubby children developing at young ages contributing to them always being heavy since the fat pockets developed at those younger ages.

Genetic factors

Both the physicians and the nurse practitioners associated genetic factors to obesity prevalence in the Rio Grande Valley. Since there is a strong influence of Mexican heritage in the population and there is a high percentage of northern Mexican residents who have settled in the area, both the physicians and nurse practitioners stated that there is a strong genetic relationship with the indigenous Native Americans in the area. As a migratory group, they survived by stocking up with food during periods of plenty and then during lean periods would live off their body fat. However, with the advent of modernization, food is readily available and thus, there is not the need to work off the body fat as was customary before the introduction of modern amenities. Yet, the population has not learned nor has changed their values associated to food and being chubby as a baby.

The four counties of Hidalgo, Cameron, Starr, and Willacy are tied into agriculture. Some of the participants contributed changing agricultural patterns to the obesity problem. Some identified the high levels of fertilizers and growth enhancing chemicals used in agriculture as a contributing factor. One participant stated, “the hormones that are injected into the animals that we eat, and the fertilizers that are used to grow the vegetables … (depletes the food) of all the minerals and stuff that is not being allowed to develop in the food so that it grows faster.”

Climate

Another difference that participants identified that leads to obesity in the Rio Grande Valley differently than the rest of the United States is the climate. Almost everyone felt that the climatic conditions, particularly in the summer, contribute to people staying in air conditioning much of the time. They state that it is just too hot and humid to be outdoors in the summer. Thus, children stay inside and become sedentary watching television or playing video games. Participants state, “The heat is what’s keeping the kids inside, they don’t want to be outside because it is too hot.” They also state, “there is a lack of recreational activities for the children, we don’t have theaters, there is really nothing here to do, and we are too far away from anything.” They continue with the idea that the heat and the lack of outdoor recreational activities are major contributing factors that differentiate the area from other parts of the Untied States.

Safe recreational areas

All the participants stated that there were very few places to be able to exercise and even when there were hike and bike trails, there were differences between those in the more affluent areas compared to those that went through poorer areas. One of the physicians talked about the differences between the two hike and bike trails in McAllen with the one on 2nd Street being more appealing since it was a more affluent area of town. Other participants identified unsafe parks and not wanting their children to play in the parks. Everyone identifies the need for recreational activities in order to burn calories but there is the need to have safe places for that to take place.

This area demonstrates that it is not just an individual factor relating to obesity but there are also community infrastructure concerns and thus changes within the larger community need to take place to create safer places for participants to recreate and burn calories.

Socio-economic factors

When asked if there was a correlation between socio-economic issues and obesity, there was some disparity between the groups. In general, the professionals saw that obesity cuts across all economic classes, but they did feel that those who have means have access to more recreational opportunities. For example, the health educators stated that there is a physical education alternative in the schools. Usually the upper class students apply for it because they are participating in extracurricular activities like dance or athletics whereas the lower class students did not seem to participate in those outside activities. This was particularly important as the educators felt that since "No Child Left Behind" was initiated, there has been a reduction in the amount of physical education within the school day and it was necessary for children to obtain their physical education through extracurricular activities that supported the more affluent children.

On the other hand, the parents and paraprofessionals truly saw that there was a strong correlation between class and obesity. They stated that when resources are tight, families would choose to purchase the cheaper foods that are higher in carbohydrates, fats, and sodium. Only the more affluent families could afford the organic foods. Thus, a relationship between obesity, class and poverty does exist.

In addition, many of the participants felt that there was a correlation between obesity, class and education. There was the feeling that those who received assistance did not always know the healthy choices or how to prepare foods without high fat.

A phenomenon in the Rio Grande Valley region is also the proliferation of buffets. Many of the participants described that people would go to the all you can eat buffet and load up and over eat, thus relating to portion size.

Another phenomenon in the area is the number of people who live in colonias, which are undeveloped housing communities. The participants stated that it is difficult to purchase groceries at the local supermarkets since they are far away. One participant stated, "I need to take two buses to shop at HEB or Globe (two of the local supermarket chains). If I buy milk it will spoil by the time I get home because of the heat, and that leaves out any frozen items. I usually buy canned goods or dry goods and supplement at the local store, which does not have as nice or fresh food as HEB or Globe and it is more expensive."

A number of participants talked about the differences between being poor in the United States compared to Mexico. They stated that in the US, the government provides food stamps whereas in Mexico there are no handouts. They said that they would use the food stamps to buy food inappropriately. One participant stated, "I believe that the people that don't get food stamps only buy what they really need. The people with food stamps or that get them sometimes misused their food stamps by buying lots of food. We have never qualified for food stamps and the little money that we have, we try to use it as best as possible." A number of individuals stated that they had grown up in Mexico. They stated that, "in Mexico there were no food stamps and one had to walk everywhere in order to get food for the day. With food stamps, people have become lazy and do not have to walk everywhere just to get food for the day."

Portion size

Everyone agreed that portion size has gotten out of control and that, it and lack of exercise, were the biggest contributors to obesity. Focus group participants stated that this was not a Rio Grande Valley phenomenon but was happening everywhere and went along with lifestyle changes over the past twenty years.

In the Rio Grande Valley region, this is exacerbated by the lack of eating a balanced diet and the proliferation of fast food restaurants where people would prefer to eat out and they get more food for the dollar than by preparing it themselves. The participants stated that people just do not understand that they do not need to eat that much.

Even those individuals receiving WIC stated that they do not understand portion sizes. One participant stated, "WIC shows you the pyramid, and tells you this and that but does not tell you how much of each group you should eat. Like they tell you that you need to eat six fruits for example, to me six apples would be too much, but they don't explain that it could be throughout the day like if you have cereal with fruit, that is one, or eating ice cream with different fruits or vanilla then you are already having some more fruit. Some people don't realize that the fruit is already in there as part of the fruit servings and even maybe two."

Interventions recommended from the focus groups:

There were four intervention suggestions that emerged from the focus groups. All the participants felt that childhood obesity was a problem, not only nationally, but also more so in the Rio Grande Valley. They proposed the need for doing a multidisciplinary and multi-systemic intervention. Some related specifically to individual changes while others would need to be community changes. Based on the data, the individual changes relate to nutrition education conducted for parents, children, and grandparents (since extended family is very important within the culture and with parents working, many times grandparents are providing daycare). As one participant said, "I believe like for me there should be more groups on education but also that involve children together. This way the parents can deal with their children and the children will be able to understand why their parents are changing their eating habits."

Second intervention is to increase exercise opportunities and things that can be done inter-generationally. It was felt that if the parents learn something but the children are not involved, then there is a possibility that it will be sabotaged by the non-participating group. Thus, there needs to be consistent in the content that is shared and presented. One of the health educators shared, "Last year my program got a grant for diabetes awareness and we started the program with youth, and the youth are ages 4-15 and the physical activity we did with them was folk dance. When the moms would come out to the program and saw what the kids were doing, they would ask why are you dancing? We would tell them that was our physical activity. They did not even think, they are having fun jumping around they are just having a ball and did not even think that was exercise and the dads would say why are you teaching them how to dance, we say its just a form of exercise or physical activity. So, when the parents saw what we were teaching the children and the nutritional information we were giving them, the parents started to want to come so they could learn, too. The kids would even tell the parents what they should and should not eat. Mom you should not be cooking with that Manteca." Thus, if educational experiences become part of a family experience, then they will be supported by all members of the family and more easily incorporated into part of a more permanent lifestyle change.

The third intervention was how to engage the professionals more in the process. The suggestion was for the need for public education that involved the professionals in the process. Much of the responsibility seemed to rest with the physician. Two physicians shared these comments, "Physicians are very busy and sometimes only spend less than 20-30 minutes with our patients some of us do spend 30 minutes, I am sure. In my practice, I have enough help to be able to do that. If I was by myself there is no way I would have an interest in trying to study a problem much less spend less than ½ an hour talking to someone." While the other physician stated, "We are just overwhelmed trying to handle their immediate problem without thinking about other problems." With part of the problem being that obesity is not covered as part of the reimbursable diagnosis and thus it is hard to bill for it. As one physician stated, "if you call it obesity they don't pay for it." While another physician stated, "talk about reimbursement we cannot make a diagnosis of obesity even when it is so pathological. You have to use a different type of wording like hypercholesterolemia glycemia, but you cannot mention the world obesity that is a bad word for Medicaid." However, if a multi-professional intervention strategy can be employed, then it is possible to have these professionals working together. As one physician stated, "I belong to the step and stride committee and there they get to be seen by the doctor, but not by himself, they are always seeing other people, like speech therapist, but they are having OT because they have developmental delays, but they have weekly visit from our office." Thus, a multi-professional team is important in addressing all aspects of the patient including a nutritionist to assist in the nutritional factors for the patient.

The fourth area of intervention is to work with community leaders to create safe parks and recreational areas to enhance more activity. Currently, places like McDonalds have play areas, but as one participant stated, "The lack of recreational places, you go to McDonalds and yes they have the playground but first you have to get the food there, so there is not a place that doesn't have food without a safe recreational area for the kids." There is the need to work closely with community leaders to create safe places for families to be able to interact and burn calories.

DISCUSSION

It is evident from the data that childhood obesity is multifaceted and it would necessitate a comprehensive intervention in order to address this public health issue. It is also evident that there are geographic differences so that an intervention in one part of the country may not work the same as in other parts of the country. There are some basic similarities that can be surmised, though. The need for an increase in safer recreational areas, particularly those that are affordable seems to be a recurrent theme, in not only the Rio Grande Valley, but other parts of the country, too. Also, the issue of the accessibility of fast food and lifestyle changes is another factor that is not endemic to the Lower Rio Grande Valley.

Factors associated with culture and genetic factors may be endemic to the Rio Grande Valley area. It suggests the need for intergenerational educational programming since the involvement of grandparents in the raising of their grandchildren seems to be an important factor to take into consideration. As stated above, the older generation felt that the use of vegetable oil harmed the integrity of the tacos, tamales, and tortillas. Thus, there is a need for introducing different dietary factors and how they relate to health.

Perceptions about fat is beautiful may have been important considerations when child mortality rates were high, but with the advent of current medical practices, the health of the child is not necessarily linked to gaining tremendous amount of weight during the first year of life. Lifestyle changes have meant that it is weight that will most likely carry with the child throughout his or her life. Thus, the need for some prenatal education on just what are healthy lifestyles and eating habits.

The comments about the entitlement programs of WIC and Food Stamps were somewhat of a shocker as to their contributing factor to obesity. On the one hand, there is the desire to provide basic food needs for the population. However, as was mentioned, with the lack of education associated with the distribution of both WIC and Food Stamps, then it is possible that people will use them inappropriately striving for quantity rather than choosing appropriately. There is the need for more education and proper nutrition in relationship to the entitlement programs.

The mention of schools reducing the amount of physical education time to focus on academics was also disconcerting. As it has been identified that a healthy nutritional diet is important for education, hence the federally funded school breakfast and lunch programs, it is equally important for children to have a healthy body in order to enhance education. Physical education helps to relieve some of the academic stressors to enhance concentration on academic subjects. Thus, the practice that some schools have adopted to provide more hours of instruction in the school day in exchange for reduced physical education hours seems to be short sighted and a reversal of policies in the 1960s where the focus was on keeping fit.

Limitations

The study used a mixed method approach in collecting data. The quantitative data was more of a convenience sample as there was only a single mail survey sent to primary care physicians and pediatricians and as such only the data from those returned surveys was tabulated. It was perceived that there was sufficient randomness to represent the population but it was not known for certain.

The same held with the survey of physician assistants. The focus of the study was to get some baseline data from the quantitative aspect but then to drill deeper using qualitative methods to identify more specifics about attitudes and perceptions.

In collecting the qualitative data, one of the problems was that none of the principle investigators were Spanish speaking and as such there was a reliance on research assistants to provide translation and assist with the focus groups and the transcription of recorded discussions. With the population reflecting a high percentage of Spanish as the first and many times the only language, that was a deficit for the team. However, it was compensated for with good research assistants and a strong relationship with community partners through the community based organizations.

Next steps

As the participants from the focus groups identified, the issue is a multifaceted one that will take a number of interventions. This is not an individual problem but one that involves all aspects of the community. On the one hand, there is the need for inter-generational education to help address perceptions and attitudes about obesity and lifestyle. In addition, there needs to be some corporate interventions as well to help reduce the level of consumption and to create a well-balanced diet.

Schools and municipalities need to be engaged in order to see what can be done to improve opportunities for expanded recreation. It is important to not only look at providing walking trails, but to guarantee their safety for individuals who choose to use them.

With health reform being a major issue and obesity being identified as a major public health problem, there needs to be a way to integrate the two. In addition, the reliance for addressing the problem does not solely rest on the shoulders of the medical community, but there is a need to break down the 'silos' and work in interdisciplinary teams to fully address this public health concern.

CONCLUSION

Obesity and childhood obesity will continue to grow as a public health problem. Obesity leads to a number of health problems that can be addressed if there are proper steps taken to address them as a comprehensive lifestyle change when a child is born. However, the issue needs to be taken seriously and involves a number of stakeholders covering all aspects of society. It is also evident that one size does not fit all, but there are specific cultural and geographic factors that need to be considered. In addition, socio-economic factors also play an important factor and it is not easily addressed by providing entitlements such as WIC and Food Stamps. There needs to be a comprehensive educational approach to help individuals understand the implications of what is being put into our mouths and how that affects our well-being and overall health.

This study demonstrated the need for engaging community partners to help identify solutions. It is not something that can come from major research institutions that dictate the changes that need to be made but it necessitates the involvement and engagement in community members in a collaborative process to arrive at solutions. Although this study reflected the needs of the Lower Rio Grande Valley area, there are lessons learned that can be replicated elsewhere.

ACKNOWLEDGMENT

This project was funded by National Institute of Health Grant # 5U13HD052415-02

REFERENCES

[1] Centers for Disease Control and Prevention. US obesity trends by state 1985 – 2008. URL: http://www.cdc.govobesity/data/trends.html.
[2] Wang Y, Beydoun MA. The obesity epidemic in the United States. Gender, age, socioeconomic, racial/ethnic, and geographic characteristics: A systematic review and meta-regression analysis. Epidemiol Rev 2007; 29: 6-28.
[3] Caprio S, Daniels SR, Drewnowski A, Kaufman FR, Palinkas LA, Rosenbloom AL, et al. Influence of race, ethnicity, and culture on childhood obesity: implications for prevention and treatment. Diabetes Care 2008; 31(11): 2211-21.
[4] US Census. URL: http://www.census.gov/2010 census.
[5] Ebbeling CB, Pawlak DB, Ludwig DS. Childhood obesity: Public-health crisis, common sense cure. Lancet 2002; 360: 473-482.
[6] Henry J, Warren J. Causes of obesity. Lancet 2001; 357: 1978.
[7] Mayer J. Glucostatic mechanism of regulation of food intake. N Engl J Med 1953; 249: 13–6.
[8] Ludwig DS, Peterson KE, Gortmaker SL. Relation between consumption of sugar sweetened drinks and childhood obesity: A prospective observational analysis. Lancet 2001; 357: 505–8.
[9] Novella S. Calories in- calories out. Public Health Comments 2008; 202: 1-58.
[10] Hunt LM, Schneider S, Comer B. Should 'acculturation' be a variable in health research? A critical review of research on US Hispanics. Soc Sci Med 2004; 59: 973–86.
[11] Poston WSC II, Foreyt JP. Obesity is an environmental issue. Atherosclerosis 1999; 146: 201–9.
[12] Reilly JJ, Armstrong J, Dorosty AR, Emmett PM, Ness A, Rogers I, et al.
[13] Early life risk factors for obesity in childhood: cohort study. BMJ 2005; 330(7504): 1357.
[14] Epstein LH, Gordy CC, Raynor HA, Beddome M, Colleen K, Kilanowski CK et al. Increasing fruit and vegetable intake and decreasing fat and sugar intake in families at risk for childhood obesity. Obes Res 2001; 9(3): 171-8.
[15] Sharma AJ, Grummer-Strawn LM, Dalenius K, Galuska D, Anadappa M, Borland E, el al. Obesity prevalence among low-income, preschool-aged children. United States, 1998-2008. MMWR 2009; 58(28): 769-96.
[16] Stulberg B. The shrinking middle class of physical activity. Huffington Post 2-14 Sept 17.
[17] Flanagan JC. The critical incident technique. Psychol Bull 1954; 51(4): 1-33.

In: Public Health Yearbook 2016
Editor: Joav Merrick
ISBN: 978-1-53610-947-4

Chapter 22

IMPACT OF EMERGENCY REFERRALS TO PRIMARY CARE ON HEALTH CARE USE AND COSTS

Amanda W Roberts*, MSSW
School of Social Work, Abilene Christian University,
Abilene, Texas, US

ABSTRACT

Uncompensated care in US hospitals totals billions of dollars annually, and is influenced to some degree by uninsured patients utilizing emergency rooms (ER). This quasi-experimental study analyzed the rate of usage and cost savings resulting from the availability of a nonprofit primary care (PC) facility for uninsured patients in lieu of ER care in a small southwestern metropolitan area. ER data were gathered retroactively for 205 uninsured patients seen at one hospital that were referred to a local PC clinic; and PC clinic data were additionally gathered for the 82 of them that received medical care at the PC clinic. Two years of ER data before initiation of PC clinic referrals (2008-2010) and two post initiation (2011-2012) were gathered. Usage of the ER and PC clinics and their costs were compared for each group pre and post-referral. For patients that used PC services (n = 82), there was an average of six ER visits pre-referral and 3.5 ER visits post-referral. ER costs averaged $2,260 per visit, of which $1,733 was uncompensated, while PC visits averaged $213. The 40% of patients (82/205) that utilized PC services resulted in a projected hospital savings of $350,000+ from uncompensated care. ER visits are considerably more costly than PC clinics and PC availability coincides with decreases in ER utilization and financial losses from uncompensated care. However, the findings also illustrate the continued utilization of ERs by the uninsured, even when other alternatives are available. A full analysis of the issues are presented with implications for administrators and clinicians.

Keywords: health, primary care, emergency rooms, social work, uncompensated care

* Correspondence: Professor Amanda Wallander Roberts, MSSW, School of Social Work, Abilene Christian University, Abilene, Texas 79699, United States. E-mail: arw08c@acu.edu.

INTRODUCTION

Health care spending and outcomes in the United States are considerably different from other countries with similar wealth. In 2012, the United States (US) had the highest health care expenditures of the 193 World Health Organization member nations (1) and notably inferior health outcomes than countries with comparable wealth. Outside of the US, the most expensive system of health care costs only about two-thirds as much as in the US (2), while, of the countries with similar resources, the US ranks last in mortality rates from preventable deaths (3, 4).

The high expense and poor outcomes in the US health care system bring into question whether the government is responsible for providing health care to its citizens. The issues of the government's role in health care have been debated recently, as the Obama Administration is working to address the health care problems in the US through new and controversial legislation in the Affordable Care Act.

One of these problems the Obama Administration is aiming to address is the lack of health insurance. The percentage of uninsured individuals living in the US has grown considerably in recent years, with rates increasing at double the growth of the population between 1980 and 2010 (5-8).

In addition to the high rates of the uninsured in the US, there are increasing percentages of the population using services of hospital emergency departments (9). The Emergency Medical Treatment and Labor Act (EMTALA) was enacted in 1986 by the US Congress, and mandates hospitals evaluate and treat emergency patients regardless of their ability to pay (10). Many studies suggest this may be a major contributing factor in the increase in emergency department utilization (11-13).

Issues surrounding emergency room (ER) crowding, use for non-urgent reasons, and frequent use are found in the literature to be contributing to health care expenses and problems in the health care system (14-16). Characteristics of frequent emergency department users have been identified, but there is still controversy surrounding whether these patients are more likely to be uninsured or simply underutilizing primary care (PC) services (17).

The high percentages of uninsured and increased use of emergency departments are problems with serious consequences, including increasing rates of uncompensated care. In 2004, hospitals in the US provided uncompensated medical care valued between $25.6 and $26.9 billion (18, 19). In 2008 that number grew to an estimated $35 billion for hospitals, and $54.3 to $57.4 billion for all health care settings (20, 21). Emergency departments have decreased viability and the quality of emergency services is suffering due to these unpaid medical expenses (22).

This problem is putting individuals without insurance at increased medical risk. With limited and sometimes no other access to medical care outside of emergency department settings, the quality of those services and maintaining viability of hospitals is crucial to their health.

Social workers often work with individuals facing disadvantages or lacking personal resources, including people without health insurance, and this is directly affecting some of the individuals social workers help. As social workers intend to assist clients from a holistic perspective (23), helping them find appropriate, if not affordable, medical care is important, regardless of the context in which the social work interventions occur.

The role social work serves in hospital settings specifically is affected by cost factors (24). Cost-benefit ratios are important to social work programs within hospitals, and have been calculated as these programs develop and evaluate services (24). As Kadushin and Kulys (25) predicted, the challenge for hospitals is to incorporate cost containment with the humanitarian objectives of providing medical services to individuals.

The social work profession emphasizes promoting equality, including equality in health (23). Health inequalities for people with low income have been documented (26-28) and it is important that social workers recognize this issue and identify interventions. These interventions would not only help those facing disadvantages, but also reduce negative consequences of the issue, including uncompensated care.

While many interventions have attempted to solve these problems, few have been proven effective. Interventions implemented aimed at reducing uncompensated care through decreased ER usage include assessing patient emergency status before admittance to the hospital; the availability of telephone consultation with health care professionals; increased cost sharing, whether through higher co-pays or co-insurance, to discourage unnecessary use of emergency services; educational interventions informing people of how to properly utilize health care services; increasing the hours of available PC services; and, promoting access to PC through increasing the number of PC doctors that serve the uninsured population (15,29).

Among the effective interventions, increased access to and utilization of PC for the uninsured have shown to decrease the use of emergency departments for PC needs (29). The current study evaluates this approach, analyzing the change in use of health care services and associated cost savings for uninsured individuals who utilized ER referrals to a non-profit medical clinic providing free or low cost PC services to uninsured individuals.

It is hypothesized that the patients utilizing PC services will have decreased use of the ER and will, therefore, have decreased health care costs. For the purpose of this study, health care costs are broken down into the overall costs for both primary and emergency medical care, charges patients are responsible for paying to the PC clinic and ER, and the amount of unpaid medical fees in the primary and emergency care settings.

METHODS

The design of this study was based on the concepts and work of Fertig, Corso, and Balasubramaniam (21). The changes made to their methods include data collection from a longer time frame for the study period (four years of total data rather than two), the selection of patients based on a referral to the PC clinic rather than enrollment in the clinic, and the exclusion of categorizing visits as urgent or non-urgent when calculating ER costs for study feasibility.

This study is a quasi-experimental content analysis of existing data from a non-profit PC clinic for the uninsured and a community-based emergency department in a small southwestern metropolitan area. ER data were gathered for two years before and after the documented PC referral, and PC clinic data were gathered for the two years following the referral. This four-year total time frame was used to take into account patient behavioral changes in health care use over a longer time than two years. The months for the referral time frame were chosen to align with the fiscal year of the PC clinic in order for increased accuracy of financial information.

Population and sampling

The population of interest for this study was the uninsured who use emergency services at the community-based hospital ER. The sampling frame included uninsured individuals aged 20 to 62 years at the time they received referrals from the ER to the PC clinic during July, August and September of 2010. This age group was chosen to exclude those with potential eligibility for public health insurance through children's Medicaid or Medicare during the time frame of the research.

Cases believed to fit the criteria from the time frame were listed alphabetically according to the month the patient received a referral. From this list every other patient was chosen for the study, which originally yielded 210 patients. One patient was determined ineligible due to insurance status unknown prior to sample selection and four were excluded due to lack of data from the ER. These five cases were believed to be insignificant to the study and exclusion of these cases was determined unlikely to influence the findings.

Human subjects protections

This study used only existing data of patient files, and did not include contact with patients. Confidential patient information was not included in this study. All information was de-identified before data were analyzed, posing minimal risk to patients whose files are included in this study. Review of study procedures was conducted by Human Subjects Institutional Review Boards of both the hospital and the university through which this study was completed, and approval from both boards was granted prior to data collection and analysis.

Total sample demographics

Patient demographic information was found through the ER records, and race reported in the current study directly reflects race indications in the patient ER files.

Table 1. Gender and race, total sample

Demographic	Percent	N
Gender		
Female	62	127
Male	38	78
Patient Race		
White	54.1	111
Hispanic	30.2	62
Black	14.1	29
Asian	0.5	1
Other	0.5	1
Missing	0.5	1

The total patient sample included 205 individuals, of which 127 (62%) were female and 78 (38%) were male. White patients comprised 54.1% of the sample while 30.2% were Hispanic, 14.1% were black and 1.5% were Asian, other, or unknown (see Table 1). The patients ranged in age from 18 to 63 on the date of their first visit to the ER, and 67.8% were 40 years old or younger (data not shown).

Patient group demographics

Patients were divided into three groups in order to analyze differences in ER usage based on use of the PC referral. Groups were divided based on number of PC visits and categorized into a non-utilization group (Group 1), a minimal utilization group (Group 2), and a utilization group (Group 3). Group 1 included the ER patients that did not utilize their referral by attending a PC appointment in the two years following receipt of the referral. Group 2 included the ER patients that minimally utilized their referral by having one to three PC appointments in the two years following receipt of the referral. Group 3 included ER patients that utilized the referral by having four or more visits to the PC clinic in the two years following the receipt of the referral.

Table 2. Gender and race percentages by patient group

Demographic	Group 1	Group 2	Group 3
Gender			
Female	60.2	56.0	78.1
Male	39.8	44.0	21.9
Race			
White	56.9	42.0	62.5
Hispanic	26.0	42.0	28.1
Black	16.3	12.0	9.4
Other	0.8	4.0	0.0

Group 1. Group 1 included 123 patients, 60% of individuals included in the study. This group had 74 females (60.2%) and 46 males (39.8%); 70 patients were white (56.9%), 32 were Hispanic (26.0%), 20 were black (16.3%); and 1 patient race was missing (0.8%); (see Table 2).

Group 2. Group 2 included 50 patients (24.39% of the total sample) who minimally utilized the referral by having between one and three PC visits during the two years after receiving the referral. This group had 28 female patients (56.0%) and 22 male patients (44.0%). In Group 2, 21 patients were white (42.0%), 21 were Hispanic (42.0%) and 6 were black (12.0%); (see Table 2).

Group 3. Group 3 included 32 patients (15.6% of the study sample) that had four or more PC visits during the two years following receipt of the referral. This group had 25 female patients (78.1%) and 7 male patients (21.9%); (see Table 2). Group 3 had 20 patients that were white (62.5%), 9 that were Hispanic (28.1%), and 3 that were black (9.4%).

Instrumentation and procedures

Data were collected from the ER and PC clinic to determine the impact use of a referral from the ER to the PC clinic had on patient use of medical care and associated health care costs.

ER data collection

Data were gathered retroactively from ER patient files for over a four year time period, July 1, 2008 through September 30, 2012. Data gathered from the ER files included patient demographics such as gender, age during first visit, and race; ER utilization information including number of visits, the cost per visit as seen in the financial statement associated with the ER visit; the amount of the billing covered by the ER Charity Care program; the dollar amount collected from the patient for each visit at the time of the visit or during the time of the study; and the amount paid on the patient's behalf from the county health assistance program Indigent Health Care (IHC).

PC data collection

Additional patient information for those who participated in PC services was gathered beginning with the date of the patient referral (between July 1 and September 30, 2010). Data for these PC patients was collected for the two years following their first PC appointment after receiving the referral from the ER. Data gathered from the PC files included PC clinic utilization information such as the number of visits, the cost per visit to provide PC services as determined through analysis of PC clinic financial statements for the fiscal years associated with the visit (2010-12); the amount charged to the patient for each visit; the dollar amount collected from the patient for each visit at the time of the visit or during the time of the study; and the amount paid on the patient's behalf by IHC.

The ER in this study discounts a portion of ER visit costs for patients without health insurance as a part of their charity care program. Additionally, some patients without health insurance are eligible to have a portion of their medical expenses paid for by IHC. These were included as factors in the study to more accurately calculate the uncompensated care for visits to the hospital and PC clinic.

Data analysis

PC data from paper patient files were gathered in Excel spreadsheets and combined with the data received from the ER in Excel spreadsheets. The data were then entered into the Statistical Package for the Social Sciences (SPSS Version 20) for analysis. Descriptive statistical analyses were conducted in SPSS, and additional data calculations were computed through Excel.

Analyzing costs

PC clinic financial statements were used to determine the cost per visit for provision of PC services for fiscal years 2010, 2011 and 2012. An average estimated cost per visit was found for each of the three fiscal years and applied to the individual patient visit costs based on the fiscal year of the PC visit date.

Total costs

The cost of ER visits for individual patients was calculated for the pre-referral and post-referral time periods based on total visit change indicated in patient files. Additional costs of the visit, such as administrative costs, were not included due to lack of data availability. The ER visit costs for the two years prior to receipt of the referral served as the total health care cost for the pre-referral years. To evaluate the overall health care costs for the post-referral years, the ER visit costs were added to the PC clinic provider costs for PC visits for each patient. The sum, average mean and difference of the costs were used in descriptive analyses.

Charges to patients

The total health care charges per patient were calculated for pre-referral and post-referral years for each patient. The ER Charity Care write-offs and IHC payments were subtracted from the total ER billing for the pre-referral years. The same process was used for the post-referral years, and that number was added to the total patient charges from the PC clinic in order to create the total health care charges for the post years.

Uncompensated care

The pre-referral uncompensated care was represented by subtraction of the ER Charity Care write-offs, IHC payments and patient payments from the total ER visit costs for each patient visit in the two years prior to receiving the referral. For the post-referral years, unpaid PC patient charges were added to the ER uncompensated care for each patient.

RESULTS

The 205 patients in this study had a total of 1773 ER visits during the four year time period of the study, with a mean of 8.59 visits per patient. The patients that utilized the PC referral (n = 82) had an ER visit mean of 9.51 for the four year time period, with a mean of 5.96 visits to the ER before the referral date and 3.54 ER visits after the referral date (data not shown).

Group 1

Group 1 had a mean of 7.98 ER visits over the four year time period (see Table 3). The visit mean for the first two years in the study was 4.89 visits, while the mean for the two year post referral period was 3.09. This change in means includes the 38 individuals who did not have any ER visits during the two year post-referral time period.

Within Group 1 there was a sub-group of 85 individuals who had at least one visit to the ER during the two years after the referral period (data not shown). The mean of their ER visits was 5.80 for the pre-referral time period and 4.47 for the post-referral time period. For this subgroup, the total four year visit mean was 10.27 visits. Group 1 had no visits at the PC clinic.

Group 2

The mean ER visits for Group 2 was 8.48 for the four year time period, with a mean of 5.58 visits to the ER during the two years before the referral and a mean of 2.90 visits for the two years after the referral (see Table 3). The average decrease in ER visits after the referral for Group 2 was 2.68. These patients had a mean of 1.68 visits to the PC clinic and a total of 84 clinic visits in the two years following the referral.

Group 3

The overall mean for ER visits for this group of patients was 11.13 for the four year study period, with a mean of 6.56 visits during the two years prior to receiving the referral and a mean of 4.56 visits during the two years after receiving the referral (see Table 3). The average decrease in ER visits was 2.00 (1 per year) for Group 3. These 32 patients had four or more PC clinic visits each with in the two years post-referral, with a total of 237 PC visits and a mean of 7.41 visits per patient.

Table 3. ER and PC visit totals and averages by patient group

Provider	Group 1 n = 123 Avg./Total	Group 2 n = 50 Avg./Total	Group 3 n = 32 Avg./Total
ER			
Total (4 year)	7.98/982	8.48/424	11.13/356
Pre-Referral (2 year)	4.89/602	5.58/279	6.56/210
Post-Referral (2 year)	3.09/380	2.90/145	4.56/146
PC Clinic	0/0	1.68/84	7.41/237

Total costs

The total billing for the 1773 ER visits was $4,007,276 (see Table 4). The average cost per patient was $19,548 and per visit was $2,260. Patients contributed $5,680 towards the total billing, less than 0.15% of the total cost. IHC reimbursed the hospital $32,550 for these visits (0.81% of the total billing), and the ER Charity Care Program discounted $895,016 (22.33%) of the total cost.

Table 4. Four year ER billing for total sample

Category	Total	Average Per Person	Average Per Visit	Percent of Total
Total Billing	$4,007,276	$19,548	$2,260	100%
ER Charity Discount	$895,016	$4,366	$505	22%
IHC Payments	$32,550	$159	$18	<1%
Patient Payments	$5,680	$28	$3	<1%
Uncompensated Care	**$3,074,030**	**$14,995**	**$1,734**	**76%**

The uncompensated care totaled $3,074,030 for these 1773 visits, 76.71% of the total billing. The uncompensated care averaged of $1,734 per visit and $14,995 per patient in the four year time period. Per year, each patient had an average of $3,749 in uncompensated care.

Group 1 had ER costs totaling $883,030 for the two years prior to receiving the PC referral and $1,304,786 for the two years post-referral (see Table 5). Group 2 had total ER costs of $474,417 for the two pre-referral years and $720,587 for the post-referral years. The sum of Group 3 total ER costs was $228,559 for the two years prior to receiving the PC referral and $395,895 for the two post-referral years.

PC clinic costs

For FY2010, the estimated cost of each PC visit was $213.43 (data not shown). This amount was similar for FY2011 and FY2012, which cost a per visit average of $208.53 and $213.31 respectively. The 321 PC patient visits cost the clinic a total of $63,778 (for some visits patients only picked up medications and did not visit with physicians or physician assistants and, therefore, were not included in clinic costs). The 82 PC patients (Groups 2 and 3) were charged a total of $5,288 (8.29% of the total cost), of which they paid $2,924 (55.30% of their charges, 4.58% of the total cost). The average total uncollected balance was $29 per patient during this two year time period. For these patient visits, the PC clinic received a total of $1,152 from IHC (1.8% of the total cost).

Group 1 did not attend the PC clinic, and, therefore did not have any PC costs.

Group 2 PC visits cost the clinic a total of $17,750 (see Table 5), and the patients were charged a total of $1,753 (9.88% of the cost). The average total charge was $35 per patient. During the study time period, patients paid a total of $1,031 (58.81% of their total charges and 5.81% of the total cost); (data not shown).

The total cost to the clinic for the Group 3 PC visits was $46,028 (see Table 5), and patients were charged a total of $3,535 (7.68% of the cost to the clinic), with an average of $110 in charges to each patient. Of the patient charges, patients paid $1,893 (53.55% of their total charges and 4.11% of the total cost); (data not shown).

Pre-referral and post-referral cost comparisons

The sum of the health care costs after subtracting the pre-referral ER costs from the post-referral ER and PC cost sum was $421,756 higher for Group 1, $263,920 higher for Group 2 and $213,364 higher for Group 3 during the two years following the receipt of the referral (see Table 5).

For the average overall costs per patient, Group 1 had $7,179 in pre-referral ER costs and $10,608 in post-referral costs, averaging a $3,429 increase in post-referral costs (see Table 6). Group 2 had a $9,682 average in pre-referral health care costs and $14,447 in post-referral health care costs (ER and PC costs for post-referral years). This shows a $4,765 increase in average post-referral costs for Group 2. Group 3 had $7,142 in pre-referral health care costs and $12,482 in post-referral costs (ER and PC costs for post-referral years), indicating a $5,340 increase in post-referral costs.

Table 5. Health care cost totals by group

Provider	Group 1 n = 123	Group 2 n = 50	Group 3 n = 32
ER			
Pre-referral	$883,030	$474,417	$228,559
Post-referral	$1,304,786	$720,587	$395,895
PC Clinic Post-referral	$0	$17,750	$46,028

Patient charges

Group 1 had an average of $6,328 in ER charges per patient they were responsible for paying in the pre-referral years (see Table 6). In the post-referral years, Group 1 was responsible for paying an average of $10,199 to the ER (they did not utilize the PC and had no PC patient charges). This shows an average increase in $3,871 in patient charges for the post-referral years when compared to the pre-referral years.

Table 6. Health care cost mean averages by group

Category	Group 1 n = 123	Group 2 n = 50	Group 3 n = 32
Total Health Costs			
Pre-referral	7,179	9,682	7,142
Post-referral*	10,608	14,447	12,482
Patient Charges			
Pre-referral	6,328	6,904	4,424
Post-referral*	10,199	6,163	8,076
Uncompensated Care			
Pre-referral	6,297	6,897	4,415
Post-referral*	10,189	6,143	8,012

*For groups 2 and 3, this number includes the associated PC clinic and ER costs.

Group 2 was responsible for paying an average of $6,904 in ER charges per patient during the two pre-referral years and $6,163 in ER and PC charges in the post-referral years (see Table 6). This shows a mean decrease of $741 in medical charges in the two years following the receipt of the referral when compared with the pre-referral years.

Group 3 was responsible for paying an average of $4,424 per person in patient charges from the ER in the two pre-referral years and $8,076 in ER and PC charges in the post referral years (see Table 6). Group 3 had a mean increase of $3,652 in health care charges they were responsible to pay in the post-referral years when compared to the pre-referral years.

Uncompensated care

Group 1 had an average of $6,297 in uncompensated ER care per patient in the pre-referral period, and $10,189 during the post-referral period (Group 1 had no PC visits and no PC uncompensated care); (see Table 6). This shows an average increase in $3,892 in uncompensated care for the two years pre-referral compared to the two years post-referral.

The average uncompensated ER care per patient for Group 2 was $6,897 for the two years pre-referral (see Table 6). For the two years post-referral, Group 2 had an average of $6,143 in uncompensated ER and PC care. Group 2 had an average of $754 less in uncompensated care per patient in the two years following receipt of the referral when compared to the pre-referral period.

Group 3 had an average of $4,415 in uncompensated ER care per patient pre-referral, and an average of $8,012 per patient in uncompensated ER and PC care in the post-referral period (see Table 6). This shows Group 3 had an average increase of $3,597 per patient in total uncompensated care from the two years prior to the referral to the two years after receiving the referral.

Discussion

It was hypothesized that patients who utilized the PC referral by attending the PC clinic (groups 2 and 3) would have decreased health care costs as described by total costs, charges they were responsible for paying, and uncompensated care in the two years post-referral compared to the two years before the referral.

The total health care cost average per patient for the post-referral period (ER and PC costs) was not lower for the patients that utilized the PC clinic (Groups 2 and 3) when compared to the pre-referral health care costs (ER costs); (see Table 6). This finding does not support the hypothesis, as total health care costs increased post-referral for patients utilizing the PC clinic. Group 1 also had an increase in post-referral total health care costs.

For the charges patients were responsible for paying, Group 2 had a decrease in the average charge per patient in the post-referral period when compared to the pre-referral period while Group 3 had an increase in charges (see Table 6). This finding partially supports the hypothesis, as Group 2 charges decreased, but does not fully support the hypothesis, as Group 3 patient charges increased. Group 1 also had an increase in patient charges post-referral.

It was hypothesized that Groups 2 and 3 would have lower amounts of unpaid medical service fees during the two years following the receipt of the referral compared to the two years prior to the receipt of the referral. The uncompensated care averages per patient were higher for Group 3 in the post-referral years when compared to the pre-referral years, but lower for Group 2 (see Table 6). These findings support the hypothesis in part, as Group 2 uncompensated care averages decreased post-referral, but not in full, as Group 3 uncompensated care averages were higher. Group 1 also had an increase in uncompensated care.

Although the total number of ER visits decreased for the group utilizing the PC clinic, the sum of the costs increased. The strongest precursor of the use of heath care is health, 30 and this increase in cost despite the reduced ER usage may be due to poor health within the sample chosen. Health inequalities for individuals with low income exist in the US (26-28) and the sample chosen was low income, as income is an eligibility factor at the PC clinic studied. If the sample chosen had poor health at the beginning of the study, improved health outcomes might not be seen in two years of patients receiving PC, and ER care may still be necessary. In this case, PC may have been used to provide remedial rather than preventative care, indicating the sample studied may have had more severe health issues that another sample with higher income may not have been experiencing. However, had a more affluent sample been available, their access to PC and use of emergency services may have been different.

The increase in costs may also be due to a decrease in health status within the sample during the study time-frame. A closer look at this sample's individual usage may help in understanding if a subset of a few individuals had serious health issues during the study that altered the findings. For example, of the total $413,506 increase in ER costs for groups 2 and 3 in the post-referral years (Groups 2 and 3 summed post-referral costs subtracted from the summed pre-referral costs, see Table 5), almost $300,000 was from one individual. The 6.6% inflation between 2008 and 2012, 31 may also have contributed to the increase in health care costs as well.

For the 40% of patients that utilized PC clinic services (82 of the 205 patient sample), they continued to use the ER at a mean of 1.77 visits per year (average of 3.54 for the two year post-referral period). Utilization of the clinic one or more times did not stop use of the ER, but decreased it by almost 60% (5.96 pre-referral visit average compared to the 3.54 post-referral visit average). Without this decrease in visits, it is reasonable to expect that the health care costs for the post-referral years would have increased even more.

Extrapolations

Based on these findings, information concerning the decrease in ER visits and associated ER costs and uncompensated care can be extrapolated.

Decrease in visits. Of the total patients who received a referral (205 patients), 40% of them (n = 82) utilized the referral by attending a medical appointment at the PC clinic at least one time. If over 1,900 referrals to the clinic are given at the ER in a year (as was the case between October 1, 2009 through September 30, 2010), then there is a potential that 760 patients (40% of 1,900) utilize the referrals to PC each year, based on the findings of this study.

For the patients that utilized the PC referral in this study (Groups 2 and 3), there was a 2.41 mean decrease (59.51%) in the number of ER visits over the two year post-referral period, or 1.205 visits per year (data not shown). For these 82 patients, that resulted in over 98 visits less in a one year period. If those numbers are applied to the projected 760 patients who utilize their PC referral and decrease their ER utilization by 1.205 visits in a one year period, then the ER would have about 915 less visits from those patients in that year.

Decrease in ER cost. In this study, the average cost of an ER visit was $2,260 (see Table 4). As the ER had a decrease in 98 visits for the 82 patients (Groups 2 and 3) utilizing the PC referral in a one year period, the ER had $221,480 less in expenditures for these 82 patients in a one year period (number of visits multiplied by average cost per visit); ($442,960 for the 2 year period). If the same numbers are applied to the projected 760 patients, PC referrals in a given year result in a savings of $2,067,900 in a year period due to the projected decreased ER usage (decrease in 915 visits multiplied by the $2,260 average visit cost).

Decrease in uncompensated care. Seventy-six percent of the total ER billing in this study was uncompensated care (see Table 4). As the 82 PC clinic patients had a decrease in 98 ER visits per year, the ER saved $169,932 in uncompensated care per year ($339,864 for the two year period). For the 760 patients that are likely to have a reduction of 915 visits in a year, the uncompensated care decrease is extracted to be $1,586,610 (915 multiplied by average uncompensated care per visit) in a one year period for these patients.

PC Clinic Costs. The cost for the medical program at the PC clinic totaled $2,053,961.15 for fiscal year 2012, and that year they provided the uninsured population with 9,629 visits. If each of those 9,629 visits was at the ER rather than the clinic, it would cost $21,761,540 (based on the $2,260 average visit cost). This average includes the costs of emergent as well as non-emergent visits, so the actual cost of non-emergent visits was not determined, thus this savings number should be used with caution. The cost of the PC clinic per patient visit was an estimated $213.31 for fiscal year 2012, or 9% of the $2,260 ER visit average cost. For the average $1,734 in uncompensated care per ER visit, an individual could have more than 8 visits to the PC clinic.

Projected cost savings of the PC clinic

Recent research32 of the same hospital shows from December 1, 2011 through November 30, 2012, the ER had 61,472 visits to the emergency department. Of the 61,472 visits, 19,970 were by the uninsured (32.49% of the total visits), 2,613 visits were by those with pending assistance (4.25%), 581 visits were by people receiving IHC assistance (0.95%), and 182 visits were by the uninsured in an ER Med Pay program (0.30%). The total number of visits for those without private or public insurance was 23,346, or 37.99% of the total visits (32).

Of these 23,346 visits, 2,283 (9.7%) showed the patient claimed the PC clinic as the individual's PC provider. If each of these 2,283 ER patient visits was by a separate individual (with no repeat visits), then there would result in 6,217 PC patients (73.14% of the 8,500 total active patients utilizing the PC clinic) that did not use the ER during that time period. If these 6,217 PC clinic patients had one visit to the emergency department a year at the average cost of an ER visit found in this study ($2,260, see Table 4), it would cost the ER $14,050,420 in a one year time period for these patients. This would likely result in $10,778,077 in uncompensated care, based on the 76.71 percentage of total costs being uncompensated found in this study. As PC clinic costs about 10% of what it would cost the ER for non-urgent and PC treatable medical needs ($2,260 ER visit cost compared to $213 PC visit cost), it is clear the most cost-effective PC treatment is found in a PC clinic setting.

Implications for practice and policy

Based on these findings and extrapolations, implications can be made concerning practice and policy. For the issues of the uninsured and uncompensated care to be improved, communication and coordination between the PC clinic and the ER, as well as the county IHC program, are important. Additionally, the expanded role of social work in addressing patient challenges could enhance health equality with this population.

Implications for practice in setting studied. In this study, 40% of individuals utilized referrals, and improved communication and coordination between the PC clinic and the emergency department about referred patients would be helpful in increasing this percentage. This should include expanding the existing sharing of patient contact information for those referred, the sharing of real time ER usage information for potential and existing clinic patients, and increased communication for a more formalized referral process.

For those ER patients referred increased follow up with the PC clinic concerning health and use of the emergency department could help change the use of the health care system on an individual level. Hiring a case manager for the clinic client base would be helpful in identifying which patients are likely to use the ER for non-urgent or PC treatable reasons and increasing follow up for those patients. If the case manager hired was also a social worker, a holistic perspective in working with patients would be useful to identify other reasons patients utilize the ER rather than the PC setting (i.e., lack of transportation and child care). Additionally, providing patients with reminders for follow up appointments, yearly physicals, and appointments after hospital discharges could prevent need for patients to use the ER for non-emergent reasons. For patients with chronic conditions that need continual care, charts should be provided to the patients to track health information at home on paper or online so there is increased personal patient responsibility for their health.

As the PC clinic can meet the PC needs of the uninsured at 9% of the cost of the ER, increased funding for the clinic and similar programs would increase the ER savings in uncompensated care. The issues this uninsured population in the study county faces should be identified for further recommendations concerning the changes that need to be made. Potential changes include increasing the hours the clinic serves the uninsured, increasing the volunteer providers at the clinic to meet specialized needs of the population, streamlining the interview process for clinic patients, and opening a new facility in another part of the county.

Implications for social work practice. The profession of social work is aimed at addressing social problems, which includes health inequalities. As the literature suggests, higher income is associated with better health outcomes (26-28). While findings of this study show the increased use of PC in a PC setting as opposed to an emergency setting can decrease health costs and uncompensated care, the use of a PC setting did not result in actual decreased costs to the ER. As discussed earlier, this may indicate that the population studied had a poor health to begin with, and the use of PC over two years served to treat existing conditions rather than prevent conditions. A variety of social factors contribute to an individual's health status (28) and social workers can engage with populations experiencing health disparities to increase health equality through addressing social needs of individuals and communities.

The World Health Organization Social Determinants of Health unit identifies community empowerment and collaboration as important to improving policies for health equality (28). Social workers can address health inequalities while putting professional values into practice through multiple avenues, including increasing access to services, advocating for evidence-based program models, and developing services that have the capacity to address diverse needs for specific populations (33). Integration of social work in the PC setting may assist in promoting health equalities, as social workers can address social determinants of health before conditions become acute. These and other methods may be employed to address health inequalities, which findings of this study suggest may contribute to the substantial amount of uncompensated care in ERs.

For social workers helping individuals that do not have insurance, recognizing the affordability of medical services in PC settings when compared to ERs can be important in helping clients access to appropriate and more affordable medical care. Knowledge of available resources for clients that are uninsured or underinsured is important for helping clients from a holistic perspective, regardless of the type of social work services provided.

For social workers in ER settings, recognition of the uncompensated care correlated with use of the ER by uninsured and taking measures to mitigate this problem can be influential in gaining programmatic support. By integrating communication with other local resources for the uninsured or underinsured and encouraging patients to receive follow up care in those facilities, social workers in hospitals can reduce the overuse of the ER for PC needs, ultimately saving the hospital from financial losses while potentially influencing hospital decision makers in favor of continuing social work services in the ER.

Implications for policy. Based on this study, it is clear that uncompensated care and use of the ER for non-emergent and PC treatable reasons is costly when compared to treatment provided in PC settings. While the EMTALA requires hospitals to provide the uninsured with the opportunity to receive health care without being turned away, preventative care is less available for the uninsured population. Focusing policies and funding on preventative care for the uninsured or underinsured is important in order to decrease overall costs of health care for this population and increase their health status. While options such as the expansion of Medicaid availability under the Affordable Care Act for this population seem costly, there may be higher costs to hospitals, counties and the state if nothing is done to help alleviate this problem.

Limitations

There were several limitations in this study. One of these limitations was the lack of differentiation between urgent and non-urgent ER visits when evaluating ER costs. The numbers included in the study include both, however, the PC clinic would only be able to alleviate costs for non-urgent or preventable ER visits, as they are not equipped nor available to handle emergent situations.

Another limitation in this study is the time period and limited control factors. As the liturature (34) suggests, the change in ER usage may take longer to be realized than four years. Issues related to chronic conditions, time of visits, and need for hospital admissions could account for some of the findings. Costs were not differentiated for urgent and non-urgent visits, which is likely to alter the calculations made concerning the amount the ER could save. Factors such as severity of visit and whether it resulted in hospital admission could have also altered findings, as individuals with serious health problems have higher treatment costs than individuals with less serious or no health problems. If the sample chosen had severe health problems, as may be the case due to health inequalities, then the amount of money the PC clinic could save the ER would be less than extrapolations suggest as individuals would still need to utilize emergency services.

The research also did not include hard data concerning the overall costs and visits of the uninsured to the PC clinic during the pre-referral periods, which may have influenced the results. If patients utilizing the PC clinic after receiving the referral were also utilizing the clinic before the referral, health care use differences and costs could be influenced.

Implications for further research

The implications for further research include use of more factors to control for anomalies and classification of the ER visits as urgent or non-urgent to determine more reliable savings numbers. Unusually high or low ER usage or expenditures could influence and potentially distort group means, and urgency of visits can help in determining the number of visits more appropriate for the PC setting. Factors concerning whether visits were made during the time the PC clinic was open, whether visits increased due to chronic conditions and others could also be analyzed in order to better understand the nature of ER usage. In other words, there is a lot more that needs to be known before an intervention model can be designed to more effectively address this complex problem.

Inclusion of social determinants of health in similar studies could more specifically identify what factors may be affecting health, which may inform social work interventions. Additionally, further research can help in understanding the use of social work in PC settings for populations with significant psychosocial needs. As a holistic perspective of care is fundamental to social work, integration of social work services in these PC settings could help address some of the health inequalities experienced by these populations through focus on social determinants of health.

ACKNOWLEDGMENTS

I would like to express my very great appreciation to Dr. Thomas Winter, Dr. Wayne Paris and Dr. David Dillman for their encouragement and constructive suggestions during the planning and development of this research. I would also like to thank the non-profit medical care clinic in this study for the opportunity to conduct this research, as well as the community-based hospital for the provision of and access to valuable data.

REFERENCES

[1] Lachman VD. Ethical challenges in the era of health care reform. Medsurg Nurs 2012;21(4):248-51.

[2] Igiede AE. Health care reform: Sociopolitical perspective. Race Gender Class 2010;17(3/4):288-97.

[3] Blacksher E, Rigby E, Espey C. Public values, health inequality, and alternative notions of a "fair" response. J Health Politics Policy Law 2010;35(6):889-920. doi: 10.1215/03616878-2010-033.

[4] Gable L. The patient protection and affordable care act, public health, and the elusive target of human rights. J Law Med Ethics 2011;39(3): 340-354. doi:10.1111 /j.1748-720X.2011.00604.x.

[5] Fronstin P. Sources of health insurance and characteristics of the uninsured: Analysis of the March 2011 current population survey. EBRI Issue Brief 2011;362:1-34.

[6] Gertz A, Frank S, Blixen, C. A survey of patients and providers at free clinics across the United States. J Commun Health 2011;36(1):83-93. doi:10.1007/s10900 -010-9286-x.

[7] US Census Bureau. General population characteristics: 1980 census of population. URL: http://www2.census.gov/prod2/decennial/documents/1980/1980censusofpopu8011u_bw.pdf.

[8] US Census Bureau. Population and distribution and change: 2000 to 2010. URL: http://www.census.gov /prod/cen2010/briefs/c2010br-01.pdf.

[9] Marco C, Weiner M, Ream S, Lumbrezer D, Karanovic D. Access to care among emergency department patients. Emerg Med J 2012;29(1):28-31. doi:10.1136 /emj.2010.103077.

[10] Moskop JC., Skylar DP, Geiderman JM, Schears RM, Bookman KJ. Health policy and clinical practice/concept: Emergency department crowding, part 1—concept, causes, and moral consequences. Ann Emerg Med 2008;53(5):605-11. doi:10.1016/j.annemer gmed.2008.09.019.

[11] Assid PA. Clinical: Emergency medical treatment and active labor act: what you need to know. J Emerg Nurs 2007;33(4):33324-6. doi:10.1016/j.jen.2007.01.007.

[12] Hoot NR, Aronsky D. Health policy and clinical practice/review article: Systematic review of emergency department crowding: Causes, effects, and solutions. Ann Emerg Med 2008;52(2):126-36. doi:10.1016/j .annemergmed.2008.03.014.

[13] McDonnell WM, Gee CA, Mecham N, Dahl-Olsen J, Guenther E. Does the emergency medical treatment and labor act affect emergency department use? J Emerg Med 2013;44(1):209-16. doi:10.1016/j.jemermed.2012 .01.042.

[14] Asplin BR, Magid DJ, Rhodes KV, Solberg LI, Lurie N, Camargo CA. A conceptual model of emergency department crowding. Ann Emerg Med 2003;42(2):173-80. doi:10.1067/mem.2003.302.

[15] LaCalle E, Rabin E. Health policy and clinical practice/review article: Frequent users of emergency departments: the myths, the data, and the policy implications. Ann Emerg Med 2010;56(1):42-8. doi:10.1016/j.annemergmed.2010.01.032.

[16] Morgan SR., Smith MA, Pitts SR, Shesser R, Uscher-Pines L, Ward MJ, Pines JM. Measuring value for low-acuity care across settings. Am J Manag Care 2012;18(9):e356-63.

[17] Weber E, Showstack J, Hunt K, Colby D, Callaham M. Does lack of usual source of care or health insurance increase the likelihood of an emergency department visit? Results of a national population-based study. Ann Emerg Med 2005;45(1):4-12.

[18] Hearld LR, Alexander JA. Patient-centered care and emergency department utilization: A path analysis of the mediating effects of care coordination and delays in care. Med Care Res Rev 2012;69(5):560-80. doi:10.1177/1077558712453618.

[19] Stephens JH, Ledlow GR. Real healthcare reform: Focus on primary care access. Hosp Top 2010;88(4):98-106. doi:10.1080/00185868.2010.528259.

[20] Hadley J, Holahan J, Coughlin T, Miller D. Covering the uninsured In 2008: Current costs, sources of payment, and incremental costs. Health Affairs 2008;27(5):399-415. doi:10.1377/hlthaff.27.5.w399.

[21] Fertig AR, Corso PS, Balasubramaniam D. Benefits and costs of a free community-based primary care clinic. J Health Hum Serv Adm 2012; 34(4):456-70.

[22] Coustasse AP. Uncompensated care cost: A pilot study using hospitals in a Texas county. Hosp Top 2009;87(2):3. doi:10.3200/HTPS.87.3.3-10.

[23] Lyons K. The SAGE Handbook of international social work [monograph on the Internet]. London: Sage, 2012.

[24] Dziegielewski S, Holliman D. Pracitce of social work in acute health care settings. In: Dziegielewski, contributors. The changing face of health care social work, 2nd ed. New York: Springer, 2004:243-66.
[25] Kadushin G, Kulys R. Patient and family involvement in discharge planning. J Gerontol Soc Work 1994;22(3/4):171-99.
[26] Martinson M. Income inequality in health at all ages: A comparison of the United States and England. Am J Public Health 2012;102(11): 2049-56.
[27] McGrail K, van Doorslaer E, Ross N, Sanmartin C. Income-related health inequalities in Canada and the United States: A decomposition analysis. Am J Public Health 2009;99(10):1856-63.
[28] Solar O, Irwin A. A conceptual framework for action on the social determinants of health. Social determinants of health discussion, Paper 2 (policy and practice). Geneva: World Health Organization, 2010.
[29] Flores-Mateo G, Violan-Fors C, Carrillo-Santisteve P, Peiro S, Argimon J. Effectiveness of organizational interventions to reduce emergency department utilization: A systematic review. Plos One, 2012;7(5):1-7. doi:10.1371/journal.pone.0035903.
[30] Lepolstat R, Golbeck K, Kostelnik D, Mandyam S, Montero D, Brown S. Impact of managed health care on the United States: Implications for universal health care system. J Hum Behav Soc Environ 2009;19(7): 805-19. doi:10.1080/15433710902922284.
[31] Inflation Calculator. US inflation calculator. Accessed 2015 Feb 01. URL: http://www. usinflationcalculator .com/.
[32] Hardcastle W. Characteristics of emergency department users in a small metropolitan area hospital. Dissertation. Abilene, TX: Abilene Christian University, 2013.
[33] Coren E, Iredale W, Rutter D, Bywaters P. The contribution of social work and social interventions across the life course to the reduction of health inequalities: A new agenda for social work education? Soc Work Educ 2011;30(6):594-609.
[34] Zahradnik AG. Does providing uninsured adults with free or low-cost primary care influence their use of hospital emergency departments? J Health Hum Serv Adm 2008;31(2):240-58.

Section three - Adolescents in English speaking Caribbean

In: Public Health Yearbook 2016
Editor: Joav Merrick

ISBN: 978-1-53610-947-4

Chapter 23

PAN AMERICAN HEALTH ORGANIZATION APPROVES NINE-YEAR REGIONAL STRATEGY AND PLAN OF ACTION TO REDUCE THE VULNERABILITIES OF CARIBBEAN ADOLESCENTS AND YOUTH

***KizzyAnn M Abraham**, BSc**
School of Arts and Sciences, University of St George's, Grenada, West Indies

ABSTRACT

The vulnerabilities of adolescents and young people in the Caribbean to HIV infection cannot be overemphasized. Especially, considering the fact that their sexual and reproductive health needs have been grossly neglected in the global HIV/AIDS response. Although HIV rates of infection are on the decline, adolescents and young people face many difficulties accessing related health care services and information. Recognizing this gap PAHOs (Pan American Health Organization) member states have approved an Adolescent and Youth Regional Strategy and Plan of Action 2010-2018. Over a period of nine years PAHO will endeavour to assist member states with implementing the seven strategic areas and its key objectives.

Keywords: adolescents, young people, Caribbean, HIV and AIDS, PAHO, health

INTRODUCTION

Unprotected heterosexual intercourse has been recognized as the main route of HIV transmission, which accounts for 79.3% of AIDS cases in the English, Dutch and French speaking Caribbean, whereas, men who have sex with men (MSM) account for merely 12.6%

* Correspondence: KizzyAnn Abraham, Research Assistant, St George's University, School of Arts and Sciences, Grenada, West Indies. E-mail: kabraham@sgu.edu.

of AIDS cases (1-3). Not surprisingly HIV prevalence is much higher in Caribbean countries that criminalize same-sex practices, in comparison to countries where it is legalized.

According to UNAIDS at the end of 2011, statistics showed that an estimated 230,000 persons were living with HIV in the Caribbean (4). Moreover, some 10,000 people had died from AIDS related deaths; meanwhile an estimated 13,000 were newly infected with HIV. CARICOM (the Caribbean Community) has reported that around 70% of AIDS cases in the region are diagnosed among persons in the 15 to 44 years old age bracket, with half of the disease burden concentrated among the 25 to 34 year old demographic (5). Considering the time it takes an HIV infection to progress to a fully diagnosed AIDS case, it can be justly deduced that these persons were infected during their adolescence (10 to 19 years old) and youth (15 to 24 years old) (6).

UNFPA, UNICEF and UNAIDS have reported that at 1.8 billion this is the largest generation of young people in human history (6, 7). As for the Caribbean approximately 40% of populaces are under the age of 24 years old (6). Thus the potential to realize "demographic dividends" from this large working population may never again be realized if governments and policymakers fail to act now, to ensure that adolescents and young people are equipped with the wherewithal to reduce their risk to sexually transmitted infections, including HIV (8).

Adolescents and Young People Neglected in HIV and AIDS Response

Although great progress has been made in the global HIV/AIDS response the sexual and reproductive health needs of adolescents and young people (10 to 24 years old) have been grossly neglected in critical health and social programmes throughout the region. The most significant reasons for this oversight are as follows: 1) few organizations are equipped with the wherewithal to focus on adolescents with a comprehensive, medium or long-term approach; 2) socio-cultural factors, associated with conservative attitudes towards pre-marital sex and the use of contraception, pose barriers to implementing policies to further adolescents' well-being and 3) the poor use of available scientific evidence and the lack of adolescent and youth participation in the development and implementation of targeted interventions (6-8).

This of course should be a major cause for concern among policymakers since the Caribbean, after sub-Saharan Africa, has been long recognized as one of the most heavily affected regions in the HIV epidemic (6). Moreover, in the Caribbean "AIDS is among the five leading causes of death among young people" (8). Anecdotal evidence suggests that among the smaller island states HIV testing levels are relatively low, especially among male, rural and younger youth (9). Thus, regardless of the lack of quantifiable data AIDS related deaths among young people in the Caribbean pose a severe threat to countries economic growth and stability.

In 1995 the Health Economics Unit, UWI (University of the West Indies) approximated the economic impact of HIV/AIDS on the region at US$20M, and projected it would reach US$80M by the year 2020, which at that time, will account for roughly 6% of the region's gross domestic product (GDP) (5). Thus, as CARICOM member states look beyond the eight

Millennium Development Goals (MDGs) towards the ICPD (International Conference on Population and Development) post-2015 agenda, and its newly set target to end the HIV epidemic by 2030, it is imperative that strategic investments are made to safeguard the SRH (sexual and reproductive health) rights of adolescents and young people in development.

VULNERABILITIES OF CARIBBEAN ADOLESCENTS AND YOUNG PEOPLE

Scientific findings suggest that health promoting or health-compromising behaviours, such as tobacco and alcohol consumption and unsafe sex are learned and reinforced during adolescence and youth (8). Ideally the health care sector is responsible for essentially meeting the needs of its citizens throughout their lifespan. In 2010, PAHO (Pan American Health Organization) reported that in most countries in Latin America and the Caribbean, several young people encounter legal and financial barriers and unfriendly environments when they utilize health services, including breaches in confidentiality, judgmental and disapproving attitudes relating to sexual activity and substance use, and discrimination (8). For these reasons, among others young people are considered a vulnerable group to HIV infection in the Caribbean.

Additionally, young people who engage in commercial sex work, and men (including adolescents) who have sex with men (MSM) are at heightened risk of contracting HIV. Other factors driving the transmission of HIV among young people include the early initiation of sexual activity, the common practice of having multiple sex-partners, and age mixing of older men with younger girls (1). According to Inciardi and colleagues (1), geography may also be a factor in the spread of HIV among adolescents, as one study of 913 girls aged 14 to 17 years old in Jamaica revealed. The study found that adolescents residing in rural areas were more likely to be uneducated or misinformed about HIV transmission when compared to their peers living in more developed communities.

In 2014, UNAIDS reported that in the Caribbean, WHO Global School-Based Student Health Survey (GSHS), fifty-six percent of girls and 79% of boys on average had sex before the age of 14 years old (10). Moreover, approximately 38% of adolescents responded that they did not use a condom at last sexual intercourse. Furthermore, general knowledge and awareness of HIV among girls and boys in the region scored 43% and 42% respectively (10). Though there has been a 35% drop in HIV prevalence amongst Caribbean young people between 2001 and 2011, the face of HIV has become disproportionally young and female. Nearly half of all new HIV infections in the Caribbean Basin occur among young people between the ages of 15 to 24 years old (1).

THE WAY FORWARD

The investment in health, education and the alignment of economic policies in favour of the SRH rights of young people cannot be overemphasized. Considering the vulnerabilities of the Caribbean's adolescents and young people to reproductive ill health, PAHO's commitment to improve their health and wellbeing has been long standing. In 2008 and 2009 the organization's member states at the 48th and 49th meetings of the Directing Council approved a Regional Strategy for Improving Adolescent and Youth Health and a Plan of Action on Adolescent and Youth Health, respectively. According to PAHO, the strategy and plan are not only designed to develop and strengthen member states national health sector's integrated response, but more importantly to respond to the needs and improve the health of vulnerable adolescents and youth (8).

Recognizing the increasing vulnerabilities of Caribbean adolescents and young people, PAHO avers that during the current economic downturn national health budgets will be constrained in meeting the health care needs of its populaces (8). Thus, making it further impossible for the most vulnerable young people to access health services, including sexual and reproductive health. Hence, additional efforts at the international, and local levels (stakeholders) will be necessary to protect the triumphs to date in adolescent and youth health, and also to strengthen the performance of national and local health systems across the region.

In retrospect PAHO's Regional Strategy and Plan is structured within a life course, gender, and human rights framework, and based on the Health Agenda for the Americas 2008-2017 and, also the Strategic Plan 2008-2012 for the Pan American Sanitary Bureau. Notably the Plan of Action takes into consideration seven strategic areas for joint alliance: 1) strategic information and innovation; 2) enabling environments for health and development using evidence-based policies; 3) integrated and comprehensive health systems and services; 4) human resources capacity-building; 5) family, community, and school-based interventions; 6) strategic alliances and collaboration with other sectors and 7) social communication and media involvement (8). The strategic areas for action will be executed over a period of nine years 2010 to 2018. Furthermore, each strategic area incorporates specific objectives and proposals for action that are based on evidence and best practices recognized by PAHO.

PAHOs STRATEGIC AREAS OF ACTION

The need for reliable information is critical to the decision making process. However, the obtainability of social and health data on young people is still very difficult, given in many instances it is either incomplete, inaccurate, and/or inconsistence where obtainable. For this reason strategic information and innovation is the first of the seven strategic areas in the Regional Strategy. The key objective is to not only strengthen the capacity of countries to generate quality health information on adolescents and youth health, but more importantly the collection, analysis, and dissemination of information will provide PAHO with necessary tools to establish priorities, guide its Plan of Action, and aid the development of policies, planning and evaluation of programs.

The second strategic area health and development enabling environments using evidence-based policies speaks for itself. Additionally, it attempts to promote the implementation of comprehensive, sustainable, and evidence-based policies on adolescent and youth health. Strategic area three seeks to facilitate and support strengthening the capacity of the health care system to respond to adolescent and youth needs. Human resources capacity-building, as strategic area number four, strives to upkeep the development and strengthening of comprehensive adolescent and youth health human resources training programs, especially those in health sciences and related fields (schoolteachers, university professors, and community health promoters). Thus, contributing to the creation of multidisciplinary teams and the development of effective policies and programs for adolescent and youth health promotion, prevention, and care.

Taking into consideration that behaviour change in adolescents and youth is influenced strongly by the socio-economic environment, a favourable one is essential for young people to achieve positive health and education outcomes. Thus strategic area number five family, community, and school-based interventions seek to develop and support adolescent and youth health promotion and prevention programs through community-based interventions. On the other hand, strategic alliances and collaboration with other sectors stands out as area number six. Understanding that the implementation of adolescent and youth health programming requires a concerted multi-sectorial approach this strategic area seeks to facilitate dialogue and alliance building between strategic partners in order to advance the adolescent and youth health agenda. Thus, ensuring that key actors participate in the development of policies and programs for this demographic. Appreciating the significant impact of the mass media and new technologies on the health and lifestyles of young people, strategic area number seven attempts to support the inclusion of social communication interventions and innovative technologies in national adolescent and youth health programs. Moreover, it is vital that stakeholders work with mass media platforms to promote a positive image of adolescents and youth, and to also incorporate new technologies in health promotion interventions.

CONCLUSION

Ensuring that adolescents and young people in the Caribbean are equipped with the knowledge and skills needed to safeguard their reproductive lives is a population and development issue. Governments and policymakers are not only hard pressed to act in a manner that is cognizant of the vulnerabilities of Caribbean adolescents and young people, but more importantly to respond to their needs and improve their health and wellbeing. Throughout the region adolescents and young people have been grossly neglected in critical health and social programmes that would impact their overall health and wellbeing. PAHO acknowledges that nearly 50% of new HIV infections occur among young people who are also confronted with a host of other health challenges. In light of these findings PAHO's member states in 2008 and 2009 approved a nine year Regional Strategy and Plan for improving adolescent and youth health. The Strategy and Plan is designed to develop and strengthen member states national health sector's integrated response and also respond to the needs and improve the health of vulnerable adolescents and youth via seven strategic areas, which have specific objectives and proposals for actions.

REFERENCES

[1] Inciardi JA, Syvertsen JL, Surratt HL. HIV/AIDS in the Caribbean basin. *Aids Care 2005*;*17*(1),9-25.

[2] World Health Organization. Global report: UNAIDS report on the global AIDS epidemic 2013. Geneva: WHO, 2013.

[3] Pan American Health Organization. Improving acccss of key populations to comprehensive HIV health services: Toward a Caribbean consensus. Washington, DC: PAHO, 2011.

[4] Joint United Nations Programme on HIV/AIDS. Fact sheet UNAIDS. URL: http://www.unaids.org/en/resources/campaigns/20121120_globalreport2012/factsheet.

[5] Caribbean Community (CARICOM) Secretariat. Model CARICOM youth summit: HIV/AIDS in the Caribbean. URL: http://www.caricom.org/jsp/community_organs/ai ds.jsp?menu=cob.

[6] United Nations International Child Emergency Fund and UNAIDS. *All in! Towards ending the AIDS epidemic among adolescents*. New York: UNICEF, 2014.

[7] United Nations Fund for Population Activities. *The power of 1.8 billion: Adolescents, youth and the transformation of the future*. New York: United Nations Population Fund, 2014.

[8] Pan American Health Organization. *Adolescent and youth regional strategy and plan 2010-2018*. Washington, DC: PAHO, 2010.

[9] World Health Organization. Global report: UNAIDS report on the global AIDS epidemic 2012. Geneva: WHO, 2012.

[10] Mugumya F. *The gap: risk and vulnerabilities for young people*. Geneva: Joint United Nations Programme on HIV/AIDS, 2014.

In: Public Health Yearbook 2016
Editor: Joav Merrick
ISBN: 978-1-53610-947-4

Chapter 24

HUMAN PAPILLOMAVIRUS (HPV) AND CERVICAL CANCER HEALTH SYSTEM PREPAREDNESS IN SAINT LUCIA: A POLICY BRIEF

Krystal Austin, MPH, Anyka Clouden, MPH, Dalia Rassier, MPH and Praveen Durgampudi*, MBBS, MPH, MSPH

Department of Public Health and Preventative Medicine,
St. George's University, Grenada, West Indies

ABSTRACT

This policy brief focuses on Chronic Disease Preparedness in St. Lucia, focusing specific interventions on cervical cancer and human papillomavirus (HPV) prevention. There is a need to implement a policy to raise awareness of cervical cancer through education and to implement a vaccination program in order to reduce the disease burden of cervical cancer on the St. Lucian population. The policy therefore comprises of two levels. The first is a vaccination campaign targeting girls and boys ages nine to thirteen, in accordance with the World Health Organization guidelines for vaccinating children between the ages of nine and thirteen to protect against HPV infection. The second is through education and screening. There should be implementation of a state wide campaign for the education of the public on HPV: what it is, what it causes and how it can be prevented, and routine screening (Pap smears) for women over twenty for the early identification of abnormal cells of the cervix which are a precursor to cervical cancer. With this two level policy, there is hope of reducing the disease burden of cervical cancer on St. Lucia, while raising the awareness of HPV and promoting prevention strategies.

Keywords: HPV, cervical cancer, Saint Lucia, public health

* Correspondence: Praveen Durgampudi, MBBS, MPH, MSPH, St. George's University Department of Public Health and Preventive Medicine, St. George, Grenada, West Indies. E-mail: pdurgampudi@sgu.edu.

INTRODUCTION

The Human Papillomavirus (HPV) is a double stranded DNA virus of the papillomavirus family. It is thought to be the most common sexually transmitted infection (STI), so common that nearly 100% of sexually active men and women are infected at some point in their lives (1). While most HPV infections are transient, with approximately 90% of infections being cleared by the body's immune system within one to two years (2), persistent infection by high risk strains is a major risk factor for the development of cervical cancer (3, 4).

Cervical Cancer is the second most common cause of cancer related deaths in women (5, 6) and the second most common non-skin cancer in females (7), accounting for 9.8% of cancer in women worldwide (4). 85% of all diagnosed cases of cervical cancer occur in developing countries, with 11% of these cases occurring in the Caribbean (4, 5, 7). Cervical cancer is a major public health concern with the Caribbean and neighboring Latin America showing some of the highest incidence and mortality rates in the world (4).

There are over thirty different strains of HPV, including low and high-risk strains. Low risk strains are not associated with cancer development, but instead cause sexually transmitted genital warts (8). High-risk strains are those that are associated with cancer development; at least fourteen oncogenic (cancer causing) genotypes have been identified (4). Persistent infection with high-risk strains of HPV is the most important risk factor for the development of cervical cancer. In fact, research has shown that virtually all cervical cancers, including both squamous cell carcinomas and adenocarcinomas, and their respective precursor lesions, have a strong causal relationship to cervical infection with HPV (4, 7).

Who is affected and how?

The Caribbean accounts for approximately 11% of incident cases and deaths due to malignant cervical neoplasms every year (5). Although HPV infection is the major risk factor for cervical cancer, there are several other risk factors involved, such as the age of sexual debut, multiple sexual partners, smoking, high parity, persistent sexually transmitted infections, lower socioeconomic status and long term oral contraceptive use (8). Research has shown an inverse relationship between levels of education and risky sexually practices which could lead to HPV infection (9). Women of a lower socioeconomic standing and decreased level of education are more likely to have more sexual partners and less likely to practice safe sex (7, 9)

Analysis of data

The data obtained from the St. Lucian health system showed that over a five-year period, 2008 to 2012, eighteen percent (18%) of the all deaths were due to cancer and 9.6% of all cancers were found to be cervical cancer. When the results where stratified by gender, 18.2% of female deaths and two percent (2%) of the total cancer deaths were due to cervical cancer. Cervical cancer was the second most prevalent cancer that caused deaths among women during that period (see Figure 1).

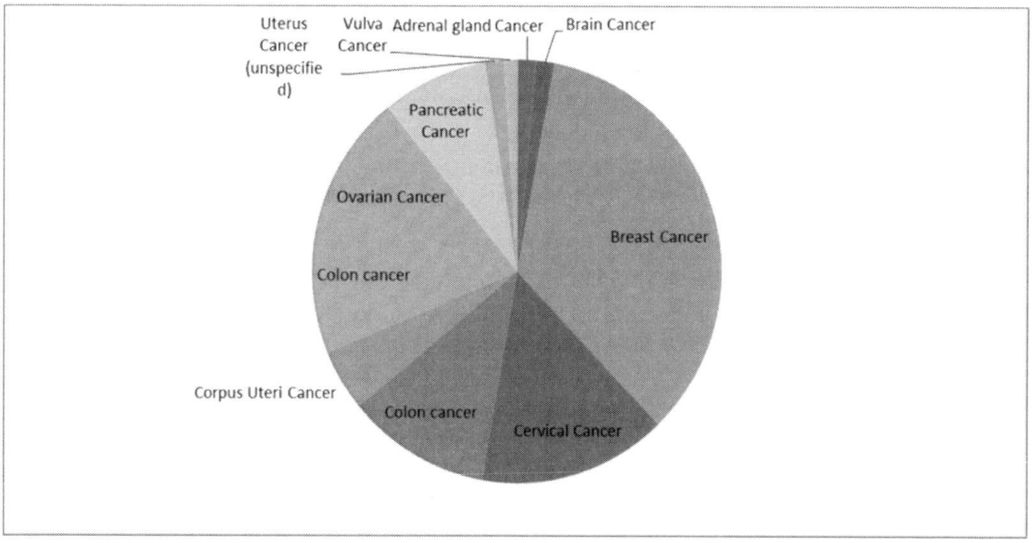

Figure 1. Distribution of cancer deaths in women.

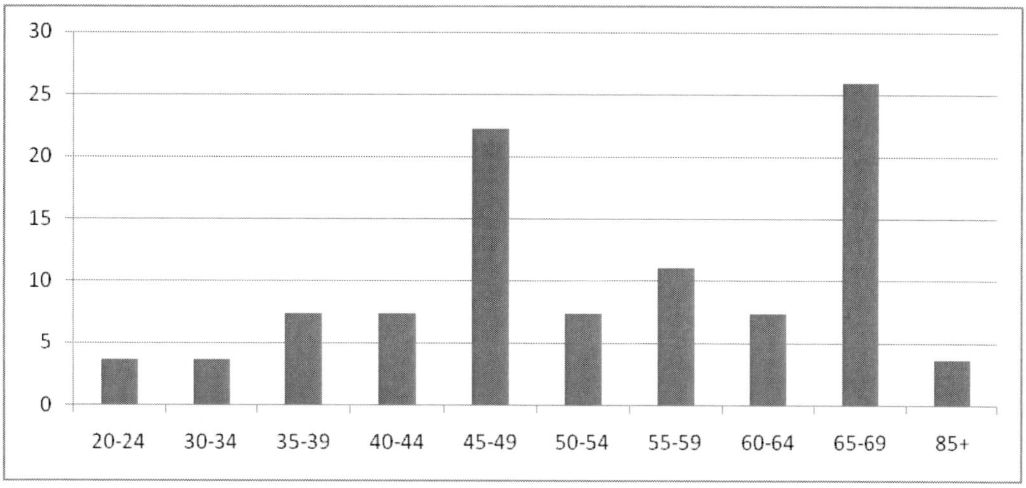

Figure 2. Morbidity of cervical cancer by age group: Percent.

From the morbidity data, i.e., people living with cervical cancer, the age groups that showed the biggest proportion of person where 65-69 and there was another peak for the age group 45-49. This double peak, while unusual for other cancers, is often seen with cervical cancer (Figure 2), corroborating research done by the Cancer Research of the United Kingdom in the UK in 2013 (10).

In both the morbidity and the mortality data, it was seen that there is a greater percentage of prevalence and death among women outside of childbearing age (Figure 3, 4).

The largest percentage of patients that died due to cervical cancer was from the capital of St. Lucia, Castries.

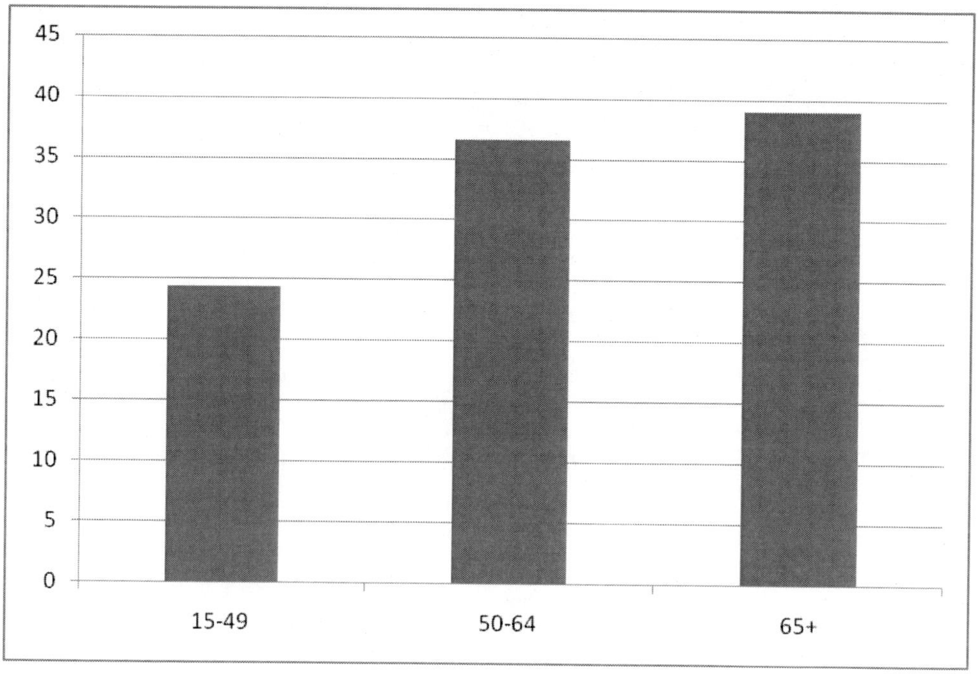

Figure 3. Age distribution of Morbidity of cervical cancer: Percent.

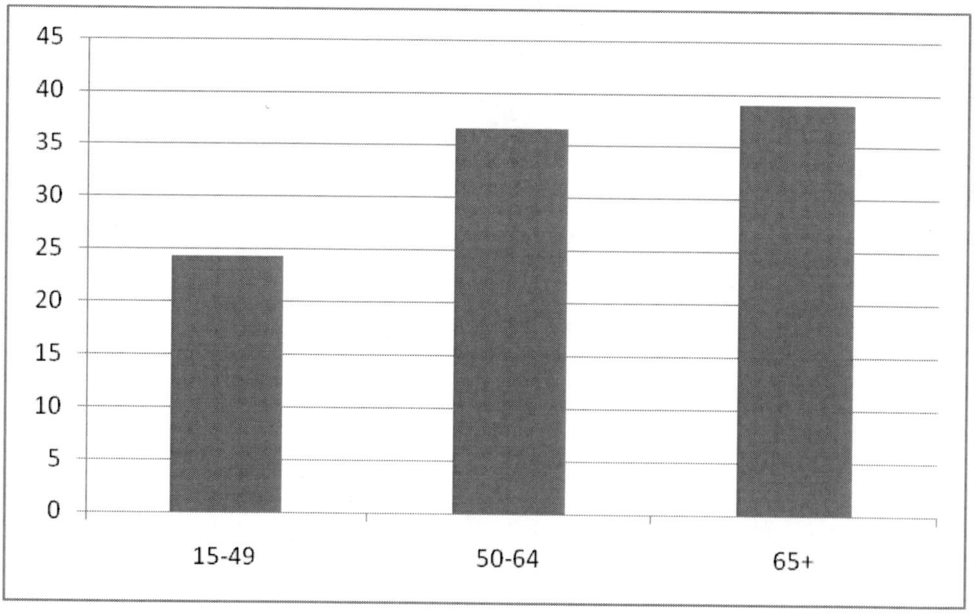

Figure 4. Age distribution of Morbidity of cervical cancer: Percent.

Distribution in the population and risk factors

Although cervical cancer is highly preventable due to early detection through screening programs and organized cytology based screening programs have been shown to decrease cervical cancer morbidity and mortality rates by as much as 80% (7), the developing world has not seen the same decrease that more developed countries have (9). This is due in part to a lack of awareness about HPV, mode of transmission, and its link to cervical cancer, as well as the lack adequate screening programs (2). Despite the rising incidence of the disease in the Caribbean, well-organized screening programs are not usually readily available and are least likely to be accessed by women who need them most (9).

How it is related to the functioning utilization of services and cost of providing care

Research has shown that in more developed countries the incidence rates of cervical cancer have declined as much as 70% in the past few decades due to routing screening (i.e., PAP smears). However, cervical cancer still presents a major public health concern in developing countries due in part to the failure of prevention programs. Although the high-risk HPV strains 16 and 18, which are seen in most cervical carcinoma in situ and invasive cervical cancers worldwide, are seen at a reduced rate in the Caribbean, they are still present (2). Research has shown that high-risk types 66, 52 and 45 may be more prevalent than 16 and 18 (3). However, it has been concluded that HPV vaccines targeting 16 and 18 may protect against persistent HPV infections by the most commonly occurring high risk strains and contribute to decreasing the burden of cervical cancer in the Caribbean (2).

Public health significance of the issue

Like many other chronic diseases, cervical cancer can place significant burdens on the society, especially in countries with limited resources like St. Lucia. The most common form of the cancer, responsible for eighty percent (80%) of cases, affects the squamous epithelial cells (11). Unlike other cancers, cervical cancer has an unusual incident pattern where there are two peaks as opposed to a gradual increase with age. According to research done by the Cancer Research of the United Kingdom, there is an increased incident rate among women aged thirty (30) to thirty–four (34) and another increase among women aged eighty (80) to eighty-four (84) (10). The policy framework should be designed is to decrease the incidence and prevalence rates of cervical cancer and HPV infection among St. Lucian women with special emphasis to target children at the secondary school level by implementing HPV vaccinations. Additionally, the intent is to raise awareness as well as empower the community to be involved in the reduction of cervical cancer.

Population affected

Cervical cancer affects woman primarily in the thirty (30) to eighty-five (85) age range. However the vaccination available targets girls aged nine (9) to twenty six (26) (12).

Policy Interventions

The problems chronic disease cervical cancer poses on St. Lucia has been recognized and corroborated by the data obtained. To address this problem two policies are proposed. The first is through vaccination in order to decrease the occurrence of HPV, a major risk factor for the development of cervical cancer, and the second is through screening to allow early detection of premalignant cells, thus reducing the disease burden on the country.

Policy 1 –Vaccination

Human Papilloma Virus (HPV) vaccines should be made available to the public. All children, both boys and girls, should be required to be fully vaccinated before entering secondary school. This is in accordance with World Health Organization (WHO) recommendations that children between the ages of 9-13 years should be vaccinated against HPV infection (6, 13).

This age group is specifically targeted because vaccination against HPV is most effective before one's sexual debut (i.e., the first time an individual has sexual intercourse). Sexually active individuals can still benefit from vaccination; however, the vaccine less effective after their first sexual experience because the vaccine does not treat existing HPV infections. None the less, the Advisory Committee on Immunization Practices recommends routine HPV vaccination between the ages of nine (9) and twenty-six (26) regardless of sexual activity or previous HPV infection (8). Therefore, the vaccination should still be made available for persons nine (9) through twenty-six (26) (1).

The vaccines presently on the market do not protect against all the strains of HPV, however, they protect against the high-risk strains that are almost always associated with cervical and anogenital cancers and the low risk strains associated with genital warts (1).

Implementation

Girls should be vaccinated in order to prevent infection with high-risk strains of HPV, which have been shown to be a major risk factor in the development of cervical cancer later in life. Boys should also be vaccinated against HPV because even though they are not at risk for developing cervical cancer (lacking the anatomy), they are often asymptomatic carriers of the virus. Vaccinating the boys will help reduce the incidence of infection in girls and women since females contract the virus from their (male) sexual partners.

A school based program, similar to those carried out in schools in Latin America (5) and those currently being carried out in schools in Barbados, may initially be most effective in implementing the vaccination policy. In a school based program, nurses would visit primary schools and administer the vaccine specifically to children in their final year of elementary education, as well as other children within the target age group who have received written consent from a parent or guardian. Nurses would also visit secondary schools to vaccinate children in forms one (1) to three (3) who received written parental consent. In this way children who are within the target age group but who are already enrolled in secondary school would also be able to receive the vaccination, as well as any other eligible children who want to be immunized.

Having the vaccine administered within the school setting would ensure a higher rate of compliance, especially if the HPV vaccine being administered is one that must be administered in three (3) doses over a six (6) month period.

Policy 2 – Education and Screening

The second policy is a two-stage process, which involves educating the public on cervical cancer, and its risk factors and screening at risk persons, women aged twenty (20) to sixty-five (65), in order to identify early cases of cervical dysplasia.

Implementation

The education campaign would include informing both males and females on what HPV is, how it is transmitted/ contracted, how to prevent infection and its link to the development of cervical and anogenital cancers. This could be added to existing STI prevention and safe sex education campaigns.

The CDC recommends that women should start having regular Pap smear from the age of twenty-one (21) or from the age of sexual debut and every three years after. However, Pap smears are not recommended for females under the age of twenty (20) or over the age of sixty-five (65) if they have undergone previous screening and are not at risk for cervical cancer. Screening is not recommended for women who have had a hysterectomy if they do not have a familial history of cervical cancer. It is recommended against HPV testing, alone or in combination with cytology, in women younger than age 30 years. It is also important to note that Pap smears should be given routinely even after the onset of menopause or discontinuation of sexual activity (14, 15).

Mass media campaigns, such as television and print advertisements, distribution of informative materials, and community workshops targeted at women should be utilized to inform them about appropriate screening methods (i.e., Pap smear) – when they should get it, at what age and how often. Women should be informed of the benefits of screening and the treatability of precancerous lesions before the development of invasive squamous cell carcinoma.

REFERENCES

[1] Center for Disease Control. HPV vaccine information for young women. URL: http://www.cdc.gov/std/hpv/stdfact-hpv-vaccine-young-women.htm.

[2] Hosein F, Mohammed W, Zubach V, Legall G, Severini A. Human papillomavirus genotypes in invasive cervical squamous cell carcinoma in Trinidad. Rev Panam Salud Publica 2013;33(4):267-70.

[3] Andall-Brereton GM, Hosein F, Salas RA, Mohammed W, Monteil MA, Goleski V, et al. Human papillomavirus genotypes and their prevalence in a cohort of women in Trinidad. Rev Panam Salud Publica 2011;29(4), 220-6.

[4] Ciapponi A, Bardach A, Glujovsky D, Gibbons L, Picconi MA, Ra. Type-specific HPV prevalence in cervical cancer and high-grade lesions in latin america and the caribbean: Systematic review and meta-analysis. Plos One 2011;6(10):1-15.

[5] Ladner J, Besson MH, Hampshire R, Tapert L, Chirenje M, Saba J. Assessment of eight HPV vaccination programs implemented in lowest income countries. BMC Public Health 2012;12(370):1-8.

[6] Luciani S, Prieto-Lara E, Vicari A. Providing vaccines against human papillomavirus to adolescent girls in the Americas: Battling cervical cancer, improving overall health. Health Affairs 2011;30(6):1089-95.

[7] Pereira-Scalabrino A, Almonte M, dos-Santos-Silva I. Country-level correlates of cervical cancer mortality in Latin America and the Caribbean. Salud Publica Mex 2012;55(1):5-15.

[8] Read DS, Joseph MA, Polishchuk V, Suss AL. Attitudes and perceptions of the HPV vaccine in Caribbean and African-American adolescent girls and their parents. J Pediatr Adolesc Gynecol 2010;23:242-5.

[9] Chekuri A, Bassaw B, Affan AM, Habet G, Mungrue K. Knowledge, attitudes, practice on human papillomavirus and cervical cancer among Trinidadian women. J Obstet Gynaecol 2012;32:691-4.

[10] Cancer Research UK. Cervical cancer incidence statistics. URL: http://www.cancerresearchuk.org/ cancer-info/cancerstats/types/cervix/incidence/uk-cervical-cancer-incidence-statistics.

[11] Godfrey CC, Michelow PM, Godard M, Sahasrabuddhe VV, Darden J, Firnhaber CS, et al. Improving diagnostic capability for HPV disease internationally within the NIH-NIAID division of aids clinical trial networks. Am J Clin Pathol 2013;140(6):881-9.

[12] Merck Pharamceuticals. Gardasil recommendations. URL: https://www.erckvaccine.com/Products/ Gardesil/Pages/recpmmendation.

[13] Samson LM, Bortolussi R, Moore DL, Robinson JL, Rousseau-Harsany E, Samson LM. Human papillomavirus vaccine for children and adolescents. Paediatr Child Health 2007;12(7):599-603.

[14] Center for Disease Control. Cervical cancer statistics. URL: http://www.cdc.gov/cancer/cervical/ statistics.

[15] Vesco KK, Whitlock EP, Eder MA, Burda BU, Senger CA, Lutz K. Risk factors and other epidemiologic considerations for cervical cancer screening: A narrative review for the US Preventive Services Task Force. Ann Intern Med 2011;155(10):698-705.

In: Public Health Yearbook 2016
Editor: Joav Merrick

ISBN: 978-1-53610-947-4

Chapter 25

SEXUAL AND REPRODUCTIVE HEALTH EDUCATION: A CASE FOR INCLUSION IN THE CURRICULUM OF PRIMARY SCHOOLS IN THE CARIBBEAN

Satesh Bidaisee**, DVM, MSPH, EdD
St George's University, School of Medicine,
Department of Public Health and Preventive Medicine,
St George, Grenada, West Indies

ABSTRACT

Sexual and reproductive health (SRH) education is defined as information that develops the capacity of people to understand their sexuality in the context of biological, psychological, socio-cultural and reproductive dimensions. SRH Curriculum for Primary Schools: For effective SRH programs, specific consequences of unprotected sexual intercourse, attitudes and knowledge regarding sexual intercourse, contraception, delaying the age of sexual debut, peer pressure and gender specific information need to be addressed in a culturally specific manner. Sexual violence, coercion and transactional sex also need to be a focus. The development of such a curriculum requires the involvement of human sexuality and behavioral experts and its successful implementation is a collaborative effort. Discussion: The economic burden of those affected by adverse SRH consequences is considerable. School-based SRH education programs present a significant economic commitment to develop, train, implement, monitor, evaluate and maintain the program. In addition to the development of community health support services and investment in research is required. However, when compared to the cost of treatment of HIV/AIDS and other STIs, this preventive approach is more cost effective. Barriers to successful implementation SRH programs include gender/sexuality stereotyping, homophobia, religion and political support. Conclusion: STIs and premature pregnancies is an increasing SRH burden for the Caribbean. The young child and adolescent population are particularly at risk of unhealthy SRH behavior, which requires an evidence based SRH education at a critical time in their development.

* Corresponding author: Satesh Bidaisee, EdD, Department of Public Health and Preventive Medicine, St George's University, St George, Grenada, West Indies. E-mail: sbidaisee@sgu.edu.

Keywords: sexual reproductive health, health education, school health, Caribbean

Introduction

Early sexual activity as noted by Duncan et al. (1) has a detrimental effect on the lives of young people leading to complications such as STIs and premature pregnancy. STIs and premature pregnancy in the young population adversely affects health, life expectancy and quality of life from personal, social and economic cost in the immediate and long term. It is therefore argued that sexual and reproductive health (SRH) education can be effective in making the young primary school population aware of the risks and prepare them for preventive strategies.

Children and adolescents are disproportionately vulnerable to adverse consequences of early sexual behavior when compared to adults (2). The increased vulnerability is critical during the period of biological, behavioral and emotional development. This is linked to biological and behavioral factors including hormonal changes at puberty, immature reproductive morphology, immunological naivety, sexual experimentation, imperceptions of risk, and alcohol and illicit drug use (3). Additionally, social factors including social disruption, economic deprivation and freedom of mobility, which reduces parental and adult supervision and unregulated behavior, are also among the determinants of STIs and premature pregnancy (3). These challenges also inhibit the educational opportunities and continued professional development for both sexes, which serves as an economic burden to the individuals, their families and society. The collective burdens of STIs and premature pregnancies as described by Johnson et al. (4) found that the burden attributed to STIs in South Africa included death, lost years of life and significant resource expenditure from living with STIs. The United Nations Educational, Scientific and Cultural Organization (5) summarize these socio-cultural challenges by stating:

> Few young people receive adequate preparation for their sexual lives. This leaves them potentially vulnerable to coercion, abuse and exploitation, unintended pregnancy and sexually transmitted infections (STIs) including HIV.

The deficiency in SRH education noted by UNESCO (5) indicates the importance of measures to develop knowledge and skills to inform healthy behavior and practices towards SRH. This knowledge gap is also noted in the UNAIDS 2008 Report (6)on the Global AIDS epidemic where among the age group 15-24 years, including those from the Caribbean, 60% did not correctly identify HIV prevention strategies. Effective SRH education as a collaborative effort on the part of schools and their stakeholders including parents, teachers, Ministries of Education and Health, non-governmental organizations and the community according to WHO (7) can provide opportunities to inform attitudes and perceptions regarding their SRH and encourage the practice of healthy behavior concerning their sexual health. This education, according to UNESCO (5), would be required to reduce misinformation, increase correct knowledge, clarify and strengthen positive values and attitudes and enhance self-efficacy. The education can also serve to improve peer group and social norm perceptions while increasing communication with parents and the community. According to Glanz, Rimer and Lewis (8), both the Theory of Reasoned Action (TRA) and the Theory of Planned Behavior (TPB) focus on educational constructs to influence attitude, social normative perceptions and perceived control respectively to explain and inform behavior. Thus, with STIs and premature pregnancies described as being behavioral in nature, they become challenges in SRH that are ncow preventable if changes in behavior are targeted. Therefore, a cost effective, accessible and culturally oriented approach for combating STI's and premature pregnancies lies with effective and early education.

Sexual and Reproductive health education is defined by the WHO (9) as:

> "Information that develops the capacity of people to understand their sexuality in the context of biological, psychological, socio-cultural and reproductive dimensions."

SRH education promotes healthy outcomes by encouraging delayed sexual activity, responsible sexual behavior and increased contraceptive use in order to reduce the number of unprotected sexual activity, sexual partners, the rate of STIs and the number of premature pregnancies. School based SRH Education programs are an effective means of addressing significant child and adolescent health issues such as STIs and premature pregnancies. Education is considered one of the important determinants of health; higher levels of education are associated with improved socio-economic status resulting in healthier behavior selection and outcomes. Independent from socio-economic status, accessible school based SRH education can provide and improve fundamental and specific skills among children and adolescents, to cost-effectively manage and prevent adverse SRH outcomes. The WHO (7) advocates for the establishment of SRH educational centers for adolescents, where all members of the school community work to provide students with integrated and positive experiences and structures that promote their sexual health and reproductive well-being.

BACKGROUND

Johns Hopkins School of Public Health, Population Information Program, (10) identify children and adolescents living in developing countries to be the most at-risk group for STIs. This emphasizes the significance of the burden reported by UNAIDS (11) to developing regions such as the Caribbean which are most vulnerable to SRH challenges. The Caribbean region is second to Sub-Saharan Africa in terms of HIV/AIDS prevalence (12). As of 2007, an estimated 230,000 people were infected with HIV in the Caribbean with national prevalence rates ranging from 3% in the Bahamas, to 0.1% in Cuba (13). In the Caribbean, the 15 - 24 age group had the highest prevalence of HIV infection and women are two to three times more likely to become infected (13).

Almost 50% of adolescents in the Americas have their sexual debut before the age of 15 which was noted in the Declaration from the 1st Meeting of Latin America and the Caribbean Ministers of Health and Education to stop HIV and STIs in the region Latin America and the Caribbean (14). The Declaration (14) also noted that approximately 20% of all births in the region were to women between the ages of 15-19 years.

Additionally, the majority of overall sexual activity reported by the declaration as not being consensual but due to incest, coercion and transactional sex. The burden therefore reflects a significant challenge for the young and adolescent population and by extension, the entire society.

SRH knowledge, attitudes and behavior among youth

The lack of SRH knowledge is compounded by inconsistent attitudes and perceptions towards SRH that may correlate to risky behaviors. O'Toole et al. (15), surveyed 2000 young people aged 12-20 years, and found that among sexually active 12-14 year olds, only 40% reported using condoms. The sexual knowledge and attitudes of the participants were influenced by religious teachings, gender and age characteristics. Younger males were identified as displaying more unhealthy behaviors, decreased knowledge and risky attitudes towards SRH. Brathwaite (16) studied the perceived STIs risk amongst youth in Haiti, Trinidad and Tobago and Jamaica and identified an attitude of invincibility, which exacerbate unhealthy behavioral patterns. In a study aiming to understand the sources and content of SRH information among Jamaican adolescents, Holder-Nevins, Eldemire and McCaw-Binns (17) concluded that electronic media was the leading source of SRH influencing messages. Brathwaite (16) further suggested psychological factors including depression, confusion, low self-esteem and frustration as contributing to early onset of sexual activity.

SRH education in the Caribbean

In many cultures, puberty represents a time of social as well as physical change for both males and females and also signifies the initiation to sexually active life (9). The period of puberty is therefore the important phase for the acquisition and/or reinforcement of healthy attitudes towards SRH. This argument suggests that SRH education should come prior to the onset of puberty, which further emphasizes the need for the educational intervention at the primary school level. However, sexual education in the Caribbean has not traditionally been part of the education system, but is rather confined to religious teachings. This restriction in SRH education can also lead to absenteeism from schools that teach SRH topics, ban on condom usage as well as contraceptive education and the option of abortion. Additionally, SRH is not discussed between adults and children in the Caribbean as the topic of sex education is taboo among Caribbean society.

An analysis of the SRH education curriculum materials from 27 countries in Latin America and the Caribbean revealed a lack of important sexual education topics such as sexual orientation, human rights, STIs other than HIV and other SRH issues (18). In the Caribbean, Health and Family Life Education (HFLE) is a critical curriculum component for teacher training in the Eastern Caribbean (19). HFLE according to UNICEF (19) is developed with teachers at their training institutions and includes core curriculum guides to equip students with life skills to promote SRH. The current SRH education system in the Caribbean appears focused on secondary school education and is considered deficient in effectively developing young persons and especially among young males to manage their SRH challenges (20). While there is evidence of teacher education in SRH, the dissemination of information to the students is not effective; this challenge is seen as one of the factors for increasing the incidence of STIs and premature pregnancy among the Caribbean youth.

As a result of inadequate or non-existent SRH education programs and the taboo associated with sex related conversations within the Caribbean culture, the youth of the Caribbean are considered under educated in matters related to SRH. This therefore, presents a further need for effective and immediate SRH education for the sexually active young population found within the primary school system of the Caribbean.

Justification for SRH education in Caribbean primary schools

Sex education in general has been introduced at secondary school level; however, this paper presents a proposal for effective and appropriate SRH education in the primary school system of the Caribbean. Coward (21) identified that 45% of all STIs in the Caribbean occur in the age group of 15-24 years. HIV is known to have an incubation period of 10 years for young adults as noted by Osmond (22) which when applied to the 15-24 year old age group suggests that the average age of infection is pre-teen to early teenage years of life.

The structure of the education system places these at-risk students aged 5 - 9 years in primary schools. Therefore, any form of effective SRH education targeted towards informing healthy sexual behavior should start at the level of primary schools. The WHO (9) report also identified puberty as the important developmental period for acquisition of relevant knowledge and forming healthy attitudes towards SRH. Rosenfield et al. (23) reported that the onset of puberty is occurring earlier than previously reported ages of 8 and 9 years. Comparative studies conducted among median ages of 8.8 and 11.3 years for Afro-Caribbean girls and boys respectively in the Caribbean are serviced by primary school curriculums, again exemplifying the need for timely and effective SRH education in Caribbean primary schools (24). Regional governments and international organizations have also recognized the need for school-based SRH education. The Ministerial Declaration at the 1st Meeting of Ministers of Health and Education to stop HIV and STIs in Latin America and the Caribbean (14) documents this as goal 4.1 of their report which states:

> By the year 2015, we will have reduced by 75% the number of schools that do not provide comprehensive sexuality education, of schools administered by the Ministries of Education.

The WHO (9) reporting on UNESCO's policy on Education for all by 2015 also recognized the importance of education, indicating that schools are the avenues to reach the majority of the world's children between the ages 10-15 years.

There is evidence demonstrating that early SRH educational programs have a positive impact. Bearing et al. (2) reported based upon a review of 85 school-based SRH education programs, 65% noted a positive effect while 7% found a negative effect on reported SRH behaviors amongst the students in the respective schools. Another study by Paul-Ebhohimhen et al. (25) also identified significant changes in knowledge and attitudes regarding STIs based on a systematic review of school-based SRH education in sub-Saharan Africa. Effective SRH education has been demonstrated to be a successful tool for informing the developing knowledge and attitudes of young persons. The vulnerable groups of pre-teen students are all situated in primary school systems where school based SRH education program interventions would be most relevant and effective in addressing the current SRH burden amongst youths in the Caribbean.

Curriculum teaching of SRH education should therefore be occurring in Caribbean primary schools because the average age of on-set of puberty currently falls within the primary school students' age range.

SRH education curriculum for primary schools

In a joint report by UNAID/UNFPA/UNIFEM on Women and HIV/AIDS (26), it is noted that educated adolescent women are more likely to take measures to prevent STIs. There is a need to challenge the traditional gender stereotyping as well as power dynamics in the male and female relationships. For an effective primary school SRH education beyond imparting knowledge, there needs to be an approach considering challenges of gender stereotypes and inequity. Curriculum content should therefore reflect the varying gender issues and should be included in the following categories of SRH curriculum content as noted by UNAIDS/UNFPA/UNIFEM (26):

1. Correcting misinformation on SRH
2. Promoting SRH
3. Measures for preventing STIs
4. Measures for preventing premature pregnancy

Curriculum development

Kirby, Rolleri and Wilson (27) identify the overall scope of a SRH education curriculum to include the increasing of knowledge and also clarifying values and attitudes, as well as increasing skills and impacting fundamental behaviors. This development requires the involvement of experts in research on human sexuality, behavior change and related pedagogical theory. Theory and research will therefore inform the instructional methods to be used (28). UNESCO (5) also supports the recommendations put forth by Kirby, Rolleri and Wilson (27) and Senderowitz and Kirby (28) and advocates for the use of a four-step approach which is to:

1. Identify health goals such as reducing premature pregnancy
2. Identify specific behaviors that need to be changed including early sexual debut
3. Identify cognitive factors that affect behavior, for example, knowledge and normative beliefs/attitudes.
4. Create instructional activities for each identified cognitive factor which can include teaching, peer-group discussion, and theatre production

However, UNESCO (5) further calls for community based SRH needs assessments citing differences that may be present across communities and education programs that identify and addressed these differences in the curriculum. It is also important that whatever is developed be sensitive to the characteristics of the community, even if the communities values represent what needs be to be changed as part of the program. Additionally, the developed curriculum should remain within the resource availability for the community to ensure its sustainability.

Prior to curriculum development and full-scale implementation is a pilot test of the design. This according to Senderowitz and Kirby (28) is to obtain practical feedback on its effectiveness as well as revise the design of the program if needed.

In the context of Caribbean primary schools, the responsibility for the SRH education program to be integrated in schools curriculum is the responsibility of the various Ministries of Education. The SRH education component must be positioned appropriately to meet the objectives of preventing STIs and premature pregnancies as well as support or at least not inhibit the delivery of the established curriculum in primary schools.

Curriculum content

For SRH education programs, the focus should include specific consequences such as HIV or other STIs, premature pregnancies or unprotected sexual intercourse. The curriculum would then also focus on informing knowledge, attitudes and beliefs towards delaying the age of sexual debut as well as managing peer pressure and attitudes regarding sexual activity and contraceptive use. UNESCO (5) notes that an effective SRH curriculum would incorporate strategies useful against specific situations where pressure exists to engage in risky behavior. The situations referenced could include those such as sexual violence, coercion and transactional sex along with drug and alcohol use. In order for messages to be cogent, they should be culturally specific to the audience, thereby addressing challenges. For example, the transactional sex practice of gift offerings in return for sexual favors by older men towards young females is a Caribbean cultural practice which promotes risky behavior. In the context of primary school SRH education, the curriculum should focus on the internal cognitive factors such as academic knowledge along with providing information and opportunities to access said SRH services at schools and within the community. It is also imperative that curriculum content be derived from scientifically and medically accurate information that is evidence based.

The inclusion of gender specific information is also important as gender inequity for both females and males is an identified determinant of SRH outcomes. UNESCO (5) recommends that issues of susceptibility and attitudes regarding risk be addressed. Participatory teaching methods and instructional strategies, such as the use of role play to develop self-efficacy to manage risky sexual behavior is also noted by UNESCO (5) as being particularly effective.

The final component of curriculum content development noted by Kirby (29) surmises the logical coverage of appropriate SRH topics. The components of the curriculum include an emphasis on first, strengthening motivation to avoid STIs and early pregnancy, then emphasizing the susceptibility and severity of adverse SRH consequences. Finally, addressing the specific knowledge, attitudes and skills that are required for effective outcomes of an SRH education program are to be developed.

Curriculum implementation

An assurance measure for the successful implementation of any community or school based program requires awareness, involvement and support of all relevant stakeholders. The presence of conservative, political, religious and cultural influences as noted by Glasier et al.

(30) is examples of factors that can impact the implementation of SRH education especially among primary schools in the Caribbean. Stakeholder consultation and collaborative partnerships are therefore needed in any approach and should be considered in curriculum development and are critical for its implementation and longevity.

The selection of educators to deliver the curriculum is essential to the success of the SRH school based program (5). The educators may include specially trained teachers in the existing system and/or personnel specialized in SRH life skills training. Kirby, Obasi and Laris (31) recommend having both types of educators as the teacher can be the source of regular updated information while the specialist SRH educators can more effectively cover sensitive topics. The continued training of teachers at the primary school level will ensure the sustainability of these programs, which together with a community based participatory approach through stakeholder support, will foster an environment that will allow for the achievement of the program's goals and bridge cultural sensitivity. In order to maximize learning and behavioral impacts, two to three years of curriculum exposure within a classroom setting is recommended (28). The integration of these findings to the primary education setting within the Caribbean indicates the last three years of primary schools comprised of 8-11 year olds, participating in said curriculum.

In addition to SRH education, WHO (9) advocates that there is a need to integrate school based SRH education with community health services especially for the vulnerable pre-teen population. There is also a need on the part of Ministries of Education in the Caribbean region to develop their own policies for SRH education and specifically for the primary school curriculum. Finally, the SRH education program would need to be monitored and evaluated throughout its implementation to determine its effectiveness in meeting the proposed goals and objectives as well as to assist in the continued development and refinement of SRH education curriculums.

DISCUSSION

The proposed intervention of SRH education in primary schools represents a preventive approach to address the increasing burden that STIs and premature pregnancies place upon the vulnerable young child and adolescent population in the Caribbean. While the risky behaviors, developmental, and psychosocial factors regarding SRH are established - this proposed approach of primary schools SRH education is new.

The Social Cognitive Theory (SCT) noted by Glanz, Rimer and Lewis (8) explains that among the many crucial factors in determining behavior, one of the most prominent is the individual's capability to symbolize the behavior that is intended to be promoted. Pre-teenage students between ages 8-11 years are not capable of symbolizing behavior. However, these are the very age groups that are symbolizing and practicing high risk SRH behaviors which justify a behavior intervention approach among 8-11 year olds. By using a SRH education program that informs correct knowledge and healthy attitudes, the students' abilities to self-determine or self-realize their behavior are supported (8). Similar successful strategies that have been developed to address the growing epidemic of obesity in several developed and developing countries include prevention programmes targeted specifically to children at preschool institutions and after-care services which include the age group from 5-11 years of age (32).

Within the context of this proposed approach, there exist systemic challenges in the Caribbean that need to be discussed and addressed to establish meaningful SRH education programs. The socially mediated taboos, gender/sexuality stereotyping as well as inequalities and misinformed values about SRH exist as part of the society and in the legal framework of the Caribbean. Jamaica, Barbados, St Lucia and other Caribbean islands still criminalize consensual same-sex relationships (13). These laws reflect widespread homophobia and lack of understanding towards different sexual orientations. The UNAIDS/UNFPA/UNIFEM (26) report on "Women and HIV/AIDS" showed that more than half of all young women in the Caribbean reported that their first sexual encounter was forced or coerced. The report further commented that schools were the places where girls first experienced discrimination, sexual harassment and abuse from either fellow students and/or adults (13). There is therefore a need for societal and legal reform in the Caribbean towards sexuality and SRH. There is also a need to combat homophobia and other stigmas by providing information and services that are essential to preventing the sexual violence and gender based victimization/abuse. This change has the potential to occur through the SRH education approach for primary schools in the region.

Religion plays a significant role in the family life of the Caribbean; numerous primary and secondary schools in the region are denominational schools. Religious fundamentalism and lack of support from religious institutions for effective SRH education is another societal barrier to its implementation. Moral and religious beliefs hamper AIDS education even among Caribbean immigrants in Canada as it is associated with "a biblical plague and as Christians and good people, they will never get AIDS so are not concerned about it" (33). This barrier further demonstrates the importance of SRH education among children and adolescents before they become adults and blinded with fundamental dogmas. While these challenges require education to facilitate a change, it is these very barriers that apply to the implementation of SRH programs in the first place.

The most critical support for SRH education in primary schools is the political support from the region. UNESCO (5) reports the growing number of countries in Latin America and the Caribbean whose Ministries of Education have supported the increase in sexuality education programs. However, this political support remains limited by the societal paralysis of uninformed knowledge, attitudes, gender/sexual orientation inequalities and the significant burden of STIs and premature pregnancies.

Involvement of researchers and the research activities are critical to provide evidence that will support the design and implementation of the SRH programs for primary schools (28). Specific research should focus on increasing the evidence of the burden among the young adolescent population as well as the social, demographic, knowledge level and attitudes as well as behavioral risk factors attributed to the burden. Research should specifically guide policy makers to develop relevant programs to address identified knowledge gaps, inform change in attitudes and assess behavioral and SRH burdens over time. An understanding of the societal, religious and political barriers of early sexual education, analysis of stakeholders and research into strategies to gain support from the region will also be informed by research and more likely to achieve positive outcomes. Another concern that was identified previously by WHO (9) was the need for SRH education to be complemented with access to community health care services. It would stand to reason that with early SRH education in primary schools, there would be a need for counseling, medical and preventive services. The infrastructure for community would therefore also need to be part of the developmental plan for SRH education.

The proposed SRH education programs for primary schools put forth a significant economic commitment to develop, train, implement, monitor, evaluate and to maintain the program in addition to the development of community health support services. This proposed preventive approach requires an initial investment of resources. However, when compared to the cost of treatment for HIV/AIDS in the Caribbean, should create an immediate consideration for the preventive approach. It is estimated by Wilcox (34) that the cost for one HIV positive person per year is 500 United States Dollars (USD). With an estimated 230,000 persons living with HIV in the region in 2009, the total annual cost of HIV/AIDS treatment is estimated to be 1.15 Billion USD (35). The high annual cost supercedes the cost of any long-term SRH education program. Additionally, the cost of HIV/AIDS treatment does not capture the total cost of adverse SRH consequences, which includes morbidity from other STIs, decreased quality of life, mortality and the economic cost of loss of human resource capital. An early SRH education program is therefore more cost effective than the current efforts to manage the complications of SRH. Additionally, if SRH education programs are expanded to include similar information and behavioral change structures, several lifestyles based chronic diseases including cardiovascular diseases, obesity and metabolic disorders just to name a few can also be prevented. The cost benefit analysis is therefore in favor for early SRH education as a preventative approach.

Limitations

The available literature including statistics and published work focused primarily on HIV/AIDS while this paper's emphasis was on STIs and premature pregnancy. HIV/AIDS is considered the most sensitive and significant in terms of impact and while it is the major reported STI, it does not represent the overall burden of SRH complications. This therefore required generalizations to be accepted about STIs and premature pregnancy from work done primarily on HIV/AIDS.

Conclusion

The increasing burdens of SRH include high prevalence of STIs and premature pregnancies among the young adolescent population. There is also a lack of knowledge and high-risk sexual behavior as well early onset of sexual activity, low usage of contraception, multiple partners and influence of coercion. These negative societal positions towards different sexual orientation will only increase the SRH consequences.

Transforming the society will require SRH education that is collaborative, sensitive and targeted to the at-risk population, which includes children and adolescents. These groups must be provided with information that is evidence based before they are likely to engage in high-risk behaviors, providing strong support for the implementation of SRH education in the primary schools.

With this transition, the region as a whole will progress to an understanding and acceptance of differing sexual orientations, mitigation of sexual violence/abuse and strengthen legislative and systematic infrastructure towards a better SRH well-being for the Caribbean.

REFERENCES

[1] Duncan ME, Peutherer JF, Simmons P, Young H. First coitus before menarche and risk of sexually transmitted disease. Lancet 1990; 335(8685): 338-40.

[2] Bearing L, Sieving J, Ferguson V, Sharma V. Global perspectives on the sexual and reproductive health of adolescents: patterns, prevention and potential. Lancet 2009; 369: 1220-31.

[3] Cowan FM. Adolescent sexual health. Adolescent reproductive health interventions. Sex Transm Infect 2008; 78: 315-8.

[4] Johnson L, Bradshaw D, Dorrington R, South African Comparative Risk Assessment Collaborating Group. The burden of disease attributable to sexually transmitted infections in South Africa in 2000. S Afr Med J 2007; 97(8): 658-62.

[5] UNESCO, 2009. International Technical Guidance on Sexuality Education: An evidence-informed approach for schools, teachers and health educators. URL: http://unesdoc.unesco.org/images/0018/001832/ 183281e.pdf.

[6] Joint United Nations Program on HIV/AIDS[UNAIDS]. Report on the global AIDS epidemic. Geneva: UNAIDS, 2008.

[7] World Health Organization. Health promoting schools: a healthy setting for living, learning and working. Geneva: WHO, 1998.

[8] Glanz K, Rimer BK, Lewis FM. Health behavior and health education. Theory, practice and research, 3rd ed. San Francisco, CA: Jossey-Bass, 2002.

[9] World Health Organization. Promoting adolescent sexual and reproductive health through schools in low income countries: an information brief. Geneva: WHO, 2008.

[10] Johns Hopkins School of Public Health, Population Information Program. Meeting the needs of young adults. Population Reports 1995; Series J(41). URL: http://www.infoforhealth.org/pr/j41/j41creds.shtml.

[11] Joint United Nations Program on HIV/AIDS [UNAIDS]. Report of the global AIDS epidemic. Presentation to the Joint United Nations Programme on HIV/AIDS. Geneva: UNAIDS, 2004.

[12] Kaiser Family Foundation. Fact Sheet: The HIV/AIDS Epidemic in the Caribbean, 2009. URL: http://www.kff .org/hivaids/ upload/ 7505-06.pdf.

[13] International Profiles, 2007. Region: The Caribbean. URL: http://www. amplifyyourvoice.org/main.cfm?actio nId=globalShowStaticContent&screen.

[14] Ministerial Declaration from 1st Meeting of Ministers of Health and Education to Stop HIV and STIs in Latin America and the Caribbean. Mexico City, 2008.

[15] O'Toole BJ, McConkey R, Casson K, Goetz-Goldberg D, Yazdani A. Knowledge and attitudes of young people in Guyana to HIV/AIDS. Intl J STD AIDS 2007; 18: 193-7.

[16] Brathwaite B. An exploration of youth risks in the Caribbean, through the voices of youth. Faculty of Medical Sciences, University of the West Indies, February 2009. URL: http://sta.uwi.edu/conferences/09 /salises/documents/B%20Brathwaithe.pdf.

[17] Holder-Nevins D, Eldemire-Shearer D, McCaw-Binns A. Competition for adolescents sexual and reproductive health values: is the media wining? West Indian Med J 2009; 58: 326-30.

[18] Demaria LM, Galarraga O, Campero L, Walker DM. Sex education and HIV prevention: an evaluation in Latin American and the Caribbean. Rev Panam Salud Publica 2009; 26: 485-93.

[19] United Nations International Children Emergency Fund. HFLE in Caribbean Schools. New Approaches, Prospects and Challenges, 2006. URL: http://www.unicef.org/ barbados/ cao_unicefeco_hfle(1).pdf
[20] Wood A. Sex education for boys. Health Educ 1998; 98(3): 95-9.
[21] Coward S. UN calls for more sex education in the Caribbean schools to curb spread of HIV/AIDS. Caribbean Press Release, 2008. URL: http://www. caribbeanpressreleases. com/articles/3723/1/UN-Calls-for-More-Sex-Education-in-Caribbean-Schools-to-Curb-Spread-of--HIVAIDS/Page1.html.
[22] Osmond DH. Epidemiology of Disease Progression in HIV. HIV InSite Knowledge Base Chapter. University of California San Francisco, 1998. URL: http://www. hivinsite.usf.edu/InSite?page=kb-03-01-04.
[23] Rosenfield RL, Bachrach LK, Chernausek SD, Gertner JM, Gottschalk M, Hardin DS, et al. Current age of onset of puberty. Pediatrics 2000; 106: 622-3.
[24] Boyne MS, Thame M, Osmond C, Fraser RA, Gabay L, Reid M, et al. Growth, body composition and the onset of puberty: Longitudinal observations in Afro-Caribbean children. J Clin Endocrinol Metab 2010; 95(7): 3194-3200.
[25] Paul-Ebhohimhen V, Poobalan A, Teijlingen E. A systematic review of school-based sexual health interventions to prevent STI/HIV in sub-Saharan Africa. BMC Pub Health 2008; 8(4). URL: http//:www.biomedcentral.com/1471-2458/8/4.
[26] Joint United Nations Program on HIV/AIDS [UNAIDS], United Nations Population Fund [UNFPA], United Nations [UNIFEM]. Women and HIV/AIDS: Confronting the Crisis. Geneva: A Joint Report by UNAIDS/UNFPA/UNIFEM, 2010.
[27] Kirby D, Rolleri L, Wilson MM. Tools to access the characteristics of effective sex and STD/HIV education programs. Washington, DC: Health Teen Network, 2007.
[28] Senderowitz J, Kirby D. Standards for curriculum-based reproductive health and HIV education programs. Arlington, VA: Family Health International/YouthNet, 2006.
[29] Kirby D. Recommendations for effective sexuality education programmes. UNESCO Evidence-informed approach for schools, teachers and health educators. Paris, France: UNESCO, 2009.
[30] Glasier A, Gulmezoglu AM, Schmid GP, Moreno CG, Van Look PFA. Lancet 2006; 368(9547): 1595-607.
[31] Kirby D, Obasi B, Laris B. The effectiveness of sex education and HIV education interventions in schools in developing countries. Preventing HIV/AIDS in young people: A systematic review of the evidence from developing countries. Geneva: World Health Organization, 2006.
[32] Dehghan M, Akhtar-Denesh N, Merchant AT. Childhood obesity prevalence and prevention. Nutrition J 2005; 4(24): 1475-91.
[33] Gilpin A. AIDS and Multiculturism. Can Med Assoc J 1997; 156(10): 1446-8.
[34] Wilcox T. How concerned should Americans be about HIV/AIDS in the Caribbean? Helium, 2008. URL: http:helium.com/items/867987-how-concerned-should-americans-be-about-HIVAIDS-in-the-Caribbean. NationsNews.com. HIV/AIDS cases still high in the region. Thursday 2 December, 2010. URL: http://www.nationnews.com/articles/ views/hiv-aids-cases-still-high-in-region.

In: Public Health Yearbook 2016
Editor: Joav Merrick

ISBN: 978-1-53610-947-4

Chapter 26

"HORNING" AND THE EMERGENCE OF FEMALE EMPOWERMENT: TRANSLATION OF GENDERED SEX PRACTICES

Scott Hutton[1], MPH, Cecilia Hegamin-Younger[1,*], MPH, PhD and Rohan D Jeremiah[2], PhD, MPH

[1]Department of Public Health and Preventive Medicine,
St George's University, Grenada, West Indies
[2]School of Public Health, University of Illinois, Chicago, Illinois, US

ABSTRACT

Horning in Grenada is considered a product of masculinity in which men customarily and frequently stray outside of a designated relationship to engage in extra sexual relations with a female other than his partner. No known research has ever explored the same practices known as female horning in Grenada. The purpose of this study was to determine if female horning exists as well as attempted to understand the rationale for the practice. One hundred and fourteen females were surveyed. The results suggest that women in Grenada are more likely to horn if they themselves have been the victims of a horning relationship. Additionally, the research concluded that female horning was occurring out of retaliation against men. Lastly, the study showed a contradiction between morality and personal desires, as 100 percent of those practicing horning reported that both male and female horning was wrong.

Keywords: Caribbean, Grenada, horning, cheating, female retaliation, sex practices

---

* Correspondence: Professor Cecilia Hegamin-Younger, PhD, Department of Public Health and Preventive Medicine, St George's University, University Centre, Grenada, West Indies. E-mail: chegamin-younger@sgu.edu.

INTRODUCTION

Promiscuity, serosorting and cultural practices, such as horning, increase the likelihood of heterosexual transmission of HIV and other infectious diseases between couples (1, 2). Additionally, these infectious diseases have "begun to reverse the developmental gains for many of the world's most vulnerable groups, nations and regions as well as [created] an additional source of instability" (3, 4). Horning in Grenada, defined as extra sexual relations with someone other than a primary partner, is traditionally considered a product of masculinity in which men customarily, and frequently stray outside of a designated relationship. As Grenada finds itself continuously progressing towards complete gender equality (5), the once well-defined societal role of men is now "marked by uncertainties over social roles and identity, sexuality, work and personal relationships" (6). These uncertainties allow the female social role to gain flexibility, power and momentum. However, as the gender roles are restructured, more females are potentially practicing horning, possibly as a way of retaliation for decades of subjectivity to "damaging dominant models that emphasize aggression" (7). The practice of horning coupled with unsafe sex practices could contribute to the elevated rates of infectious disease and HIV transmission in the Caribbean, making rates "... second to only Sub-Saharan Africa" (8). The prevalence of female horning has not been extensively studied although much has been done on the role gender equality plays in Caribbean society (5, 9) and in disease transmission throughout the world (2). The purpose of this study is to examine the cultural components behind female horning. Specifically, this study will examine whether horning exists in Grenada and will attempt to understand the rationale for the practice.

It is customary that in most conversations with Grenadian men, they will assert their practice of horning. Additionally, the notion that horning is becoming increasingly popular with women was a construct developed during the same discussion, with most men indicating that female horning was a form of retaliation due to the female genders societal advances. In conjunction with the current knowledge on masculinity, Caribbean men often define and compare themselves in regards to relationship status with other men and more increasingly, women (10). For example, a Caribbean man that is capable of having more horning relations than another is deemed more powerful and masculine than one that does not. Take for example, a cultural aspect of "the calypso"—popular genre of local music, Caribbean men were once socially taught to follow the folklore-based tale of "the Mighty Shadow" (10). As a young man, the Shadow encourages "looking for horn" to ensure ones masculine place in society and dominance over women (10). However, as the paternal role in Caribbean society becomes less defined (11), the Mighty Shadow has been squandered with it, allowing for the uprising of females (12); it is this uprising and the blurring of gender divisions that place the female gender at the forefront of horning retaliation.

If in fact female horning is utilized as retaliation, horning in both the male and female populations may contribute to the increase in disease transmission Grenada is encountering (13). As with any infectious disease, the likelihood of transmission increases with the number of times one comes into contact with an infected person. Couples are becoming infected with HIV and sexually transmitted diseases (STD's) at far higher rates due to the unknown status of their partners, with the most common method of transmission in Grenada being heterosexual intercourse (14). Additionally, around the world "there is a consistent trend of more women living with HIV than men due to the fact that women are physically more susceptible to HIV infection than men, and gender-based violence makes them even more vulnerable" (15). "Grenada recorded its first case of HIV in 1984 and has a cumulative total of 464 cases at the end of 2011" (14). Similarly, STD's throughout the country have also steadily increased, with the most affected population being those aged 15 to 44 years (16).

As past heterosexual HIV transmission in Grenada has been related to a number of factors including male pleasure superceding female pleasure, dominant male sexual relationship control, and gender roles as defined by society (7), Grenadian females now have the motivating factors to retaliate. Specifically in Grenada the "impact of US media has resulted in the disintegration of norms and values" (16), further demoting masculinity, replacing it with materialism and a lessened gender divide. The lack of relationship commitment that Grenada as a developing nation observes being heavily practiced in Western society, places greater desire to align with the assumed modern ideals and practices. For example, laws banning prostitution, and thus promiscuity, in New Zealand have recently been reversed as the industry argued that sex outside of a committed relationship is synonymous to masturbation (18). With the modern world devaluing the stability of a relationship, developing nations will mistakenly observe the fact that horning is not only accepted but also practiced by the Western world.

With the emphasis on HIV research turning to the climbing rates of heterosexual disease transmission, science narrows in on the social aspects of transmission, such as the dynamics of the relationship itself. Research conducted by Pulerwitz et al. (19) revealed that unequal gender power in sexual relationships prevented women from encouraging partners to wear condoms, and as the power begins to be equally shared, condom usage rises. It is not until this power equality distribution occurs that sexually transmitted disease rates fall. If gender equality has truly begun to reach homeostasis in Grenada, then condom negotiation should be taking place between couples, ultimately driving disease trends down. However, Grenada's disease profile has yet to reflect this, indicating that other potential influences may play an important role. Additionally, as common quoted percentages place half of committed heterosexual relationships ending in separation or divorce (20), researchers focus on the increasing number of partner sharing events that may occur subsequent to high divorce rates. Mah and Halperin reported (21):

> Concurrent sexual partnerships (CSP, defined as overlapping partnerships where sexual intercourse with one partner occurs between two acts of intercourse with another partner)—compared to serial partnerships—can increase the size of an HIV epidemic, the speed at which it infects a population, and its persistence within a population.

Additionally, according to Pinkerton (1) individuals of unknown serostatus predominantly assume their negative disease state, as well as that of their partners, establishing the concept of serosorting. Pinkerton further hypothesized that it was these individual assumptions in regards to serostatus that allow for more lax safe-sex practice requirement (1). Furthermore, if serostatus is continuously assumed to be negative, then the more time a couple spends in a relationship the more likely disease transmission is to occur (22).

As literature focusing primarily on horning in Grenada does not exist, the importance of gender relations and constructs is essential to any new and developing research on the island.

Early anthropological theories of the 1970's describing Caribbean sexuality indicate that polygyny is "informally accepted" (23), and thus is learned and subconsciously passed on to subsequent generations. However, Kempadoo (23) pointed out that with the Mighty Shadow falling victim to modern acculturation, a greater emphasis should be placed on the importance of family and child rearing; but this is absent in Grenada. Instead, the working class population is routinely associated with "loose" sex practices (23), but research is unable to postulate why. Possible reasons for the current limitations stem primarily from the lack of research focusing on gender roles in Grenada since the formation of the original theoretical framework. The research behind these constructs and theories fails to account for potential changes in the social ideology of Grenada. Kempadoo again mentioned that the frequently used social and behavioral theories applied to Grenadian society are now considered obsolete, as women are increasingly able to match the behavior of men (23). Furthermore, it is now feared that as female promiscuity increases, exposure will corrupt the future views and sexual behaviors of young boys, further increasing the incidence of promiscuity (23); again, a cultural influence not accounted for in early theoretical frameworks, as men were the sole influence on young boys.

METHODS

In order to better understand the behaviors and social relations related to cultural practices like horning, the focus of this cross-sectional study was females in Grenada, aged 18 to 60 years. This age group was selected based on government disease surveillance that previously indicated those within the age range of 15 to 44 years suffer most from HIV and STD's in Grenada (16). Those that were currently involved in a relationship as well as those with past relationship experience were surveyed in order to assess for current or past horning experiences. A total of 114 women age 18 to 60 years participated in this study.

The inclusion criteria for this study was the following: 1) female, 2) between the ages of 18 and 60 years of age and 3) be of Grenadian citizenship. Women were identified through verbal and/or electronic recruitment from convenience sampling around popular everyday destinations, as well as through Facebook groups which were closed to the general public and only include women of Grenadian descent, within the target population. Paper-based surveys were used at public locations. All surveys sent out electronically were completed and returned via the SurveyTool anonymous survey site. Each participant targeted through Facebook was provided with the electronic survey URL, which was generated upon creation of the survey in SurveyTool, with one survey attempt per IP address being allowed.

Participation in the study included taking an anonymous printed or electronic survey, after giving informed consent, composed of 17 items that measured perceptions on horning, experience with a partner who horned, personal experience with horning practices, personal reasons for practicing horning and acceptability of horning. "Horning" was defined as cheating on a partner in their current relationship, OR on their partner of a past relationship, OR having cheated after finding out their partner cheated first. In addition to horning, participants were asked about the number of sexual partners in the last 12 months, indicating if promiscuity is widely practiced. All variables from the survey were summarized and used for assessment of trends and themes. EpiInfo 3.5.3 was the software providing data record keeping as well as analysis.

RESULTS

A total of 114 female Grenadians were recruited to participate in the study. Of the 114, 54 (47.4%) filled out the electronic-based survey, with the remaining 60 (52.6%) completing the paper-based survey. The demographic characteristics collected from the survey respondents have been summarized in Table 1.

Table 1. Distribution of participant characteristics (n = 114)

	Overall	Horn	Do Not Horn	Sig.
Mean Age (std dev)	26.3 (8.28)	24.7 (5.35)	27.4 (9.81)	Ns
Mean Sexual Debut Age (std dev)	17.2 (2.44)	16.5 (2.32)	17.9 (2.38)	**
Relationship Status				
Married (%)	10 (8.8)	4 (40.0)	6 (60.0)	Ns
Dating (%)	71 (62.3)	34 (47.9)	37 (52.1)	Ns
Single (%)	33 (28.9)	14 (42.4)	19 (57.6)	Ns
Level of Education Completed				
Primary School (%)	10 (9.1)	2 (20.0)	8 (80.0)	Ns
Secondary School (%)	28 (25.5)	11 (39.3)	17 (60.7)	Ns
Post-Secondary (%)	57 (51.8)	25 (43.9)	32 (56.1)	Ns

** = Statistically significant. Ns = Not statistically significant.

The mean age of the sample population was 26 years old, with a majority of the women having completed some sort of Post-Secondary degree (52%). Of the 114 respondents, 50 (43.9%) reported practicing horning, as per the studies definition. The response rate for the paper-based survey was 97 percent, as two females declined to participate. The response rate for the electronic survey cannot be calculated, as the investigators do not know how many females received links to the survey due to the use of snowball sampling amongst local females.

Multiple analyses were conducted using horning status as the stratified variable under study. Of particular interest was the significant difference ($t = 2.95$, $df = 1$, $p = 0.004$) between ages of sexual debut for those that horn, versus those that do not horn. Women who practiced horning, on average, had a sexual debut age 1.4 years younger than women who did not practice horning. The stratified sample also revealed that 40 percent of married women practiced horning. Likewise, for women involved in a non-married relationship, totaling 71 women, 34 (47.9%) reportedly practiced horning. There was no statistical difference between the two above mentioned horning groups ($t = 0.89$, $df = 1$, $p = 0.37$). Furthermore, of the 64 women that did not horn, 5 (7.8%) reported that they would cheat if they knew their partner would never find out. Lastly, 100% of the women that reportedly practiced horning, indicated that horning was wrong for both men and women, yet 3 (4.7%) of non-horning women reported that horning was acceptable.

Level of education between these two groups was not a factor in determining the likelihood of horning when stratified into having completed primary school only, secondary school only, being currently enrolled in post-secondary school, or having completed post-secondary school (Chi square = 1.58, df = 1, p = 0.21; Chi square = 0.12, df = 1, p = 0.73; Chi square = 1.84, df = 1, p = 0.18; and Chi square =0.04, df=1, p = 0.85). Furthermore, there was no difference between obtaining a public or private education between women who horn and women who do not horn (Chi square = 0.71, df = 1, p = 0.39 and Chi square = 0.02, df = 1, p = 0.90). There was also no relationship found between women who obtained a mix of public and private education and horning status (Chi square = 0.59, df = 1, p = 0.44). On average, women who practiced horning reported having greater than 3 partners in the past 12 months (52%). Conversely, 38 (59.4%) non-horning women reported having only 1 partner in the past 12 months, and another 11 (17.2%) reported only having 2 partners in the past 12 months.

Common themes amongst women who reported horning were also identified. A majority of the women (52%) who indicated a partner had cheated on them reported leaving the relationship after retaliating. However, a slightly smaller portion of women (34%) indicated that they strayed from the relationship out of their own curiosity and attraction for another partner. Very few women indicated they horned out of necessity (2%), i.e., money to pay bills. Very few women also reported violent outbursts after becoming victims of a horning relationship. These results are summarized in Table 2 below.

Table 2. Reasons for horning (n = 50)

	n (%)
Bored	6 (12)
Retaliation	26 (52)
Attraction (experience)	17 (34)
Money	1 (2)

DISCUSSION

This study demonstrated that female horning is a cultural phenomenon occurring in Grenada, which historically observed only the practice of male horning. Overall, women practicing horning are doing so as a method of retaliation against men, as many Grenadian men hypothesized. As Grenadian history has shown, the island community was once driven by masculine ambitions and desires (5). However, as women have stepped into a more influential economic role by dominating the public sector workforce (5), owning their own home at rates equivalent to men (5), becoming increasingly educated, and having entered the world of politics, traditional masculine ideals are being cast out. Grenada's modern woman is making leaps towards complete gender equality, and is not allowing a history of oppression to get in the way of progress.

Although an unarguably important advancement for Grenadian society, female empowerment and its subsequent effect on horning may have dire consequences in regards to disease transmission in this isolated population. Epidemiologists from the Ministry of Health of Grenada have indicated increasing rates of both HIV transmission and STD transmission (13). This research supports the hypothesis that female horning may be a new contributing factor to these disease transmission trends. Possibly contributing to these increasing rates is the study finding that women who horn in Grenada report their first sexual experience at a younger age than women who do not horn, alluding to a greater lifespan of years possibly devoted to risky sexual behavior and exposure. Having sex at an earlier age could potentially correlate with the likelihood of improper contraceptive use, exposing either of the participants to the damaging effects of living with HIV or STDs in a society where both are still linked with pejorative outcomes. In combination with a lack of sexual education courses available beyond primary school, and an inherent cultural notion to ignore the problem, Grenadian women may continue to have sex at an earlier age.

A significant finding from this study involves the relationship between horning women and non-horning women. With demographic variables such as level of education and relationship status normally influencing risky behavior, this study concluded that the women in the sample were equally likely to horn. The experience of a public or private educational background unexpectedly had no influence on the decision to horn, as private educational programs in Grenada are highly integrated with the church. Ultimately, the sample showed that women who horn are just as educated as women who do not horn, they are just as likely to receive a private or public education, and are just as likely to be married, when compared to non-horning women, indicating that there is truly no "high-risk" group to target.

These culminating effects indicate that Grenadian females are caught in a struggle between morality and personal desire; a debate unexplainable by this study's findings. Having discussed the findings with educated professionals on the island, these unanticipated results go against the reported religious obligations of Grenadian society. Possibly for reasons other than retaliation, but beyond the scope of this study, Grenadian female's personal desires are superseding religious beliefs and morality, causing them to temporarily promote actions that they know to be wrong. This moral debate establishes the impact between disease transmission and cultural influences further demonstrating the need for disease transmission reduction programs to take into account historical customs and values passed along by society which may influence the outcome of risky behaviors.

As with many cross-sectional study designs it is difficult to capture and describe the entire inner workings of horning and sexual behaviors. Extending research into rates of contraceptive use in the horning population is a necessity, in order to determine the association between horning and disease transmission in Grenada. Research also needs to be directed towards the moral struggle that is occurring, as religiosity is reportedly high in Grenadian society. Investigations into how and why the construct of horning is still disseminated throughout Grenada can shed new light on the phenomena, as research in the field is borderline archaic. Lastly, establishing the temporal relationship between exposure to a partner cheating and the subsequent cheating actions of the exposed will further strengthen the argument that horning as a form of retaliation is an emerging practice in Grenada.

Participation in the study was based on a convenience sampling methodology, indicating that the participants may not be representative of the entire island population. However, with St. George's being the business and social hub for the island, survey respondents could have possibly come from regions across the island. By using shop, roadside stands, and the open-air market venders, as well as the many customers visiting these sites, as potential respondents, the breadth of geographical distribution of survey respondents could possibly be greater than expected. Another possible shortcoming of the study comes with any survey-based research, especially those dealing with sensitive topics like sexual behavior. It is quite possible that survey respondent's under- or over-reported their actions, leading to an under- or over-reporting of horning results. Among those abovementioned limitations, the study did have some strengths, one of which being the positive response to the topic. Survey respondents were engaged in the purpose of the study and were empowered to share their opinion, possibly leading to a higher likelihood of accurate results. Respondents often approached the survey distributor and requested to partake in the study, revealing a population eager to have their voice heard. Additionally, the study was the first of its kind, potentially opening the door for research much like it in the near future.

Having determined the damaging effects male and female horning may have on an isolated population, it must be reiterated how important public health is to island society. Often lacking resources to promote safe sex education and practices, Caribbean nations like Grenada are plagued by increasing rates of HIV and STD's. With the world of research turning to the impact chronic disease has on society, it is important to remember the role infectious disease play on the same population. Even more important is to understand the influences cultural practices play on disease transmission. By learning what we can about the culture, immersing ourselves in its customs and values, and truly striving hard to aid in an unbiased manner, public health will change the face of disease transmission in Grenada.

REFERENCES

[1] Pinkerton S. Acute HIV infection increases the dangers of serosorting. Am J Prev Med 2009;35(2):184.

[2] Inciardi JA, Syvertsen JL, Surratt HL. HIV/AIDS in the Caribbean Basin. AIDS Care 2005;17(1);S9-25.

[3] Allen C, McLean R, Nurse K. The Caribbean, HIV/AIDS and security. In: Griffith IL, ed. Caribbean security in the age of terror: Challenge and change. Jamaica: Ian Randle Publishers, 2004:219-251.

[4] Periago MR, Fescina R, Ram?n-Pardo P. Steps for preventing infectious diseases in women. Emerg Infect Dis 2004;10(11):1968–73.

[5] Economic Commission for Latin America and the Caribbean, United Nations Development Fund for Women. Gender dimensions of socio-economic conditions in Grenada. Port of Spain: ECLAC, 2005.

[6] Frosh S, Phoenix A, Pattman R. The trouble with boys. Psychologist 2003;16:1-7.

[7] Gupta GR. Vulnerability and resilience: Gender and HIV/AIDS in Latin America and the Caribbean. Washington, DC: International Center Research Women, 2002.

[8] United States Agency for International Development. HIV/AIDS health profile: Caribbean. Washington, DC: USAID, 2011:1-6.

[9] 9. Foster VEB. The construct of a postmodernist feminist theory for Caribbean social science research. Soc Econ Stud 192;41(2):1-43.

[10] Lewis L. Caribbean masculinity: Unpacking the narrative. In: Lewis L. The culture of gender and sexuality in the Caribbean. Gainesville, FL: University Press Florida, 2003:94-97.

[11] Lindsay K. Is the Caribbean male an endangered species? In: Mohammed P, ed. Gendered realities: Essays in Caribbean feminist thought. Jamaica, West Indies: University West Indies Press, 2002: 56–82.

[12] United Nations Global Action Special Session. UNGASS country progress report – Grenada. New York: UNGASS, 2010:1-17.

[13] Ministry of Health. HIV, AIDS, and STI report. Grenada: National Infectious Disease Control Unit, 2011.

[14] Joint United Nations Programme on HIV/AIDS. Monitoring countries status: Grenada progress report. New York: UNAIDS, 2011:1-3.

[15] World Health Organization. Women and AIDS: Have you heard us today? Geneva: WHO, 2009.

[16] Pan American Health Organization. Grenada. Health in the Americas. URL: http://ais.paho.org/hia_cp/en/2007/Grenada English.pdf.

[17] Teelucksingh J. The United States media and Caribbean gender relations. In: Korieh CJ, Okeke-Ihejirika P, eds. Gendering global transformations: Gender, culture, race, and identity. New York: Taylor Francis, 2009:72-82.

[18] Farley M. Bad for the body, bad for the heart: Prostitution harms women even if legalized or decriminalized. Violence Against Women 2004;10(10): 1087–125.

[19] Pulerwitz J, Amaro H, Jong WD, Rudd R. Relationship power, condom use and HIV risk among women in the USA. AIDS Care 2002;14(6):789-800.

[20] Centers for Disease Control and Prevention. Births, marriages, divorces, and deaths: Provisional data for 2009. Natl Vital Stat Rep 2010;58(25):1-6.

[21] Mah TL, Halperin DT. Concurrent sexual partnerships and the HIV epidemics in Africa: evidence to move forward. AIDS Behav 2010;14(1):11-6.

[22] Wang L, Ge Z, Luo J, Shan D, Gao X, Ding G, et al. Transmission risk among serodiscordant couples: A retrospective study of former plasma donors in Henan, China. J Acquire Immune Defic Syndr 2010;55(2):232-8.

[23] Kempadoo K. Past studies, new directions: Constructions and reconstructions of Caribbean sexuality. In: Kempadoo K. Sexing the Caribbean: Gender, race, and sexual labor. New York: Psychology Press, 2004:15-22.

In: Public Health Yearbook 2016
Editor: Joav Merrick

ISBN: 978-1-53610-947-4

Chapter 27

VIOLENCE AMONG ADOLESCENTS IN 13 CARIBBEAN ISLANDS

Shantel Peters-St John*, MPH, Doneal Thomas, MPhil and Shelly Rodrigo, PhD
Department of Public Health and Preventive Medicine,
School of Medicine, St George's University, Grenada, West Indies

ABSTRACT

Cross-national data from 13 Caribbean countries that participated in the Global School-Based Student Health Survey between 2007 and 2010 were analyzed to determine the prevalence of violence and examine associations between violence and risk factors in adolescents. Adolescents who reported physical violence were compared with those who did not in relation to the reported risk factors. Odds ratios (ORs) and their 95% confidence intervals (CIs) for the risk factors were estimated. Being in a physical fight and being physically attacked during the 12 months preceding the survey was reported by 39.7% and 36.6% of the adolescents studied in the 13 countries, respectively. Moderate to strong associations were observed between exposure to physical violence and gender, loneliness, suicidal ideation, school truancy, substance use (alcohol, tobacco and drugs), lack of parental supervision and close friends ($p \leq 0.05$ for all associations). Violence-related behaviors in childhood and adolescence are common in the Caribbean and are associated with risky behaviors such as smoking, drug use and truancy. The potential for poor health outcomes and continued violence in adulthood is high and therefore violence in childhood and adolescence requires urgent attention. There is a critical need for interventions targeting high-risk adolescents at the school and community levels.

Keywords: adolescents, violence, injury, risk factors, truancy

---

* Correspondence: Shantel Peters-St John, MPH, Instructor, St. George's University, Grenada, West Indies. E-mail: speters@sgu.edu.

INTRODUCTION

Violence is noted to be a global public health problem, with early aggressive behavior in childhood being a risk factor for violent behavior in adults (1). Violence causes more than 1.6 million deaths worldwide every year, with more than 90% occurring in low- and middle-income countries and being one of the leading causes of death globally for persons ages 15 to 44 years (2. In addition to death, such early exposure have been associated with poor health outcomes since risky health behaviors such as smoking and substance abuse are often found to be associated with violence (3).

Violence in childhood and adolescence has been reported in numerous studies worldwide (4-6) and also in the Caribbean (7, 8). However, no study has compared violence in adolescents across the Caribbean English speaking Caricom member states since data has been lacking for many of the countries. Understanding the burden of violence has implications for policy and programme planning at the wider Caribbean level. This paper estimates the prevalence of physical violence among adolescents using data from the Global School-based Student Health Survey (GSHS).

METHODS

Data were obtained from the multi-stage cluster designed Global School-based Student Health Survey (GSHS) developed and initiated in 2001 by the World Health Organization in collaboration with several United Nations' groups with technical assistance from the US Centers for Disease Control and Prevention (CDC). The aim of the ongoing self-administered survey is to obtain data on the heath behaviors and protective factors among school-aged adolescents that would assist countries in the development of programs, polices and interventions for school and youth health (World Health Organization). Further details of the GSHS can be obtained at http://www.who.int/chp/gshs and http://www.cdc.gov/gshs.

To date, for the Caribbean region, data sets are publicly available for Anguilla, Antigua and Barbuda, British Virgin Islands, Cayman Islands, Dominica, Grenada, Guyana, Jamaica, Montserrat, St. Kitts and Nevis, Saint Lucia, St. Vincent and the Grenadines, Suriname and Trinidad and Tobago. For this paper data from Suriname was not used since it is Dutch-speaking country in mainland South America, which would provide a different dynamic. Comparison of cross-country data is enabled by the use of a standardized scientific sample selection process, common school-based methodology and core questionnaire modules (9).

A total of 11 core questionnaire modules were administered, in addition to core-expanded questions and country-specific questions, one of which addressed violence and unintended injuries. This paper focuses on physical violence based on two items with binary outcomes (physically attacked and participation in a physical fight). Risk factors included: tobacco use; alcohol abuse; drug use; skipping school; loneliness; and suicidal ideation (each being based on a single item and recoded to a binary variable). Other factors included in the study are parents rarely or never check homework, did not understand problems, and did not know what the child is doing in the past 30 days, which were recoded on a binary scale.

CDC cleaned the data for inconsistencies in responses, with the usable data being made available to counties and for public access. The combined dataset contained information on

16, 406 students from the 13 countries; however 372 (2.27%) were excluded due to nonresponse to age, gender and the outcome variables (participation in a physical fight or being physically attacked).

Data were analyzed using the Statistical Package for Social Sciences (SPSS, version 22) at alpha = 0.05. Chi-square analyses were used to compare differences in the proportions of risk factors reported by students who were physically attacked or had been in a physical fight with those who did not report such outcomes. Associations of the risk factors with exposure to being physically attacked or being in a physical fight were examined using logistic regression.

RESULTS

Overall data were analyzed for 16,034 students having a mean age of 13.8 years (±0.99 years), with 54.5% being male. The overall prevalence of being physically attacked was 36.6% and being in a physical fight was 39.7% across the region. Males were more likely to be engaged in violence compared with females (20.3% versus 16.2% for being physically attacked and 23.5% versus 16.2% for being involved in a physical fight of the entire dataset), the differences being statistically significant ($p < 0.001$). When country was considered, a similar pattern was noted with the differences being statistically significant ($p < 0.001$) (see Table 1).

Table 1. Prevalence of violence among Caribbean adolescents aged 12 to 15 years

	Physically attacked		In a physical fight	
	n (%)	p-value	n (%)	p-value
Age				
12	606 (33.0)	0.001	700 (38.1)	<0.001
13	1584 (36.8)		1754 (40.7)	
14	1982 (38.2)		2165 (41.7)	
15	1689 (35.9)		1747 (37.2)	
Gender				
Male	32.58 (44.6)	<0.001	3775 (51.7)	<0.001
Female	2603 (29.8)		2591 (29.7)	
Location				
Anguilla	198 (29.0)	<0.001	243 (35.6)	<0.001
Antigua and Barbuda	470 (40.1)		537 (45.8)	
British Virgin Islands	353 (30.4)		406 (34.9)	
Cayman Islands	406 (36.4)		469 (42.1)	
Dominica	444(34.9)		463 (36.4)	
Grenada	524 (41.3)		477 (37.6)	
Guyana	759 (39.1)		706 (36.4)	
Jamaica	474 (39.8)		519 (43.6)	
Montserrat	49 (32.0)		56 (36.6)	
St Kitts and Nevis	490 (34.1)		529 (36.8)	
Saint Lucia	373 (35.0)		435 (40.8)	
Saint Vincent	417 (35.5)		513 (43.7)	
Trinidad and Tobago	904 (37.6)		1013 (42.2)	

In the univariate analysis, significant associations were noted with all risk factors except age (see Table 2). Of interest is the finding that for those who considered suicide, there was a 1.84 (95%CI: 1.70 – 2.00) chance of being physically attacked compared with those who did not consider suicide in the past 12 months. Truancy, alcohol use and suicidal ideation were all associated with statistically higher odds of being in a fight.

When location was considered, adolescents in Grenada were 1.17 (95% CI: 1.02 – 1.34, $p = 0.03$) more likely to be physically attacked than those in Trinidad and Tobago. Statistically significant lower odds were noted for adolescents in Anguilla (OR = 0.68, 95% CI: 0.57 – 0.82, $p < 0.001$), British Virgin Islands (OR = 0.72, 95% CI: 0.62 – 0.84, $p < 0.001$) and St Kitts (OR = 0.86, 95% CI: 0.75 – 0.98, $p = 0.03$) when compared with those in Trinidad and Tobago. There was a statistically higher odds of being in a physical fight for adolescents in Antigua and Barbuda (OR = 1.16, 95% CI: 1.01 – 1.33, $p = 0.04$) compared with the Trinidadian counterparts. Statistically significant ($p < 0.05$) lower odds were observed for adolescents in Anguilla (OR = 0.76, 95% CI: 0.64 – 0.91), British Virgin Islands (OR = 0.74, 95% CI: 0.64 – 0.85), Dominica (OR = 0.79, 95% CI: 0.68 – 0.90), Grenada (OR = 0.83, 95% CI: 0.72 – 0.95), Guyana (OR = 0.78, 95% CI: 0.69 – 0.89) and St Kitts (OR = 0.80, 95% CI: 0.70 – 0.91).

Table 2. Associations between physical violence indicators in a sample of Caribbean boys and girls aged 12 – 15

	Physically attacked		In a physical fight	
	OR (95% CI)	p-value	OR (95% CI)	p-value
Age	1.03 (0.99 - 1.06)	0.13	0.97 (0.94 - 1.00)	0.09
Gender[a]	0.53 (0.49 - 0.56)	<0.001	0.39 (0.37 - 0.42)	<0.001
Smoked ≥ 1 cigarette in the past 30 days	1.40 (1.30 – 1.50)	<0.001	1.42 (1.32 – 1.52)	<0.001
Drank alcohol ≥ 1 time in the past 30 days	1.43 (1.32 – 1.54)	<0.001	1.66 (1.53 – 1.79)	<0.001
Used drugs in lifetime	1.33 (1.23 – 1.49)	<0.001	1.28 (1.19 – 1.38)	<0.001
Often felt lonely in the past 12 months	1.47 (1.38 – 1.57)	<0.001	1.16 (1.08 – 1.23)	<0.001
Seriously considered attempting suicide in the past 12 months	1.84 (1.70 – 2.00)	<0.001	1.50 (1.39 – 1.62)	<0.001
Parents rarely/never check homework	1.12 (1.08 – 1.23)	0.001	1.08 (1.01 – 1.15)	0.027
Parent rarely/never understand problems	1.24 (1.16 – 1.32)	<0.001	1.09 (1.02 – 1.16)	0.014
Parents rarely/never know what child is doing	1.34 (1.25 – 1.43)	<0.001	1.40 (1.30 – 1.50)	<0.001
Absence from school without permission ≥ 1 day in the past 30 days	1.58 (1.48 – 1.68)	<0.001	1.68 (1.58 – 1.80)	<0.001
Has less than 2 close friends	1.21 (1.08 – 1.35)	0.001	1.14 (1.02 – 1.28)	0.021

[a]Male is the reference category for gender.

Discussion

This paper contributes to the understanding of violence in Caribbean adolescents. Currently there is a paucity of published data addressing this vulnerable group. The data showed that 36.6-39.7% of Caribbean adolescents were involved in physical violence in the 12 months prior to the survey. These figures may be an underestimate of the actual since other forms of physical violence such as parental; teacher; and intimate partner were not captured by the survey. These figures are however lower than the 42% reported by Brown et al. (5) in a study of the GSHS data for five African countries. The higher figure for the African countries may be a reflection of the conflict occurring in that region.

It was interesting to note that Grenadian adolescents were more likely to be physically attacked than those in Trinidad and Tobago where crime is high. One reason for this may be the high alcohol consumption per capita in Grenada (10). Alcohol consumptions had long since been linked to violent behavior and this analysis showed that alcohol consumption in the past 30 days was significantly associated with an increased likelihood of being physically attacked and being in a physical fight.

There exists a high likelihood of poor health outcomes and continued violence in adulthood since studies have shown an association between violence and health. Violence in childhood and adolescence is therefore a public health problem that requires urgent attention. Early integrated interventions targeting high-risk adolescents at the school and community levels are required to address the problem.

References

[1] Mytton JA, DiGuiseppi C, Gough D, Taylor RS, Logan S. School-based secondary prevention programmes for preventing violence (Review). Cochrane Database Syst Rev 2006;(3):CD004606.

[2] Krug EG, Dahlberg LL, Mercy JA, Zwi AB, Lozano R. World report on violence and health. Geneva: World Health Organization, 2002.

[3] Chartier M, Walker J, Naimark B. Childhood abuse, adult health, and health care utilization: Results from a representative community sample. Am J Epidemiol 2007;165(9):1031-38.

[4] Alwan H, Viswanathan B, Rousson V, Paccaud F, Bovet P. Association between substance use and psychosocial characteristics among adolescents of the Seychelles. BMC Pediatr 2011;11: 85.

[5] Brown DW, Riley L, Butchart A, Meddings DR, Kann L, Harvey AP. Exposure to physical and sexual violence and adverse health behaviours in African children: results from the Global School-based Student Health Survey. Bull World Health Organ 2009;87(6):447-55.

[6] Brener ND, Simon TR, Krug EG, Lowry R. Recent trends in violence-related behaviors among high school students in the United States. JAMA 1999; 282(5):440-6.

[7] Halcon L, Blum RW, Beuhring T, Pate E, Campbell-Forrester S, Venema A. Adolescent health in the Caribbean: a regional portrait. Am J Public Health 2003;93(11):1851-7.

[8] Le Franc E, Samms-Vaughan M, Hambleton I, Fox K, Brown D. Interpersonal violence in three Caribbean countries: Barbados, Jamaica, and Trinidad and Tobago. Rev Panam Salud Publica 2008;24(6): 409-21.

[9] World Health Organization. Global school-based student health survey (GSHS). URL: http://www.who .int/chp/gshs/en/.

[10] World Health Organization. Global status report on alcohol and health. Geneva: WHO, 2014.

In: Public Health Yearbook 2016
Editor: Joav Merrick
ISBN: 978-1-53610-947-4

Chapter 28

SOCIO-CULTURAL FACTORS INFLUENCE VULNERABILITY TO HIV INFECTION: AN OUTREACH TO MEN WHO HAVE SEX WITH MEN (MSM) IN GRENADA

Trent R Worrell[1], MPH, Peter E Gamache, PhD[2], Rohan D Jeremiah[3,*], PhD, MPH and Kamilah B Thomas-Purcell[4], PhD, MPH, MCHES

[1]School of Medicine, St George's University, Grenada, West Indies
[2]Turnaround Achievement Network, Tampa, Florida, US
[3]School of Public Health, University of Illinois, Chicago, Illinois, US
[4]Nova Southeastern University, College of Osteopathic Medicine, Center for Interprofessional Education and Practice and the Master of Public Health Program, Ft Lauderdale, Florida, US

ABSTRACT

The purpose of this study was to explore the socio-cultural factors that influence vulnerabilities associated to HIV infection for men who have sex with men (MSM) in the small Caribbean nation, Grenada. Forty-seven Grenadian MSM ages 16 to 42 years provided data regarding homophobia, stigma and discrimination, sexual behaviors, HIV/AIDS, and sexually transmitted infections (STIs). Results indicated that MSM who participated in a formal educational program were significantly more likely than non-participants to obtain HIV testing every 10-12 months. Since stigma and discrimination were found to affect both groups, successful HIV interventions within communities that seek to engage MSM need to focus on ensuring confidentiality, creating safe spaces, and enhancing cultural and linguistic competence.

Keywords: MSM, HIV/AIDS, intervention, grenada, caribbean, stigma, discrimination

---

* Corresponding author: Rohan D Jeremiah, PhD, MPH, Assistant Professor, Division of Community Health Sciences, School of Public Health, University of Illinois, 1603 West Taylor Street, MC 923, SPH1, Room 658, Chicago, IL 60612, United States. E-mail: rjerem@uic.edu.

INTRODUCTION

Two hundred and fifty thousand people live with human immunodeficiency virus (HIV) in the Caribbean in 2013 (1). Second to sub-Saharan Africa, the Caribbean and Eastern Europe are considered priority intervention areas because their recorded HIV prevalence rates are at least 1% (1, 2, 3). Unlike Sub-Saharan Africa where the majority of HIV transmission is observed among women, a disproportionate percentage of HIV transmission in the Caribbean is through unprotected sex between men. It is estimated that the prevalence of HIV among men who have sex with men (MSM) is the highest (25.4%) in the world (2, 4).

Rampant stigma, homophobia, and cultural taboos about sex between men are major barriers to reaching this group with prevention campaigns (5, 6). These social-cultural beliefs are products of ingrained views on gender roles, religion, and national identity within the Caribbean culture, thus making it more difficult for interventionists to address the root behaviors of HIV transmission and to implement potentially efficacious sexual health interventions (7). These interlocking realities of Caribbean culture and the recognition of sexual and gender diversities must be addressed at the systematic and structural levels (5).

Moreover, about 83% of the Caribbean countries that have submitted data for the UNAIDS global report since 2006 have maintained outdated colonial European (mainly British-derived) laws, wherein HIV risk behaviors are criminalized. These laws include bans on sex between men and policies against syringe exchange, which prohibit outreach and education to high-risk populations (6, 8, 9, 10). Researchers seeking to test and measure the effectiveness of these interventions can experience institutional challenges when these bans are in place, particularly regarding vulnerable populations such as prisoners.

According to the International HIV/AIDS Alliance and the Commonwealth HIV and AIDS Action Group (11), English-speaking Caribbean countries that criminalize same-sex practices have a higher HIV prevalence than Spanish-speaking Caribbean countries (12).

HIV/AIDS STIGMA

According to UNAIDS, "HIV/AIDS-related stigma and discrimination rank among the biggest—and most pervasive—barriers to effective responses to the AIDS epidemic" (13). This stigma negatively affects preventive behaviors, such as condom use, HIV test-seeking behavior and care-seeking behavior following an HIV positive diagnosis. Stigma also adversely impacts the quality of care provided to HIV-positive patients, in addition to the perception and treatment of people living with HIV/AIDS (PLWHA) by communities, families, and partners (14-19).

To understand how stigma is defined and perpetuated, theorists of HIV stigma frequently give credit to Goffman (20), who conceptualized stigma as a spoiler of identity (i.e., a mark of discredit and rejection). Under Goffman's definition, stigmatization is a dynamic process that arises from the perception that there has been a violation of a set of shared attitudes, beliefs, and values. Society thus labels an individual or group as different or deviant. Stigmatization can lead to prejudicial thoughts, behaviors, and/or actions on the part of governments, communities, employers, health care providers, coworkers, friends, and families (21-23).

Others have defined stigma as a set of social processes that are linked to societal power structures (24). Sources of stigma are often layered and intertwine with rigid opposition to marginalized minority groups and behaviors such as injection drug use and sex outside of marriage. These layers of stigma unfortunately help to extend and deepen stigma-related trauma among those who are infected and affected by HIV/AIDS, such as family members of those who are infected (15, 25, 26). Within the Caribbean context, much of the stigmatization of HIV infection is attached to myths and misperceptions regarding homosexual men or men who have sex with men.

Homosexuality and Men Who Have Sex with Men in the Caribbean

According to extensive research within Latin America and the Caribbean led by Caceres (26, 27) homosexuality refers to a series of constructs and ideas such as the orientation of sexual desire, sexual behavior, sexual identity, and sexual socialization (28-30), none of which are mutually exclusive. For example, although there is general knowledge of male homosexual behavior within in the region, the acceptance of homosexual or bisexual identities can vary greatly (29, 26, 31-33).

Caceres (29) emphasized that there is fluidity among the labels of homosexuality and men who have sex with men (MSM) in the Caribbean because a large proportion of MSM in the region do not identify as gay or bisexual (29, 34, 35). Diverse forms of gay identities (i.e., from local/traditional forms of homosexuality to newer, globalized patterns that share meanings and language with counterparts in North America and Europe) exist in larger urban areas within the Caribbean (26, 29, 32, 33). Such identities normally emerge from, and help consolidate, gay subcultures in these places. These subcultures do not determine unitary constituencies of gay men (and lesbians) in each locality; rather, they are heavily influenced by general social stratification in relation to class, age, and ethnicity, which mostly replicate the power relations among the larger population (29). Members of these core gay subcultures interact sexually among themselves and with men who do not share a gay identity in any of its forms. The latter also constitute a diverse group according to class, age and ethnicity (29).

HIV in the English-Speaking Caribbean

The interrelationship between HIV/AIDS stigma, identity, desire, behavior, and sex roles among MSM in this region is complex, because homosexuality is a target of discriminatory actions, human rights violations, political avoidance, and punitive policies toward men who share this identity (36). Thus, many MSM do not disclose this identity, and some may outwardly maintain that they have sexual relations with women to avoid this association. For example, in Trinidad and Tobago, one in four MSM said that they regularly have sex with women (6). Given the need to address HIV infection among MSM and their sexual networks, HIV risk reduction strategies in the Caribbean need to consider this psychosocial context of a given region (37).

The Grenadian context

Given the challenging circumstances surrounding MSM and the social, cultural, and political barriers that contribute to MSM vulnerability to HIV infection in the English-speaking Caribbean, the Grenada Chapter of the Caribbean HIV/AIDS Partnership (GrenCHAP) was established. GrenCHAP is a non-profit community-based organization that provides HIV prevention services for MSM in Grenada. GrenCHAP's objective is to promote the health of marginalized populations, including MSM, through prevention education and skills building (38).

GrenCHAP has worked closely with MSM in Grenada since 2007 by providing a program called the Men's Forum, a biweekly meeting where MSM engage in safe and candid discussions about critical topics and issues affecting their lives. Discussion topics include healthy relationships, cultural and internalized homophobia, factors and behaviors that place MSM at increased risk for HIV/STIs, methods to decrease risk of HIV/STI transmission, and how to overcome stigma and discrimination toward MSM. A trained facilitator presents topics and questions for discussion, encourages participation, and provides scientifically correct information.

Non-governmental organizations such as GrenCHAP are necessary for targeted HIV linkage and engagement in Grenada because discriminatory laws, stigma, and homophobia block HIV prevention interventions from adequately reaching the MSM population. To further understand the issue affecting MSM in Grenada, researchers worked with the GrenCHAP Men's Forum in Grenada to provide a safe space to conduct this cross-sectional, exploratory study of MSM. The study participants include MSM who participated in previous Men's Forum meetings (group A) and MSM who did not (group B). The study collected data regarding homophobia, stigma, discrimination, sexual behaviors, HIV/AIDS, and STIs, in addition to specific socio-cultural factors influencing vulnerability to HIV infection.

Methods

The population in Grenada comprises approximately 103,930 individuals (39). Grenada is the most southern of the Windward Islands of the Caribbean and consists of three islands forming an archipelago—Grenada, Carriacou, and Petit Martinique. The largest island, Grenada, is the seat of government and home to the largest population base of the country (40).

In 2011, GrenCHAP estimated at least 280 MSM reside in Grenada. More accurate HIV prevalence data for MSM in Grenada are unavailable, because MSM is not a tracking variable for the Grenadian Ministry of Health. Due to the difficulty in obtaining accurate MSM population data and the need to recruit participants among trusted networks, snowball sampling was conducted to garner as many participants as possible (41, 42).

Participants were recruited by means of client outreach and referrals from friends of GrenCHAP clients. Because the majority of MSM in Grenada do not outwardly express this identity, GrenCHAP's outreach personnel played an active role in the recruitment of individuals who wanted to keep their sexual orientation confidential. Outreach personnel had experience working with MSM through past outreach efforts and personally met with participants to administer a hardcopy of the survey at a mutually established location.

The study was also advertised in online media used by MSM in the region (i.e., GrenCHAP's Facebook page and an online chat room). Messages were posted to these media and linked potential participants to the study's online web survey. Potential study participants were required to meet the following eligibility criteria: (1) self-identification as MSM by indicating they were gay, bisexual, same gender-loving, or sexually active with other men (without identifying with a sexual orientation label); (2) a Grenadian citizen living on the island or a non-national resident; and (3) at least 16 years old (the legal age of consent in Grenada). When eligibility was established, participants were categorized into two groups: group A if they participated in GrenCHAP's Men's Forum, or group B if they did not.

Study procedures

This study was approved by the Institutional Review Board of St. George's University in Grenada and thus subject to stringent ethical protocols to protect human research participants. Potential participants were provided information with the use of a fact sheet about the study prior to providing consent and completing their survey. Due to the sensitive nature of this topic, a waiver of written and signed consent was granted to ensure that participant names were not linked to study data. The survey took approximately 15 minutes to complete for most participants, and in some cases participants opted to take additional time to provide a hard copy.

Survey measures

Data were collected from a combination of 47 written and online surveys. The survey included demographic characteristics, whether they participated in the GrenCHAP's Men's Forum, general knowledge about HIV/AIDS and STIs, internal stigma about being an MSM, external stigma and discrimination toward MSM, personal attitudes regarding social stigma and discrimination against MSM, and sexual behaviors. The internal and external stigma assessment measurements were adapted from the Pan Caribbean Partnership Against HIV and AIDS (PANCAP) Regional Stigma and Discrimination Unit's survey measuring dimensions of stigma (43).

Participants reported their age, nationality, level of formal education, and monthly income in East Caribbean dollars (US$1 = EC$2.67). Participants were asked to indicate agree or disagree for each statement relating to general knowledge about HIV/AIDS and STI testing, access to testing, HIV transmission, and severity of the disease. Participants' responses of strongly agree, agree, disagree or strongly disagree measured internal stigma about being an MSM, how they felt about their community in Grenada, and stigma and discrimination toward MSM. The final portion of the survey measured participants' overall sexual behavior with women and tourists and their sexual activity and risk-taking in the past year. Participants filled in an answer where needed and indicated agree or disagree.

Data analysis

This investigation compared responses of those who participated in GrenCHAP's Men's Forum (group A) to those who did not (group B). Incomplete surveys were not included in data analyses. Quantitative data were analyzed using StatPlus® (44). The independent variable was GrenCHAP's Men's Forum. The dependent variables were general knowledge about HIV/AIDS and STIs, internal and external stigma, attitudes due to stigma and discrimination, personal behaviors about sex, and trends in STIs. Responses to these dependent and demographic variables were either continuous or categorical.

Percentages were calculated for each dependent variable to obtain an overall assessment of the study's participants. Differences between group A and group B were assessed using a two-sample t-test for continuous data and a chi-square test for categorical data. The categorical responses Strongly Agree, Agree, Disagree and Strongly Disagree were dichotomized to Agree or Disagree. Odds ratios and 95% confidence intervals were reported, and significance was defined as $p < 0.05$.

RESULTS

The demographic characteristics of the participants in group A were highly similar to the demographic characteristics of participants in group B (see Table 1). About 79% of all of the participants were Grenadian (the remainder indicated American, Canadian, Trinidadian, Barbadian, and Surinamese), and the average age was 28.2 years. Nearly 74% reached university or college education levels, and income ranged from less than EC$500 to EC$5,000 (US $187 to US $1,872) per month.

Participants' knowledge of how HIV is transmitted, risk factors for HIV transmission, and severity of the disease did not differ between MSM in groups A and B (see Table 2). No difference was found between the groups in access to HIV/STIs testing, as 93.6% knew where to get tested for HIV and STIs. However, 27.7% reported experiencing trouble accessing testing resources. The percentage of those who knew that HIV cannot be contracted through normal social contact and activities such as kissing, sneezing, and sharing utensils was 97.9%, yet only 44.7% knew that HIV can be contracted through oral sex without a condom. All participants (100%) knew that condoms can reduce chances of transmitting HIV and that untreated HIV can lead to AIDS and death.

Measurements assessing internal stigma did not differ between the MSM groups; 95.7% of all survey participants were concerned about homophobia and discrimination and believed it was too risky to let others know they were MSM (see Table 3). The findings of the study showed that nearly 92% of all participants are very cautious about who they tell about their sexual orientation, and 80.9% try to hide it. Fewer than 25% feel ashamed or guilty that they are MSM. Overall, the majority of MSM did not believe that they would be a better person if they were not an MSM and believed themselves to be just as good as other people.

Table 1. Baseline characteristics of 47 participants recruited in Grenada

Characteristic	All Participants		Group A MSM in Men's Forum (N = 20)		Group B MSM Not in Men's Forum (N = 27)		p-value+
	N	Mean	N	Mean, (range)	N	Mean, (range)	
Age *(years)*	47	28.2	20	26.8, (16 – 39)	27	29.2, (19 – 42)	0.23
Characteristic	N	%	N	%	N	%	p-value++
Nationality	47		20		27		
Grenadian	37	78.7	15	75	22	81.4	0.59
American	2	4.3	2	10	0	0	0.09
Canadian	3	6.4	1	5	2	7.4	0.74
Trinidadian	3	6.4	1	5	2	7.4	0.74
Barbadian	1	2.1	0	0	1	3.7	0.38
Surinamese	1	2.1	1	5	0	0	0.24
Education	46		20		26		
Primary School	1	2.2	1	5	0	0	0.25
Secondary School	9	19.6	4	20	5	19.2	0.95
College	16	34.8	8	40	8	30.8	0.52
University	18	39.1	6	30	12	46.2	0.27
Post-Graduation	2	4.3	1	5	1	3.85	0.85
Monthly Income[a] *(XCD)*[b]	12		8		4		
Less than \$500	2	16.7	1	12.5	1	25	0.58
\$500 - \$1,500	6	50	4	50	2	50	1
\$1,500 - \$3,000	3	25	3	37.5	0	0	0.16
\$3,001 - \$4,000	0	0	0	0	0	0	n/a
\$4,001 - \$5,000	0	0	0	0	0	0	n/a
More than \$5,000	1	8.3	0	0	1	25	0.14

Note: +two-sample t-test; ++chi-square test; [a]Indication of monthly income was optional; [b]Eastern Caribbean Dollar; n/a = not applicable, values too small.

Table 2. Participants' general knowledge about HIV and STIs

	All Participants (N = 47)		Group A MSM in Men's Forum (N = 20)		Group B MSM Not in Men's Forum (N = 27)			
	N	%	N	%	N	%	OR	95% CI
Know where to get tested for HIV/STIs	44	93.6	19	95	25	92.6	1.5	0.1-18.03
Have trouble accessing HIV/STI testing	13	27.7	5	25	8	29.6	0.8	0.21-2.92
Know that HIV cannot be contracted through normal social contact/activities	46	97.9	19	95	27	100	n/a	
Know that having fewer sex partners can reduce the chances of getting HIV	43	91.5	17	85	26	96.3	0.2	0.02-2.3
Know that STIs can increase the chances of getting HIV during sex	44	93.7	19	95	25	92.6	1.5	0.1-18.03

Table 2. (Continued)

	All Participants (*N* = 47)		Group A MSM in Men's Forum (*N* = 20)		Group B MSM Not in Men's Forum (*N* = 27)			
	N	%	N	%	N	%	OR	95% CI
Know that condoms can reduce the chances of contracting HIV	47	100	20	100	27	100	n/a	
Know that HIV can be contracted through oral sex without a condom	21	44.7	12	60	9	33.3	3.0	0.9-9.96
Know that lubricant can reduce the chances of condom breakage	37	78.7	18	90	19	70.4	3.8	0.71-20.3
Know that untreated HIV can lead to AIDS and death	47	100	20	100	27	100	n/a	

Note: n/a = not applicable, values too small.

Table 3. Participants' internal stigma

	All Participants (*N* = 47)		Group A MSM in Men's Forum (*N* = 20)		Group B MSM Not in Men's Forum (*N* = 27)			
	N	%	*N*	%	*N*	%	OR	95% CI
Feel ashamed that they are MSM	10	21.3	4	20	6	22.2	0.9	0.21-3.63
Feel guilty because they are MSM	11	23.4	5	25	6	22.2	1.2	0.3-4.54
Feel like they are a bad person because they are an MSM	5	10.6	1	5	4	14.8	0.3	0.03-2.94
Try to hide that they are an MSM	38	80.9	15	75	23	85.2	0.5	0.12-2.26
Believe that letting others know they are an MSM is risky	45	95.7	18	90	27	100	n/a	
Worry about others discriminating against them because they are an MSM	45	95.7	19	95	26	96.3	0.7	0.04-12.44
Very cautious about who they tell that they are an MSM	43	91.5	18	90	25	92.6	0.7	0.09-5.6
Feel that they are not part of their community in Grenada because they are an MSM	14	29.8	5	25	9	33.3	0.7	0.18-2.42
Feel that they are not as good as other people because they are an MSM	3	6.38	1	5	2	7.4	0.7	0.06-7.81
Believe that they would be a better person if they were not an MSM	5	10.6	1	5	4	14.8	0.3	0.03-2.94

Table 4. Participants' external stigma and discrimination

	All Participants (*N* = 47)		Group A MSM in Men's Forum (*N* = 20)		Group B MSM Not in Men's Forum (*N* = 27)			
	N	%	*N*	%	*N*	%	**OR**	**95% CI**
Believe that most MSM are rejected when others find out about them	38	80.9	17	85	21	77.8	1.6	0.35-7.45
Believe that where they live in Grenada, MSM are treated like outcasts	38	80.9	16	80	22	81.5	0.9	0.21-3.93
Believe that most people feel MSM are bad individuals	18	38.3	10	50	8	29.6	2.4	0.71-7.92
Believe that most people feel uncomfortable being around someone who is an MSM	30	63.8	15	75	15	55.6	2.4	0.68-8.5
Believe that friends and family are afraid others will reject them if they find out that they are an MSM	36	76.6	15	75	21	77.8	0.9	0.22-3.34

Participant beliefs about their public image and how they were treated by others who knew they were MSM did not differ between groups A and B (see Table 4). In fact, more than 80% of all participants believed that MSM in Grenada are treated like outcasts and that most MSM are rejected when others find out about them, yet more than 60% believed that most people feel MSM are not bad individuals. In addition, 76.6% of the participants believe that friends and family are afraid that MSM will be rejected by others who find out about their sexual practices.

The impact of stigma and discrimination on participants' attitudes on sexual behaviors and risk-taking did not differ between groups A and B (see Table 5), with one exception; MSM in group A, those who participated in GrenCHAP's Men's Forum, were significantly more likely to feel that they had to go the extra mile to connect with other MSM, compared to the group B MSM, who did not participate in GrenCHAP's Men's Forum. In fact, 80.9 to 85.1% of all participants believed that homophobia, stigma, and discrimination make it difficult to meet other MSM, and that they have to put in more effort to connect with other MSM in Grenada. Fewer than 30% of the MSM surveyed resort to risky sexual behavior to regain control over their sex lives or behave in risky ways because of the law banning sex between men. Moreover, fewer than half believe that greater acceptance of MSM in Grenada and removing the law banning sex between men would change their sexual behaviors.

MSM in group A were significantly more likely to get tested for HIV every 10 to 12 months than MSM in group B (see Table 6). Other sexual behaviors did not differ between groups. More than 90% of the MSM surveyed were sexually active in the past year. In both groups, MSM reported having sex with men and women as well as with tourists or individuals outside of Grenada. More than half took what they considered to be desperate measures to have sex with other MSM, with 44.7% engaging in sex without a condom in the past year.

Table 5. Participants' attitudes due to stigma and discrimination

	All Participants (*N* = 47)		Group A MSM in Men's Forum (*N* = 20)		Group B MSM Not in Men's Forum (*N* = 27)			
	N	%	*N*	%	*N*	%	OR	95% CI
Feel like they cannot be themselves because of homophobia and discrimination in Grenada	25	53.2	13	65	12	44.4	2.3	0.7-7.64
Believe that homophobia, stigma, and discrimination make it difficult to meet other MSM	40	85.1	19	95	21	77.8	5.4	0.6-49.29
Feel that because they are an MSM in their community in Grenada, they have to go the extra mile to connect with another MSM	38	80.9	19	95	19	70.4	8.0*	0.91-70.35
Behave in risky ways because of the laws and stigma against MSM	14	29.8	5	25	9	33.3	0.7	0.18-2.42
Feel desperate when it comes to finding another sexual partner as an MSM in their community in Grenada	33	70.2	14	70	19	70.4	1.0	0.28-3.48
Resort to risky sexual behavior to regain control over sex life because of the laws banning sex between men and resistance against MSM	11	23.4	6	30	5	18.5	1.9	0.48-7.37
Believe that removing the law banning sex between men would change their sexual behaviors	19	40.4	11	55	8	29.6	2.9	0.87-9.71
Believe that greater acceptance of MSM in Grenada would change their sexual behaviors	20	42.6	10	50	10	37.0	1.7	0.53-5.50

Note: *significance at the $p < 0.05$ level, chi-square.

DISCUSSION

Examinations of internal and external stigma among MSM and attitudes regarding community discrimination directed toward them are essential to understanding challenges to HIV prevention in Grenada. While group A and group B had equal desires to avoid HIV infection, and both indicated that stigma and discrimination are shared realities among MSM in Grenada, MSM from the Men's Forum (group A) felt stronger about their difficulty in meeting other MSM in Grenadian communities than MSM who did not partake in the Men's Forum (group B).

Table 6. Participants' sexual behaviors

	All Participants (*N* = 47)		Group A MSM in Men's Forum (*N* = 20)		Group B MSM Not in Men's Forum (*N* = 27)			
	N	%	*N*	%	*N*	%	OR	95% CI
Have sex with men and women	19	40.4	6	30	13	48.1	0.5	0.14-1.56
Have sex with tourists or individuals outside of Grenada	33	70.2	16	80	17	63.0	2.4	0.61-9.04
Have been sexually active in the past year	44	93.6	20	100	24	88.9	n/a	
Have engaged in sex without a condom in the past year	21	44.7	8	40	13	48.1	0.7	0.22-2.31
Have taken what they consider desperate measures to have sex with other MSM in the past year	24	51.1	9	45	15	55.6	0.7	0.2-2.09
Had an STI in the past year	2	4.3	1	5	1	3.7	1.4	0.08-23.29
Got tested for HIV in the past year[a]	38	80.9	14	70	24	88.9	0.3	0.06-1.35
N/A	12	25.5	5	25	7	25.9	1.0	0.25-3.6
Every 1 – 3 months	2	4.3	1	5	1	3.7	1.4	0.08-23.29
Every 4 – 6 months	14	29.8	3	15	11	40.7	0.3	0.06-1.09
Every 7 – 9 months	11	23.4	5	25	6	22.2	1.2	0.3-4.54
Every 10 – 12 months	8	17.0	6	30	2	7.4	5.4*	0.95-30.18
	N	**Mean**	*N*	**Mean**	*N*	**Mean**	***p*-value**	
Amount of sexual partners in the past year	47	5.38	20	4.85	27	5.8	0.35	

Note: *significance at the $p < 0.05$ level, chi-square test; n/a = not applicable, values too small; aNot all participants who answered this question specified how often they got tested.

The primary protective factor against the spread of HIV was that members of the Men's Forum were more likely to get tested for HIV than non-members. This is ideal in terms of HIV prevention, because the Center for Disease Control (CDC) reports that sexually active MSM have an increased risk for HIV infection and thus recommends that MSM be tested for HIV infection at least annually (45). Moreover, knowing one's HIV status is one of the most important components of HIV prevention because the knowledge provides MSM the choice to remain negative, if they are negative, and for those who are positive, to seek access to treatment to reduce the risk of HIV transmission to future partners (46). However, the influence of community perception and the perpetuation of stigma and discrimination remain dominant community health issues that influence MSM health.

Conclusion

This study elucidated underlying socio-cultural factors that contribute to MSM vulnerability to HIV infection in Grenada. It is one of the first evidence-based knowledge-building investigations of HIV-related stigma and discrimination in Grenada. According to USAID (8), building this foundation is one of the first steps toward the successful reduction of stigma and discrimination.

This study also gave voice to a sample of at-risk MSM who largely remain hidden and demonstrated the need for more targeted interventions to the MSM community in Grenada. Based on the study findings, one strategy to tackle the challenges experienced by MSM is to streamline and link awareness and prevention efforts to available HIV/AIDS testing services in ways that are culturally and linguistically competent.

Due to the advancement of HIV/AIDS testing that can facilitate private and confidential ways to get tested, non-governmental organizations such as GrenCHAP that focus on the MSM community can become testing sites for MSM. This integration of testing services and social services can improve the frequency and continuity of MSM social network-building and population health in Grenada.

Strengths and limitations

The strengths of this study include data collection methods that were tailored specifically for the study's target population, respecting MSM privacy, confidentiality, and anonymity. GrenCHAP's preexisting relationship with some members of the MSM community facilitated recruitment of potential participants, especially those with a preference for undisclosed MSM identities. Innovative strategies, such as use of a popular online website designed especially for MSM to recruit individuals who are particularly sensitive about exposing their MSM identity, allowed anonymous access to the study's web survey. These recruitment strategies provided MSM the privacy to confidently answer survey questions freely and honestly. Web surveys yield data of comparable quality to that of hard-copy surveys (47). The findings generated from this study will prove useful because HIV prevention programming for MSM has never been systematically examined in Grenada.

Limitations of this study were unavoidably inherent during participant recruitment. Although ensuring participant confidentiality and anonymity prompted the use of innovative recruitment strategies, some recruitment strategies were eliminated due to the threat of exposing MSM to discrimination in a homophobic society. Any public advertising such as street outreach, mailings, telephoning, and the distribution of flyers were several recruitment strategies that were eliminated because the majority of MSM are largely hidden among others in the general population; likewise, many MSM keep their sexual orientation secret due to fear of discrimination. No public establishments exist for gay men in Grenada, which negated the use of venue-based sampling. Therefore, limited recruitment strategies may have contributed to the comparatively small sample size.

Other limitations include selection bias in the study's target population. There is a slight chance that the majority of recruited participants who agreed to participate are empowered MSM; they may be comfortable with their sexual orientation, not necessarily open, and thus more inclined to voice their opinions and attitudes via the study's survey. MSM who choose not to participate due to fear or unwillingness to accept their sexual orientation are the most ideal candidates for this type of study.

Another limitation is the fact that the majority of men recruited were comparatively young MSM with an average age of 28 years. Their views may not reflect the views of older

MSM. Overall, the study sample may not be representative of the greater MSM community in Grenada.

Future studies of this nature will benefit from the qualitative subject matter of focus group interviews. Quantitative and qualitative data combined can provide further insight and more in-depth analysis of the relationship between societal homophobia, stigma, and discrimination to MSM behavior and sexual risk-taking in Grenada and throughout the Caribbean. It is evident from this study that targeting non-gay-identified MSM would pose a unique challenge for implementing HIV prevention for MSM. Therefore, interventions should go beyond traditional models that have been based solely on information or skills-building to address individual risk behaviors, and moved toward approaches that address the community stigma and discrimination that are perpetuated towards Grenadian MSM (29).

REFERENCES

[1] Joint United Nations Program on HIV/AIDS [UNAIDS]. Fact sheet 2014. Geneva: WHO, 2014.

[2] Henry J. Kaiser Family Foundation. Fact sheet: The global HIV/AIDS epidemic. Accessed 2014 Dec 10. URL: http://www.kff.org/hivaids/upload/3030-17.pdf.

[3] PEPFAR-Caribbean. Caribbean regional HIV and AIDS partnership framework. Five-year strategic framework to support implementation of Caribbean regional and national efforts to combat HIV and AIDS. New York; PEPFAR 2012. URL: http://www.pepfar. gov/documen ts/organization/143196.pdf.

[4] Beyrer C, Baral S, van Griensven F, Goodreau S, Chariyalertsak S, Wirtz A, Brookmeyer R. Global Epidemiology of HIV infection in men who have sex with men. Lancet 2012; 380(9839): 367-77.

[5] Altman D, Aggleton P, Williams M, Kong T, Reddy V, Harrad D, Reis T, and Parker R. Men who have sex with men: stigma and discrimination. Lancet 2012; 380(9839): 439-45.

[6] Joint United Nations Program on HIV/AIDS [UNAIDS]. Report on the global AIDS epidemic. Geneva: WHO, 2010.

[7] Huedo-Medina TB, Boynton MH, Warren MR, LaCroix JM, Carey MP, Johnson BT. Efficacy of HIV prevention interventions in Latin American and Caribbean nations, 1995-2008: A meta-analysis. AIDS Behav 2010; 14(6): 1237–51.

[8] Joint United Nations Program on HIV/AIDS [UNAIDS]. Report on the global AIDS epidemic. Geneva: WHO, 2006.

[9] Joint United Nations Program on HIV/AIDS [UNAIDS]. Report on the global AIDS epidemic. Geneva: WHO, 2008.

[10] Joint United Nations Program on HIV/AIDS [UNAIDS]. World AIDS day report. Geneva: WHO, 2012.

[11] International HIV/AIDS Alliance and Commonwealth HIV and AIDS Action Group. Enabling legal environments for effective HIV responses: A leadership challenge for the Commonwealth. Hove, United Kingdom: International HIV/AIDS Alliance, 2010.

[12] United States Agency for International Development [USAID]. HIV/AIDS health profile: Latin America and the Caribbean. Washington, DC: USAID, 2011.

[13] Brown L, Macintyre K, Trujillo L. Interventions to reduce HIV/AIDS stigma: What have we learned? AIDS Educ Prev 2003; 15(1): 49–69.

[14] Gerbert B, Maguire BT, Bleecker T, Coates TJ, McPhee SJ. Primary care physicians and AIDS: Attitudinal and structural barriers to care. JAMA 1991; 266(20): 2837–42.

[15] Herek GM, Glunt EK. An epidemic of stigma: Public reactions to AIDS. Am Psychol 1988; 43(11): 886-891.

[16] Herek GM, Glunt EK. Interpersonal contact and heterosexuals' attitudes toward gay men: Results from a national survey. J Sex Res 1993; 30(3): 239–44.

[17] Macintyre K, Brown L, Sosler S. It's not what you know, but who you knew: Examining the relationship between behavior change and AIDS mortality in Africa. AIDS Educ Prev 2001; 13(2): 160–74.
[18] Malcolm A, Aggleton P, Bronfman M, Galv?o J, Mane P, Verrall J. HIV-related stigmatization and discrimination: Its forms and contexts. Crit Public Health 1998; 8(4): 347–70.
[19] Muyinda H, Seeley J, Pickering H, Barton T. Social aspects of AIDS-related stigma in rural Uganda. Health Place 1997; 3(3): 143–7.
[20] Goffman, E. Stigma: Notes on the management of a spoiled identity. Englewood Cliffs, NJ: Prentice Hall, 1963.
[21] Cameron E. Legal rights, human rights and AIDS: The first decade. Report from South Africa 2. AIDS Anal Afr 1993; 3(6): 3–4.
[22] Jayaraman KS. Indian state plans compulsory HIV testing, segregation and branding. Nature 1998; 4(4): 378.
[23] Zierler S, Cunningham WE, Andersen R, Shapiro M, Nakazono T, Morton S. Violence victimization after HIV infection in a US probability sample of adult patients in primary care. Am J Public Health 2000; 90(2): 208–15.
[24] Link BG, Phelan JC. Conceptualizing stigma. Annu Rev Sociol 2001; 27(1): 363-85.
[25] Parker RG, Aggleton P. HIV and AIDS-related stigma and discrimination: A conceptual framework and implications for action. Soc Sci Med 2003; 57(1): 13-24.
[26] Caceres CF, Rosasco AM. The margin has many sides: Diversity among gay and homosexually active men in Lima. Cult Health Sex1999; 1(3): 261–75.
[27] Rushing WA. The AIDS epidemic: Social dimensions of an infectious disease. Boulder, CO: Westview Press, 1995.
[28] Douglas CJ. Homosexuality in the Caribbean: Crawling out of the closet. Grenada: Mayzoon Press, 2013.
[29] Aggleton P. Bisexualities and AIDS: International Perspectives. London: Taylor Francis, 1996.
[30] Caceres CF. HIV among gay and other men who have sex with men in Latin America and the Caribbean: A hidden epidemic? AIDS 2002; 16(Suppl 3): 23–33.
[31] Stein E. Forms of desire: Sexual orientation and the social constructionist controversy. New York: Routledge, 2013.
[32] Carrier J. De los otros: Intimacy and homosexuality among Mexican men. New York: Columbia University Press, 1995.
[33] Lancaster RN. That we should all turn queer? Homosexual stigma in the making of manhood and the breaking of a revolution in Nicaragua. In: Parker R, Gagnon J, eds. Conceiving sexuality: Approaches to sex research in a postmodern world. New York: Routledge, 1995: 135-56.
[34] Parker R. Beneath the equator: Cultures of desire, male homosexuality, and emerging gay communities in Brazil. New York: Routledge, 1999.
[35] Parker RG, Caceres C. Alternative sexualities and changing sexual cultures among Latin American men. Culture, Health Sex 1999; 1(3): 201–6.
[36] Parker R. Sexuality, culture and society: Shifting paradigms in sexuality research. Cult Health Sex 2009; 11(3): 251–66.
[37] amfAR: The Foundation for AIDS Research. MSM, HIV, and the road to universal access - How far have we come? AmfAR special report. New York: Foundation AIDS Research, 2008.
[38] Garcia Calleja JM, Walker N, Cuchi P, Lazzari S, Ghys PD, Zacarias F. Status of the HIV/AIDS epidemic and methods to monitor it in the Latin America and Caribbean region. AIDS 2002; 16(3): S3–S12.
[39] Mathlin N, Charles K, Ross K. GrenCHAP: Organization information. Saint George, Grenada: GrenCHAP, 2012.
[40] United States Department of State. Grenada. Accessed 2014 Dec 10. URL: http://www.state.gov/r/pa/ei/bgn/2335.htm.
[41] Government of Grenada. Grenada national strategic plan for health (2008-2012): Health for economic growth and human development. St. George's, Grenada: Government Grenada, 2008.
[42] Denzin NK, Lincoln YS. Handbook of qualitative research. London: Sage, 2000.

[43] Schensul J, LeCompte M. Ethnographer's toolkit. Walnut Creek, CA: Altamira Press, 1999.

[44] Pan Caribbean Partnership Against HIV and AIDS [PANCAP], Regional Stigma and Discrimination Unit. The stigma community response baseline: Marginalized groups assessment instrument. Georgetown, Guyana: PANCAP, 2010.

[45] AnalystSoft Incorporated. StatPlus:mac - statistical analysis program for Mac OS. Vancouver, BC: AnalystSoft Incorporated, 2010.

[46] Branson BM, Handsfield HH, Lampe MA, Janssen RS, Taylor AW, Lyss SB. Revised recommendations for HIV testing of adults, adolescents, and pregnant women in health-care settings. MMWR 2006; 55(RR14): 1–17.

[47] United Nations Population Fund [UNFPA]. HIV prevention now – programme brief #5: Voluntary counseling and testing (VCT) for HIV. New York: United Nations Population Fund, 2002.

[48] Trau RNC, Härtel CEJ, Härtel GF. Reaching and hearing the invisible: Organizational research on invisible stigmatized groups via web surveys. Br J Manage 2012; 24(4): 532-41.

In: Public Health Yearbook 2016
Editor: Joav Merrick
ISBN: 978-1-53610-947-4

Chapter 29

CHILD SEXUAL ABUSE IN SAINT LUCIA

Lamese Basilyous*[1,*]*, MPH
and Praveen Durgampudi*[2]*, MBBS, MPH, MSPH
[1]School of Medicine, St. George's University, Grenada, West Indies
[2]Department of Public Health and Preventative Medicine,
St. George's University, Grenada, West Indies

ABSTRACT

The purpose of this secondary data analysis was to assess the prevalence of child sexual abuse (CSA) in Saint Lucia. A total of 1,526 primary and secondary school students completed the 2000 Youth Health Survey. Several questions within the survey specifically targeted: adolescent sexual behavior and experiences, quantifying sexual experience and the age of first intercourse, the appeal of sex, number of sex partners, contraception, and sexually transmitted diseases. The majority (62%) of female students and 24% of male students reported that their first sexual intercourse was forced against their will. Female children had a 5.1 times higher likelihood of becoming victims of sexual abuse over male children (CI: 3.31 – 7.85). Further findings showed that the same female students who reported that their first sexual encounter was forced, 56% of them further responded that they had not been sexually abused. Similarly, of the male students who also reported that their first sexual encounter was forced, 77% responded that they had in fact not been sexually abused. While many students were victims of CSA, most did not recognize the criminality of the abuse. The potential for sexually transmitted infections and HIV apart from mental agony and trauma is daunting.

Keywords: child sexual abuse, St. Lucia, HIV, STI

---

* Correspondence: Lamese Basilyous, MPH, St. George's University School of Medicine, St. George, Grenada. E-mail: l.basilyous@yahoo.com.

INTRODUCTION

Worldwide, sexual violence against children is an enormous problem. According to the UNICEF in 2002, there were an estimated 223 million girls and boys under the age of 18 who experienced some form of sexual abuse (1). This is a massive problem because those children grow to be defective individuals in their communities with many psychological problems, which overall, weakens the society (2, 3).

Child sexual abuse (CSA) is especially prevalent in the Caribbean region. According to the WHO, "In several Caribbean countries, the first sexual experience of young girls is often forced; studies have shown that this was the case for 42.8% of girls below age 12 years" (1). This is due to the fact that the community does not see CSA as against the norm and some men believe it is their right to have sexual contact with girls within their household (4). In many cases, CSA is viewed as the mistake of the victim and, this is more prevalent if the victim is a female (4, 5). In most of the reported cases of CSA, the victims are females. However, although it is less frequent, males can also fall victims to CSA (4).

Saint Lucia is one of many islands in the Caribbean that is facing a potential problem of CSA epidemic. Fear and limited trust in the legal structure both contribute to CSA underreporting by victims and their families (6). This could be due to the cultural misunderstanding of the consequences of sexual abuse toward children and the population perspective regarding this issue (6). According to the Pan American Health Organization (7), between the years of 1990 to 1995, there has been on average 100 cases of child abuse annually, from which 35% are CSA related. Between 2005/2007, there was a yearly increase in the number of reported CSA cases in Saint Lucia (8).

According to the Royal Saint Lucian Police Force (RSLPF), there has been an incremental increase in the number of reported CSA cases starting from the year 2000 until current; unfortunately these numbers do not take into account CSA underreporting. The reason for unreported cases is due to the fact that most of the sexual abuse happens within the household, so both the victim and the mother are afraid to report because the abuser is usually the family breadwinner (5). The second factor that contributes to underreporting when it happens outside of the household is that many of the victims' families are willing to accept settlements like cash in exchange for their vow of silence (9).

From this perspective, it can be inferred that CSA should not be classified as an isolated crime with limited consequences. Instead the negative and harmful effects of CSA incidence in any given community have a far wider reach. UNICEF has suggested a multiple level approach to understanding and accounting for the negative impact of CSA on society, particularly in the Eastern Caribbean (5).

In contributing to progressive public health policy in St. Lucia, this study will choose to focus on addressing the issue of childhood rape of children between the ages of 10 and 17. Child sexual abuse is largely categorized by child rape, which involves any act of forced violence, manipulation, coercion, physical penetration of the victim, or a combination of the latter (5, 6). For the purpose of this research, rape is defined as forcibly penetrating a child's mouth, anus, or vagina, with the penis or any other object (5, 6). Additionally, CSA is also inclusive of sexual acts involving children, such as transactional sexual abuse, child pornography, and forcing children to participate in sexual acts. All the above stated acts qualify as sexual violence because they are committed against a child who is unable to or deprived of their ability to consent or refuse (5).

Therefore the objective of this research is to assess the prevalence of CSA in Saint Lucia and to better understand the circumstances correlated with CSA incidence. This will help in creating a plan to address the issue in Saint Lucia where education programs can be created to change societal perspectives in order to prevent CSA.

METHODS

Under the direction of the World Health Organization (WHO) and the Pan American Health Organization (PAHO), the health ministries of nine CARICOM nations participated in a data sampling effort designed to address many of the health factors (10, 11). Adolescents between the ages of 10 and 19 were of particular interest in this health policy shift due to their higher likelihood of engaging in or being exposed to the risk factors that would compromise their health (10, 11). Conducted from 1996-1998, questionnaire style surveys were administered throughout student classrooms and were completed under the decree of confidentiality and voluntary choice (10, 11).

Although not part of the initial data collection effort, recognition that many of St. Lucia's youth population morbidity and mortality rates were trending towards social causes led PAHO to obtain funding to administer the questionnaire in St. Lucia as well (10). Regarded as the Youth Health Survey of 2000, a total 1,526 students between the ages of 10 and 19 were sampled from a combination of 29 primary and secondary academic institutions (12). Demographically, slightly over half of the respondents were female and 80% of the total respondents were of African descent (12).

Several questions within the survey specifically targeted: adolescent sexual behavior and experiences, quantifying sexual experience and age of first intercourse, the appeal of sex, number of sex partners, contraception, and sexually transmitted diseases (11). While briefly addressed, the survey also singled out the topic of intercourse in order to determine how many students felt that they were unprepared or forced into it against their will (11). This strongly compelling and disquieting question would soon become the root objective of another comprehensive study regarding CSA prevalence and incidence throughout the CARICOM region.

RESULTS

Analysis of the data collected from the St. Lucian Youth Health Survey of 2000 revealed a stunning trend in terms of the understanding young students had regarding the criminality of sexual abuse. Of the 136 (17%) female students between the ages 10 and 17 who had sexual intercourse, 62% of them reported that their first sexual intercourse was forced against their will (Figure 1). Of the 318 (46%) male respondents reporting having sexual intercourse also between the ages of 10 and 17, nearly 24% of students reported that their first sexual intercourse was forced against their will (Figure 2). In assessing the strength of association between being either male or female and CSA, an odds ratio calculation indicated a strong association of female children having a 5.1 times higher likelihood of becoming victims of sexual abuse over male children (CI: 3.31 – 7.85). From a policy perspective, the reality that female victims would outnumber male victims would at the very least require sensitivity to be exercised by both police forces and healthcare providers in instances of reported cases.

In further findings from the St. Lucian Youth Health Survey of 2000, of female students who reported that their first sexual encounter was against their will, 56% of them further responded that they had not been sexually abused (Figure 3). Similarly, of the male students who also reported that their first sexual encounter was against their will, 77% responded that they had in fact not been sexually abused (Figure 4). A chi-squared test was utilized to obtain a p-value of less than 0.001 for both male and female students, thus supporting regional findings that there are a significant number of children who are victims of CSA but do not recognize the criminality of the abuse.

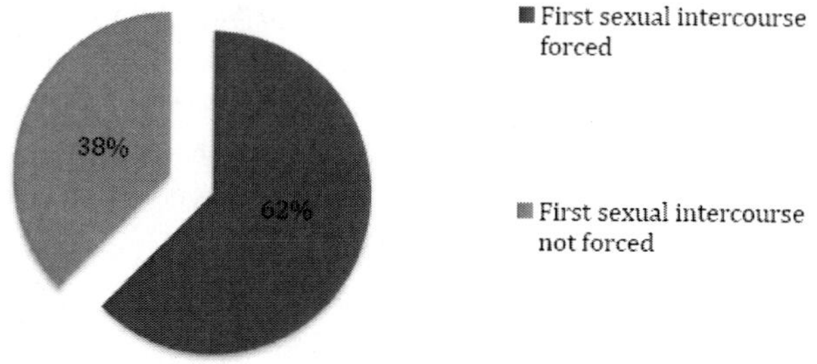

Figure 1. Female students' first sexual intercourse.

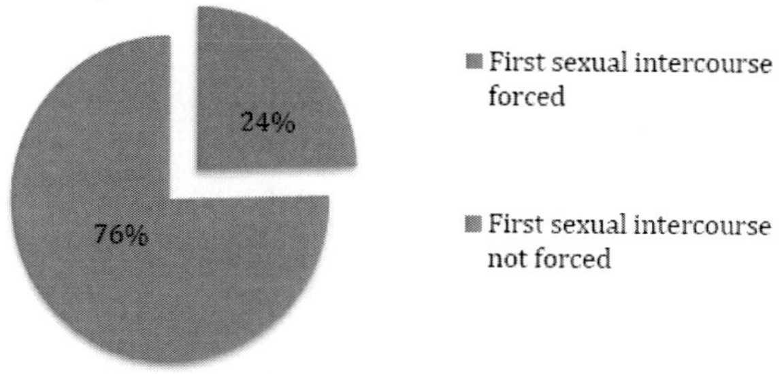

Figure 2. Male students' first sexual intercourse.

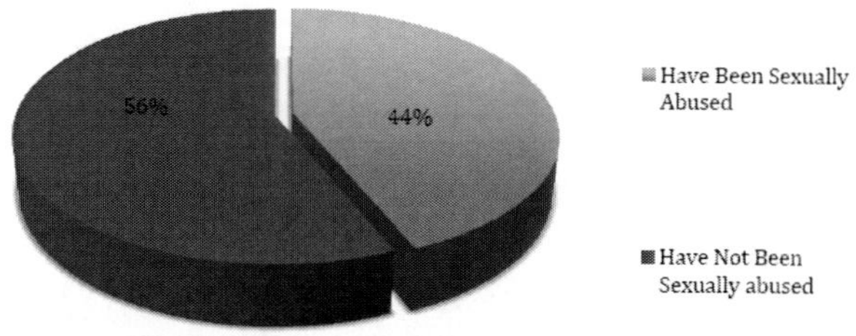

Figure 3. Female students who recognize first forced sexual intercourse as abuse.

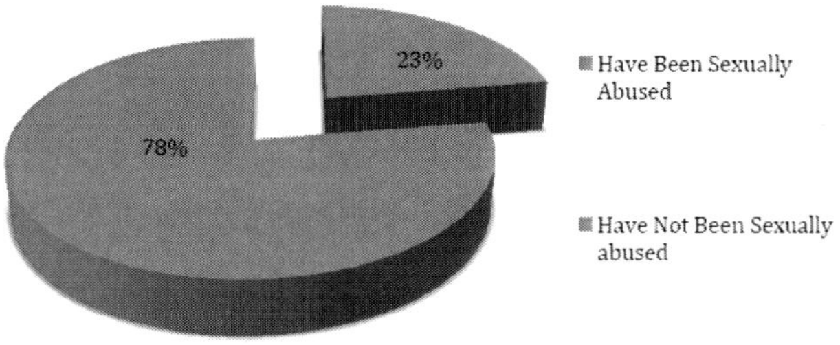

Figure 4. Male students who recognize first forced sexual intercourse as abuse.

Discussion

Although young boys are showing increasing potential to become victims, CSA most commonly impacts females (5). Interviews with victims and survivors suggested that girls of all ages were at high risk from intra-familial abuse (5). Many affected females were first victimized under the age of ten, and abuse persisted until mid-adolescence, either when their abuser found a new target or they left the home (5). In addition, young females being viewed as potential targets for transactional CSA is also of growing concern (5).

There are a significant number of children who are victims of CSA but do not recognize the criminality of the abuse. This revelatory analysis suggested a strong correlation to the findings by WHO, in that children within the Eastern Caribbean largely do not understand or perceive sexual violence as criminal abuse and thus do not understand the necessity to report the crime itself. Essentially, while victims are able to process a sense of violence to them, they are unable to link that very violence to a criminal act. This issue in perception is largely tied to the education sector in St. Lucia, where a greater policy emphasis and enforcement is critical to convey the criminal nature of sexual abuse and the benefits of reporting the crime.

Children who are victims of CSA suffer many consequences including: academic shortcomings, behavioral issues, and both physical and psychological problems (2). According to nine studies that focused on the consequences of CSA, "CSA was not only associated with posttraumatic stress but also with delinquency, academic difficulties, conduct disorders, substance abuse, depression, anxiety, suicidal ideation, and personality disorders" (13). CSA does not just affect the victims but it also affects the community as a whole (2) CSA should be prevented at the community level, which has shown to be a more effective prevention level compared to the individual level.

In order to create effective educational programs at multi-sectorial levels to prevent CSA in Saint Lucia, the culture and beliefs of the society has to be examined carefully. Therefore a study is recommended to assess the level of social awareness of child sexual abuse in Saint Lucia. After fully understanding the cultural beliefs and perceptions toward CSA in Saint Lucia, educational programs will be created to change societal perspectives in order to prevent CSA. These educational programs will be created for children, teachers, parents, healthcare workers, and police forces to target their main perceptions and beliefs regarding CSA in Saint Lucia and incorporate culturally appropriate material.

Conclusion

The most effective measure for CSA prevention is education at both the school and community levels in a multi-sectorial approach to increase the awareness of CSA. Many studies have discussed the importance of education in prevention of CSA (2, 14, 15). In many cases, the lack of education acted as a barrier for seeking help (14). The WHO recommends measures to prevent CSA including education at almost every level, from children and adolescences in school based programs, to educating parents, healthcare providers, police forces, and the entire community (16). Therefore, it is postulated that improved awareness through community education shall serve as means to reduce the incidence of child sexual abuse in St. Lucia and, prevention can be achieved through multi-sectorial collaboration between the Ministries of Education, Health and Royal St. Lucian Police Force.

Recommendations

A qualitative study is recommended to measure the knowledge and identify the perception of CSA in Saint Lucia. The study is based on the socio-ecological model where community level intervention is a more effective measure to change the perception of Saint Lucian regarding CSA. The study population will be citizens from Saint Lucia who are knowledgeable about the problem and the culture and, those who can provide insight to be used in creating community based educational programs that can influence the target population to recognize the problem and take action to prevent it. The study population will include: teachers who can influence children and their families by teaching them about CSA (2, 17), doctors and healthcare workers who can recognize risk factors in patients as well as identify victims and protect them from further abuse (18, 19, 20), and police officers who can take quick action to protect victims and reduce the incidence in areas with high risk factors. By identifying the perception of CSA, the knowledge, and risk factors in Saint Lucia, effective programs can be implemented to prevent CSA. Educational programs could be created to target the cultural perceptions and beliefs regarding CSA in Saint Lucia and incorporate culturally appropriate material.

References

[1] Fact sheet: Child sexual abuse. UNICEF, 2010: URL: http://www.unicef.org/lac/Break_the_Silence_Initiative-Fact_sheet(1).pdf.

[2] Wurtele, S. Preventing sexual abuse of children in the twenty-first century: preparing for challenges and opportunities. J Child Sex Abus 2009;18(1):1-18.

[3] De Bellis M, Spratt E, Hooper S. Neurodevelopmental biology associated with childhood sexual abuse. J Child Sex Abus 2011;20(5):548-87.

[4] United Nations Children's Fund. Violence against children in the Caribbean Region regional assessment. Panama: UNICEF, 2005.

[5] United Nations Children's Fund. Unmasking child sexual abuse. Barbados: UNICEF, 2009.

[6] Jemmott ET, Jones AD. Child sexual abuse in the Eastern Caribbean: perceptions of, attitudes to, and opinions on child sexual abuse in the Eastern Caribbean. United Nations Children's Fund: UNICEF, 2011.

[7] Pan American Health Organization. Health in the Americas 1998, volume II. Washington, DC: PAHO, 1998.
[8] Pan American Health Organization. Health in the Americas 2007, volume II. Washington, DC: PAHO, 2007.
[9] Eugene C. Child sexual abuse: women and human development in Caribbean islands. Proceedings of the 2nd Caribbean Small Islands Developing States Conference, Curacao, 2012 Jan 8-9.
[10] Halcon L, Blum R, Beuhring T, Pate E, Campbell-Forrester S, Venema H. Adolescent health in the Caribbean: a regional portrait. Am J Public Health 2003;93(11):1851-7.
[11] Blum R, Halcon L, Beuhring T, Pate E, Campbell-Forrester S, Venema A. Adolescent health in the Caribbean: risk and protective factors. Am J Public Health 2003;93(3):456-60.
[12] Hornick JP, Matheson J. (2007). Child Development and Children at Risk in St. Lucia Volume I: A Review of the needs and services for children. Calgary: International Centre, University of Calgary, 2007.
[13] Cromer L, Goldsmith R. Child sexual abuse myths: attitudes, beliefs, and individual differences. J Child Sex Abus 2010;19(6):618-47.
[14] Smith K, Bryant-Davis T, Tillman S, Marks A. Stifled voices: barriers to help-seeking behavior for South African childhood sexual assault survivors. J Child Sex Abus 2010;19(3):255-74.
[15] Dhawan J, Gupta S, Kumar B. Sexually transmitted diseases in children in India. Indian J Dermatol Venereol Leprol 2010;76(5):489-93.
[16] United Nations Human Rights Council. National report submitted in accordance with paragraph 15 (a) of the annex to Human Rights Council resolution 5/1: Saint Lucia. Geneva: UNHRC, 2010.
[17] Walsh K, Rassafiani M, Mathews B, Farrell A, Butler D. Teachers' attitudes toward reporting child sexual abuse: problems with existing research leading to new scale development. J Child Sex Abus 2010;19(3):310-36.
[18] Newton A, Vandeven A. (2010). The role of the medical provider in the evaluation of sexually abused children and adolescents. J Child Sex Abus 2010;19(6); 669-86.
[19] Rew L, Bowman K. Protecting youth from early and abusive sexual experiences. J Pediatr Nurs 2008;34(1): 19-25.
[20] McDonald K. Child abuse: approach and management. Am Fam Physician 2007;75(2):221-8.

In: Public Health Yearbook 2016
Editor: Joav Merrick

ISBN: 978-1-53610-947-4

Chapter 30

THE THREAT OF HIV AND HEPATITIS C TRANSMISSION AMONG GRENADIAN ADOLESCENTS FROM INJECTION DRUG USE

Cecilia Hegamin-Younger[1,*], PhD, Rohan Jeremiah[2], PhD, Praveen Durgampudi[1], MBBS, Jonathan Waller[3], MPH, and Abdul Seckam[4], MPH, MSc

[1]Department of Public Health and Preventive Medicine, St George's University, Grenada, West Indies
[2]School of Public Health, University of Illinois, Chicago, Illinois, US
[3]School of Medicine, St. George's University, Grenada, West Indies
[4]Cardiff School of Health Sciences, Cardiff Metropolitan University, Wales, United Kingdom

ABSTRACT

The objective of this paper was to describe the prevalence in injecting drug use and post injecting behaviors in Grenadian adolescents. A nationally represented random weighted sample of 5,570 Grenadian secondary school students completed a drug prevalence survey developed by the Grenadian Drug Secretariat and Inter-American Drug Abuse Control Commission. Although 3% of the secondary school students reported injecting drugs 53% had unprotected sexual intercourse, 54% had more than 1 concurrent partner and 32% exchanged sex for drugs, money and other services. In a small island nation where injecting drug use has not been identified as an issue, such practices in adolescents raise concerns about the risk for transmission of HIV/AIDS, hepatitis C, sexually transmitted infections and other blood-borne diseases.

Keywords: injection drug use, HIV, hepatitis C, Grenada

---

* Correspondence: Cecilia Hegamin-Younger, Professor of Biostatistics, Department of Public Health and Preventive Medicine, St. George's University, Grenada, West Indies. E-mail: chegamin-younger@sgu.edu.

INTRODUCTION

When HIV penetrates a network of injecting drug users who share needles there is a possibility that 50% of the network of drug users will get infected within a few months" (1). Due to how transmissible diseases occur amongst injection drug users (IDUs), the spread of HIV and Hepatitis C is of serious concern in the Caribbean, particularly small island nations such as Grenada. Injectable drug use has not been identified as an issue in Grenada (Dave Alexander, personal communication, June 4, 2013 Office of Drug Control Secretariat; Francis Martin, personal communication, April 3, 2015, Government of Grenada Ministry of Health). However, given the drug trade routes using the Caribbean islands to transport drugs from South America to West Africa, Europe and the United States (2), where injectable drugs are a serious problem (3), islands comprising the Eastern Caribbean route are vulnerable to the introduction of injectable drugs.

Injection drug use is linked to many serious health complications. Drug use increases the probability that a user will engage in other risky behaviors, such as unsafe sexual practices and the sharing of drug paraphernalia, which in the case of injection drug use includes syringes. These two risk behaviors are major contributors to the spread of diseases, such as HIV and Hepatitis C and were responsible for more new cases of Hepatitis C than any other practice and were a major reason for the spread of HIV in Canada (4). In Canada, the Public Health Agency of Canada found that approximately 17% of new cases of HIV and 70-80% of new cases of Hepatitis C were due to these types of risky behaviors (5). Within the United States, approximately 8% of the new cases of HIV infection each year are due to injection drug use (6).

The spread of HIV and Hepatitis C among adolescent IDUs is concerning because this group is more likely to partake in certain risky behaviors. Such activities include, having sexual relations with multiple partners, engaging in unprotected sex, and sharing syringes (7). Adolescent injecting drug users tend to have an earlier age-onset of sexual activity, multiple sexual partners, sex while under the influence of a substance, and inconsistent use of protection (8). In 2008 Plüddermann and colleagues reported that among the IDUs, 67% sometimes used a condom and 5% never used a condom with their regular partner and 63% sometimes used a condom and 1% never used a condom with a non-regular or casual partner (9).

The sharing of needles and syringes is also a concern for adolescents receiving and transmitting these diseases. Although HIV and Hepatitis C are spread through both unsafe sexual practices and sharing of syringes, the transmission of Hepatitis C is more related the sharing of non-sterile needles among IDUs (10). Plüddermann et al. (9) found that 89% of IDU reported that they had shared syringes within the past month. In addition, Matthews found that transmission of Hepatitis C through injection drug use occurred for 73% of subjects, with sexual transmission occurring for 18% (10).

Whilst vast amounts of data has been collected and analyzed on injection drug use in other countries, such as the United States (12), however there has been no research conducted in Grenada related to injection drug use among adolescents. The purpose of this study was to examine the prevalence of injection drug use, unsafe sexual practices, and improper syringe use in Grenada adolescents. The aims of this study were to: (1) determine the prevalence of injection drug use among secondary school students; (2) examine the patterns of syringe use among students that admit to using injectable drugs; and (3) compare the health risk behaviors between students that are IDUs and those that are not IDUs.

METHODS

As part of monitoring and evaluating the prevalence of adolescent drug use in Grenada, an anonymous questionnaire developed by the Drug Control Secretariat of Grenada and the Inter-American Drug Abuse Control Commission (CICAD) was administered to a random sample of secondary school students. This questionnaire contained 105 questions representing drug use, parental involvement, consequences of drugs and health risk behavior. The questionnaire has been administered twice prior to the current administration, in 2005 and 2008. The current questionnaire introduced several questions about injection drug use and sexual behavior.

To estimate the prevalence of drug use, a random sample of 1,490 students in forms 2, 4 and 5 from seventeen public and private secondary school students throughout the island of Grenada and Carriacou were selected to participate in this questionnaire to evaluate and monitor the prevalence of adolescent drug use. A two-stage sampling frame was used to select the participants. The first stage randomly sampled the secondary schools. Sixteen schools were randomly selected from twenty secondary schools on the island of Grenada. The second stage included a random selection of students in forms 2, 4 and 5 within each of the selected secondary schools. All students (n=1,490) in the selected classrooms were asked to participate. A total of 1,460 students participated, representing an 80% response rate. A weighted sample was used in analysis to represent the national population of 5,570 students.

To examine the prevalence of injection drug use and patterns of behavior the following questions were analyzed: (1) have you ever used injected drugs such as Heroin, cocaine, crack or steroids; (2) When you last injected, what was done with the used syringe/needle; (3) Do you clean used needles/syringes that were given to you; (4) If so, how often do you clean them; (5) Do you and/or your partner use a condom every time you have sex; (6) with how many different partners did you have sexual intercourse in the last 12 months; (7) Have you had sex with someone of the same sex; (8) Have you ever experimented with anal sex; (9) have you ever exchanged sexual services for money, drugs or other goods; (10) do you have a regular partner that you have sex with; (11) did you use a condom at the last sexual intercourse with your regular partner; (12) have you ever had sex with someone that you don't usually have sex with; (13) did you use a condom with the person that you usually don't have sex with; and (14) did you have sexual intercourse in the last 12 months. All items were summarized using frequencies and percentages for the total sample and separately for females and males. Odds ratios and 95% confidence intervals were calculated to examine at-risk sexual behaviors of IDU with non-IDU.

RESULTS

One thousand four hundred and ninety students from across seventeen public and private secondary schools participated in the third secondary school drug prevalence survey. This sample represents a population of 5,570 students, as illustrated in table 1 (13), the majority of this population were between 15 and 16 years old (41.5%) followed by students 12 to 14 years old (31.2%) and 17 years old and older (16.8%). Approximately 37.5% of the students were in the 2nd Form, 35.5% in the 4th Form and 27% in the 5th Form. There were slightly more females (51.3%) than males (48.3%).

A total of 140 (3%) secondary students reported using injecting drugs such as Heroin, cocaine and steroids and 60% were males. Odds ratios were calculated to compare IDU and non-IDU students. Overall, IDUs were more likely to engage in activities that could potentially lead to the spread of HIV and Hepatitis C when compared with non-IDU students. IDUs were 1.84 (95% CI: 0.90-3.76) times as likely to have sex with someone they don't usually have sex with, 3.5 (95% CI: 1.70-7.24) times as likely to have unprotected sexual intercourse in the last month, 16.5 (95% CI: 5.44-50.20) times as likely to have been diagnosed with a sexually transmitted infection, 18.7 (95% CI: 8.50-41.02) times as likely to have been taken sexually advantage of, and 23.5 (95% CI: 11.02-50.19) times as likely to have taken sexually advantage of someone else.

Table 1. Demographic summary of the sample

Demographic indicator	Number (%)
Type of school	
Public	5409 (97.1)
Private	161 (2.9)
Age (in years)	
11-14	1739 (31.2)
15-16	2312 (41.5)
17+	938 (16.8)
Gender	
Female	2857 (51.3)
Male	2690 (48.3)
Form in school	
2nd	2090 (37.5)
4th	1976 (35.5)
5th	1505 (27)

Injecting use behavior: Of the 3% of students reported injecting drugs, 21% reported throwing their needles/syringes away and 54% cleaned needles/syringes given to them (Table 2). Of the students who reported cleaning needles given to them, 52% always cleaned them, while 48%frequently or infrequently cleaned needles given to them.

Examining gender differences of injecting use, males were equally likely as females to report injecting drug use such as Heroin, cocaine or steroids (3% vs. 2%, respectively). Females were more likely to throw their needles away after use (38% vs. 13%) and clean their needles given to them (69% vs. 49%).

Post use behavior. Over half (51%) the students reporting injecting drug use also reported having sex in the past year (Table 3). The majority of these students (53%) reported having unprotected sex in the past month and 43% of the students reported not using a condom with a person they do not usually have sex with.

Table 2. Summary of injecting drug use behavior

	Total %	Females %	Males %
Ever injected heroin, cocaine or steroids? (n(%))	140 (3%)	49 (2)	84 (3)
What was done with the needle after use?			
Threw it away	21	38	13
Kept to reuse it	17	16	19
Gave it to someone else	1	0	22
Something else	16	0	27
Do not know	5	16	0
Did you clean a needle/syringe given to you?	54	69	49
How often do you clean needles given to you?			
Always	52	68	40
Frequently	42	21	60
Infrequently	6	12	0

Table 3. Summary of post injection use behavior

	Total (%)	Females (%)	Males (%)
Total	51	49	61
Had unprotected sex in past 30 days	53	50	54
Used a condom with non-regular sex partner	43	35	46
Used condom with regular sex partner	52	66	46
Number of concurrent partners			
1	26	67	7
2	16	0	23
3	16	16	16
4+	22	17	38
Sex with more than one person at a time	32	0	46
Does partner inject drugs?	37	17	46
Same gender sex	48	51	47
Anal sex	16	0	24
Sex with someone older	42	49	49
Exchange sex for drugs money or services	32	17	39
Does partner inject drugs?	37	17	46

In addition to not using protection, the majority (54%) of students have multiple sexual partners and many engage in sex with more than one person at a time (32%).

The majority of males (85%) and females (67%) reported having a regular sex partner. However, 77% of the males and 30% of females reported having more than one sexual partner. In addition, 46% of males and no women reported engaging in-group sex. Sexual behavioral patterns also exhibited gender differences (Table 3). Males were more likely to have anal sex (24% vs. 0%) and exchange sex for drugs, money and services (39% vs. 17%) than females. In contrast, females were more likely to have sex with an older person (49%) than males (39%).

Discussion

Injecting drug users are more likely to engage in sexual behavior, which puts them at risk to receive and spread HIV HCV and STIs than students who do not inject drugs. In addition, the use and reuse of needle practices of adolescents indicated that youth are at heightened risk of disease transmission. Although the injecting behavior is a concern, post injecting behaviors underscores the risk of transmitting STI, HIV and HCV. The Caribbean sex network is more complex than the developed world and more often than not it is not exclusive (14, 15). As seen with secondary school students the number of sexual partners is not one to one. While only 7% of the males have 1 partner, 67% of the females have one partner, suggesting non-exclusivity, which one would expect in secondary school students (14). Intergenerational sex partners exacerbates the HIV risks for young women, as it not only exposes them to higher HIV prevalence age cohorts, but also because of the power differentials and transactional nature of these relationships which may explain the low uptake of regular condom use in females (16).

Moreover, the exchange sex for drugs, money or service increases the risk of transmission of HIV HCV and STIs. This finding must be understood in the context of an ever-growing economy based on tourism (70% of GDP) and high percentage of people (40% unemployed) and in particular young people who are unemployed. These economic issues along with drug use have driven increasing numbers of people into transactional sex (17). The reality of men being unemployed and in a heavily tourism economy that can provide space for unregulated transactions between visitors and local communities makes a very volatile situation for such exchange.

Conclusion

There is considerable evidence that is indicative that IDUs are at elevated risk of communicable disease. The combined exposure of reuse and sharing of needles, inconsistent condom use, multiple partners, same sex relationships with these findings a major intersectional public health challenge amongst Caribbean adolescents. Such patterns raise concerns about increased risk for HIV/AIDS, Hepatitis C, STI and other blood-borne diseases.

While 3% of secondary students reported injecting drugs, the use of injecting drugs is not common in Grenada. It is typically introduced into Grenadian community through foreign persons or experiences outside Grenada (Francis Martin, personal communication, April 3, 2015, Government of Grenada Ministry of Health). This study represents the first measure of IDU in Grenadian secondary school students, providing baseline information and new directions for surveillance, health systems, health promotion and health education strategies in addressing this phenomenon. Once these aforementioned areas have been addressed through further exploration, clearer pathways and policies may be formulated for Grenada.

REFERENCES

[1] Swe LA, Rashid A. Prevalence of HIV and the risk behaviours among injecting drug users in Myanmar. Int J Collab Res Intern Med Public Health 2012;4(1):56-70.
[2] United States Department of State. Bureau for International Narcotics and Law Enforcement Affairs. International Narcotics Control Report Strategy: volume I drug and chemical control. Washington, DC: US Department State, 2013.
[3] Strathdee SA, Stockman JK. Epidemiology of HIV among injecting and non-injecting drug users: current trends and implications for interventions. Curr HIV/AIDS Rep 2010;7(2):99-106.
[4] Public Health Agency of Canada. HIV/AIDS Epi Updates, November 2007. Ottawa, ON: Surveillance Risk Assessment Division, Centre Infectious Disease Prevention Control, Public Health Agency Canada, 2007.
[5] Remis RS. Modelling the incidence and prevalence of hepatitis C infections and its sequelae in Canada 2007: final report. Ottawa, ON: Community Acquired Infections Division Centre Communicable Diseases Infection Control Infectious Disease and Emergency Preparedness Branch, Public Health Agency of Canada, 2007.
[6] CDC. Monitoring selected national HIV prevention and care objectives by using HIV surveillance data—United States and 6 dependent areas—2012. HIV Surveillance Suppl Rep 2014:19(3).
[7] Mitchell MM, Latimer WW. Unprotected casual sex and perceived risk of contracting HIV among drug users in Baltimore, Maryland: evaluating the influence of non-injection versus injection drug user status. AIDS Care 2009;21(2):221-30.
[8] Chan YF, Passetti LL, Garner B., Lloyd JJ, Dennis M. (2011). HIV risk behaviors: Risky sexual activities and needle use among adolescents in substance abuse treatment. AIDS Behav 2011;15(1):114-24.
[9] Plüddermann A, Parry CD, Flisher AJ, Jordaan E. Heroin users in Cape Town, South Africa: Injecting practices, HIV-related risk behaviors, and other health consequences. J Psychoactive Drugs 2008;40(3):273-9.
[10] Bhunu CP, Mushayabasa S. Assessing the effects of intravenous drug use on Hepatitis C transmission dynamics. J Biol Syst 2011;19(3):447-60.
[11] Matthews GV, Pham ST, Hellard M, Grebely J, Zhang L, Oon A, White PA. Patterns and characteristics of Hepatitis C transmission clusters among HIV-positive and HIV-negative individuals in the Australian trial in acute hepatitis C. Clin Infect Dis 2011;52(6):803-11.
[12] Johnston LD, O'Malley PM, Bachman JG, Schulenberg JE. Monitoring the future national survey results on drug use, 1975-2010. Ann Arbor, MI: Institute Social Research, University Michigan, 2011:744.
[13] Hegamin-Younger C. Grenada secondary school drug prevalence survey 2013. St George's, WI: Government Grenada, 2014.
[14] Kempadoo, K. Caribbean sexuality: Mapping the field. Caribbean Rev Gender Stud 2009; 3:1-24.
[15] Hegamin-Younger C, Jeremiah R, Bilbro N. Patterns of Caribbean masculinity among males in Grenada. Am J Mens Health 2014;8(4):335-8.
[16] Mathers BM, Degenhardt L, Phillips B, Wiessing L, Hickman M, Strathdee SA, Wodak A, Panda S, Tyndall M, Mattick RP. Global epidemiology of injecting drug use and HIV among people who inject drugs: a systematic review. Lancet 2008;372(9651):1733-45.
[17] Kempadoo K. Freelancers, temporary wives and beachboys: Researching sex work in the Caribbean. Fem Rev 2001;67:39-62.

In: Public Health Yearbook 2016
Editor: Joav Merrick
ISBN: 978-1-53610-947-4

Chapter 31

PROVISION OF TUBERCULOSIS SERVICES IN PUBLIC FACILITIES TO HIV/AIDS INFECTED CLIENTS IN THE EASTERN CARIBBEAN

Martin S Forde[1,*], ScD, St Clair M Forde[2], PhD, Anika Keens-Douglas[1], MPA and Altrena G Mukuria[3], DrPH

[1]Department of Public Health and Preventive Medicine,
St. George's University, Grenada, West Indies
[2]Research Management Consultant,
St. Augustine, Trinidad, West Indies
[3]Constella Futures, Washington, DC, US

ABSTRACT

The capability to provide supportive management practices and resources for diagnosing and treating HIV and AIDS patients who may also be co-infected with tuberculosis (TB) was assessed in healthcare facilities of six Eastern Caribbean island states. Of the islands reviewed, only half had a national TB treatment strategy. In islands that had facilities that followed a national TB treatment strategy, such as Direct Observed Treatment Short-course (DOTS), only a third kept a data register record. Further, limitations in the ability of facilities within this region to provide TB diagnoses were found. The lack of on-site treatment protocols, testing materials, and supplies, and updated training were also challenges in TB service provision in all six countries.

Keywords: Caribbean, HIV, AIDS, tuberculosis, support services

* Correspondence: Martin S Forde, Professor, St. George's University, Department of Public Health, PO Box 7, St. George's, Grenada, West Indies. E-mail: martinforde@mac.com.

Introduction

The incidence of HIV and AIDS in the Caribbean region which ranges from 1.5 to 4.1% is second only to sub-Saharan Africa (5.9%) (1). Additionally, in the Western hemisphere, the Caribbean region is the most severely affected region with approximately half a million people living with HIV/AIDS (1).

Tuberculosis (TB) is one of the most common opportunistic infection associated with HIV and AIDS. An estimated 360,000 out of 1.5 million persons who died from this infection in 2013 were HIV-positive (2). For HIV infected persons, TB is now the leading cause of death (3). Globally, HIV infected persons are 29 times more likely to be infected with TB than those who are HIV-negative (2). Within the Caribbean region, although significant strides have been made in the diagnosis and preventing of the spread of TB among HIV infected persons, the true burden of TB remains underestimated based on currently used diagnostic protocols (4).

The ability and capacity to diagnose and treat TB is considered an essential component of care for HIV and AIDS clients. WHO advocates the use of the Direct Observed Treatment Short-course (DOTS) strategy for TB treatment to improve compliance with full treatment. Other generally accepted standard elements for providing quality TB services include: diagnosis based on sputum smear with backup or confirmation using X-ray; a recording system that clearly indicates newly identified cases and monitoring their course of treatment and adherence to treatment protocol; written guidelines and protocols for TB diagnosis and treatment; and a continuous supply of the TB treatment regime for each TB patient (5).

Within the Caribbean region, TB has been found to be a major co-infection of HIV and AIDS persons (6). Given the high incidence rate of HIV and AIDS in the Caribbean region, having the capacity and capability to provide supportive management practices, resources and supplies for diagnosing and treating HIV and AIDS co-infected TB patients is essential in order to stem the morbidity and mortality associated with HIV and AIDS persons who also are infected with TB. With funding support from the US Agency for International Development (USAID), the HIV and AIDS Service Provision Assessment (HSPA) Survey was developed to assess the quality and capacity of HIV- and AIDS-related services in the Caribbean region (5, 7-11). The main objective of this paper is to report on the findings of this survey as to the capacity and capability within seven Eastern Caribbean islands to provide TB treatment and related services to HIV and AIDS persons.

Methods

Public health facilities in seven islands—Antigua and Barbuda, Grenada, Dominica, St Kitts, Nevis, St Lucia, and St Vincent and the Grenadines—which are members of the inter-governmental, regional Organization of Eastern Caribbean States (OECS), were visited between December 2005 and March 2006. For the purpose of this report, the country of St Kitts and Nevis is separated into two, and data are reported for each island individually.

In this study a 'facility' refers to any major health service center which would include a hospital, district health center, laboratory, etc. A 'site' refers to any service area within a facility, so that a hospital (facility) could have several sites or areas where services are provided. Facilities included both public (government managed) and private (non-government entities such as faith-based organizations and other non-profit organizations and private laboratories). A list of all governmental and non-governmental facilities that provide HIV and AIDS related services was obtained from the Ministry of Health and the National AIDS Program Coordinator in each Caribbean country. Data were collected and analyzed at each service site within a facility and then aggregated to present facility-level data.

Data collection protocol

A team of nursing, National AIDS Programs service providers, epidemiologists, and other health staff were recruited from each of the islands in this study to collect the data. A two-week training was conducted for survey interviewers that included practical training and actual survey conduct in health facilities of different types. A training manual was developed and distributed to all survey interviewers to support standardized data collection.

A list of facilities to be visited was given to each island survey team. Data collection took one day in most facilities, with two days being allocated to hospitals, if required. In addition, if one of the observed services such as Voluntary Counseling and Testing (VCT) was not offered the day of the survey, or the health facility was closed, the teams returned on a day when the service was offered or the facility was open for clients.

The team leader was instructed to ensure that the informant for each component of the facility survey was the most knowledgeable person for the particular health service or system component being addressed. Where relevant, the data collector indicated whether a specific item being assessed was observed, reported available but not observed, not available, or whether it was uncertain if the item was available. Equipment, supplies, and resources for specific services were required to be in the relevant service delivery area or in an immediately adjacent room to be accepted as available. Informed consent was taken from the facility director and from all other interviewed respondents and interviewed providers.

Data collection questionnaires

Data were collected using structured printed questionnaires. The content areas covered by the questionnaires included all categories of service and care for HIV and AIDS: voluntary counseling and testing, prevention of mother-to-child transmission, antiretroviral therapy, post-exposure prophylaxis, basic and advanced-level clinical services for HIV and AIDS (inpatient and outpatient), tuberculosis, sexually transmitted infections, and malaria. For each type of service, information was collected on the availability of systems, resources, and infrastructure to support quality services. Additionally, a review was made of systems, guidelines, referrals, service records, individual client records, staff supervision, resources, laboratory diagnostics, equipment, pharmaceuticals and supplies, staff training, and infrastructure. This paper describes only the data gathered on the capacity of health facilities to provide tuberculosis service for the seven islands surveyed.

Statistical analyses

Since HIV and AIDS services are not typically offered across all facility types, and services are relatively scarce, the sampling design employed emphasized collecting data from all known sites where HIV and AIDS services were offered (typically advanced care facilities) thus resulting in a sample that is disproportionately representative of these services. To account for the overrepresentation of these facilities in the sample, for the data analysis weights were constructed. Given that the data for Antigua and Barbuda, Dominica, St. Kitts, Nevis, St. Lucia, and St. Vincent and the Grenadines are all census data of all facilities present on these islands, no weights were applied to these data sets. The data for Grenada, however, represent a sample of the HIV and AIDS service facilities present on that island, which was then weighted. The weighting of Grenada's dataset allowed the generation of regional totals that are representative of the distribution of facilities within each country and ensures that facilities from each country are proportionally represented for the seven islands. Weighting resulting in decimals were rounded to the closest whole number.

All survey questionnaire data were entered into CSPro (12) using double data entry to ensure accurate keying of results. Once a final dataset was completely entered and cleaned, the statistical software program Stata (13) was used to do all subsequent analyzes.

RESULTS AND DISCUSSION

The supportive management practices required to ensure the provision of a quality tuberculosis care and support service for HIV and AIDS clients are presented by an evaluation of recent pre- or in-service training of providers and regular supervisory visits to service providers. The availability of services for TB treatment or diagnosis in each country is presented as well as the components for management of tuberculosis (including treatment strategies), resources and supplies for diagnosing tuberculosis.

Availability of services

Care and support services (CSS) for People Living with HIV (PLHIV) include any services that are directed towards improving the life of PLHIV. Other CSS may include palliative care and socio-economic and psychological support services. Tuberculosis (TB) and sexually transmitted infections (STIs) are both illnesses associated with HIV and AIDS. Programs to "RollBack Malaria" are being addressed in conjunction with those addressing HIV and AIDS, TB, and STIs, to decrease the most serious underlying causes of death and disease. Facilities that provide CSS should also offer services for TB, STIs and malaria (if appropriate).

From Table 1, it can be seen that of the 95 public facilities surveyed on the seven islands, 45 offer CSS to HIV and AIDS clients. Among them, 36 have an HIV testing system in place, 38 offer STI services, 29 offer diagnosis or treatment of any kind for tuberculosis, and 12 offer malaria treatment services.

Table 1. Basic HIV/AIDS-related service provision by public facilities that offer any care or support services (CSS), CHSPA[1], 2005/2006

Country	Total number of facilities	Number of facilities offering CSS for HIV/AIDS clients	Among facilities offering CSS for HIV/AIDS clients:			
			Number with HIV testing system	Number offering STI services	Number offering any TB diagnostic or treatment services	Number offering malaria treatment services
Antigua and Barbuda	9	4	4	2	2	1
Dominica	16	12	11	11	10	3
Grenada[2]	20	2	2	2	1	1
Nevis	7	1	1	1	1	0
St. Kitts	13	3	3	3	3	1
St. Lucia	12	10	3	7	2	2
St. Vincent and the Grenadines	18	13	12	12	10	4
	95	45	36	38	29	12

[1] Caribbean HIV and AIDS Service Provision Assessment (CHSPA) conducted for Antigua and Barbuda, Dominica, Grenada, Nevis, St. Kitts, St. Lucia, and St. Vincent and the Grenadines.
[2] Weighted numbers.

Supportive management

In addition to the provision of services, supportive management practices are required to ensure the quality of those services (Table 2). This includes recent pre- or in-service training of providers and regular supervisory visits to service providers. In 33 of the 95 facilities, at least a half of the interviewed providers of TB, malaria, or STI services had received pre- or in-service training during the past 3 years, while in 36 of the facilities at least half of the interviewed providers of TB, malaria, or STI services were personally supervised at least once during the past 3 months. In countries with some human resource constraints for HIV and AIDS services and possible lack of consistent funding, this could be an area to look at scaling-up. For example, a study of public and private physicians in Barbados found that some (especially those who graduated in or before 1984) had not received recent training in HIV and AIDS care and support (14).

Tuberculosis services and service-related conditions

A total of 48 facilities with 68 service sites offer any TB services (Table 3). Only 25 of the 48 facilities offer DOTS. The DOTS treatment strategy is either directly observed 2 months, follow-up 6 months, or directly observed 6 months, which can be an effective strategy in treating the disease if the infrastructure and medication are available. Another strategy includes follow-up treatment only, in which clients receive follow-up after intensive treatment for TB by a different clinical site/facility. Only 18 of 48 facilities report that they perform only follow-up treatment.

Table 2. Number of facilities with supportive management practices for health service providers who treat infections relevant to HIV/AIDS,[1] 2005/2006

Country	Total Number of facilities	Number of facilities with: At least half of the interviewed providers of TB, malaria, or STI services received pre- or in-service training related to one of these topics during the past 3 years	At least half of the interviewed providers of TB, malaria, or STI services were personally supervised at least once during the past 3 months
Antigua and Barbuda	9	3	2
Dominica	16	9	8
Grenada	20	3	4
Nevis	7	2	5
St. Kitts	13	4	4
St. Lucia	12	5	5
St. Vincent and the Grenadines	18	7	8
	95	33	36

[1] Number of public facilities having the indicated conditions to support health service providers.

Table 3. Tuberculosis services,[1] 2005/2006

Country	Number of facilities offering any TB services	Number of TB Un-weighted service sites	Among facilities offering any TB services, number reporting they follow indicated treatment strategy[2]			Among facilities offering any TB services, number with:			
			DOTS[3]	Follow-up treatment only[4]	No direct observation component[5]	Observed client register at any site where TB treatment is offered	Observed TB treatment protocol at all sites where TB treatment is offered	All first-line TB medicines available[6]	All items for TB indicator[7]
Antigua and Barbuda	2	2	0	1	1	0	0	1	0
Dominica	11	16	2	9	2	1	2	3	0
Grenada[8]	3	7	1	0	2	0	0	0	0
Nevis	7	8	7	0	0	0	2	1	0
St. Kitts	8	11	8	0	1	1	6	2	0
St. Lucia	4	7	4	1	0	3	0	2	0
St. Vincent and the Grenadines	13	17	3	7	3	1	2	2	0
	48	68	25	18	9	6	12	11	0

[1] Number of public facilities having the indicated components for management of tuberculosis (TB).
[2] More than one treatment strategy may apply if facility offers TB services from multiple sites.
[3] Treatment strategy followed is either direct observe 2 months, follow up 6 months, or direct observe 6 months.
[4] Follow-up clients after intensive treatment offered elsewhere.
[5] Provides initial TB treatment but no direct observation component.
[6] Any combination of isoniazid (INH), rifampicin, ethambutol, and pyrazinamide. If medicines provided are prepackaged for individual DOTS clients, medicines had to be available for all DOTS clients.
[7] Observed client register for DOTS in any service site, TB treatment protocols in all relevant sites, and all first-line TB medicines available in facility.
[8] Weighted.

In resource-constrained settings, diagnosing co-infection or simply diagnosing TB without explicit training (and follow up for providers) can be complicated. Table 3 further shows that among the facilities offering any TB services, only six of the 48 facilities where

TB treatment is offered had an observed TB treatment protocol at all sites, and only 11 facilities offering any TB services had all first-line TB medicines available (this includes any combination of isoniazid (INH), rifampicin, ethambutol, and pyrazinamide). If medicines provided are pre-packaged for individual DOTS clients, medicines had to be available for all DOTS clients. First-line treatment is important to treat the disease fully and to assist in preventing multi-drug resistant TB. Further, only 6 facilities of the 48 offering any TB services had an observed client register at any site where TB treatment is offered; yet 18 facilities offering any TB services reported that they provide follow-up treatment. Registers would be helpful to any follow-up system for TB.

Tuberculosis treatment and/or follow-up using DOTS

Of the 48 public facilities surveyed that offer any TB diagnostic or treatment services, 36 report that they are part of the National DOTS program (Table 4). As noted earlier, DOTS is one strategy to treat patients with TB that is fairly effective as it necessitates the direct observation of a client taking medication administered by a provider. Only 24 facilities report they follow the DOTS strategy, and 29 DOTS strategy service sites were found across these facilities. However, only eight facilities, following the DOTS strategy, had all first-line TB medicines available. Only nine of the facilities, following the DOTS strategy, had an observed client register for DOTS or an observed TB treatment protocol in all eligible service sites. In terms of the protocol, if it is available in certain service sites within the facility, but not all, the facility would be ineligible for this count. Further, of the 24 facilities following the DOTS strategy, only four facilities are able to maintain a client register record.

Table 4. Tuberculosis treatment and/or follow-up using Direct Observed Treatment Short-course (DOTS)[1], 2005/2006

Country	Number of facilities	Number of facilities with indicated TB activities			Among facilities following DOTS strategy, number with:				Number of DOTS strategy service sites
		Any TB diagnostic or treatment services	Report they are part of national	Follow DOTS strategy[2]	Observed client register for DOTS	Observed TB treatment protocol in all eligible	All first-line TB medicines available[2]	All items for TB indicator[3]	
Antigua and Barbuda	9	2	0	0	0	0	0	0	0
Dominica	16	11	9	2	1	0	1	0	4
Grenada[4]	20	3	0	0	0	0	0	0	1
Nevis	7	7	7	7	0	2	1	0	8
St. Kitts	13	8	8	8	1	6	2	0	8
St. Lucia	12	4	4	4	2	1	2	1	4
St. Vincent and the Grenadines	18	13	8	3	0	0	2	0	4
	95	48	36	24	4	9	8	1	29

[1] Number of public facilities having the indicated components for management of tuberculosis (TB).

[2] Treatment strategy followed is either direct observe 2 months, follow up 6 months, or direct observe 6 months.

[3] Any combination of isoniazid (INH), rifampicin, ethambutol, and pyrazinamide. If medicines provided are prepackaged for individual DOTS clients, medicines had to be available for all DOTS clients.

[4] Observed client register for DOTS in any service site, TB treatment protocols in all relevant sites, and all first-line TB medicines available in facility.

[5] Weighted.

Table 5. Resources and supplies for diagnosing tuberculosis[1], 2005/2006

Country	Number of facilities	Number of facilities with any TB diagnostic or treatment services[2]	TB diagnosis using sputum: Among facilities diagnosing TB using sputum, number with: All items for conducting sputum test for TB[3]	Observed record of sputum test results	All items for indicator[4]	Number of facilities diagnosing TB using sputum test	TB diagnosis using X-ray: Among facilities diagnosing TB using X-ray, number with X-ray capacity[5]	Number of facilities diagnosing TB using X-ray
Antigua & Barbuda	9	2	2	2	2	1	0	1
Dominica	16	11	1	1	1	9	1	6
Grenada[6]	20	3	2	1	1	3	1	2
Nevis	7	7	0	0	0	2	3	2
St. Kitts	13	8	1	0	0	8	1	8
St. Lucia	12	4	2	2	2	3	2	3
St. Vincent and the Grenadines	18	13	1	1	1	9	1	9
	95	48	9	7	7	35	9	31

[1] Number of public facilities with the indicated tuberculosis (TB) diagnostic elements, by country.
[2] Unit follows up TB patients, or prescribes initial therapy, or conducts TB test.
[3] Includes sputum microscopy, culture, or rapid test.
[4] All items for conducting test with observed record of test results.
[5] Facility reports performing X-rays for diagnostic purposes.
[6] Weighted.

Resources and supplies for diagnosing TB

Of the 48 facilities that provide any TB diagnostic or treatment services, 35 use a sputum test for TB diagnosis (Table 5). Only nine, however, included sputum microscopy, culture, or rapid test, with seven having observed records of sputum test results. Thirty-one of the facilities reported diagnosing TB using X-ray, although only nine facilities among them had X-ray capacity (i.e., reported performing X-rays for diagnostic purposes).

CONCLUSION

The WHO reports that TB is the leading cause of death among PLHIV with one in four deaths among HIV-infected persons occurring due to TB (15). Further, this same report points out that PLHIV are facing the emerging threat of multidrug- and extensively drug-resistant TB with an estimated 440,000 multidrug-resistant TB cases in 2009 alone.

TB infection control measures are still not implemented in many HIV service settings. The HSPA Survey findings provide information on both basic- and advanced-level HIV and AIDS services within the Caribbean region and the capability of systems within this region to provide quality TB care and support for HIV and AIDS infected persons.

Efforts to provide basic care and support services have been made throughout Eastern Caribbean countries. Shortcomings, however, are still evident in the areas of standard protocol implementation, training and supervision for clinical services staff, an adequate resources and supplies for diagnosing TB and maintenance of records. In resource-constrained settings such as those exemplified in these small island states in the Eastern Caribbean, basic diagnosing co-infection and treatment of TB as part of HIV and AIDS services appears to be a challenge. There is a real need to have appropriate guidelines on hand for diagnosing TB at HIV testing and treatment sites. It is imperative that functioning resources, medicines and supplies for diagnosing TB are widely available. In order to maximize the benefit from existing TB diagnoses protocols, training and refresher training and primary record keeping of client information are important for all health workers responsible for HIV clients. Training should focus on standardize procedures particular the use of the WHO recommended DOTS strategy and meticulous follow-up to ensure adherence to treatment by TB clients.

There is a real need to have appropriate guidelines on hand for diagnosing TB and HIV and treating the two as co-infections, since provision of Antiretroviral Therapy (ART) and TB medication in these situations would need special attention. Further, providers of HIV and AIDS services need to stay abreast of new information and indications for preventing and treating opportunistic diseases that reflect the breadth of co-infection concerns.

Accurate record-keeping systems are also resource-dependent, as they require trained staff and a well-maintained health information system. These are significant challenges for many TB facilities in the Caribbean. Without a good health information system, however, it is very difficult for epidemiologists to follow the patterns and trends in the HIV/AIDS and TB epidemics.

It is imperative that functioning resources and supplies for diagnosing TB are available. As the data in Table 5 illustrates, the resources that are available among facilities with any TB diagnostic or treatment services are limited. It is difficult to clinically diagnosis TB patients who may be co-infected with HIV or AIDS with only one diagnostic tool: x-ray diagnosis, bacteriologic diagnosis, blood culture or nucleic acid amplification assays (6, 16). Thus, it is important to assess what is available in each country to understand best where the gaps might occur to facilitate the scaling-up of services.

To scale-up services to diagnose and rapidly treat patients for TB, it might be beneficial to consider the feasibility of modeling the Haiti system, in which TB testing and diagnosis is performed if patients present for an HIV test with a cough. If possible, clients are treated the same day and co-infected persons were followed up and treated with the appropriate medication. Linking these two services (TB diagnosis and HIV testing and counseling) would provide a beneficial opportunity to identify and co-treat the two infections (16).

ACKNOWLEDGMENTS

Data collection for this study was made possible by support from the U.S. Agency for International Development (USAID) through Cooperative Agreement GPO-A-00-03-00003-00. The authors would also like to thank MEASURE Evaluation, the University of North Carolina, and Macro International Inc. who were all very instrumental in the design and execution of this survey. In particular, the authors deeply appreciate the governmental cooperation given in all the islands visited in the conduct of the Caribbean HIV and AIDS Service Provision Assessment. We also wish to thank the Department of Public Health and

Preventive Medicine at St. George's University, in Grenada, which provided extensive management and logistical support throughout the duration of this study.

REFERENCES

[1] Pan American Health Organization. Report of the Caribbean Commission on Health and Development. Washington, DC: PAHO, 2006.

[2] World Health Organization. Global tuberculosis report 2014. Geneva: WHO, 2014.

[3] Silversides A. HIV/TB co-infections rising. CMAJ 2006;175(7):725.

[4] White YG. Tuberculosis in HIV: making good with what we have. West Indian Med J 2013;62(2):107-8.

[5] US Agency for International Development (USAID) ME. Dominica Caribbean Region HIV and AIDS Service Provision Assessment Survey 2005. Grenada: St Georges University, TR-07-48, 2006.

[6] Kaplan J. Diagnosis, treatment, and prevention of selected common HIV-related opportunistic infections in the Caribbean region. Top HIV Med 2005;12(5):136-41.

[7] US Agency for International Development (USAID) ME. Saint Lucia Caribbean Region HIV and AIDS Service Provision Assessment Survey 2005. Grenada: St Georges University, TR-07-47, 2006.

[8] US Agency for International Development (USAID) ME. St. Vincent and The Grenadines Caribbean Region HIV and AIDS Service Provision Assessment Survey 2005. Grenada: St Georges University, TR-07-46, 2006.

[9] US Agency for International Development (USAID) ME. Antigua and Barbuda Caribbean Region HIV and AIDS Service Provision Assessment Survey 2006. Grenada: St Georges University, TR-07-50, 2007.

[10] US Agency for International Development (USAID) ME. Grenada Caribbean Region HIV and AIDS Service Provision Assessment Survey 2006. Grenada: St Georges University, TR-07-52, 2007.

[11] US Agency for International Development (USAID) ME. Saint Kitts and Nevis Caribbean Region HIV and AIDS Service Provision Assessment Survey 2006. Grenada: St Georges University, TR-07-51A, 2007.

[12] US Census Bureau. The census and survey processing system (CSPro). Washington, DC: USCB, 2006.

[13] Stata Corporation. Data analysis and statistical software. College Station, TX: StateCorp LP, 9.2 ed, 2006.

[14] Massiah E, Roach TC, Jacobs C, St John AM, Inniss V, Walcott J, et al. Stigma, discrimination, and HIV/AIDS knowledge among physicians in Barbados. Rev Panam Salud Publica 2004;16(6):395-401.

[15] World Health Organization (WHO). TB/HIV Facts 2011. URL: www.who.int/.../hiv/topics/tb/ hiv_tb_fact sheet_june_2011.pdf.

Pape JW. Tuberculosis and HIV in the Caribbean: approaches to diagnosis, treatment, and prophylaxis. Topics HIV Med 2004;12(5):144-9.

In: Public Health Yearbook 2016
Editor: Joav Merrick
ISBN: 978-1-53610-947-4

Chapter 32

THE INFLUENCE OF FAMILY STRUCTURE ON SEXUAL HEALTH BEHAVIOR IN SAINT LUCIA YOUTH

Andrea Reichert[1,*], MPH, Lydia Atkins[2], MPH, Livio Ituah[1], MPH and Richard Atkins[1], MPH

[1]School of Medicine and Department of Public Health, St George's University, Grenada, West Indies

[2]Spartan Health Sciences University, School of Medicine, Saint Lucia, West Indies

ABSTRACT

This study investigates the role of family structure on sexual health behavior in Saint Lucia Youth. This includes the role of single-parent versus two-parent households as well as maternal and paternal influences. Methods: Sexual behavior was analyzed in a population of 709 males and 817 females aged 10-19 attending school in Saint Lucia based on secondary data from a self-administered questionnaire. Data was obtained on sexual behaviors of interest such as sexual initiation, multi-partnered sexual activity and condom use. Other variables included the family structure and some socio-demographics. Questions pertinent to family structure and sexual health were cross tabulated and a 95% confidence interval was calculated for each cross tabulated variable. Youth were separated into groups based on whether they lived with both parents, one mom only, or one dad only. Results: Adolescents who lived with only one parent showed a greater likelihood of engaging in sexual activity, became sexual active at a younger age, and were less likely to use contraception. Birth control use was low overall and age at sexual onset was very young. The findings demonstrated a noticeable variation in the relationship between family structure and risk-taking sexual behavior. Conclusion: This study illustrated the need for public health policy to target sexual health behavior in Saint Lucian youth. Programs must aim to increase the presence of two-parent households and implement condom education in schools and in the community.

Keywords: Saint Lucia, sexual health, youth, family influence

---

* Correspondence: Andrea Reichert, MPH, St. George's University School of Medicine, St. George, Grenada, West Indies. E-mail:areicher@sgu.edu.

INTRODUCTION

The WHO Global School-Based Student Health Survey (GSHS) among 13-15 year olds, determined that in the Caribbean region approximately 20% of girls and 40% of boys reported to have been sexually active (1). The Caribbean GSHS reported that 56% of girls and 79% of boys on average had early debut of sex before aged 14. The Caribbean adolescents, who were sexually active, also reported high risk behaviours such as multiple partners and no condom use. Interventions aimed at reducing the risks of STIs and pregnancies among adolescents in the Caribbean need to focus prevention strategies on the factors that affect sexual risk-taking behaviours.

Multiple factors combine together to affect the health of individuals and communities. These influencing factors, which could include both social and behavioral factors, are important determinants of health outcomes in a number of medical conditions. Studies investigating the distribution of these health factors among populations are essential in public health to understand the overall health of a population and where certain preventive efforts can be directed to improve health. Sexual behavior is a particularly important determinant of health in youth populations. In addition, the correlation between sexual health outcomes and the individuals' levels of education, or socio-economic status is well documented (2-5). Sexual activity can be linked to disease risk, increased risk of maternal and infant mortality, population growth, education of women, poverty cycles and other indicators of population health (6). The Caribbean has the second highest prevalence of HIV globally (7, 8). The epidemic in the Caribbean is characterized by significantly higher rates being observed among individuals with high sexual risk-taking behaviours (7). Adequately responding to this epidemic requires research and prevention strategies that addresses the factors that affect sexual risk-taking behaviours.A number of studies have associated sexual behavior in youth with the structure and characteristics of the family unit (9-11). These studies contribute to the growing evidence that family characteristics can influence individual sexual risk-taking behaviours (12, 13). Findings from studies have also related the number of parents in the household with the child's age at sexual initiation (9, 10, 14). There is a wealth of information that exists regarding single versus multi-parental influence on the sexual activity of young adults (9, 15-18). However, there is a scarcity of research to examine the association with sexual risk-taking in adolescents, the early sexual initiation and the family structure.

This paper examines existing data on the prevalence of sexual behaviors under three broad categories: how parents influence the likelihood of youth having sex, how parents influence the age of sexual initiation among youth, and finally, how parents influence the use of birth control among adolescents.

Parents play a significant role in the decision made by children in whether or not they engage in sexual activity. Multiple studies suggest that teenagers who live with one parent are more likely to have had early sex debut than those who live with two parents (17, 19, 20). In a study by Young et al. (15), which controlled for the variables gender, age and race, the researchers proposed that the greater likelihood of youth in single-parent families having sex may be due to non-marital sexual activity being more commonly present among single parents. In addition, adolescents with both parents have two adults available to advise them on emotional and personal issues for example, as it relates to sex (17). This problem is not isolated to a particular culture or locality, but globally affects adolescents. Oman et al. (20), surveyed families living in inner-city areas of the United States and found similar results where 70% of teenagers living with two parents had never had sex, while only 55% of teenagers living with one parent had never had sex. A study in Britain found that males from single parent families were 50% more likely than those from two-parent families to have initiated sexual activity before the age of 17 years (21). In the Caribbean, a cross-sectional study of youth was conducted over nine different countries and found that parental involvement and supervision played an important role in the likelihood of sexual activity (22). Thus, being raised by a single parent has been associated with early sexual début and even when other variables such as socio-economic status and religiosity are considered, this association remains. However, in the Saint Lucian, Caribbean context, family structure has not been examined as a predictive variable of youth sexuality.

Other studies have determined that other characteristics of the family, such as the educational level of the individual parent, more significantly, that of the mother can influence the age of sexual initiation (11, 23-25). It was reported that adolescents in homes with parents with higher educational attainment delayed the age of sexual debut when compared to those coming from households with parents with little or no education (23). It was determined that higher educational levels modified the relationship between parenting practices and sex initiation among young adolescents (23).

Other studies have associated parental roles with the age of sexual onset or sexual debut (9, 16). There are various theories as to why this relationship is present, many of which discuss the roles of maternal and paternal influence on youth. The absence of the father has been associated with sexual behavior in youth. In single parent households where the father is absent, early sexual activity and teen pregnancy were shown to be significantly greater (26, 27). A study by Ellis et al. (26) measured the effect of father absence on early sexual activity. The study posited that the earlier the father left in the child's life, the greater the increase seen in early sexual activity among a cohort of girls in both the United States and New Zealand.

In another study of girls in single parent families without a father present, the likelihood that a girl came from socially troubled background was related to how early that girl's father left home (26). Socially troubled backgrounds included factors such as lower socioeconomic status, greater stress in the family, ethnic minority, young age of the mother at childbirth and strained relationships within the family (26). Consequently, the absence of the father was a risk factor for both early debut of sexual activity and adolescent pregnancy.

Less commonly discussed but still apparent is maternal influence on the onset of youth sexual activity. With fathers no longer present in a family, daughters are exposed to their mothers' behaviors. These behaviors may include dating and finding new partners, which have been shown to encourage early sexual experience in females (26).

The third factor that was investigated among youth in Saint Lucia seeks to identify how parents influence the use of contraceptives among their sexually active children. Use of condoms was looked at specifically as this method of birth control was most prevalent among the population studied.

In the Caribbean, strong parent-child relationships showed increased condom use among males and females, with the results being more significant in males (22). One particular study found that teenagers were more likely to discuss contraception and sexual activity with a parent who has the same gender (28). This has important implications for female or male adolescents who do not have a parent of the same gender at home with whom to discuss contraception options. When this is the case, adolescents tend to rely more on information from their friends than their single parent (28). Conversations with parents about contraceptives have been shown to result in increased contraceptive use in males but not in females (29). Miller (30) argues that there are many variables affecting contraceptive use among youth in addition to family influence. Parents can affect whether youth will use contraceptives, but ultimately they do not have complete control over whether this occurs. Their role lies in making contraceptive use and other sexual behaviors more or less likely (30).

From a review of the existing literature, it can be seen that parents have a multitude of effects on their children's sexual activity. The likelihood of having sexual intercourse, the age at sexual onset, and the use of contraceptives are all affected by the presence or absence of either parent. Many of the studies show evidence of earlier and riskier sexual behavior among youth living with one parent, although some studies suggest otherwise.

This paper seeks to determine the influence of family structure on the sexual behavior among Saint Lucian youth. The literature elucidates that early sexual initiation is associated with the structure of the family. The researchers aimed to determine whether adolescents from polygamous families are at greater risk of being exposed to risky sexual behavior. The study wanted to understand the social context of sexual risk-taking behaviour and focused on how family structure influences sexual behavior among youth in Saint Lucia. The study hypothesizes that there is a relationship between family structure and sexual risk-taking behavior among youths in Saint Lucia. Early initiations of sex and risk-taking sexual behaviors are functions of family structure and individual relationships (9).This analysis is an essential part of gathering more information on the overall health of this population so that appropriate preventive efforts and policies can be implemented and to guide the epidemiological surveillance of sexual transmitted infections.

METHODS

Sexual behavior was analyzed in a population of male and female youth living in Saint Lucia to uncover patterns in sexual activity in 2000 which were used to direct policy and program development. Age and gender were controlled for. This study looked specifically at the role of single-parent versus two-parent households on youth sexual activity. In addition, maternal and paternal influences on youth sexual behavior were examined.

Study population

The study population includes 709 males and 817 females aged 10-19 years living in Saint Lucia. Data from all males and females were used. Youth were separated by the age that they first had sexual intercourse. In addition, youth were separated into groups based on whether they lived with both parents, one mom only, or one dad only. Within these groups, data were analyzed based on questions about sexual health behavior indicated in the data analysis section below.

Data collection and analysis

Secondary data, from the Youth Health Survey of 2000 was used from a self-administered questionnaire that was given to a cohort of students from Saint Lucia aged 10-19 years. The questionnaire included information on socio-demographic variables as well as information on sexual practices, condom use, family characteristics, sexual debut, age at sexual initiation, number of partners, and frequency of condom use. Questions pertinent to family structure and sexual health were cross tabulated and then a 95% confidence interval was calculated for each cross tabulated variable. Multivariate analysis was done to identify the factors that predict youth risky sexual behavioural patterns. Data was analyzed using SPSS, version 21.

RESULTS

Greater than one-third of the study participants were in the fifth form and nearly 10% of them were either not in school or in Pre-form. The majority of the participants were Christians, nearly 64% of whom were Catholic. Forty-one percent of the participants came from two-parent families, and 4.2% were from single father families. Of the participants surveyed, age ranged from 10 to 19 years (see figure 1) with a mean age of 13.6 (SD 2.09).

Table 1. Distribution of respondents by their demographic characteristics

Characteristics	Male, N=709	Female, N=817	Total, N=1,526
Family Structure	332 (56.8)	387 (58.4)	7199 (47.1)
Both Parents			
Single parent, Mother	220 (37.6)	245 (37)	465 (30.5)
Single parent, Father	33 (5.6)	31 (4.7)	64 (4.2)
Mean Age (SD)	13.63 (2.07)	13.58 (2.12)	13.6 (2.09)

Sexual practices and behaviour

Greater than one third of the students surveyed reported ever having had sexual intercourse and the mean age at sexual debut was 11.87 (±2.09) years (see Table 2 and 3). Age of sexual debut was younger for males than for females. Figure 2 indicates that of the sexually active youth, 45% were 10 years or less when they first had sexual intercourse. Table 3 shows that a higher proportion of both males and females who live with one parent have had sex than the proportion of youth who live with both parents. In addition, the percentage of youth who initiated sex by age 10 was higher in both males and females who lived with single parents than males and females in two-parent families. While the mean number of partners was 2.85 (±1.85) for the students surveyed, the males students reported having almost double the number of partners than the female students.

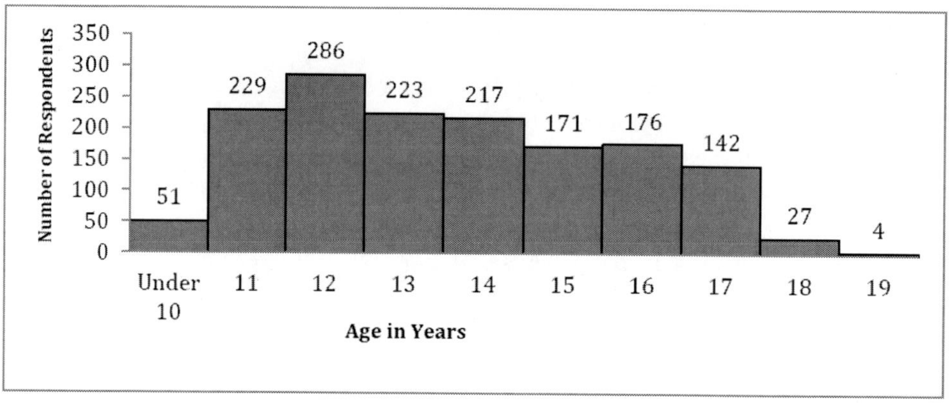

Figure 1. Age distribution of study participants.

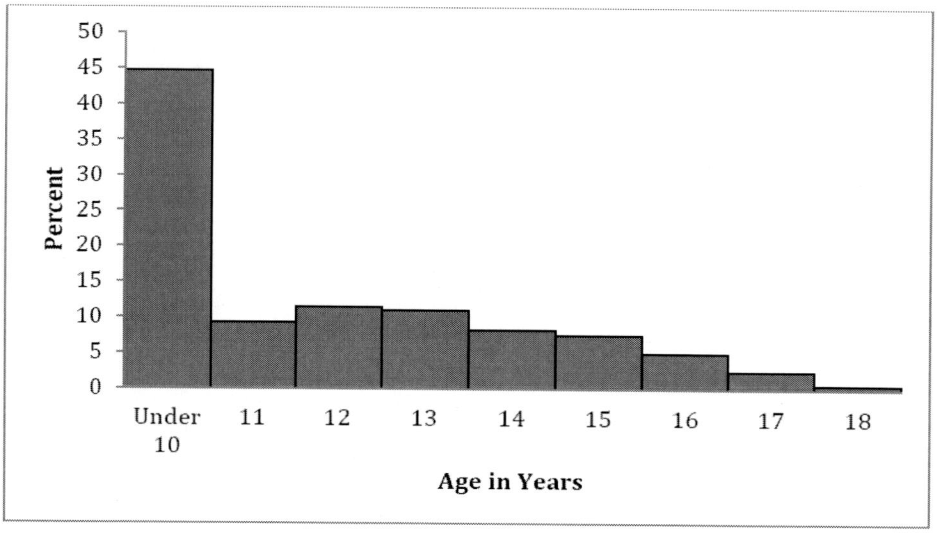

Figure 2. Age of first sexual intercourse in Saint Lucia youth in those who have had sex. (n=1526) The proportion of youth that initiated sex by age 10 is 45%. (95% CI 40.18% to 49.22%).

Table 2. Distribution of respondents by sexual practices and risk behaviours

Sexual Behavior Patterns	Male, N=354	Female, N=156	Total, N=510
Sexual debut			
Mean number of sex partners	3.21 (1.86)	1.97 (1.51)	2.85 (1.85)
Mean age at sexual debut	11.44 (1.86)	12.92 (2.44)	11.87 (2.15)
How often do you use birth control?			
Never	210 (59)	70 (45)	208 (55)
Sometimes	40 (11)	27 (17)	67 (13)
Always	74 (21)	34 (22)	108 (21)
Condom use at last sexual encounter	135 (38)	63 (40)	198 (39)
Use of oral contraceptive			
Yes	11 (3)	8(5)	19 (3.7)

Table 3. Distribution all of ages of Saint Lucia youth who have had sex and who haven't had sex by family structure

Family Structure	Have had sex			Have not had sex		
	n	(%)	95% CI	n	(%)	95% CI
Live with both parents	213	31.6	(25.36, 37.84)	461	68.40	(64.16, 72.64)
Live with one mom	173	39.3	(32.02, 46.58)	267	60.70	(54.84, 66.56)
Live with one dad	28	46.7	(28.22, 65.10)	32	53.30	(36.01, 70.59)
Total	510	36.0	(33.50, 38.50)	906	64.00	(60.88, 67.13)

Table 2 shows that among sexually active students 55% never used condoms while 13% sometimes or irregularly used. The males reported higher likelihood of non and inconsistent use of condoms than female respondents. In both sexes there was higher reporting of condom never being used or irregularly used compared to those who reported to always using a condom.

Inconsistent condom use was also reported when respondents were asked about last sexual encounter, though marginally higher use reported for females compared to males. There was a significant difference in reported consistency of condom use based on age of sexual debut, with usage more than twice as high in youth who initiated sex between 15 and 18 years compared age of initiation by 10 years, see Table 4. Generally, birth control use was especially low in youth who initiated sex before age 10, 14% reported to have always used birth control and 75% have never used birth control. Across all age groups there was low reporting of oral contraceptive use, only 5% of the female respondents reported use. Oral contraceptive use was also reported by 3% of the males, however it is unclear whether they were reporting on partner used.

Almost twice as many of the male respondents (48%) compared to females (25%) had early initiation of sex at less than 11 years (see Table 5). While respondents from polygamous families have had sexual intercourse than those from monogamous families, there is no much difference between them in age at first sex. Almost half of the respondents students from single parents home have had first sex before age 11. More of the students from monogamous and single parent homes have multiple partners and almost 20% higher in single father families than any other family structure.

Table 4. Percentage of youth who have had sex who used a condom during their last act of sexual intercourse by age at first sexual experience

Family Structure	11-14 years			15-18 years	All Ages				
	n	n	(%)	n	(%)	n	(%)	Chi-Square	P-value
Live with both parents	26 (46)	42 (56)	56	25	78.1	93	57.1	8.41	0.02
Live with one mom	21 (34)	28 (45)	45.2	13	21	62	48.4	13.76	0.001
Live with one dad	3 (6)	6 (55)	54.5	0	0	9	47.4	0.54	0.46
Total	50 (36)	76 (60)	59.9	38	73.4	164	51.2	31.86	<.0001

Table 5. Percentage distribution of survey respondents who have ever had sex, age at first sex, multi-partner sexual relations, and inconsistent condom use by selected characteristics

Characteristics	N	Age at sex <11	2+ Sex partners	Condom use at last sexual encounter
Total	510	208 (41)	308 (60)	188 (37)
Gender				
Male	354	169 (48)	253 (71.5)	135 (38)
Female	156	39 (25)	55 (35.2)	63 (40)
Family Structure				
Both parents	210	68 (32)	122 (58)	91 (43)
Single parent, mother	173	81 (47)	101 (59)	61 (36)
Single parent, father	28	12(43)	22 (79)	9 (32)

Table 6. Family structure and risky sexual behavioural patterns among youth in Saint Lucia

	Both parents	Mother only	Father only	Test statistic	p-value
Sex debut (yrs)	12.22 (2.18)	11.69 (2.19)	11.33 (1.47)	3.98	0.02
# partners	2.77 (1.82)	2.77(1.82)	3.23 (1.95)	0.78	0.46
No form of protection	83 (51.6%)	91(67.9%)	16 (66.7%)	8.67	0.01
Used condom	91 (55.8%)	61 (48%)	9 (47.4%)	1.92	0.38
Used the pill	5 (3.6%)	8 (7.5%)	2 (11.8%)	2.92	0.23

Table 7. Gender and risky sexual behavioural patterns among youth in Saint Lucia

	Females	Males	Test statistic	p-value
Sex debut (yrs)	12.92 (2.44)	11.44 (1.86)	50.11	<0.001
# partners	1.97 (1.51)	3.21 (1.86)	47.73	<0.001
No form of protection	55 (51.9%)	178 (60.8%)	2.517	0.11
Used condom	63 (55.8%)	135 (49.5%)	1.27	0.26
Used the pill	8 (9%)	11 (4.6%)	2.345	0.13

Factors predicting risky sexual behavioural patterns

In this section we examine predictors of risky sexual behaviours; age at sexual debut; multiple sexual partnerships or relationships, non-regular sexual relationships; inconsistent condom use and birth control use (see Tables 6 and 7).

Risky sexual behaviours

Gender, being male, and single father families were significant in predicting the likelihood of younger age initiation for sexual intercourse. There is a significant difference for age of sexual debut between a student living with both parents and with mother only with an average difference is 0.547 years.

Multiple sexual partner relationships (2+)

When the correlates of multiple sexual partnerships among the respondents was assessed, it showed that female respondents were less likely to have multiple sex partners than the males and that males had more sexual partners compared to females, which has been observed in other studies (9). There was a significant gender difference in the number of partners and age of sex debut, however there was no significant difference in the number of sexual partners based on family structure.

Inconsistent condom use

In this paper, inconsistent condom use is defined as not using condoms always when one has sex. While condom use was reported higher for females than males, there was no significant difference and no family variable was significant. However, the expected pattern of relationship is observed. For example, respondents from polygamous had a higher likelihood of condom use than otherwise. There was a reported significant difference in high risk behaviour in doing nothing as a form of birth control, or using no form of protection which was proportionately higher for students from single parent families compared with both parent households.

DISCUSSION

This paper describes and identifies the predicting family variables for high risk sexual behavior among students in Saint Lucia. The findings will be particularly relevant for health intervention for adolescents and youths in Saint Lucia especially as it relates to the prevention of STIs in this age cohort, as well as teen pregnancies and the introduction of Human Papillomavirus (HPV) vaccines for young girls.

In Saint Lucia and other Caribbean nations, positive parent-teen relationships were identified as protective factors in preventing early sexual debut (22). In this study, data collected on sexual behavior in Saint Lucia youth indicated an early age for sexual onset as well as low use of birth control and condoms among the study population. The findings indicated earlier initiation of sexual intercourse among Saint Lucia youth compared to other studies, (9, 31). The results were also suggestive of a high level of sexual networking with increased number of sexual partners and consistent with other studies that have found that male adolescents and youths have more sexual partners than females, irrespective of age (9).

These results were especially apparent among male and female youth who lived with one parent and these adolescents were also more likely to engage in sexual intercourse. Findings from this study are consistent with existing literature citing increased sexual activity, a younger age at sexual onset and decreased condom use in youth living with a single parent (26). Given these results, health policy should aim to increase the presence of fathers in the home and increase condom use, especially in youth at young ages when they first start to engage in sexual activity.

It is important to note, that in contrast to the studies showing earlier sexual onset in youth from single parent families, the quality of the relationship between the child and mother had a greater effect (32). Relationship quality was measured by closeness, amount of love and affection given, and the level of communication between the mother and her child (32). Thus, there are multiple factors that play a role in the age of first sexual experience in youth in both single and two parent households. These should be taken into consideration in the development of policies and the design of interventions aimed at addressing sexual behavior in youth.

The findings in this study were similar to that of other studies that determined that there was a relationship between the absence of the father and sexual-related behaviors among females. There are various theories as to why this result may have occurred. Hetherington's (33) evolutionary model suggests that in the first five years of a girl's life the foundation is laid for motivational systems involved in later sexual activity. Girls from birth to five years old collect information about the reproductive strategies of their parents and this information is stored (33). Thus, the absence of a girl's father before the age of five can have a large impact on the reproductive activity that she may participate in as a teenager. Another model based on personality, suggests that certain personality traits associated with early sexual behavior in females may be a result of paternal absence (26). Stern et al. (34) suggest that fathers play an important role in passing on important values and moral actions to youth and that fathers act to deter certain negative or risky behaviors including those associated with sexual activity. The study by Stern et al. (34) looked at the relationship between father absence and social issues including sexual activity, drinking and marijuana use (34). More social issues among youth occurred when the father was not present in the adolescent's family structure to advise and guide youth and this negative effect was more apparent among males (34). Another effect seen in males living in single households is that they may not perceive marriage as an important factor in sexual interactions (17). After witnessing parents engage in extra-marital sex, this may seem normal to an adolescent (27). Males in this living situation might engage in early or regular sexual activity well before marriage (17).

The active presence of the father in the family can be increased by offering educational workshops on conflict resolution within marriage so that couples will be more likely to stay together. In addition, workshops could help fathers develop stronger parenting skills and learn from other dads. Father-child monthly events could be held in the community in an effort to strengthen the relationship between fathers and their youth. Male targeted interventions to educate males on their critical role in the family can be implemented and it can be aimed at reaching youth before fatherhood.

To increase condom use, health policy must focus on education in schools as well as in the community. In schools, a key component of providing condoms is educating youth on how to use them as well as education on other aspects of sexual health. This can be demonstrated by contrasting two studies in Seattle and Massachusetts. At a school in Seattle, condoms were given out to students with little education on how to use them. 29% of students acquired one condom from school yet only 13% of those students used the condom during sexual intercourse (35). In contrast to this, students were given condoms at a school in Massachusetts and were provided with detailed instructions on how to use them properly and how condoms are important in preventing STI transmission. Sexually active youth in the school were more likely to report using a condom during the most recent time they had sex (36).

They key difference between each of these studies is that in addition to providing condoms to youth at school, these youth must be educated on how and why to use them. While the approach in the Seattle and Massachusetts studies may not be culturally appropriate in making condoms available to students, it sets the stage for engaging the schools and parents in the need to consider making these services available to youth who are sexually active.

Although the Ministry of Health in Saint Lucia is open to a discussion about condom distribution, many school principals are opposed as they believe providing condoms may lead to youth engaging in more sexual activity (Gleaner, 2009). The Massachusetts study by Blake and colleagues (36) found that youth involved in condom programs at school were less likely to report sexual activity than youth in similar populations attending schools where condoms were not given out. Consequently there is a need for the engagement of the Ministry of Education as well as the Religious community on the need to reorient the Health and Family Life Education (HFLE) programs in schools, and using youth groups to reach the youth, providing peer support youth groups while engaging parents in the process.

Promoting the active presence of fathers in families and increasing condom education and availability can be combined to form a policy in Saint Lucia titled FOCUS: Family Oriented Contraceptive Utilization in Saint Lucia. Saint Lucia can benefit greatly from implementation of this policy by decreasing rates of STI transmission, reducing teenage pregnancy, increasing the status of women and increasing the overall health of youth living in the island nation. Cooperation of all leaders and stakeholders is essential in adopting the proposed sexual health policy to create powerful and positive change in the lives of Saint Lucia youth.

Limitations and strengths of the study

The use of secondary data from a self-administered questionnaires could have resulted in inconsistencies and missing information and did not provide an opportunity for verification where data gaps or inconsistencies existed. As a results it did not provide the investigators with the opportunity to clarify a number of issues, such as positive responses for oral contraceptive use by male respondents. However, due to the sensitivity of the data collected, the instrument conferred confidentiality of the reported data than face-to-face interviews would have.

The study would have benefited if it were possible to have obtained both quantitative and qualitative data from respondents, parents and sexual partners. In addition a longitudinal study, while more expensive and takes longer to conduct would have provided more dynamic information and would not have been prone to the responder bias introduced by the study design that relied on most of the variables being measured retrospectively. Further studies should address the socioeconomic correlates of risky sexual behavior that explores the understanding of the relationship between family characteristics, structure, poverty rating and risky sexual behaviors as sexual behavior is a multifaceted phenomenon influenced by a diverse range of variables.

The findings of this study can help guide and inform numerous child health policies and has implications not only for reproductive health policy but also social protection policies for youth in Saint Lucia.

CONCLUSION

Previous studies have established that family structure is a predictor of sexual-related behaviors among youth. It is posited that the socio-economic status influences the sexual decision-making processes of adolescents by limiting the decision-making powers of the marginalized poor, and that poverty is more prevalent in single parent households. When these constructs are applied to youth in Saint Lucia it is expected that youth from single parent households who are at greater risk for low socio-economic status are more likely to engage in risky sexual behavior.

This study confirms this position. There is a need to strengthen the findings with qualitative data to explore the patterns of sexual-related behavior exhibited by the youth in Saint Lucia.

REFERENCES

[1] World Health Organization. Global school-based student health survey (GSHS) purpose and methodology. Geneva: WHO, 2009.

[2] Rao TS, Gopalakrishnan R, Kuruvilla A, Jacob KS. Social determinants of sexual health. Indian J Psychiatry 2012;54(2):105-7.

[3] World Health Organization. Developing sexual health programmes: A framework for action. Geneva: WHO, 2010.

[4] Women's Health West. Social determinants of sexual and reproductive health. Melbourne: Western region Sexual and Reproductive Health Working Group, 2011.

[5] Devieux JG, Rosenberg R, Saint-Jean G, Bryant VE, Malow RM. The continuing challenge of reducing HIV risk among Haitian youth: The need for intervention. J Int Assoc of Provid AIDS Care 2015;14(3):217-23.

[6] Greif MJ, Dodoo FN, Jayaraman A. Urbanisation, poverty and sexual behaviour: the tale of five African cities. Urban Stud 2011;48(5):947-57.

[7] Figueroa JP. The HIV epidemic in the Caribbean: meeting the challenges of achieving universal access to prevention, treatment and care. West Indian Med J 2008;57(3):195-203.

[8] De Boni R, Veloso VG, Grinsztejn B. Epidemiology of HIV in Latin America and the Caribbean. Curr Opin HIV AIDS 2014;9(2):192-8.

[9] Odimegwu C, Adedini SA. Do family structure and poverty affect sexual risk behaviors of undergraduate students in Nigeria? Afr J Reprod Health 2013;17(4): 137-49.

[10] Bakken RJ, Winter M. Family characteristics and sexual risk behaviors among black men in the United States. Perspect Sex Reprod Health 2002;34(5):252-8.

[11] Merchan-Hamann E, Ekstrand M, Hudes ES, Hearst N. Prevalence and correlates of HIV-related risk behaviors among adolescents at public schools in Brasilia. AIDS Behav 2002;6(3):283-93.

[12] Odimegwu CO, Solanke LB, Adedokun A. Parental characteristics and adolescent sexual behaviour in Bida Local Government Area of Niger State, Nigeria. Afr J Reprod Health 2002;6(1):95-106.

[13] Fatusi AO, Blum RW. Predictors of early sexual initiation among a nationally representative sample of Nigerian adolescents. BMC Public Health 2008;8:136.
[14] Flewelling RL, Bauman KE. Family structure as a predictor of initial substance use and sexual intercourse in early adolescence. J Marriage Fam 1990;52:171–81.
[15] Biddlecom A, Awusabo-Asare K, Bankole A. Role of parents in adolescent sexual activity and contraceptive use in four African countries. Int Perspect Sex Reprod Health 2009;35(2):72-81.
[16] Peres CA, Rutherford G, Borges G, Galano E, Hudes ES, Hearst N. Family structure and adolescent sexual behavior in a poor area of Sao Paulo, Brazil. J Adolesc Health 2008;42(2):177-83.
[17] Young EW, Jensen LC, Olsen JA, Cundick BP. The effects of family structure on the sexual behavior of adolescents. Adolescence 1991;26(104):977-86.
[18] Goldberg RE. Family instability and early initiation of sexual activity in Western Kenya. Demography 2013;50(2):725-50.
[19] Miller B, Benson B, Galbraith K. Family relationships and adolescent pregnancy risk: A research synthesis. Dev Rev 2001;21:1-38.
[20] Oman RF, Vesely SF, Aspy CB. Youth assets and sexual risk behavior: the importance of assets for youth residing in one-parent households. Perspect Sex Reprod Health 2005;37(1):25-31.
[21] Devine D, Long PRF. A prospective study of adolescent sexual activity: description, correlates and predictors. Adv Behav Res Ther 1993;15(3):185-209.
[22] Lerand SJ, Ireland M, Blum RW. Individual and environmental impacts on sexual health of Caribbean youth. ScientificWorldJournal 2006;6:707-17.
[23] Roche KM, Mekos D, Alexander CS, Astone NM, Bandeen-Roche K, Ensminger ME. Parenting influences on early sex initiation among adolescents: How neighborhood matters. J Fam Issues 2005;26(1):32-54.
[24] Browning CR, Leventhal T, Brooks-Gunn J. Sexual initiation in early adolescence: The nexus of parental and community control. Am Sociol Rev 2005;70(5): 758-78.
[25] Scott-James D, White A. Correlates of sexual activity in early adolescence. J Early Adolesc 1998;1(2):221-38.
[26] Ellis BJ, Bates JE, Dodge KA, Fergusson DM, Horwood LJ, Pettit GS, et al. Does father absence place daughters at special risk for early sexual activity and teenage pregnancy? Child Dev 2003;74(3):801-21.
[27] Mendle J, Harden KP, Turkheimer E, Van Hulle CA, D'Onofrio BM, Brooks-Gunn J, et al. Associations between father absence and age of first sexual intercourse. Child Dev 2009;80(5):1463-80.
[28] Moore D, Erickson P. Age, gender, and ethnic differences in sexual and contraceptive knowledge, attitudes, and behaviors. Fam Commun Health 1985; 8(3):38-51.
[29] Jaccard J, Dittus PJ, Gordon VV. Maternal correlates of adolescent sexual and contraceptive behavior. Family planning perspectives. 1996;28(4):159-65, 85.
[30] Miller BC. Family influences on adolescent sexual and contraceptive behavior. J Sex Res 2002;39(1):22-6.
[31] Bonell C, Allen E, Strange V, Oakley A, Copas A, Johnson A, et al. Influence of family type and parenting behaviours on teenage sexual behaviour and conceptions. J Epidemiol Commun Health 2006;60(6): 502-6.
[32] Davis E, Friel L. Adolescent sexuality: disentangling the effects of family structure and family context. J Marriage Fam 2001;63(3):669-78.
[33] Hetherington E. Effects of father absence on personality development in adolescent daughters. Dev Psychol 1972;7:313-26.
[34] Stern M, Northman J, Van Slyck M. Father absence and adolescent "problem behaviors": Alcohol consumption, drug use, and sexual activity. Adolescence 1984;19(74): 301-12.
[35] Kirby D, Brener ND, Brown NL, Peterfreund N, Hillard P, Harrist R. The impact of condom availability [correction of distribution] in Seattle schools on sexual behavior and condom use. Am J Public Health 1999;89(2):182-7.
Blake SM, Ledsky R, Goodenow C, Sawyer R, Lohrmann D, Windsor R. Condom Availability Programs in Massachusetts High Schools: Relationships With Condom Use and Sexual Behavior. Am J Public Health 2003;93(6):955-62.

In: Public Health Yearbook 2016
Editor: Joav Merrick

ISBN: 978-1-53610-947-4

Chapter 33

Correlation between Self-Efficacy in Sexual Negotiation and Engagement in Risky Sexual Behaviors: Pilot Study of Adolescents Attending a Secondary School in Grenada, West Indies

Desiree Jones[1], MPH,
Kamilah B Thomas-Purcell[2], PhD, MPH, CHES,
Jacquelyn Lewis-Harris[3], PhD,
and Christine Richards[4,*], MPH, PhD

[1]School of Medicine, St George's University, Grenada, West Indies
[2]Nova Southeastern University, College of Osteopathic Medicine, Office of Research and Innovation and the Master of Public Health Program, Fort Lauderdale, Florida, US
[3]Department of Anthropology and Education, University of Missouri, St. Louis, Missouri, US
[4]Department of Public Health and Preventative Medicine, St George's University, Grenada, West Indies

Abstract

Adolescents' sexual decision making is largely determined by normative ideals of sex and self-efficacy in sexual negotiation. The goal of this current research is to examine whether there is a correlation between self-efficacy and the likelihood to engage in risky sexual behavior among a sample of Grenadian adolescents. It is aimed to determine whether self-efficacy serves as a protective factor for risky sexual behavior. With this information, it can be better understood how interpersonal skills can facilitate positive

* Correspondence: Christine Richards, MPH, PhD, St George's University, Department of Public Health and Preventative Medicine, St. George, Grenada, West Indies. E-mail: chriscrich@hotmail.com.

sexual health discourse and better inform sexual decision making in youth. Thirty-seven students in grade 9 from a high school in Grenada participated in this pilot study. Within grade 9, 10 (27%) students reported being sexually active. Of those, 70% were males and 30% were females. In addition, males with poor self-efficacy represented 18.9% of the total student sample, and males with high self-efficacy represent 32.4% of the total student sample. Females with poor self-efficacy represented 8.1% of the total student population, and females with high self-efficacy represent 40.5% of the total student population. There was a positive correlation between non-sexual activity and positive self-efficacy (OR: 8.63, 95% CI: 1.65, 44.99). Overall the data shows that risky sexual behavior is correlated, though minimally, with negative self-efficacy. On average students who were not sexually active displayed a more positive self-efficacy. Adolescents with positive self-efficacy tend to have more positive sexual behavioral outcomes. In addition there were gendered trends of males tending to have higher levels of self-efficacy and increased likelihood to engage in risky sexual behavior.

Keywords: self-efficacy, risky sexual behavior, Grenada, adolescents, Caribbean youth

INTRODUCTION

Globally HIV/AIDs continues to be a pressing concern among public health practitioners, researchers and educators. Many individuals have an increased risk of susceptibility due to their social vulnerability, which is influenced by the larger structural constructs of education, poverty, and gender inequity (1). Although HIV/AIDS is a growing concern among all age groups, research has shown that adolescents are among the most vulnerable, due to their engagement in risky sexual behaviors (2). World Health Organization (3) defines "adolescence" as young people between the ages of 10 and 19 years old. They are often the age group most influenced by external structural and interpersonal determinants, both positively and negatively. Indeed, the most effective manner in addressing this critical health epidemic will be addressing the attitudes and behaviors of youth (2).

The Caribbean region has an adult HIV prevalence of approximately 1.0 percent, which is second to Sub-Saharan Africa. The number of people living with HIV (PLHIV) in the Caribbean is approximately 240,000, and has not varied much since the latter half of the 20th century. AIDS is now the foremost cause of death for individuals 15-45 years and total incidences are growing exponentially, with prevalence rates as high as 3.2% (4). In Grenada, more than 70% of HIV/AIDS cases and 76% of AIDS-related deaths occur among individuals between 15-44 years old (2).

People between 10-24 years old constitute nearly 30% of the Caribbean population (1). Since youth constitute such a large segment of the population, it is essential to develop a comprehensive report of health trends to improve overall community health. Many gaps remain in knowledge of adolescent sexual behavior—motives for early sex initiation, multiple sexual partners, and lack of contraception use. Halcon (1) reported that this current transition from communicable diseases to "social morbidities" among adolescents could largely be attributed to intrapersonal risk behaviors and perceptions influenced by social environmental factors.

In order to foster the enactment and enforcement of effective policies and program initiatives that can adequately address adolescents' risky sexual behavior, it is necessary to understand the multi-dimensional determinants that influence intention and performance of such behavior. Within Grenada and the broader Caribbean, there is a need to create and strengthen community support dynamics and promote healthy sexual discourse to facilitate behavior change among adolescents in an enabling environment. Recent studies have shown that there is a correlation between risky sexual health behavioral choices and self-efficacy (5). Among Grenadian adolescents, positive self-efficacy, delineated by positive peer-to-peer sexual health communication and actions, may be correlated with decreased levels of participation in risky sexual behaviors such as reduced contraceptive use and multiple sexual partners. The following brief review of the literature expounds upon the association between self-efficacy in sexual negotiation and likelihood of youth to engage in risky sexual behavior.

When assessing sexual health trends among adolescents within the Caribbean, it is evident that there is a continual perpetuation of risky sexual practices among adolescents. Of approximately 5,231 sexually active and Caribbean adolescents, 75% reported that they did not use any form of contraceptives consistently (1). With data such as this, there is an emerging transnational concern to determine motives and intentions behind youth's inconsistent use of contraceptives during sexual intercourse. Research has assessed the determinants and consequences of sexual behavior among adolescents to be largely associated with self-efficacy, normative ideas, and familial and peer influence. Self-efficacy can be defined as a personal assessment of one's ability to organize and execute behaviors that lead to successful outcomes (6). Contraceptive self-efficacy is essential to understanding contraceptive behavior among adolescents because self-efficacy largely motivates behavioral modification. Specifically, many researchers have begun looking at the link between self-efficacy and the likelihood of sexually active adolescents to engage in risky sexual behavior across gender and age groups, including multiple concurrent partners and lack of contraception use. Bandura (7) defined self-efficacy as belief in one's own capabilities to systematize and perform specific behaviors required to manage various situations. He discusses four core constructs of self-efficacy: mastery experience, vicarious experience, social persuasion and the somatic/emotional state. The most interpretive of the four constructs is mastery experience, which is where an individual personally gauges one's own perceptions and how they influence his own behaviors. The second most important construct is the vicarious experience. When individuals have limited prior experiences or are uncertain of their own capabilities, a vicarious experience through another representative model becomes very influential (8). Schunk (9) elucidated that this representative model is often a peer that possess powerful persuasion over self-perceptions of conception. An individual's perception of his or her capabilities can significantly influence feelings, thoughts, motivation, and behavior in performing tasks and negotiating needs and wants with others (10). Traen (11) further illustrated this concept by pointing out how an adolescent's belief in his ability to behave in a certain manner can affect the initiation or further performance of the behavior through a quantitative investigation of the relationship between past contraceptive behavior, and self-efficacy among Norwegian adolescents. Traen (11) expounded on the notion that past behaviors can influence communication self-efficacy by evaluating various emotional responses, such as shame, emotional intimacy, and guilt. Assessment of these emotional responses were illustrated through the positive correlation between adolescents' self- efficacy during a setting in which they were expected to communicate with their partner about contraception use, and self-efficacy within a scenario where they deter an unwanted coital engagement.

Other studies have also explored sex negotiation skills among youth. Longmore (12) argues that the highly unplanned nature of adolescent sexual activity is due to negative contraceptive self-efficacy. The researchers define contraceptive self-efficacy as the "conviction that one can control sexual and contraceptive situations to achieve contraceptive protection" in terms of conditional responses to perceptions of motivational barriers. They found that efficacy regarding the negotiation of condom use predicted safer sex practices. Adolescents who inconsistently used contraception had lower condom self-efficacy scores than adolescents who consistently use contraception. Logistic regression analysis of adolescents in Burkina Faso also revealed that there was a positive correlation between the use of contraceptives and self-efficacy in the use of condoms (13). Kalichman (14) also found a positive correlation between self-efficacy and frequency of unprotected sex. It was determined that self-efficacy was the best predictor of the likelihood a student would engage in safe sexual practices. The effects of self-efficacy on condom use even exceeded the effects of gender, age, or group normative values. In addition, it was found that the ability to effectively use contraception was also influenced by external social norms and intrapersonal attitudes, beliefs, and perceptions.

The link between perceptions and actual elicitation of behavior can be greatly determined by healthy sex communication. Van Campen (5) reports evidence of healthy sexual communication being a protective factor in engagement of risky sexual behaviors among Mexican-American adolescents in the southwestern region of the United States (5). Lack of positive condom-use negotiation can often be difficult due to fears of the other partner sensing mistrust in the relationship. Healthy communications can also be difficult due to emotions of obligations and embarrassment (13).

In summary, evidence suggests that self-efficacy and healthy communication skills are associated with the likelihood to engage in risky sexual behaviors. The investigation of risky sexual behavior in relation to youth self-efficacy is of importance because of the increasing need to promote and ensure sexual health knowledge and reproductive rights. In addition, there is the need to reduce negative outcomes of risky behavior, such as the spread of HIV/AIDs and other STD/STIs, pregnancy and poor mental health.

The goal of this secondary analysis is to determine whether there is a correlation between self-efficacy and the likelihood to engage in risky sexual behavior among a sample of Grenadian adolescents. Specifically, this study examined the following objectives (1) determine the influence of gender on self-efficacy and risky sexual behavior; (2) assess how self-efficacy influences risky sexual behavior; and (3) examine contraception usage in relation to self-efficacy and risky sexual behaviors.

METHODS

This study was conducted in St. Georges, Grenada in the southeastern Caribbean Sea. The current population is 103,328 individuals. Grenada's educational school is compulsory from age 5-14 and based on the British educational system. There are both public and private secondary schools, with a total of 22 secondary schools.

Study design

The current study is a secondary analysis of adolescents' self-efficacy and likelihood to engage in risky sexual behavior. The initial study, conducted in 2013, included the use of a questionnaire used to assess student's knowledge, attitudes and behaviors concerning sexual health literacy, school conduct, drug use, HIV knowledge, self-efficacy, perceived susceptibility, and sexual performance. This cross-sectional study utilized standardized methodology and was developed through collaborative effort and consensus of the Ministry of Education and St. George's University Department of Public Health and Preventative Medicine. This survey was part of a larger intervention study—Focus on Youth Caribbean-Grenada (FOYC-G)— which was an evidence-based culturally appropriate curriculum that was implemented with Grenadian secondary-school students. The primary objective of this program implementation was to assess students' knowledge, attitudes and behaviors and to understand any potential barriers that exist to students having healthy sexual negotiation skills and appropriate understanding of sexual and reproductive health. FOYC-G was a 10-session educational program targeting adolescents 9-15 years old. Negotiation and communication skills were exhibited and practiced through vignettes, role-playing, and games. Formative research from this pilot-study would be used to tailor the FOYC-G curriculum targeted to a larger Grenadian population.

Sample

For this study, the target population was a group of 37 students at a pilot secondary school in northern Grenada. Eligibility criteria for students included males and females in grade 9 that have attended school for at least one year.

A purposive sampling methodology was used. The principal recruited a group of students generated from the inclusion criteria mentioned above. He then sent introductory letters to a sample of parents of students in grade 9. Each letter included a parental consent form and a telephone number for interested parents to call for additional information or to decline their child's participation in the study.

Data analysis

Analyses included frequencies, odds ratio, and confidence intervals. For the purposes of this analysis, the alpha level was set to 0.05. In order to analyze the data, some questions were collapsed to encompass a group idea. The dependent variable, risky sexual behavior was assessed by analyzing results of the number of coital partners, contraception use, age at first intercourse, and frequency of sexual activity. Each response was determined to have a specific point value. *High Risk Sexual Behavior* was defined as having a score of 10 or higher. *Low Risk Sexual Behavior* was defined as having a score below 10.

The independent variable of interest is self-efficacy and was assessed by analyzing results of sexual negotiation of condom use and sexual boundaries. Each response was determined to have a specific point value. *Positive Self-Efficacy* was defined as responding positively (score of 4 or lower) to discussing and expressing sexual boundaries in regards to sexual negotiation, condom usage, consensual sexual engagement with minimum embarrassment and hesitation. *Negative Self-Efficacy* was defined as responding negatively (score of 5 or above) to discussing and describing sexual boundaries in regards to talking about sex, condom usage, consensual sexual engagement with minimum embarrassment, and hesitation. *Contraception Use* was defined as any student that responded with a yes (1) to the usage of contraceptives (birth control pill, condom, diaphragm, foam, depo provera, etc.) during the last sexual intercourse.

RESULTS

During the 2013 cross-sectional study, 37 students in grade 9 from a pilot-secondary school participated in the study. The average age was 14.16 years. Nineteen (51.4%) students were male and 18(48.7%) female. Fifteen (40.5%) students lived in a single-parent household; 17 (45.95%) students lived in a double-parent household; and 5 (13.51%) students lived in a household with other relative. Within grade 9, there were 10 students with sexual intercourse experience (27%). Of these 10 students, 7 (70%) were male and 3 (30%) were female. Of the 10 sexually active students, 7(70%) used contraception during the last coital engagement. The only form of contraception mentioned was a condom. Of the total sample, 16.2% were sexually active males and 8.1% were sexually active females (see Figure 1). Of the sexually active students, 8 (80%) engaged in high risky behavior (6 males and 2 females). The median sex initiation age ranged between 13-15 years. Males with poor self-efficacy represented 18.9% of the total student population, and males with high self-efficacy represent 32.4% of the total student population (see Figure 2). Females with poor self-efficacy represent 8.1% of the total student population, and females with high self-efficacy represent 40.5% of the total student population.

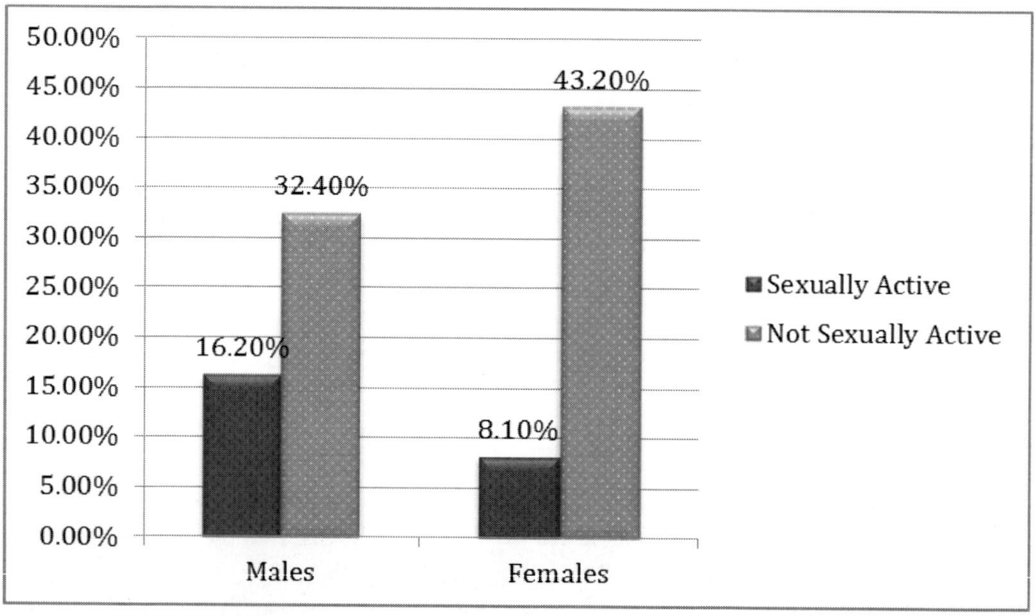

Figure 1. Frequency of sexually active students by gender.

Table 1. Summary of self-efficacy: Total sample

	Self-Efficacy			
Characteristic	Positive n (%)	Negative n (%)	Odds Ratio	95% CI
Sexually Active				
No	23 (65.16)	4 (10.81)	8.63	(1.65, 44.99)
Yes	4 (10.81)	6 (6.22)		
Sexual Behavior Risk				
High	3 (30)	5 (50)	0.6	(.03, 13.58)
Low	1 (10)	1 (10)		

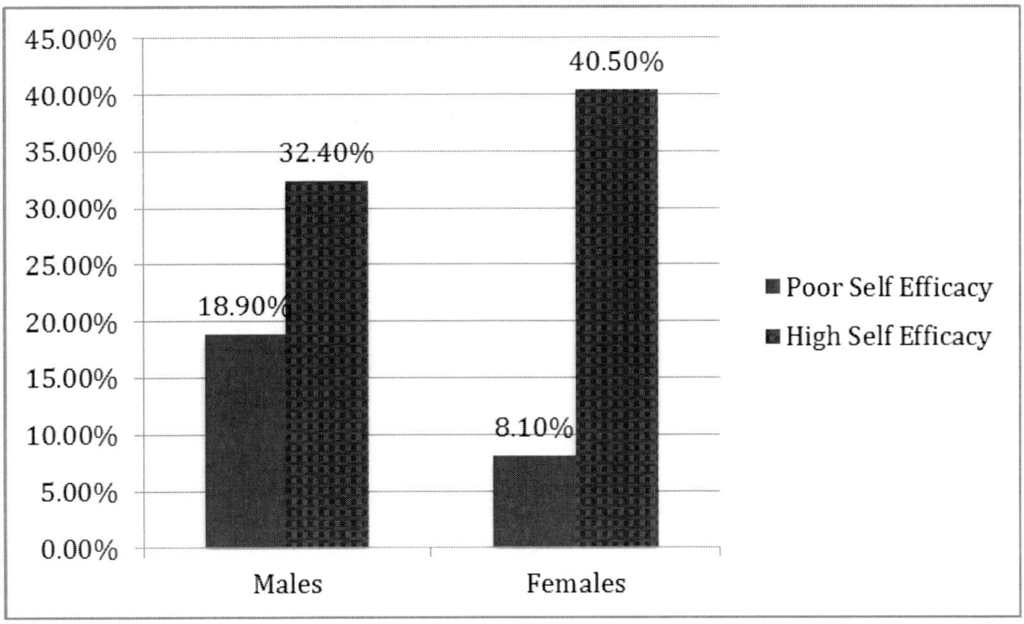

Figure 2. Distribution of frequency of self-efficacy.

Table 2. Summary of condom usage

	Condom Use			
	Yes n (%)	No n (%)	Odds Ratio	95% CI
Self-Efficacy				
Positive	3 (30)	1 (10)	1.5	(0.09, 25.39)
Negative	4 (40)	2 (20)		
Sexual Behavior Risk				
High	6 (60)	2 (20)	3	(0.2, 73.64)
Low	1 (10)	1 (10)		

There is a negative correlation between the likelihood to engage in sexual intercourse and positive self-efficacy. Indicated by Table 1, an odds ratio of 8.63 (95% CI: 1.65, 44.99) indicates that those students who had positive self-efficacy were 8.63 times more likely to be students who are not sexually active. This indicates that the variables sexual activity and self-efficacy are likely dependent on one another.

Students with positive self-efficacy were 1.67 times (95% CI: 0.07, 37.73) more likely to engage in low risky sexual behavior as opposed to high-risk sexual behavior. Students that used condoms were 1.5 times more likely (95% CI: 0.09, 25.39) to be students who possessed positive self-efficacy (see Table 2). In addition, students that used condoms were 3 times more likely (95% CI: 0.2, 73.64) to be students that engaged in high-risk sexual behavior.

DISCUSSION

The purpose of this research was to determine whether there was a correlation between self-efficacy and the likelihood to engage in risky sexual behavior among a sample of Grenadian adolescents. With this information, it could be better understood how interpersonal skills can facilitate positive sexual health discourse and better inform sexual decision making in youth. The data revealed an interplay among major themes of early sex initiation, gendered patterns of self-efficacy, and gendered patterns of high-risk sexual behavior.

Gender, normative ideals, and self-efficacy largely influence youth cognitive processes and behavior in sexual performance and decision-making. The data revealed there were more males engaging in high-risk sexual behavior in comparison to females. In addition, there were more males exhibiting poor self-efficacy. The relationship among gender, self-efficacy, and risky sexual behavior has been explored in recent studies. Studies have shown that the young adult male is more apt to engage in risky activities when self-efficacy is low (15). Males who underestimate the skills they possess are less likely to make appropriate healthy sex decisions. Regardless of the motives, the findings of this study suggest that there is a need to consider gender specific approaches while developing HIV/AIDS preventive and sexual health literacy programs for Grenadian adolescents.

Risky sexual behavior is correlated, though minimally, with negative self-efficacy. On average, students who were not sexually active displayed a more positive self-efficacy. Thus suggesting that students who are not engaging in sexual practices are better equipped to resist peer pressure and make healthy sexual health decisions in terms of condom use intentions, attitudes, and norms. In addition, adolescents with positive self-efficacy tend to have more positive sexual behavioral outcomes, such as an affirmative condom usage. Although not statistically significant, this was indicated by a possible correlation between students with high-risk sexual behavior having a higher likelihood of having negative self-efficacy than students with low-risk sexual behavior. The data also indicated a possible correlation of condom usage with high self-efficacy and a greater likelihood of engaging in high-risk sexual behavior. Many past studies have shown that these optimistic beliefs in one's capability to negotiate safer sex practices can be the most important predictor of protective behaviors and positive outcomes (16, 17, 18).

The previously mentioned data coupled with an early sex initiation range of 13-15 years indicates the importance of incorporating more sexual health educational opportunities for all students, both sexually active and non-sexually active.

Limitations of study

Due to the use of a pilot study with only 37 students, there is much selective and information bias. External validity is limited and it is difficult to make generalizations that reflect current trends of the larger Grenadian populations. With such a small sample size, confidence intervals are wide and it is difficult to observe variance in gradients of self-efficacy and high-risk behavior. Since the current study was a cross-sectional study, no causal associations or effects of confounding variables can be determined. In addition, the dependent variable is a behavior and sole assessment of such through a questionnaire can lead to a possible overestimation of correlations. Some additional qualitative research methods should be added to future quantitative studies with a larger sample of students to raise the validity of the study findings. There are assumptions within the study of honest responses from participants, heuristic value of certain theory, and normal distribution of the data collection. In addition there are areas outside the scope of the study, which could enhance the research.

CONCLUSION

"Self-efficacy instigates the adoption, initiation, and maintenance of health-promoting behaviors" (6). The findings of the current study highlighted the importance of eliciting further research and refined current understanding of the multi-dimensional factors influencing risky sexual behavior among Grenadian adolescents. Psychosocial dynamics in addition to sexual education can greatly influence the likelihood of youth to engage in risky sexual behavior. In order to start paving a path to ameliorate the adverse effects of such behavior, it is necessary to improve sexual health literacy of among youth. This data could be used to inform the Grenadian government how to reevaluate current sexual health interventions and how to implement more evidence based interventions. By exploring the predictive values of self-efficacy on actual sexual behavior, the Ministry of Education can use better-informed educational practices to support youth in cultivating healthy self-perspective and interpersonal skills in sexual negotiation. There are currently programs to reduce HIV/AIDs cases and the negative consequences of risky sexual behavior. In 2013, Grenada Planned Parenthood launched a new manifesto, known as Vision 20-20, with a renewed focus on increasing sexual health literacy. Goals included: securing sexual and reproductive health rights; halving the unmet need of contraceptives; and making comprehensive sex education available to all. This study can possibly enhance the aims of Vision-20/20 and further stimulate and contribute to development of more successful ways of educating adolescents about HIV/AIDs and risky sexual behavior prevention.

Recommendations include a longitudinal follow-up project and implementation of new curricula. This follow up would include adolescents representative of all 22 secondary schools in grades 9, 10 and 11. An expansion of this study to include students from every

Grenadian secondary school could be very informative in providing more information about how the concept of self-efficacy can be pivotal in positive sexual health promotion activities. Furthermore, additional research should be done to explore other potential underlying motives behind sexual behaviors, norms, and intentions, such as familial dynamics, personal culture, school performance, extracurricular activities, and sexual health curriculums. Van Campen (5) demonstrated that family involvement is an important dynamic to consider in intervention with minority adolescents. Future research in Grenada should examine to what extent parent-child sexual communication and parental monitoring influences adolescent sexual risk beliefs and behaviors.

Formation of innovative curricula would include the creation of an attractive program with stimulating didactical lessons that take into account cultural nuances and gender differentiation. Because the majority of students exhibiting negative self-efficacy displayed a high likelihood in engaging in high-risk sexual behavior, one goal of the program should be to focus on increasing the student's perceived perception of making informed healthy sexual decisions. Upon designing a novel curriculum, a thorough assessment is needed to effectively address the problem at hand. The educational objectives should be clearly delineated and differentiated by sex. The program should be an attractive and dynamic program with stimulating didactical lessons and activities. With possible evidence that self-efficacy influences the likelihood to engage in risky sexual behavior, it may be necessary to examine how external factors may influence the target groups concerning healthy decision making and sexual health literacy. Koestner (19) supported this notion that long-term program implantation can be more sustainable if adolescents' self-efficacy and autonomy is considered and elevated.

REFERENCES

[1] Halcón L, Blum R, Beuhring T, Pate E, Campbell-Forrester S, Venema A. Adolescent health in the Caribbean: A regional portrait. Am J Public Health 2003;93(11):1851-7.

[2] National Infectious Disease Control Unit. Ungass report of Grenada. New York: UNAIDS, 2010. URL: http://www.unaids.org/en/dataanalysis/knowyourresponse/countryprogressreports/2010 countries/grenada_2010_country_progress_report_en.pdf.

[3] World Health Organization. Adolescent health. Geneva: WHO, 2014. URL: http://www. who.int/topics/adolescen t_health/en/.

[4] Joint United Nations programme on HIV/AIDS (UNAIDS). UNAIDS Report on the Global AIDS Epidemic 2010. Geneva: UNAIDS, 2010.

[5] Van Campen K, Romero A. How are self-efficacy and family involvement associated with less sexual risk taking among ethnic minority adolescents? Fam Relat 2012;61(4):548-58.

[6] Luszczynska A, Scholz U, Schwarzer R. The general self-efficacy scale: Multicultural validation studies. J Psychol 2005;139(5):439-57.

[7] Bandura, A. Social foundations of thought and action: A social cognitive theory. Englewood Cliffs, NJ: Prentice-Hall, 1986.

[8] Pajares F, Johnson M. Self-efficacy beliefs and the writing performance of entering high school students. Psychol Sch 1996;33:514-32.

[9] Schunk DH. Peer models and children's behavioral change. Psychol Sch 1987;22:208-23.

[10] Bandura, A. Self-efficacy. In: Ramachaudran VS, ed. Encyclopaedia of human behavior. New York: Academic Press, 1994;4:71-81.

[11] Traeen B, Kvalem I. Investigating the relationship between past contraceptive behavior, self-efficacy, and anticipated shame and guild in sexual contexts among Norwegian adolescents. J Commun Appl Soc Psychol 2007;17:19-34.
[12] Longmore M, Manning W, Giordano P, Rudolph J. Contraceptive self-efficacy: Does it influence adolescents. J Health Soc Behav 2003;44(1):45-60.
[13] Guiella G, Madise M. HIV/AIDS and sexual-risk behaviors among adolescents: Factors influencing the use of condoms in Burkina Faso. Afr J Reprod Health 2003;11(3):182-96.
[14] Kalichman S, Stein JA, Malow R, Averhart C, Devieux J, Jennings T. Predicting protected sexual behavior using Information-Motivation-Behavior Skills model among adolescent substance abusers in court ordered treatment. Psychol Health Med 2002;7:327-38.
[15] Chandler C. A study of perceived self-efficacy on sexual risk-taking behaviors in young men. Anchorage, AK: University of Alaska, ProQuest, 2008.
[16] Basen-Engquist K. Psychosocial predictors of "safer-sex" behaviors in young adults. AIDS Educ Prev 1992;4:120-34.
[17] Kasen S, Vaughn RD, Walter HJ. Self-efficacy for AIDS preventive behaviors among tenth grade students. Health Educ Q 1992:19;187-202.
[18] Wulfert E, Wan C. Condom use: A self-efficacy model. Health Psychol 1993;12:346–53.
[19] Koestner R, Jochum R, Salter N, Horberg EJ, Gaudreau P, Powers T, et al. Bolstering implementation plans for the long haul: The benefits of simultaneously boosting self-concordance or self-efficacy. Pers Soc Psychol Bull 2006;32:1547-58.

In: Public Health Yearbook 2016
Editor: Joav Merrick

ISBN: 978-1-53610-947-4

Chapter 34

RISKY SEXUAL BEHAVIORS AND MARIJUANA USE AMONG GRENADIAN ADOLESCENTS

Olufunmilola Ajala*[1,*]*, MPH, Christine Richards*[1]*, MPH, PhD, Leselle Pierre*[1]*, MSc, Nanette Hegamin*[2]*, PhD and Tessa Alexander-St Cyr*[1]*, MSc

[1]Department of Public Health and Preventative Medicine, St George's University. Grenada, West Indies
[2]Global Health Collaboratory, St Louis, Missouri, US

ABSTRACT

Adolescent risky sexual behaviors and marijuana use have been widely researched. There is, however, limited research on the association between adolescents' risky sexual behavior and marijuana use in other Caribbean countries and none in the tri-island state of Grenada. This study took the form of a secondary school data analysis of the 2013 Grenada Secondary school Drug Prevalence Survey. In this cross-sectional study, using a two stage cluster sampling method (randomization was done based on school and classroom selection), a total of 1490 Grenadian school adolescents from 17 public and private schools were surveyed. This study found there was an association between Grenadian adolescents' risky sexual behavior and Marijuana use. Adolescents who used marijuana were more likely to be sexually active, to have sex with someone other than their 'partner', to have sex with multiple partners at a time and to exchange sex for money. The association between Grenadian adolescents' risky sexual behaviors and marijuana use is consistent with that of other Caribbean states. This association is a serious public health issue in Grenada considering the health and economic impacts on the state.

Keywords: risky sexual behaviors, sex, marijuana, adolescents, public health, Grenada

---

* Correspondence: Olufunmilola Ajala, Department of Public Health and Preventive Medicine, St George's University, St George, Grenada, West Indies. E-mail: oajala@sgu.edu.

INTRODUCTION

Adolescents have a high chance of contracting sexually transmitted infections and HIV/AIDS because of substance abuse and risky sexual behaviors such as engaging in unprotected sex, early age of sex initiation, and having multiple sexual partners. Worldwide, five million young people have HIV and 40% of new STIs are among young people between 15-24 years of age (1). The issue of HIV/AIDS and STIs is important in the Caribbean because Caribbean countries have high rates of sexually transmitted disease, HIV/AIDS transmissions, and substance abuse and thirty percent of Caribbean countries' populations are made up of people between the ages of 10-24 (2).

Research studies in Caribbean countries have shown that there is a relationship between adolescents' substance use and risky sexual behaviors. A National Adolescent Health survey was done in Anguillan adolescents aged 10-18 years, examined the associations of sexual behaviors, alcohol use, and drug use among females and males and found that 40% of the adolescents used alcohol and that males initiated sexual activity at younger ages than females, and were twice as likely to have sexual intercourse and multiple partners (3). Only, 22% of the sexually active Anguillan youth less than 12 years of age reported using a condom (3). Similarly, a survey by the World Health Organization (WHO) found that only 53.3% of all sexually active adolescents reported that they always used a condom during sexual intercourse (2).

In addition to analyzing the association between early substance use and risky sexual behaviors, further studies have been done on adolescents of Antigua, Bahamas, Barbados, Dominica, and Jamaica to analyze the associations of marijuana use, alcohol use, smoking cigarettes, and early initiation of sexual intercourse (4). The Caribbean Youth Survey showed that there was a strong association between early sexual intercourse and being female. The survey also showed an association between early sexual intercourse and the consumption of large amounts of alcohol, cigarettes, and marijuana (odds ratio (OR) = 50.7) (4). Among the 16-18 year old males, the use of marijuana was strongly associated with early sexual encounters and the use of alcohol was associated with early sexual encounters among 10-15 year old males (4). The results of a cross-sectional study questionnaire completed by Bahamian adolescent students showed that more adolescent males than females participated in risky behaviors which supported the results of the Caribbean Youth (5). In addition, another cross sectional study completed by 2206 adolescents of Trinidad, showed that those who ingested large amounts of alcohol had high associations with marijuana use and engaged in unprotected sex, which is comparable with the results of the Caribbean Youth Survey (OR = 13.2) (6).

To address the association of adolescents' risky sexual behaviors and substance use, several educational interventions have been implemented in several Caribbean countries. The purpose of the educational interventions is to raise awareness and educate people about substance use and risky sexual behaviors and to promote safe sex practices. 'Focus on Youth in the Caribbean' is an example of an intervention that took place in the Bahamas, to educate adolescents about STIs, HIV/AIDS, and the proper use of condoms (7). A survey was administered to the participants of the intervention to evaluate the effectiveness of the intervention. The survey results showed that the intervention did not have a strong impact on the knowledge of youth between ages 10-15 years and suggested that the younger population were not interested in the intervention or they were not worried about contracting STIs or HIV (7). A similar survey completed by Puerto Rican participants to assess the effectiveness of an intervention showed that the participants' home environments and family structure can have an impact on how participants respond to interventions (8).

Although research has been done in the selected Caribbean countries to analyze the association between adolescents' risky sexual behaviors and substance use, there is a lack of research about the association in Grenada. In addition, the drug and sexual health policies that have been implemented in certain Caribbean countries and throughout the world have addressed the association in a way that is culturally sensitive to the people of the specific region. However, the drug and sexual health policies of Grenada have not been effective at addressing substance use and sexual health because the rate of using substances such as alcohol and marijuana remains high and the HIV and STIs rate has increased over the past ten years in Grenada (9). The purpose of the project is to assess Grenadian school adolescents' risky sexual behaviors and relate them to patterns of marijuana use.

The goal of the project is to create effective drug and sexual health policies in Grenada. The objectives of the project were to determine whether or not there was a statistically significant difference in adolescents who consume marijuana and those who do not consume marijuana when it comes to risky sexual behaviors and to identify the relationship between adolescents' risky sexual behaviors and marijuana consumption.

METHODS

For this study, a secondary data analysis of the Grenada Secondary School Drug Prevalence Survey of 2013 was conducted. A total of 1,490 Grenadian school adolescents who were enrolled in public and private Grenadian secondary schools participated in this study. Of the students participating, 537 (36%) were in grade 8, 533 (36%) in grade 10 and 420 (28%) in grade 11 (see Table 1). Ages ranged from 11 to 18 years. Seventeen public and private Grenadian schools were included in the sample size. The majority of students (97%) attended public schools. A two stage cluster sampling design was used to collect the data. The secondary schools were randomly selected to participate in the first stage. Classrooms of the schools of the selected schools were randomly sampled in the second stage. All students in the selected classrooms were administered questionnaires. The questionnaires were anonymous and participation was voluntary.

Table 1. Summary of demographic variables

	N (%)
Total Students	1490
Public school students	1447 (97.1)
Private school students	43 (2.9)
Students enrolled in 2nd form	537 (36)
Students enrolled in 4th form	533 (35.8)
Students enrolled in 5th form	420 (28.2)
Females	767 (51.7)
Males	717 (48.3)

To examine marijuana consumption in adolescents the following variables were used to describe risky sexual behaviors: 1) The use of condoms and/or contraceptives during sexual intercourse; 2) same gender sexual intercourse; 3) exchanging sex for money or drugs; 4) having two or more sexual partners; 5) had sex with someone you usually do not have sex with and 6) had sex with more than one person at a time.

Data analysis

Descriptive statistics, including means and frequency, were used to describe the population in this study. The outcome of interest is to determine how strongly associated the use of marijuana among Grenadian adolescents is with risky sexual behaviors. Multivariate statistical analysis was used. The chi-square test, odds ratio, and logistic regression analysis were used to analyze the categorical independent and dependent variables.

RESULTS

Overall, the study showed that there was an association between Grenadian adolescents' risky sexual behaviors and marijuana use (see Tables 2-4). There was a statistically significant difference among the adolescents who have consumed marijuana and the adolescents who have not consumed marijuana when it comes to risky sexual behaviors. Eighteen percent of the students who participated in the study stated that they have consumed marijuana in their lifetime and 32% of the students who participated in the study stated that they were sexually active.

The average age of students who consumed marijuana was 15 years, which is the age group for 10th grade students. Students in Grade 10 had the highest number of adolescents to state that they have consumed marijuana at least once in their lifetime and students in Grade 10 also had the highest number of adolescents who stated that they were sexually active. Students in Grade 8 had the lowest amount of adolescents who stated that they were sexually active and the lowest amount of adolescents who stated that they have consumed marijuana in their lifetime.

Adolescents who consumed marijuana were 3.6 times more likely to be sexually active, 3.08 times more likely to have had sex with someone that they usually do not have sex with, twice more likely to have sex with more than one person at a time, and 5.11 times more likely to have exchanged sex for money or drugs.

Gender, grade level of education, and marijuana consumption were significant to whether or not an adolescent engaged in risky sexual behaviors. Accounting for gender, age, and form level of education, adolescents who consumed marijuana were about three times more likely to be sexually active and twice more likely to have sex with someone of the same sex. Adolescents who has consumed marijuana in their lifetime were three times more likely to have two or more sexual partners, 6.4 times more likely to have sex with more than one person at a time and approximately three times more likely to have exchanged sex for money or drugs. There were more males than females who stated that they have consumed marijuana in their lifetime and were sexually active. There were also more males than females to have engaged in sexual intercourse with more than one person at a time, to have not used a condom, and to have exchanged sex for money or drugs.

Table 2. Summary of risky sexual behaviors and marijuana use

Sexual Health Risk Behavior	Consumed Marijuana		Chi-square	p-value
	Yes N (%)	No N (%)		
Sexually active			74.123	<0.001
Yes	120 (33.1%)	243 (66.9%)		
No	96 (11.9%)	709 (88.1%)		
Had sex with someone you usually do not have sex with			46.979	<0.001
Yes	88 (37.6%)	146 (62.4%)		
No	117 (16.4%)	598 (83.6%)		
Condom use			11.755	0.001
Yes	46 (26.4%)	128 (73.6%)		
No	69 (32.7%)	142 (67.3%)		
Exchanged sexual intercourse			35.645	0.001
for money or drugs	23 (54.8%)	19 (45.2%)		
Yes	224 (19.2%)	945 (80.2%)		
No				
Number of sexual partner			0.623	0.430
1	113 (29.2%)	274 (70.8%)		
2+	38 (33%)	77 (67%)		
Had sex with more than one			2.598	0.107
person at a time	31 (37.8%)	51 (62.2%)		
Yes	147 (29%)	360 (71%)		
No				

Table 3. Summary of sexual health risk behaviors by gender

Sexual Health Risk Behavior	Male N (%)	Female N (%)	Chi-square	p-value
Sexually active			51.71	<0.001
Yes	258 (61.5)	161(38)		
No	350 (40)	520 (59.7)		
Had sex with more than one			36.552	<0.001
person at a time	91 (90)	10 (8)		
Yes	341 (58.7)	240 (41.3)		
No				
Exchanged sex for money or			11.810	<0.001
goods	37 (72.5)	14 (27.4)		
Yes	603 (48)	653 (51.9)		
No				
Always use a condom			120.161	<0.001
Yes	137 (65.5)	72 (34.4)		
No	152 (61.7)	94 (38.2)		
Consumed marijuana			17.374	<0.001
Yes	135 (56.7)	103 (43.2)		
No	442 (41.8)	614 (58.1)		
Number of sexual partners			31.144	<0.001
1	233 (53.8)	200 (46.2)		
2+	116 (80)	29 (20)		

Table 4. Summary of sexual risk behaviors by grade level

Sexual Health Risk Behavior	Grade 8 N (%)	Grade 10 N (%)	Grade 11 N (%)	Chi- square	p-value
Sexually active				50.38	<0.001
Yes	96 (23)	176 (42)	148 (35)		
No	377 (43)	275 (31)	222 (25)		
Sex with more than one person at a time				2.538	0.04
Yes	28 (28)	45 (45)	28 (28)		
No	155 (27)	221 (38)	207 (36)		
Exchanged sex for money or				3.162	0.02
goods	14 (26)	24 (45)	15 (28)		
Yes	465 (37)	437 (35)	358 (28)		
No					
Always use a condom				22.01	<0.001
Yes	70 (33)	83 (40)	57 (27)		
No	84 (34)	80 (32)	84 (34)		
Consumed marijuana				43.02	<0.001
Yes	41 (17)	106 (44)	92 (38)		
No	420 (40)	343 (33)	297 (28)		
Number of sexual partners				4.196	0.002
1	121 (28)	153 (35)	160 (37)		
2+	45 (31)	60 (41)	40 (28)		

Analysis of current Grenadian policies

Grenada has followed guidance set by WHO, PAHO and other health organizations in formulating policies relating to the use of marijuana, alcohol and other drugs as well as policies on sexual health. Some of these policies will be now be analyzed.

Grenadian secondary school's drug policies

According to the Ministry of Education, the two main drug policies that are implemented in primary and secondary Grenadian schools are The Drug Prevention and Education Program and the National School Policy on Drugs. According to the document that describes the National School Policy on Drugs, the policy is implemented to provide assistance to students who are affected by drug consumption, to protect students against the harmful effects of drugs, to guide and encourage students to reduce drug consumption, and provides an alternative disciplinary action other than law enforcement for students who are caught with drugs (10). The program's goal is to give the student a opportunity to correct himself or herself by providing education, counseling, drug rehabilitation, and other helpful resources. The document that describes the National School Policy on Drugs does not address drug prevention and resistance in schools.

The Drug Prevention and Education Program is a component of the Health and Family Life Education (HFLE) program (11). The HFLE program is delivered through classes that are incorporated into primary and secondary schools' curriculums to educate students about health and fitness, the environment, sexuality, and relationships. According to the policy document, the drug prevention and education program is implemented and taught in secondary schools' health classes and social studies classes. The prevention program teaches students about the ways substances can affect the heart, nervous system, brain, and development. The prevention program does not teach students about the influence of drugs on risky sexual behaviors.

Sexual health policy in Grenadian secondary schools

The topic of sexual health is discussed in the HFLE program. According to the HFLE curriculum, sexual health is taught by health teachers and social studies teachers and educates students about sexual identity, personal hygiene, puberty, and interpersonal relationships. The program also educates and encourages abstinence from sexual intercourse. The curriculum does not discuss contraception, risky sexual behaviors, or the association of drugs, such as marijuana, with risky sexual behaviors.

Sexual health policies within the Ministry of Health

According to Grenada's law, the legal age to consent to sexual intercourse is 16 years. However, the legal age of adulthood in Grenada is 18 years of age. According to Grenada's law, healthcare providers can refuse service or resources, such as contraception, to adolescents who are under 18 years of age if they are not accompanied by an adult. There is not a policy to address confidentiality of the patient regardless of his or her age.

The Ministry of Health offers a program that focuses on prevention of HIV/AIDS. According to policy document of the program, the program's target audience includes sex workers, gay men, and HIV positive individuals. Notably, the audience of the program is not secondary school students. The program hosts educational courses, counseling, and contraception at medical clinics. However, individuals must inquire about the information. The program does not have a partnership with any Grenadian secondary schools.

Grenada's Planned Parenthood Association (GPPA) sexual health policy

Grenada's Planned Parenthood Association (GPPA) Grenada's Planned Parenthood Association (GPPA) is a non-government organization that provides sexual health information and education, pap smears, pregnancy tests, condoms, and contraceptives to people who inquire about it (12). According to GPPA's written policy, GPPA does not refuse service to anyone and is available to everyone in Grenada. Although GPPA provides sexual health counseling and education, GPPA cannot provide sexual health education and sexual health presentations to primary and secondary schools unless the school invites or inquiries about GPPA's services. The only school in Grenada that GPPA has been invited to and provides sexual health education to is the Program for Adolescent Mothers (PAM). Adolescents who are enrolled in PAM are young mothers who have already experienced sexual intercourse. GPPA provides contraceptives and sexual health exams to the young women. However, the sexual health education and prevention aspects of the service may not be very effective to these women because they have already experienced sexual intercourse and are mothers.

Discussion

Overall, prevention is not the priority of the current Grenadian drug programs and sexual health education programs in Grenadian schools and through-out the Grenadian community. Non-government organizations (NGOs), the Ministry of Education, and the Ministry of Health should collaborate together and with the Grenadian community to form sexual health education programs within secondary schools and within the community. The group collaboration may enable sexual health to be more openly discussed among adolescents and adults. Such an initiative can help decrease the negative stigma or perception of sexual health education, so that adolescents who inquire about contraceptives and sexual health education may not be perceived in a negative way. NGOs and sexual health education programs should use the media, such as television advertisements, newspapers, and magazines, to encourage the Grenadian secondary students to about sexual health education and available resources. The media, NGOs, Ministry of Education, Ministry of Health, and drug enforcement officials can emphasize the association of marijuana consumption and risky sexual behaviors in secondary schools and throughout the Grenadian community.

The sexual health education programs and drug prevention programs within the Health and Family Life Education Programs of school curriculums should be expanded. School curriculums should include classes that are dedicated only to the topics of sexual health education and drug abuse and prevention education. The sexual health education courses in schools should teach students about available contraception and the relationship that marijuana consumption has with sexual behaviors. The educational courses should discuss and encourage prevention and safe sex practices in the courses. The program can also be extended to the co-curriculum through which school-based groups and clubs can focus on sexual health and marijuana consumption as a form of peer education initiative.

Policy Recommendations

1) No healthcare professional in Grenada should refuse service to adolescents under age 18. Pharmacies, hospitals, medical clinics, and non-government organizations should keep adolescents' information confidential, educate adolescents about risky sexual behaviors and drug use, prevention, and provide service to all adolescents regardless of age.
2) Sexual health courses and drug prevention courses should be taught by health teachers. The first half of the semester should discuss the core topics of the family and life education program and the second half of the semester should discuss only sexual health and drug prevention and resistance.

3) Sexual health counseling service, similar to the current drug abuse and resistance counseling, should be made available to secondary school students.
4) The current drug resistance and prevention programs should emphasize and teach students about the association of drugs, specifically marijuana, with risky sexual behaviors. In addition to discussing drug prevention, the program should discuss that marijuana consumption can be a factor in whether or not an adolescent engages in risky sexual behaviors and that risky sexual behaviors can cause STIs and unplanned pregnancies. Sexual health behaviors should be discussed as a topic in the drug resistance and prevention program.

CONCLUSION

The association among Grenadian adolescents' risky sexual behaviors and marijuana consumption is similar to the association between risky sexual behaviors and marijuana consumption among other Caribbean adolescents. In addition, the majority of new STD cases are diagnosed in adolescents. The association between Grenadian adolescents' risky sexual behaviors and marijuana is a public health issue in Grenada because of the consequences of adolescents' risky sexual behaviors and marijuana consumption such as unplanned pregnancies. These pregnancies along with drug rehabilitation, and burden of disease related to STDs can increase health care expenses of the Grenadian government. The Grenadian government has a limited budget, so preventable health issues should be addressed in Grenadian schools and the community. Overall, the results of the study will benefit all Grenadians as they will be informed about the prevalence and association of risky sexual behaviors and marijuana consumption that exists in Grenada. The information can improve current policies and help create new interventions to target the Grenadian secondary school adolescents.

REFERENCES

[1] Konings M, Henquet C, Maharajh H, Hutchinson G, Van Os J. Early exposure to cannabis and risk for psychosis in young adolescents in Trinidad. Acta Psychiatr Scand 2008;118(3):209-13.

[2] Ohene S, Ireland M, Blum, R. The clustering of risk behaviors among Caribbean youth. Matern Child Health J 2005; 9(1):91-100.

[3] Kurtz S, Douglas K, Lugo Y. Sexual risks and concerns about AIDS among adolescents in Anguilla. AIDS Care 2005;17S:36-44.

[4] Latimer, W, Rojas, V, Mancha, B. Severity of alcohol use and problem behaviors among school-based youths in Puerto Rico. Rev Panam Salud Publica 2008;23(5): 325-32.

[5] Pinder-Butler S, Frankson M., Hanna-Mahase C, Roberts R. HIV/AIDS knowledge and sexual behaviour among junior high school students in New Providence, Bahamas. West Indian Med J 2013;62(4):318-22.

[6] Katz CM, Fox A. Risk and protective factors associated with gang involved youth in a Caribbean nation: Analysis of the Trinidad and Tobago Youth Survey. Rev Panam Salud Publica 2010;27(3):187-202.

[7] Wang B, Stanton B, Chen X, Li X, Dinaj-Koci V, Brathwaite N, Lunn S. Predictors of responsiveness among early adolescents to a school-based risk reduction intervention over 3 years. AIDS Behav 2013;17(3):1096-1104.

[8] Velez-Pastrana MC, Gonzalez-Rodriguez RA, Borges-Hernandez A. Family functioning and early onset of sexual intercourse in Latino adolescents. Adolesc 2005;40(160):777-91.
[9] Rutledge S, Abell N, Padmore J, McCann T. AIDS stigma in health services in the Eastern Caribbean. Sociol Health Illn 2009:31(1):17-34.
[10] Government of Grenada. Policy on drugs, 2012. URL: www.gov.gd/egov/pdf/ncodc/docs/national_school_policy_drugs.pdf.
[11] Grenada Ministry of Education. Health and family education curriculum: Curriculum development. St George's, WI: Government of Grenada, 2013.
[12] International Planned Parenthood Federation. Grenada Planned Parenthood Association. URL://www.ippf.org/our-work/where-we-work/western-hemisphere/grenada.

SECTION FOUR - PUBLIC HEALTH ISSUES

In: Public Health Yearbook 2016
Editor: Joav Merrick
ISBN: 978-1-53610-947-4

Chapter 35

Universal Newborn Hearing Screening in the United States

Shibani Kanungo[1,*], MD, MPH and Dilip R Patel[2], MD, MBA
[1]Metabolic Genetics and Newborn Screening, Geisinger Health System, Danville, Pennsylvania, US
[2]Department of Pediatric and Adolescent Medicine, Western Michigan University Homer Stryker MD School of Medicine, Kalamazoo, Michigan, US

Abstract

Hearing impairment or loss can be defined by the partial or total inability to hear sounds experienced in the environment, represent a wide spectrum of disease due to congenital or acquired causes and seen with various developmental disorders requiring early intervention services for optimal health outcomes. Early detection to decrease morbidity and prevent life-long disability was the principle of newborn screening adapted to Universal Newborn Hearing Screening. We explore how Universal Newborn Screening evolved, from history to epidemiology, from policy to shaping of a public health program and from cost benefits of current universal screening to possible next steps in decreasing morbidity and preventing lifelong disability nationally and internationally.

Keywords: newborn hearing screening, hearing loss, public health

Introduction

Hearing impairment or loss is the partial or total inability to hear sounds experienced in the environment. According to the World Health Organization (WHO), there are approximately 360 million people worldwide with hearing impairment (1). Hearing impairment is a diagnosis encompassing a wide spectrum of presentations and disease processes, a vital

* Correspondence: Shibani Kanungo, MD, MPH, Metabolic Genetics and Newborn Screening, Geisinger Health System, Danville, 100 North Academy Avenue, PA 17822, United States. E-mail: skanungo@geisinger.edu.

impact on human development, a major public health concern, a battleground for cultural identity and the conception of health, and a research field rich with ongoing questions. Hearing loss can be further differentiated into conductive and sensorineural hearing loss (SNHL) and can be unilateral or bilateral or differentiated by different risk factors (2). Auditory anatomical and physiological shaping begins early in embryologic development and is refined throughout early childhood, which has important implications for possible congenital and acquired hearing impairment resulting from toxic exposures to underlying genetic defects. The epidemiology of newborn hearing loss along with the ease of available technology was instrumental in the development of "Universal newborn hearing screening" (UNHS) programs in the US and worldwide. Discussion about UNHS in the United States is incomplete without understanding the history and evolution as a public health program with active participation of all stake holders–parents, specialists, professional societies and the government.

EPIDEMIOLOGY

Best evidence on national prevalence of newborn hearing loss is noted in the MMWR 2010 report (3) with CDC (Center for Disease Control and Prevention analysis of EHDI (Early hearing detection and intervention) surveillance data in United States from 1999-2007; geared to determine the status of efforts to identify newborns and infants with hearing loss. Though, data until 2005 was passively reported to CDC, 2005-2007 CDC-EHDI active data collection did not demonstrate a huge difference between prevalence of newborn hearing loss – 1.1 versus 1.2 per 1,000 screened; even though the percentage of infants screened increased from 46.5% in 1999 to 97% in 2007 and the number of States reporting increased from nine States and territories to 44 States and territories. In January 2000, Statement of the American College of Medical Genetics on Universal Newborn Hearing Screening noted that hearing loss is present at birth in 1-2 per 1,000 infants (4). The CDC-EHDI prevalence data in the US is similar to public and private institution reports in different European countries/regions, but there seems to be reports of higher prevalence of newborn hearing loss reported from developing countries as noted in Table 1.

Table 1. Prevalence of hearing loss

Country	Prevalence	Author	Published year	Pubmed reference
United Kingdom	1.8 per 1000	Watkin et al. (5)	2012	22686437
Switzerland	1.2 per 1000	Metzger-Müller et al. (6)	2013	24338080
Ireland	1.3 per 1,000	O'connor etal (7)	2013	23456183
Israel	1.3 per 1,000	Gilbey et al. (8)	2013	23122541
Belgium	1.5 per 1000	Van Kerschaver et al. (9)	2013	22452806
Turkey	2.2 per 1000	Tasci et al. (10)	2010	20015280
Brazil	0.96 per 1000	Bevilacqua et al. (11)	2010	20303604
Brazil	2 per 1000	Oliviera et al. (12)	2013	24142311
UAE	2.6 per 1000	Ur Rehman et al. (13)	2012	23301401
India	8 per 1000	Rai et al. (14)	2013	23642585

THE HISTORY OF UNIVERSAL NEWBORN HEARING SCREENS (UNHS) IN THE UNITED STATES

The history of Newborn Screening for any disorder is incomplete without mentioning Dr. Robert Guthrie's (1916-1995) work establishing PKU (phenylketon-uria) screening in 1960s as a public health program initiative in the State of Massachusetts. Though, around the same time as initial PKU screening, a varied range of efforts by different disciplines towards early detection, diagnosis and intervention for hearing loss were in the works Downs et al. (15, 16) and, initial hospital based screening for hearing loss took place as early as 1970s. By the late 1980s, Dr. C. Everett Koop (1916-2013), then US Surgeon General, pioneered that detection of hearing loss to be included in the Healthy People 2000 goals for the nation (17).

In 1988, the Maternal and Child Health Bureau (MCHB), a division of the US Health Resources and Services Administration (HRSA), funded pilot projects in Rhode Island, Utah, and Hawaii to test the feasibility of a universal statewide screening program to screen newborn infants for hearing loss before hospital discharge (18). Wide spread practice of hospital based screening did not occur until after the 1993 NIH Consensus Development Conference on Early Identification of Hearing Impairment in Infants and Young Children that recommended that all newborn infants be screened for hearing shortly after birth (19).

O March 18, 1999, Congressman James Walsh (R, NY) introduced the Newborn Infant and Hearing Screening and Intervention Act of 1999 (20). In May, 1999, Senator Olympia Snowe (R, ME) introduced the companion bill in the Senate. At the end of the legislative session, federal appropriations committees in both the House and Senate earmarked new funding for newborn hearing screening. The language was included in the Omnibus Appropriations bill President Clinton signed in November, 1999. This landmark federal legislation 'Newborn and Infant Hearing Screening Intervention Act of 1999' enacted by the federal government provided funding to states from the Health Resources and Services Administration and the Centers for Disease Control and Prevention to support the infrastructure required for planning, development, implementation, and refinement of early hearing detection and intervention (EHDI) programs and for EHDI tracking and data management systems. Universal Newborn Hearing Screening as an essential component of early detection and intervention for infants with hearing loss was adopted after support from multiple professional societies, advocacy groups, and government agencies participating in the Joint Committee on Infant Hearing (JCIH) (21, 22).

In 2007, the Joint Committee on Infant Hearing (JCIH) endorsed early detection of and intervention for infants with hearing loss through integrated, interdisciplinary community, state, and federal systems of universal newborn hearing screening, evaluation, and family-centered intervention (23). The goal of EHDI was determined to maximize linguistic and communicative competence and literacy development for children who are deaf or hard of hearing. The updated 2007 JCIH position statement delineated specifics addressing:

- Definition of targeted hearing loss;
- Hearing-screening and -rescreening protocols - separate protocols recommended for NICU and well-infant nurseries;
- Diagnostic audiology evaluation by Audi-ologists with skills and expertise in evaluating newborn and young infants and including ABR testing;

- Medical evaluation including genetics and otolaryngology consultation for every confirmed hearing loss;
- Early intervention service establishment;
- Surveillance and screening in the medical home;
- Communication between the birth hospital, State and parents;
- Information infrastructure for data manage-ment and outcome tracking.

The national resource for EHDI at the National Center for Hearing Assessment and Management (NCHAM) provides timeline, summary and details of each State specific mandates and enacted Newborn Hearing Screen legislation (24).

After 10 years of being introduced as a legislation, in December 2010, the United States Senate and the House of Representatives each voted to approve the Early Hearing Detection and Intervention Act of 2010 (HR. 1246, S. 3199). President Obama signed the legislation into law on December 22nd 2010 (25, 26).

The Early Hearing Detection and Intervention Act of 2010 amends the Public Health Service Act to: 1) expand the newborn and infant hearing loss program to include diagnostic services among the services provided and 2) require the Secretary of Health and Human Services (HHS), acting through the Administrator of the Health Resources and Services Administration, to assist in the recruitment, retention, education, and training of qualified personnel and health care providers to implement the program.

It revised program purposes to include: 1) developing and monitoring the efficacy of statewide programs and systems for hearing screening of newborns and infants, prompt evaluation and diagnosis of children referred from screening programs, and appropriate education, audiological, and medical interventions for children identified with hearing loss; 2) developing efficient models to ensure that newborns and infants who are identified with a hearing loss through screening receive follow-up by a qualified healthcare provider and 3) ensuring an adequate supply of qualified personnel to meet the screening, evaluation, and early intervention needs of children.

It amended the definition of "early intervention" to require that families be given the opportunity to obtain the full range of appropriate early intervention services, educational and program placements, and other options for their child from highly qualified providers.

It requires the Secretary to establish a postdoctoral fellowship program to foster research and development in the area of early hearing detection and intervention.

The 2013 supplement to the recommendations in the year 2007 position statement of the Joint Committee on Infant Hearing (JCIH) provides comprehensive best practices guidelines for early hearing detection and intervention (EHDI) programs on establishing strong early intervention (EI) systems with appropriate expertise to meet the needs of children who are deaf or hard of hearing (D/HH) (27).

COST BENEFIT

The varying disease burden in different parts of the world as noted under 'Epidemiology of newborn hearing loss', along with more recent data suggesting need of targeted surveillance in at-risk children who pass the hearing screen (5, 28) or school entry hearing screening as in the United Kingdom (29) requires us to take into consideration of cost benefit of universal hearing screen and its implementation as a public health program across the world. We know that implementation of any public health program includes a cost- benefit analysis of a proposed project – a process by which the costs of a program to proposed benefits to the individual and society is taken into consideration. Often such calculations are based on available literature as evidence or conducted prospectively taking outcome measures into consideration.

There is a paucity of comprehensive long term data in form of randomized control trials, or observational parallel cohorts or epidemiological evidence that takes into consideration at all probable variables and outcomes. In general, cost of universal newborn hearing screening (UNHS) include capital (cost of equipment) and operating expenses (costs for disposables and personnel), as well expenses for follow-up (diagnostic testing costs) and early intervention programs and services. Taking into consideration various model assumptions, it was shown that even though initially, the costs of UNHS exceed its benefits; but there are short term and long term reaching a maximum annual benefit of seven billion dollars 75 years after initiation of the program, which also results in the societal benefit for all years thereafter (30).

Short term cost benefits analysis projects the benefit of improved language reduced the lifetime costs associated with deafness by approximately $430 000 per deaf individual (31). Long-term benefits, both individual and societal are yet to be predetermined conclusively and understandably difficult to estimate with accuracy. With varying prevalence of newborn hearing loss in different parts of the world, the cost-effectiveness of universal newborn hearing screening (UNHS) in United Kingdom was compared to selective screening of newborns with risk factors in India (32) and demonstrated that the cost-effectiveness of a screening intervention was largely dependent upon two key factors: the cost (per patient) of the intervention drives the model substantially, with higher costs leading to higher cost-effectiveness ratios and the baseline prevalence (risk) of hearing impairment. Though, the economic limitations of developing countries or regions may warrant implementation of 'at-risk' or targeted newborn hearing loss screening more feasible than UNHS (33, 34). There are also suggested values in adding bloodspot-based genetic testing of common mutations as second tier testing for bedside newborn hearing screening (35).

CONCLUSION

Universal newborn hearing screening helps with early diagnosis and intervention of hearing impairment - a complex and multi-faceted public health concern that can have long-term impacts on health, education, and quality of life outcomes in a child and a future generation. There may be a paradigm shift requiring a second phase to UNHS with pre-school based screening to improve long term educational and quality of life outcomes. Lifetime costs associated with hearing loss per child/disabled adult far outweighs costs of UNHS or early childhood screening.

ACKNOWLEDGMENTS

This paper is an updated and revised version of an earlier publication.

REFERENCES

[1] World Health Organization. Deafness and hearing loss fact sheet, 2013. URL: http://www.who.int/mediacentre/factsheets/fs300/en/.

[2] Chung P, Kanungo S, Patel DR. Hearing impairment, In: Rubin IL, Merrick J, Greydanus DE, Patel DR, eds. Rubin and Crocker health care for people with intellectual and developmental disabilities across the lifespan, Dordrecht: Springer, 2015, in press.

[3] Gaffney M, Eichwald J, Grosse SD, Mason CA. Identifying infants with hearing loss, United States, 1999-2007. MMWR 2010;59(08):220-3.

[4] American College of Medical Genetics (ACMG). Statement of the American College of Medical Genetics on universal newborn hearing screening. Genet Med 2000;2:149-50.

[5] Watkin P, Baldwin M. The longitudinal follow up of a universal neonatal hearing screen: the implications for confirming deafness in childhood. Int J Audiol 2012;51(7):519-28.

[6] Metzger D, Pezier TF, Veraguth D. Evaluation of universal newborn hearing screening in Switzerland 2012 and follow-up data for Zurich. Swiss Med Wkly 2013;143:w13905. Doi: 10.4414/smw. 2013.13905.

[7] O'Connor A, O'Sullivan PG, Behan L, Norman G, Murphy B. Initial results from the newborn hearing screening programme in Ireland. Ir J Med Sci 2013; 182(4):551-6.

[8] Gilbey P, Kraus C, Ghanayim R, Sharabi-Nov A, Bretler S. Universal newborn hearing screening in Zefat, Israel: the first two years. Int J Pediatr Otorhinolaryngol 2013;77(1):97-100.

[9] Van Kerschaver E, Boudewyns AN, Declau F, Van de Heyning PH, Wuyts FL. Socio-demographic determinants of hearing impairment studied in 103,835 term babies. Eur J Public Health 2013; 23(1):55-60.

[10] Tasci Y, Muderris II, Erkaya S, Altinbas S, Yucel H, Haberal A. Newborn hearing screening programme outcomes in a research hospital from Turkey. Child Care Health Dev 2010;36(3):317-22.

[11] Bevilacqua MC, Alvarenga Kde F, Costa OA, Moret al.. The universal newborn hearing screening in Brazil: from identification to intervention. Int J Pediatr Otorhinolaryngol 2010;74(5):510-5.

[12] Oliveira JS, Rodrigues LB, Aur?lio FS, Silva VB. Risk factors and prevalence of newborn hearing loss in a private health care system of Porto Velho, Northern Brazil. Rev Paul Pediatr 2013;31(3):299-305.

[13] Ur Rehman M, Mando K, Rahmani A, Imran A, Ur Rehman N, Gowda K, Chedid F. Screening for neonatal hearing loss in the Eastern region of United Arab Emirates. East Mediterr Health J 2012; 18(12):1254-6.

[14] Rai N, Thakur N. Universal screening of newborns to detect hearing impairment—Is it necessary? Int J Pediatr Otorhinolaryngol 2013; 77(6):1036-41.

[15] Downs MP, Sterritt GM. Identification audiometry for neonates: a preliminary report. J Audiol Res 1964;4:69–80.

[16] Downs MP, Sterritt GM. A guide to newborn and infant hearing screening programs. Arch Otolaryngol 1967; 85(1):15-22.

[17] US Department of Health and Human Services, Office of Disease Prevention and Health Promotion. Healthy People 2000: National Health Promotion and Disease Prevention Objectives. Washington, DC: US Government Printing Office, 1991.

[18] Forsman I. Universal newborn hearing screening, 2006. URL: http://www.infanthearing.org/ncham/presentation s/2006amchpmeetig.pdf

[19] NIH Consensus Statement. Early identification of hearing impairment in infants and young children. NIH Consensus Statement 1993;11:1–24.

[20] H.R.1193 (106th). URL: https://www.govtrack.us/con gress/bills/106/hr1193.

[21] Joint Committee on Infant Hearing; American Academy of Audiology, American Academy of Pediatrics, American Speech-Language-Hearing Association, Directors of Speech and Hearing Programs in State Health and Welfare Agencies. Year 2000 position statement: principles and guidelines for early hearing detection and intervention programs. Pediatrics 2000; 106:798–817.
[22] American Academy of Pediatrics, Joint Committee on Infant Hearing. Year 2007 position statement: principles and guidelines for early hearing detection and intervention programs. Pediatrics 2007;120(4):898–921.
[23] Joint Committee on Infant Hearing. Supplement to the JCIH 2007 position statement: Principles and guidelines for early intervention after confirmation that a child is deaf or hard of hearing. Pediatrics 2013;131(4):e1324-49.
[24] National Center for Hearing Assessment and Management (NCHAM), Utah State University. URL: http://www.infanthearing.org/legislative/mandates.html.
[25] Govtrack.us. Early Hearing Detection and Intervention Act, 2010. URL: https://www.govtrack.us/congress/bills/111/s3199.
[26] Committee on Energy and Commerce. The Early Hearing Detection and Intervention Act, 2010. URL: http://democrats.energycommerce.house.gov/index.php?q=bill/s-3199-the-early-hearing-detection-and-intervention-act-of-2010.
[27] American Academy of Pediatrics. Statement of endorsement. Supplement to the JCIH 2007 Position Statement: Principles and guidelines for early intervention after confirmation that a child is deaf or hard of hearing. Pediatrics 2013 Mar 25. Doi: 10.1542/peds.2013-0008.
[28] Wood SA, Davis AC, Sutton GJ. Effectiveness of targeted surveillance to identify moderate to profound permanent childhood hearing impairment in babies with risk factors who pass newborn screening. Int J Audiol 2013;52(6):394-9.
[29] Bristow K1, Fortnum H, Fonseca S, Bamford J. United Kingdom school-entry hearing screening: current practice; Arch Dis Child 2008;93(3):232-5.
[30] Gorga MP, Neely ST. Cost-effectiveness and test-performance factors in relation to universal newborn hearing screening. Ment Retard Dev Disabil Res Rev 2003;9(2):103-8.
[31] Keren R, Helfand M, Homer C, McPhillips H, Lieu TA. Projected cost-effectiveness of statewide universal newborn hearing screening. Pediatrics 2002;110 (5): 855-64.
[32] Burke MJ, Shenton RC, Taylor MJ. The economics of screening infants at risk of hearing impairment: an international analysis. Int J Pediatr Otorhinolaryngol 2012;76(2):212-8.
[33] Huang LH, Zhang L, Tobe RY, Qi FH, Sun L, Teng Y, et al.. Cost-effectiveness analysis of neonatal hearing screening program in China: should universal screening be prioritized? BMC Health Serv Res 2012;12:97.
[34] Rai N, Thakur N. Universal screening of newborns to detect hearing impairment—Is it necessary? Int J Pediatr Otorhinolaryngol 2013;77(6):1036-41.
[35] Schimmenti LA, Warman B, Schleiss MR, Daly KA, Ross JA, McCann M, Jurek AM, Berry SA. Evaluation of newborn screening bloodspot-based genetic testing as second tier screen for bedside newborn hearing screening. Genet Med 2011;13(12):1006-10.

In: Public Health Yearbook 2016
Editor: Joav Merrick

ISBN: 978-1-53610-947-4

Chapter 36

PUBLIC HEALTH ASPECTS OF SUICIDE IN CHILDREN AND ADOLESCENTS

Ahsan Nazeer**, MD
Department of Psychiatry, Western Michigan University,
Homer Stryker MD School of Medicine, Kalamazoo, Michigan, US

ABSTRACT

Suicide in children and adolescents is a complex and devastating problem for families and society both nationally and internationally. This review considers various aspects of this phenomenon including its epidemiology, risk factors, protective factors, issues of prevention, and management. Risk factors for suicide have been reviewed including personal characteristics, psychopathology of those committing suicide, history of previous suicide attempts, sexual orientation, familial factors, and access to lethal means of suicide. Protective factors include social support and religion. Principles of prevention have been considered including school-based programs, screening tools, skills training, Gatekeeper training, community-based programs, and health-care programs. Management includes principles involved in management before and after self-harm. Also considered are family therapies and therapies aimed at specific problems such as depression, bullying, substance abuse, and others. Clinicians should be actively involved with their communities to seek prevention of suicide in children and adolescents.

Keywords: childhood, adolescence, suicide, public health

INTRODUCTION

Child and adolescent suicide is a complex global public health problem that has intrigued researchers, academicians and policy makers for decades. Suicide is one of the leading causes

* Correspondence: Ahsan Nazeer, Department of Psychiatry, Western Michigan University Homer Stryker MD School of Medicine, 1717 Shaffer Road, Suite 101, Kalamazoo, MI 49048, United States. E-mail: ahsan.nazeer@med.wmich.edu.

of death; an estimated 30,000 people in the United States and 1 million people worldwide die of suicide. Global suicide rates have increased drastically, and lost U.S. productivity due to suicide is now estimated at $12 billion per year. The World Health Organization and United States (US) government have taken numerous steps toward establishing policies and prevention strategies, including calls for expanded collection of suicide data. Suicide also is one of the major causes of death in the adolescent population.

Despite the fact that progress has been made in our understanding of risk factors for suicide, it remains a major global medical burden. Among the 4 million suicide attempts yearly, about 90,000 adolescents succeed, averaging one successful attempt every 5 minutes; the cumulative result is that suicide is the 5th leading cause of adolescent death worldwide. In the following review, we will examine the current research on prevalence, risk factors and prevention strategies.

EPIDEMIOLOGY

The U.S. adolescent suicide rate gradually increased during the 20th century, becoming more marked during the 1960s and reaching an overall peak in the 1990s, although there have been other significant peaks and troughs. Although adolescent suicide rates stabilized during the late 1990s, they had increased by 250% between 1960 and 1980 and doubled between 1960 and 2001. Since the late 1990s, the suicide rate has declined, reaching a 30-year low in 2003 (1). Numerous explanations for this reduction have been put forth, including earlier identification of at-risk teens, better and more focused delivery of mental health services to families in need and increased use of antidepressants. Unfortunately, this overall epidemiological trend shifted between 2000 and 2005, with a 14% increase in youth suicide during these years. This shift may have been due to reduced antidepressant prescribing amid the public health outcry and "black box" warnings regarding the association of antidepressant use with emergence of suicidal ideation.

The US Centers for Disease Control (CDC) recently published the National Suicide Statistics, with data updated to cover 2009, the latest year for which these numbers are available. According to the CDC, suicide rates declined in both sexes for the 1991-2000-time period but were consistently higher for 2001-2009. The CDC data also identifies numerous disturbing trends, including a 233% increase in suffocation suicide rates among females 10-24 years old. On the other hand, firearm suicide rates in females aged 10 to 24 years decreased from 1993 through 2007, while poisoning remained relatively constant at 0.48 suicides per 100,000 from 2002 to 2009. During 2005-2009, use of a firearm (29.7%) was the preferred mode of suicide among 10-24 year-old males, but suffocation (48.5%) was more common among the equivalent female cohort. For the same group, firearms and suffocations caused the largest number of fatal self-injuries, while poisoning and cutting caused the fewest.

Demographically, group differences between males and females do not exist until mid-to-late adolescence (15-19 years), at which time the rate of suicide among males increases dramatically. During 2005-2009, the highest suicide rates were among American Indian/Alaskan Natives and Non-Hispanic Whites. Suffocation was the preferred method of suicide among American Indian/Alaskan Natives while Non-Hispanic Whites preferred firearms. Asian/Pacific Islanders had the lowest suicide rates among males, while Non-Hispanic Blacks had the lowest rates among females. In 2009, more female high school students planned (13% vs 8%) and attempted (8% vs 4%) suicide, as compared to their male peers (2).

Global suicide rates

Nationally recorded data on child and adolescent suicide must be interpreted with caution, as there are differences in data reporting among different nations. In many cultures, suicide in adolescents is usually under-reported, due to the desire to protect families from the stigma of suicide and to avoid any future social repercussions. Another reason to be cautious in comparing data is that different studies use different questionnaires to assess suicidality; the resultant variability in results may be due to measurement bias. A few recent studies, including the WHO/EURO Multicenter Study on Parasuicide and the WHO Multisite Intervention Study, have used standardized measures to overcome this bias.

Because of the above-mentioned inconsistencies, global figures for teen suicide vary, but it continues to be the 2nd leading cause of death, after motor vehicle accidents (MVA). Worldwide, suicide is the 3rd leading cause of death among adolescent males, after violence and MVA; it is the leading cause of death among adolescent females. Rates are highest in Eastern Europe and the Russian Federation and lowest in Central and South America. The male-to-female ratio continues to range from 3:1 to 7:1, except in India and China, where no differences are found between genders.

Suicide in young children

Suicide in children younger than 10 years of age is considered to be a rare phenomenon. Scientific literature has reported suicidal ideation in children as young as 5 years of age; however, this is controversial. Researchers have suggested that depression and substance abuse problems, two major risk factors for suicide in adolescents, are either rare or simply not present in very young children. Others have argued that because young children engage in concrete operational thinking and have limited problem solving abilities, they are not capable of understanding the finality of death and therefore cannot plan for a suicide attempt.

On the other hand, developmental theorists agree that the common denominator in a suicide attempt is *intent* to self-harm, regardless of the child's understanding of causality, finality and lethality of attempt. Parental absence and a family history of suicidal behavior are two factors that are associated with earlier onset of suicidal ideation in children. So far, the most consistent pattern that has emerged from the literature is that the risk of suicide increases significantly at 12 years of age and peaks at 16 years of age. In the U.S., suicide mortality rates were 1.5/100,000 for 10-14 year-olds and 8.2% for 15-19 year-olds (3).

RISK FACTORS

More than 30% of youth who commit suicide have some personality traits in common. In one study, children in the 12-14 year age range who had attempted suicide were frequently described as intelligent, socially isolated, aggressive and vulnerable to criticism. A history of impulsive aggressiveness has consistently been shown to predispose to suicidal behavior. Impulsivity by itself may lead to suicide attempts, as evidenced by the fact that many adolescents with ADHD show little planning before their attempts. Low self-esteem and hopelessness also have been associated with current and future suicidal ideation and attempts. Recent loss, interpersonal conflicts and legal issues are common precipitants for suicide in conduct-disordered youth (4).

Psychopathology

Youth with psychiatric disorders carry a 9-fold increase in suicide risk as compared to their peers. More than 90% of young suicide attempters have at least one diagnosed psychiatric disorder, and increased severity and chronicity of the disorder is strongly correlated with increased suicide risk.

Mood disorders are the most prevalent psychiatric disorders among adolescent suicide victims of both genders. The odds ratio of increased suicide risk ranges between 11 and 27 among those with a mood disorder. Among the mood disorders, depression continues to be a major precipitant for suicide and disability in adolescents. In one study, more than 60% of adolescents with depression had had a history of suicidal ideation, and more than 30% of them had attempted suicide. In 2004, the US Food and Drug Administration (FDA) issued a "black box warning" for antidepressants; a decrease in the use of these medications to treat depression and a subsequent increase in completed suicides followed. Recent meta-analysis suggests that the benefits of treating depression outweigh the risks associated with these medications. Data regarding bipolar disorder and suicide is discrepant, as some studies have indicated that having bipolar disorder is a risk factor for suicide whereas others have not associated it with increased risk (5).

Substance use disorders are highly comorbid with mood disorders and are a major risk factor for suicide in older youth. It also has been noted that the diagnostic profiles of youth with suicide attempt and youth with suicidal ideation are somewhat different and that substance abuse is more closely associated with suicide attempt than with ideation. Other psychiatric disorders, including anxiety, posttraumatic stress disorder (PTSD) and conduct disorder also have been reported to be associated with increased risk of suicide.

Previous suicide behaviors

A history of previous suicide attempt is the single most important predictor of subsequent suicidal behavior, while suicidal ideation in the absence of a plan is associated with a decreased risk of suicide attempt in the future. Regarding the course of suicidal ideation, it is noted that 34% of individuals with suicidal ideation will make a suicide plan and 72% of those with a plan will make a suicide attempt.

The risk of a repeated suicide attempt is highest during the first 3-6 months following the initial attempt, with greater increased risk for male adolescents (30-fold) than for females (3-fold). In comparison to the general population, this risk remains elevated for the next 2 years. Ongoing suicidal intent and the potential lethality of the method used in the previous suicide attempt are other variables that impact the future course of suicidal risk. Youth who make highly lethal attempts and have serious suicidal intent are at extremely high risk for repeated attempts. Serious suicide intent is characterized by: 1) having certain beliefs about the suicide, 2) planning for a successful attempt, 3) taking measures to avoid detection and 4) expressing a wish to die.

Sexual orientation

Recent research has found a 2-6-fold increase in non-lethal suicidal behaviors among homosexual youth. This risk is aggravated by comorbid depressive symptoms, substance use and a sense of victimization.

Familial factors

A family history of suicide behaviors is one of the strongest predictors of suicide in youth. There is evidence that suicidal behavior is familial and transmitted irrespective of risk for other psychiatric disorders. Youth suicide is about 5 times more likely among children whose mothers have completed suicide, while first-degree relatives of suicide attempters have a 2-6-fold increased risk of suicidal behavior, compared to the general population.

Parental psychopathology, particularly depression and substance use disorder, has been associated with completed suicide and suicide attempts in youth; however, other studies have failed to find this association after controlling for the youth's psychopathology and psychosocial stressors. Loss of a parent to death or divorce before 12 years of age is a significant risk factor for completed suicide. There is also a consistent body of research linking youth suicide with family discord. Physical and sexual abuse and poor communication with the father are other risk factors for youth suicide attempts.

Access to lethal means

There is a consistent body of literature linking the presence of firearms at home with completed suicides. The availability of a gun at home makes it more likely that a gun will be used as a method of suicide. Absence of guns from the home makes it less likely that one will be used for a suicide attempt and may result in the use of less lethal means. There is also an association between stricter gun control laws and lower suicide rates.

PROTECTIVE FACTORS

Protective factors are those that decrease the likelihood of a suicide attempt, despite the presence of psychopathology.

Social support

Social support, including the perception of family cohesion, is noted to be a protective factor for suicidal behavior. Adolescents who describe family life as emotionally supportive are 3-5 times less likely to engage in suicidal behavior than peers with the same levels of mood psychopathology and life stress. Presence of young children at home is associated with *increased* risk of a *first* onset of suicidal ideation, but in the long-term this factor is protective against suicide.

Religion

Empirical research on the effects of spiritual beliefs and religious practices is in its infancy; however, the protective role of religion against suicidal behavior in African Americans is noteworthy. It has been posited that some of this beneficial effect may be mediated by meeting with like-minded people in religious services, people who can provide support during times of stress.

PREVENTION

Youth suicide prevention strategies are aimed at identifying young people who are at risk of self-harm. Traditionally these measures are implemented in school, community and health-care systems (6).

School-based programs

Suicide awareness programs were implemented on the premise that adolescents are more likely to confide in and seek support from their peers than from adults. The objective of these programs was to provide knowledge and to improve help-seeking behaviors in students. During the last two decades, several studies have evaluated these programs but so far have failed to find a positive effect. There is in fact evidence to the contrary, that these curriculum-based suicide awareness programs can cause at-risk students to become more distressed and less likely to seek care. Because of these results, emphasis has shifted from promoting "suicide awareness" to alternative strategies described below.

Screening

One strategy that has received attention is direct case finding via systematic screening. School-wide screening programs use self-report questionnaires and individual interviews and have focused on identifying youth with depression, recent or past suicidal ideation and attempts, and substance use problems. This systematic screening is sensitive (83%-100%) in finding youth at risk, but is less specific (51%-76%). In order to minimize false positive screening results, direct case finding using standardized interviews such as the Diagnostic Interview Schedule for Children (DISC) are employed.

Skills training

Skills training programs are aimed at strengthening cognitive and behavioral skills, with an emphasis on problem solving and coping skills, to both reduce the impact of suicide risk factors and enhance the effects of protective factors.

School personnel training (gatekeeper training)

Only one-tenth of high school teachers and one-third of school counselors believe that they can identify a student at risk of suicide. The purpose of this training is to increase knowledge and improve skill among school personnel with regard to identifying students at risk and making referrals when needed. These programs have shown improvement in intervention and referral skills among school personnel and are well accepted by school principals.

Community-based programs

Crisis centers and hotlines provide immediate support to youth in crisis. There is limited information about the efficacy of hotlines in the prevention of youth suicide, but about 15% of suicidal teens report having used these hotlines.

Firearms are one of the most common methods of committing suicide. Imposing restrictions on firearms as a means of preventing youth suicide is a key strategy but has shown conflicting results. Some studies have noted reduction in overall suicide rates while others have not found such an effect. While "mean-restricting measures" are a politically volatile topic in the US, providing education to parents of high-risk youth about limiting their access to firearms is less controversial and has been found to be marginally effective.

Healthcare-based programs

There is a dire need for pediatricians and primary care physicians to be trained to screen for suicide and mood disorders. In one study, 72% of primary care physician stated that they have prescribed antidepressants to adolescents, but only 8% stated that they had formal training in the treatment of adolescent depression. Educational programs for health care professionals have shown promise in reducing suicide rates, but ongoing efforts toward enhanced education are warranted.

MANAGEMENT

Despite significant public interest and public health agency concern regarding youth suicide, there is limited data available to support recommending one intervention over another. Unfortunately, it is difficult to predict suicide, but management can be broadly categorized into 'before self-harm' and 'after self-harm' groups (7).

Management before self-harm

In this phase of treatment, identification of at risk youth by screening and adequate treatment or referral is important. Physicians should use routine health care visits to screen for mental illness and suicidal thoughts. Risk factors need to be identified, but caution is advised in interpreting these risk factors, as many commonly occur and do not lead to a suicide attempt in the majority of cases. Common identifiable risk factors are noted in table 1.

Primary care physicians should feel comfortable interviewing depressed teens and estimating their level of distress and the extent of their dangerousness to self and others. Table 2 lists common warning signs for adolescent suicide that should be considered during the evaluation.

The recommended method for assessment of suicidal thoughts is a direct interview of the at-risk youth. It is recommended that confidentiality be discussed, with an explanation that the physician must act in the best interest of the youth if there is a danger to self or others. The adolescent and the parents should be interviewed separately, as important information is likely to be withheld in the parents' presence. The events preceding the suicidal intent and any self-mutilation behaviors should be assessed in detail. Self-mutilating behaviors are associated with significant psychopathology and should not be dismissed as being attention-seeking or manipulative; this behavior confers a 3-10% lifetime risk of eventual suicide.

Table 1. Common youth suicide risk factors

- Family: Separation, familial discord, impaired parent-child relationship, parental divorce, loss of a parent
- Parents: Parental mental health problems
- Psychopathology: Mood, psychosis, and sub-stance use disorders, panic disorder, history of aggression and impulsivity
- Trauma: History of past physical or sexual abuse
- History of previous suicide attempts
- Difficulty adjusting to gender identity
- Social: Difficulties in school, limited friends, bullying, not attending school, break-up with girlfriend/boyfriend, awareness of a friend's self-harm

Table 2. Warning signs of youth suicide

- Sudden negative change from baseline behavior
- Agitation
- Intoxication
- Recent stressful event
- Unprovoked episodes of crying
- Indications of youth being in an abusive relationship
- Recent onset of apathy and withdrawal
- Hopelessness, guilt and feelings of worthlessness
- Preoccupation with death
- Giving away prized possessions
- Worsening signs of depression

Physicians should ask questions to assess known risk factors as well as level of intent. Self-harming behaviors may or may not be associated with a true intent to commit suicide and should be assessed in the context of other risk factors, in order to avoid having a false sense of security. Physicians also should assess protective factors, as listed in Table 3, including the youth's reasons for living. Individuals who believe that it is acceptable to end one's life have a 14-fold increase in risk of making a suicide plan. The youth's access to lethal means, including medications and guns, should be assessed, and parents should be counseled regarding reducing access to such items.

Table 3. Protective factors

- Family cohesiveness
- Supportive family environment
- Engagement in school activities, including sports
- Good academic achievement
- Religiosity

If there is any reason to believe that an adolescent is at risk of suicide, the physician or support staff must stay with the individual until a plan is established for providing an appropriate level of care. Although data is lacking, the safest course of action in these situations is to arrange for hospitalization, which provides a safe and supportive environment for the adolescent.

Management after self-harm

In the majority of cases, and adolescent who has attempted suicide presents to an emergency room, where a psychiatrist, psychologist or psychiatric nurse assesses them. A thorough psychosocial evaluation, including assessment of protective factors, should be conducted (8). Collateral information should be taken from parents; however, in more than 80% of cases, the parents are unaware of a suicide attempt. The physician should explore the adolescent's "concept of death" by asking: "What would you expect to happen?" or "Had you thought you would still be around to see the consequences of an attempt?" Lethality of attempt also should be considered, although it is not a good indicator of suicide intent, as children may not have the cognitive skills necessary to estimate the level of lethality of their attempt. Table 4 lists the characteristics of suicide attempt that suggest high self-harm intent.

Table 4. Characteristics that indicate high suicide intent

- Planned and prepared in advance
- Told others beforehand about suicidal thoughts
- Timed to avoid discovery by parents
- Suicide note or a message left
- Others were not informed after the act

As noted above, inpatient hospitalization is usually the safest course of action following a teen suicide attempt; however, this decision must be made in conjunction with the available data about the presence or absence of factors that may indicate risk for repeated self-harm.

Table 5. Characteristics that indicate risk for repeated self-harm

- Lack of remorse and constant hopelessness after the failed attempt
- History of previous suicide attempts
- Family history of completed suicide attempt
- Social isolation
- Ongoing substance use problems
- Psychosis

If the decision is made to discharge the patient from the emergency room, it is advisable to make a referral to a child and adolescent psychiatrist for ongoing care and treatment. Among those adolescents who make a suicide attempt, there is significant heterogeneity in the clinical presentation, and treatments should be tailored according to the youth's developmental level. Goals of outpatient treatment are stress reduction and prevention of any future suicide attempts.

Problem solving

These therapies help adolescents to identify triggers of suicidal thoughts and to develop behavioral alternatives to suicide so that they can cope with such situations if they arise in the future. As learning is often context dependent, exposure tasks are usually included within cognitive therapy approaches. During exposure tasks, the adolescent is asked to reimagine the situation that led to the suicide attempt and then to imagine an alternative way of confronting such situations differently in the future in order to avoid making another attempt.

Family therapies

Therapy approaches can also be extended to the whole family. Family therapies are structured and aim to provide education and promote understanding of suicidal behaviors. Issues of validation ("no one understands me") can also be addressed within the family framework.

Other therapies

Depending upon the presenting problem (e.g., substance use issues, depression, bullying, etc.), additional approaches may be suggested by the outpatient provider.

CONCLUSION

Suicide in children and adolescents is a complex and emotional problem for families and societies nationally and internationally (9). Risk factors for suicide have been reviewed including personal characteristics, psychopathology of those committing suicide, history of previous suicide attempts, sexual orientation, familial factors, and access to lethal means of suicide. Protective factors include social support and religion. Principles of prevention have been considered including school-based programs, screening tools, skills training, Gatekeeper training, community-based programs, and health-care programs. Management includes principles involved in management before and after self-harm. Also considered are family therapies and therapies aimed at specific problems such as depression, bullying, substance abuse, and others (10). Clinicians should be actively involved with their communities to seek prevention of suicide in children and adolescents.

REFERENCES

[1] McLoughlin AB, Gould MS, Malone KM. Global trends in teenage suicide: 2003-2014. QJM 2015 Jan 31. pii:hcv026.

[2] Pena JB, Matthieu MM, Zayas LH, Masyn KE, Caine ED. Co-occurring risk behaviors among White, Black, and Hispanic US high school adolescents with suicide attempts requiring medical attention, 1999–2007: implications for future prevention initiatives. Soc Psychiatry Psychiatr Epidemiol 2012;47(1):29-42.

[3] Tishler CL, Reiss NS, Rhodes AR. Suicidal behavior in children younger than twelve: a diagnostic challenge for emergency department personnel. Acad Emerg Med 2007;14(9):810-8.

[4] Gould MS, Greenberg TED, Velting DM, Shaffer D. Youth suicide risk and preventive interventions: a review of the past 10 years. J Am Acad Child Adolesc Psychiatry 2003;42(4):386-405.

[5] Nerves MG, Leanza F. Mood disorders in adolescents: diagnosis, treatment, and suicide assessment in the primary care setting. Prim Care 2014;41(3):587-606.

[6] Kostenuik M, Ratnapalan M. Approach to adolescent suicide prevention. Can Fam Physician 2010; 56(8): 755-60.

[7] Daniel SS, Goldston DB. Interventions for suicidal youth: a review of the literature and developmental considerations. Suicide Life Threat Behav 2009;39(3): 252-68.

[8] Ougrin D, Tranah T, Shahl D, Moran P, Asarnow JR. Therapeutic interventions for suicide attempts and self-harm in adolescents: systematic review and meta-analysis. J Am Acad Child Adolesc Psychiatr 2015; 54(2):97-107.
[9] Hawton K, Saunders KE, O'Connor RC. Self-harm and suicide in adolescents. Lancet 2012;379(9834):2373-82.
[10] Shain BN. Suicide and suicide attempts in adolescents. J Pediatr 2007;120(3):669-76.

In: Public Health Yearbook 2016
Editor: Joav Merrick

ISBN: 978-1-53610-947-4

Chapter 37

A REVIEW OF SCHIZOPHRENIA IN CHILDHOOD

Ahsan Nazeer**, MD
Department of Psychiatry, Western Michigan University,
Homer Stryker MD School of Medicine, Kalamazoo, Michigan, US

ABSTRACT

This review considers childhood-onset schizophrenia which is a chronic debilitating illness presenting before 13 years of age. Schizophrenia is a complex and devastating psychiatric disorder and pediatric schizophrenia begins before 18 years of age and research suggests is a continuum with adult schizophrenia. Concepts of epidemiology and etiology are reviewed. Symptoms include delusions, hallucinations, disorganized speech, disorganized behavior, and negative symptoms. The differential diagnosis includes substance use disorders, drug intoxications, bipolar disorder, and anxiety disorders. Management includes psychosocial interventions and psychopharmacology. Medication includes atypical antipsychotics, typical antipsychotics, and depot injections. Clinicians should carefully monitor and manage the side effects of these medications. Current concepts of diagnosis and management are reviewed.

Keywords: Childhood, psychiatry, mental health, schizophrenia

INTRODUCTION

The last few years have seen a tremendous increase in the research on pediatric schizophrenia, a chronic debilitating illness that presents before 18 years of age. The term childhood-onset schizophrenia (COS) is reserved for children in whom the onset of symptoms begins before 13 years of age. There is ample evidence that pediatric schizophrenia is on a

* Correspondence: Ahsan Nazeer, Department of Psychiatry, Western Michigan University Homer Stryker MD School of Medicine, 1717 Shaffer Road, Suite 101, Kalamazoo, MI 49048, United States. E-mail: ahsan.nazeer@med.wmich.edu.

continuum with adult schizophrenia with premorbid cognitive abnormalities, chronic course and long-term morbidity and mortality (1).

Emil Kraepelin (1856-1926) differentiated between dementia praecox (i.e., schizophrenia) and manic-depressive illness and conceptualized childhood-onset schizophrenia as a rare form of adult onset illness with symptoms quite similar to the adult version (2). Eugene Bleuler (1857-1939) later categorized these symptoms and coined the term "schizophrenia." During this conceptual phase, for varied reasons, childhood developmental deficits and problems in speech, cognition and social oddities got lumped together with childhood psychosis, making childhood psychosis a part of a broader spectrum of mental illnesses of children that also included autism. Lauretta Bender's (1897-1987) work at Bellevue Hospital in New York furthered the developmental understanding of schizophrenic children, but it was not until Rutter's seminal publications that the distinctions between schizophrenia and autism were clarified. As a result, these entities were now considered to be two different sets of disorders.

Since the publication of the Diagnostic and Statistical Manual, Third Edition (DSM-III), childhood-onset schizophrenia has been diagnosed using the adult criteria established by the DSM system that carries over to the current DSM-5. The DSM requires the presence of at least two of the following symptoms: delusions, hallucinations, disorganized speech, disorganized or catatonic behavior and negative symptoms (e.g., flat affect, poverty of speech and avolition) for the major part of one month during any six-month interval. DSM-5 also cautions that although the main symptoms of schizophrenia are the same in childhood, there are also important differences. In childhood schizophrenia, delusions are less elaborate and visual hallucinations are more common. These hallucinations should also be distinguished from developmentally normal fantasies. DSM-5 has also removed the schizophrenia subtypes that were noted in DSM-IV-TR (3). The following is a brief description of these symptoms.

Delusions

Delusions refer to firmly held beliefs that cannot be accounted for by the individual's cultural and religious backgrounds. Delusions are further categorized by the nature and content of the beliefs. Some examples are: delusions of grandeur (belief that one has special powers); delusions of persecution (belief that one is being followed, spied upon or treated badly); and delusions of erotomania (belief that someone of higher status is in love with him or her).

Hallucinations

Hallucinations are false perceptions without identifiable external stimuli. In psychotic disorders, these misperceptions can occur in any of the five senses; therefore, psychotic individuals can present with auditory, visual, gustatory (taste-related), olfactory (smell-related), or somatic hallucinations.

Disorganized speech

Individuals with psychotic disorders can present with abnormalities in the form or context of speech. Their speech may become completely incomprehensible, with inventions of new words (neologisms) or *word salad* (a jumble of meaningless or illogical words and phrases).

Disorganized behavior

Examples of disorganized behaviors include impaired ability to maintain adequate hygiene, disrespect of personal space of others, intrusive behaviors, plan and achieve reasonable goals, or failure to respond in a socially appropriate manner.

Table 1. Common conditions associated with psychosis

Neurological
Delirium
Meningitis
Brain tumors
Migraines
Complex partial seizures
Illicit drugs
Inhalants
Hallucinogens
Alcohol
Cannabis
Alcohol
Stimulants
Systemic Diseases
Cirrhosis
Hypothyroidism
Hyperthyroidism
Addison's disease
Psychiatric
Post-traumatic stress disorders
Reactive attachment disorder
Pervasive developmental disorders
Bipolar disorder-manic states
Depression with psychotic features
Others
Imaginary friends
Hypnagogic, Hypnopompic hallucinations
Developmental delays
Language deficits

Table 2. Conditions that may be misconstrued as schizophrenia

Vivid imagination
Imaginary friends
Hypnagogic/Hypnopompic hallucinations
Flashbacks of traumatic memories
Mood disorders
Peculiar thinking of children with mental retardation and autism spectrum disorders
Speech, hearing and visual impairment
Drug toxicity or withdrawal

Negative symptoms

Negative symptoms usually indicate an absence of normal behaviors. Examples of these symptoms include: flat affect (lack of emotional expression); inability to experience pleasure (anhedonia); lack of or limited speech (alogia); and, lack of initiation (avolition).

Diagnosing psychotic disorders in children continues to be a challenging task for the majority of clinicians. Much of this difficulty arises from the fact that, on occasion, children at different developmental levels endorse symptoms that blur the boundaries between pathological and non-pathological behaviors. Examples include imaginary friends, hypnagogic and/or hypnopompic hallucinations, the intense and fixed interests of children with pervasive developmental disorders, and the flashbacks of traumatized children.

It is also important to note that the presence of psychotic symptoms in children is not synonymous with the diagnosis of schizophrenia (4). As the DSM criteria rely heavily on the presence of the positive symptoms of psychosis (hallucinations, delusions, disorganized speech and behavior), there is an ongoing debate on whether this criterion is appropriate for the diagnosis of schizophrenia in children. Positive symptoms, by themselves, are unreliable indicators of underlying psychopathology, as they can be present in numerous other disorders (including mood disorders). Some of the conditions that can easily be misconstrued as schizophrenia are listed in Table 2.

EPIDEMIOLOGY

Because of the challenges in effectively diagnosing this disorder in children, the exact prevalence is not known. Estimates suggest childhood schizophrenia to be quite rare before 13 years of age, constituting only about 0.1%-1% of all schizophrenic cases (5). In these cases the onset is insidious and prognosis is poor. Overall prevalence is suggested to be in the range of 1%, with EOS occurring in approximately 1/10,000 and COS in 1-2/100,000 children. Symptoms are more common in children older than 15 years of age, making this segment the bulk of pediatric schizophrenia. Most studies note an average male to female ratio of 1.5-2:1.

The predominance among males during the early adolescent years disappears in late adolescence. A recent study has argued against this trend, and has noted a continued male preponderance in later years, with a male-to-female ratio of 1.4:1. Most studies have not compared schizophrenic symptoms on the basis of race and ethnicity. One 2006 study from

United Kingdom "Aetiology and ethnicity in schizophrenia and other psychoses study" (AESOP) noted psychosis to be more common in blacks and minority ethnic groups as compared to white British population.

ETIOLOGY

Although no definitive etiology of childhood-onset schizophrenia is identified, certain factors including family history of schizophrenia, old paternal age and taking psychoactive drugs during late adolescent years, seem to increase the risk of developing schizophrenia.

Genetic factors seems to play a major role as noted by the increased prevalence of schizophrenia like symptoms among first degree relatives of children with schizophrenia. Research findings suggest that these relatives display; abnormalities in ocular smooth pursuit movements, increased expressed emotions, higher proportions of ADHD and conduct disorder and impairment in spatial working memory and executive functions.

About 10% of individuals with schizophrenia before 13 years of age also display cytogenetic abnormalities as noted among the NIMH COS sample. Studies have also noted hypoxia related complications during prenatal period among individuals with schizophrenia. On neuroimaging, enlargement of lateral ventricles is the most consistent finding but research has also demonstrated decreased volumes of frontal and temporal gray matter and hippocampus in schizophrenics as compared to health controls.

DIAGNOSIS

Because of the insidious onset of the disease, a longitudinal perspective is necessary to correctly diagnose schizophrenia. Retrospective evaluation of the symptoms may yield better and earlier diagnostic information than following the symptoms prospectively. This is because children who later develop schizophrenia have a history of impaired pre-morbid functioning and display deficits in cognition, language and development as compared to non-schizophrenic children.

Impaired sociability and social withdrawal appear to lead to a more severe form of schizophrenia, with poor premorbid functioning being more common in males than in females (6).

Speech problems, developmental delays and neurological soft signs (including primitive reflexes and coordination problems) are other clues worth noting. Deficits in full scale IQ, verbal memory, attention, sustained attention and word fluency also has been noted in neuropsychological assessments. Cannon, et al. noted the following five factors to have significant predictive validity in diagnosing schizophrenia: "a genetic risk for schizophrenia with recent deterioration in functioning, higher levels of unusual thought content, higher levels of paranoia, greater social impairment, and a history of substance abuse" (7). Table 4 presents some of the commonly used rating scales to aid with diagnosis.

Table 3. Medical and psychiatric history

Obtain history from multiple informants
Seek detailed description of hallucinations
Auditory, visual, tactile, olfactory, gustatory (last two suggest more organic pathology), quality of hallucinations, well-formed or bizarre, specific themes, thoughts of self-harm or harm to others.
Establish the age of onset
Time of the day when psychotic symptoms are more prevalent
Association with sleep-wake cycle
Associated problems with academic and social functioning
History of trauma in the past
History of headaches and vomiting
Family history of schizophrenia
Medications
Use of illicit drugs
Developmental history

DIFFERENTIAL DIAGNOSIS

As mentioned in the above text, numerous psychiatric disorders can present with psychotic symptoms as a part of broader spectrum of mental disorders. Correct diagnosis is mandatory to effectively treat the respective disorders. The following disorders can present a diagnostic challenge during the evaluation of childhood schizophrenia.

Substance use disorders (SUD) and drug intoxications

SUDs are comorbid with primary psychotic disorders and also can be the cause of psychotic symptoms. Clinically, substance induced psychotic disorders are acute, brief and are related to the episode of drug intoxication or withdrawal. The psychotic symptoms may wax and wane depending upon how long it has been since the drug(s) were ingested. Symptoms of outpatients may continue if use continues; and symptoms may vary if different drugs are ingested (either intentionally or unintentionally based on varied suppliers).

Table 4. Commonly used rating scales

Brief Psychiatric Rating Scale for children (BPRS-C)	21 item clinician based scale. Not specific for psychosis and deals with general childhood psychopathology. Very commonly used in research.
Schedule for Affective Disorders and Schizophrenia for school Age children (K-SADS)	Semi-structured interview. Common research tool. Assess overall psychopathology including mood and anxiety disorders along with psychosis.
Positive and Negative Syndrome Scale for Children (Kiddie-PANSS)	Refined version of the adult scale to be used in children. Structured interview. Studies show good Inter-rater reliability and quality of differentiate schizophrenic from non-schizophrenia children.

Symptoms due to intoxication of inpatients should gradually improve, but symptoms related to withdrawal may worsen before they improve. Since many of the hallucinogenic drugs do not appear on standard drug panels, and since urine samples may only contain metabolites of drugs for a limited few days, toxicology may not provide the full answer to the question of what caused the symptoms. Patients also present with other associated symptoms of drug intoxication that can give clues to the underlying cause of psychosis. Since SUDs can induce toxic psychotic states, drug use and withdrawal should be ruled out before making a diagnosis of schizophrenia. Table 2 lists categories of hallucinogenic drugs of abuse.

Hallucinogenic drugs derived from fungi ("shrooms"), cacti (e.g., peyote), herbs, or synthetic chemicals (e.g., LSD), appear to act mainly on the 5-HT2A receptor, altering one's perception of reality. Resulting "trips" are experiences that may be either exciting or frightening and dangerous.

Cannabinoid receptor drugs such as cannabis, hashish, and the "synthetic marijuana" products (sold as "K2," "spice," and many others; there are 450 synthetic analogues of delta-9-thetrahydrocannabinol) can cause psychosis with hallucinations. These drugs are Cb1 and Cb2 full or partial agonists. Five of these cannabinoids, JWH-018, JWH-073, CP-47,497, JWH-200, and cannabicyclohexanol sold legally over the counter for a while as non-drugs are now classified as illegal Schedule I drugs in the US.

Deliriants are cholinergic receptor antagonists derived from a variety of poisonous plants, such as datura (moonflower), deadly nightshade, mandrake, and henbane. Common antihistamines such as diphenhydramine, hydroxyzine, and dimenhydrinate (Dramamine™) also can cause hallucinations and delirium when taken in very high doses and when combined with certain other drugs. Taken in very large doses, they can cause hallucinatory experiences, with associated poor judgment, which are not recalled later due to the amnestic effect of these drugs. Clinical signs can include dilated pupils, confusion and rage, and both positive and negative hallucinations may develop. Dehydration may be severe, and death can occur.

Amphetamines and cocaine also may induce hallucinations and delusions, usually of a frightening nature. Ecstacy (MDMA) also may produce frightening hallucinations, although it has been promoted for its empathogenic effects. The so-called bath salts that contain amphetamine analogues also can cause hallucinations and delirium. Neuro-chemically, these drugs work on dopaminergic, noradrenergic and serotonergic receptors.

Table 5. Hallucinogenic drugs of abuse

Psychedelics (5-HT_{2A} receptor agonists)
Tryptamines
Piperazines
Stimulants (amphetamines)
Phenethylamines
Cannabinoids (CB-1 receptor agonists)
Dissociatives
NMDA receptor antagonists
Sigma-opioid receptor agonists
Deliriants (anticholinergics)
Withdrawal delirium from chronic use of alcohol or sedatives

Both schizophrenia and SUDs are highly heritable, and if present together, they can lead to a worsening in clinical course, morbidity and mortality. Most of the above drugs are not detected by standard ELISA drug screening tests available over the counter or in hospital laboratory drug screens; therefore, it may be necessary to send the urine samples for confirmation to toxicology laboratories where they can subject the samples to chromatography followed by tandem mass spectroscopy (LC or GC/MS/MS); it may be helpful to alert the toxicologist of what drugs may be involved especially if the ELISA test was negative. Time from last exposure usually will lead to reduction and eventual elimination of symptoms, although there is some controversial evidence of irreversible changes to brain structure as well as slower to recover reversible changes to the brain.

Bipolar disorder

Psychotic symptoms are a predominant part of early onset bipolar disorder. Youth in the acute manic phase can be misdiagnosed with schizophrenia. Evaluating the nature and quality of hallucinations and associated mood symptoms usually gives clues to the correct diagnosis. In bipolar disorder, psychotic symptoms are more mood congruent (elevated, grandiose mood). While in schizophrenia youth have a history of gradually deteriorating premorbid functioning, thought blocking, and delusions of guilt, remorse and hallucinations surrounding evil, the devil or Satan. Negative symptoms of schizophrenia (poor energy, lack of interest, limited speech) can give the impression of depression to the casual observer.

Anxiety disorder

Symptoms of anxiety are frequently present in patients with schizophrenia. These symptoms can be present in any phase of the illness, and usually are the result of poor psychosocial functioning, life stressors and comorbid substance use (8). Children with exposure to trauma can present with symptoms of psychosis or dissociation including hallucinations and paranoia. These symptoms usually occur during stressful periods of life and in the face of repeat trauma that overwhelm the already fragile coping skills of youth. Impairment in psychosocial functioning usually triggers these micro-episodes without any preceding prodrome and deterioration in functioning that usually is a hallmark of a primary psychotic disorder.

Treatment

Evaluating the acuity of the situation is the most important initial step in the management of schizophrenia. Studies have estimated a lifetime risk of suicide between 4.9-10% (9). Suicide risk is higher during the initial years of the illness and also immediately after hospital discharge. It is important to remember that despite these high-risk phases, suicidal ideation tends to persist throughout the course of schizophrenia. Some patients may be more verbal in discussing their thoughts than others. So, while interacting with these individuals, it is important to be cognizant of some of the warning signs that may include: sudden calmness, verbal or physical aggression, restlessness, pacing, muted response to auditory or visual hallucinations, and changes in mental status. If the threat is imminent, it is advisable to arrange for a supervised transfer to the emergency department, as mere reassurance is usually ineffective in psychotic people

Consultations

As mentioned above, making the correct diagnosis is the most crucial, yet daunting step. In a recent NIMH cohort, 1,300 cases were referred to the researchers with a possible diagnosis of childhood schizophrenia (10). After the structured clinical interviews, only 64 cases of those 1,300 referrals were actually diagnosed with schizophrenia. Mood disorders were found to be the most common diagnosis. This study underscores the challenges in making the correct diagnosis. Therefore, in cases where there is a suspicion of psychosis in young children, it is wise to consult with a child and adolescent psychiatrist. Despite the fact that the diagnosis is easier to make during later adolescence, in the case of an atypical presentation in an older child, it is usually helpful to also seek the opinion of a pediatric psychiatrist and a neurologist.

Psychopharmacology

Medication management and psychopharmacological interventions is the mainstay of the treatment of schizophrenia. Goals of the management include: maintenance of safety, management of acute symptoms, and the prevention of long-term deterioration in functioning. The American Academy of Child and Adolescent Psychiatry (AACAP) practice parameters recommend both typical and atypical antipsychotic agents except clozapine to be considered as the primary treatment option. This recommendation is in line with the clinical practice in which both typical and atypical antipsychotics are found to be equally efficacious, but differ significantly in their side effect profile.

Among the available options, atypicals were widely considered to be a safer and more efficacious option in the treatment protocol. Numerous recent studies including CATIE (Clinical Antipsychotic Trials of Intervention Effectiveness), CutLASS (Cost Utility of the Latest Antipsychotic Drugs in Schizophrenia) and EUFEST (European First Episode Schizophrenia Trial) have challenged this notion (11, 12). Armenteros and Davies reviewed published trials of typical (the older first generation antipsychotic drugs) and atypical (the newer antipsychotic; see Table 3) medications in order to develop an evidence base of use of antipsychotic medications. Among the published studies, they noted a response rate in the *atypical* group ranging from 13%-75% in comparison to 35%-93% in the *typical* group. Effect sizes suggested that typical antipsychotics were superior to atypicals, although both were effective even after considering other variables. Irrespective of the initial choice of the medications, significant numbers of patients remain non-adherent to the medications leading to decreased efficacy of treatment and a gradual downward course of the disease.

Table 6. Atypical antipsychotics

Medication	Dose	Side effects*
Risperidone	0.25-4 mg	Sedation, weight gain, metabolic syndrome, hyperprolactinemia
Olanzapine	2.5-20mg	Dizziness, weight gain, dry mouth, constipation
Quetiapine	25-600mg	Sedations, postural hypotension, headaches, cataracts (risk established in beagles)
Ziprasidone	20-160mg	Nausea, QTc prolongation
Aripiprazole	2.5-30mg	Nausea, vomiting, akathesia, tachycardia
Clozapine	12.5-900mg	Sedation, tachycardia, hypersalivation, agranulocytosis, seizures
Iloperidone**	12-24mg	Dizziness, somnolence, tachycardia, dry mouth, weight gain, nasal stuffiness,

* All antipsychotics-except clozapine-can cause extrapyramidal symptoms (EPS). Olanzapine, clozapine and quetiapine appears to have less risk of tardive dyskinesia.

** Recently approved atypical antipsychotic medication. So far, data is not available for its use in children.

Atypical antipsychotics

Despite the above evidence, for all practical purposes, atypical antipsychotics continue to be the initial medication choice for the majority of clinicians who treat childhood schizophrenia. Table 6 lists the available atypical medications, average dose range and common side effects.

The Food and Drug Administration (FDA) has approved risperidone, olanzapine, quetiapine and aripiprazole for the treatment of schizophrenia in adolescents 13-17 years of age. Current evidence regarding the efficacy of these medications is limited to a few double blind, randomized clinical trials and data on the long-term effects of these medications also limited at best.

The "Treatment of early onset schizophrenia spectrum disorders study" (TEOSS) was a publically funded multi-site trial in which children with schizophrenia and schizoaffective disorder were randomly assigned to risperidone, olanzapine and molindone for eight weeks (13). Over 8 weeks, response rates were best for molindone (50%), followed by risperidone (46%) and olanzapine (34%). Olanzapine was associated with most weight gain as compared to other two and reached a degree that the data safety monitoring board decided to discontinue the olanzapine arm midway through the study. Molindone was associated with more akathesia. It is disappointing that only 12% of the subjects in the study remained adherent to the treatment by 12 months. Atypical antipsychotics are associated with numerous side effects but have more propensity for developing metabolic syndrome in comparison to the typical agents. Agents differ in their tendency to develop metabolic syndrome. Olanzapine and clozapine are associated with higher risk of developing this syndrome followed by quetiapine and risperidone. Ziprasidone and aripiprazole have the least possibility of causing this side effect. Table 7 lists some of the basic characteristics of the metabolic syndrome.

Increased awareness, prevention and ongoing evaluation of metabolic syndrome has become the standard of care in the medical community. Because of the chronicity of schizophrenia, youth are subjected to these medications for many decades. Resultant side effects can cause long-term morbidity. Thus it is important to monitor, prevent and manage these side effects. Family education about healthy eating habits and in some cases dietary consult with dietitian is helpful. Preventive measures including encouraging a healthy life style in terms of eating, exercise, avoidance of smoking and drugs and alcohol while maintaining realistic goals for healthy living are also appropriate items for discussion. Routine physical activity including short periods of brisk walking, avoiding sedentary activities, and gradually adding regular activity into the daily schedule should be encouraged (14).

Choosing medications that have a lower tendency to cause metabolic syndrome is also an important decision to make at the start of the treatment. At the baseline it is recommended to take a family history for risk factors including diabetes, hypertension and hypercholesterolemia. Weight, waist circumference, blood pressure and BMI should be established at baseline. Fasting glucose, lipid panel and EKG should be ordered. Weight and waist circumference should be reevaluated at one month, three months and then annually. Fasting glucose and lipid panel should be evaluated three months after the initial visit. Fasting glucose can be repeated annually and fasting lipid panel every five years thereafter.

In the event of emergence of metabolic syndrome, a change or discontinuation of the antipsychotic, if clinically appropriate, can be considered. Caution is mandated for the risk of ketoacidosis, and the patient and family needs to be educated about the signs and symptoms. The primary care doctor or endocrinologist should be consulted for co-management of this problem in particular and of metabolic syndrome in general. In the following days and months, the metabolic profile needs to be judiciously monitored, and consideration should be given for the use of niacin, gemfibrozil or metformin.

Typical antipsychotics

The use of typical antipsychotics has fallen out of favor since the introduction of atypical antipsychotics. The typical antipsychotics carry increased risk of extrapyramidal symptoms (EPS). Recent studies, including the CATIE trial, have questioned the purported superior efficacy of the atypicals over their older counterparts. In this trial, at moderate dosages, typical antipsychotics are found to be comparably efficacious to the atypicals. Higher doses of these medications cause numerous unwanted side effects including tardive dyskinesia and risk of non-adherence. Perphenazine, haloperidol and molindone did better with perphenazine showing higher efficacy on the neuropsychological profile in comparison to the atypicals. Results of the CATIE trial were significant in showing the lack of difference in efficacy between typical and atypical agents.

Table 7. Basic characteristics of metabolic syndrome

General characteristics	Criteria specific for youth
Weight gain	Waist $\geq 90^{th}$ percentile
High blood pressure	$\geq 90^{th}$ percentile
Abnormalities in lipid metabolism	HDL ≤ 40, Triglycerides ≥ 110
Insulin resistance and hyperglycemia	Fasting glucose ≥ 110 mg/dl

Depot injections of medication

Research has consistently shown that non-adherence to the psychopharmacological treatment continues to be one of the main factors leading to relapse. About 65% of the patients relapse within one year but this rate drops to 25-30% if a patient is maintained on antipsychotic medications during this time. There are numerous reasons why individuals remain non-adherent to the medication. Side effects of the medications, a complicated dosing regimen, and perceived lack of efficacy are the few worth noting. In addition, lack of insight into the social unacceptability of positive and negative symptoms of schizophrenia may further reduce adherence. Non-adherence to the medications during teen years leads to impaired educational progress and achievement and reduced vocational potential and social skills acquisition. Frequent bouts of disease recurrence predispose individuals to life instability that can cause legal entanglements, violence and injury, drug involvement and addiction, a reputation of being mentally ill, poor employment history, financial poverty, and cognitive decline.

Two of the typical antipsychotics (haloperidol, fluphenazine) and three atypical antipsychotic medications (risperdone, olanzapine, paliperidone palmitate) are available in depot injection formulations that provide several weeks of clinical efficacy. Drug levels are steadier than with oral agents, which may reduce the prevalence of EPS side effects that arise shortly after an oral dose. These preparations are indicated in cases where medication adherence is inconsistent. For non-adherent adults, depot antipsychotic medications are used, along with case management and court-ordered outpatient treatment, to reduce the frequency of hospitalization and other morbidities that interfere with community living. For youth, especially adolescents, this approach may help when parental structure does not effectively enforce good adherence, or is unavailable.

It should be noted that smoking increases liver metabolism of neuroleptics; those who smoke as outpatients may speed up the catabolism of their medications as compared to their inpatient experiences where smoking is limited or prohibited. Consequently, dose stabilization during an inpatient hospital stay may be undermined by an increase or resumption of smoking after discharge.

Side effects of these medications are very similar to those of oral antipsychotics. Extrapyramidal side effects are usually dose dependent and are not very different in intensity and frequency than the oral counterparts. Some of the side effects of depot medications are: pain at the injection site, dizziness, blurred vision and tardive dyskinesias. Benefits of improved adherence, convenience, dependable bioavailability and better psychosocial functioning outweigh the risks associated with these preparations.

Psychosocial interventions

Managing the psychosocial aspects of treatment is an extremely important part of the management of schizophrenia. Individual and family focused psychoeducation and psychotherapies improve long-term outcomes and increase medication adherence (15). Reduction in the expression of hostility by family members has been shown in adults to markedly improve outcome. Skills training and long-term rehabilitation are other facets of psychosocial management. As schizophrenia is chronic and progressive, long-term planning for when the child reaches the age of majority should begin during adolescence. Larger communities have Assertive Community Treatment (ACT) teams that may assist in managing the more difficult cases. One should be aware that some youth with childhood schizophrenia do manage to function as adults as long as they remain treatment adherent.

CONCLUSION

Childhood-onset schizophrenia is a complex and devastating psychiatric disorder that begins before age 13 years of age. Pediatric schizophrenia begins before 18 years of age and research suggests is a continuum with adult schizophrenia. Concepts of epidemiology and etiology are reviewed. Symptoms include delusions, hallucinations, disorganized speech, disorganized behavior, and negative symptoms. The differential diagnosis includes substance use disorders, drug intoxications, bipolar disorder, and anxiety disorders. Management includes psychosocial interventions and psychopharmacology. Medication includes atypical antipsychotics, typical antipsychotics, and depot injections. Clinicians should carefully monitor and manage the side effects of these medications.

REFERENCES

[1] Jacobsen LK, Rapoport JL. Research update: Childhood onset schizophrenia: Implication of clinical and neurobiological research. J. Child Psychol Psychiat 1998; 39(1):101-13.

[2] Adityanjee, Aderibigbe YA, Theodoridis D, Vieweg VR. Dementia praecox to schizophrenia: The first 100 years. Psychiatry Clin Neurosci 1999;53(4):437-48.

[3] American Psychiatric Association. Diagnostic and statistical manual of mental health disorders: DSM-5, 5th ed. Washington, DC: American Psychiatric Publishing, 2013.

[4] Del Beccaro MA, Burke P, McCauley E. Hallucinations in children: a follow-up study. J Am Acad Child Adolesc Psychiatry 1988;27(4):462-5.

[5] McGrath JJ. Variations in the incidence of schizophrenia: data versus dogma. Schizophr Bull 2006; 32(1):195-7.

[6] Strous RD, Alvir JM, Robinson D, Gal G, Sheitman B, Chakos M, et al. Premorbid functioning in schizophrenia: relation to baseline symptoms, treatment response, and medication side effects. Schizophr Bull 2004;30(2):265-78.

[7] Cannon TD, Cadenhead K, Cornblatt B, Woods SW, Addington J, Walker E, et al. Prediction of psychosis in youth at high clinical risk: a multisite longitudinal study in North America. Arch Gen Psychiatry 2008;65(1):28-37.

[8] Muller JE, Koen L, Soraya S, Emsley RA, Stein DJ. Anxiety disorders and schizophrenia. Curr Psychiatr Rep 2004;6(4):255-61.

[9] Palmer BA, Pankratz VS, Bostwick JM. The lifetime risk of suicide in schizophrenia: A reexamination. Arch Gen Psychiatry 2005;62(3):247-53.

[10] Calderoni D, Wudarsky M, Bhangoo R, Dell ML, Nicolson R, Hamburger SD, et al. Differentiating childhood onset schizophrenia from psychotic mood disorders. J Am Acad Child Adolesc Psychiatry 2001; 40(10):1190-6.

[11] Lieberman JA, Stroup TS, McEvoy JP, Swartz MS, Rosenheck RA, Perkins DO, et al. Effectiveness of antipsychotic drugs in patients with chronic schizophrenia. N Engl J Med 2005;353(12):1209-23.

[12] Jones PB, Barnes TR, Davies L, Dunn G, Lloyd H, Hayhurst KP, et al. Randomized controlled trial of effect on quality of life of second vs. first generation antipsychotic drugs in schizophrenia: Cost Utility of the Latest Antipsychotic Drugs in Schizophrenia Study (CUtLASS 1). Arch Gen Psychiatry 2006;63(10):1079-87.

[13] Sikich L, Frazier JA, McClellan J, Findling RL, Vitiello B, Ritz L, et al. Double-blind comparison of first- and second-generation antipsychotics in early-onset schizophrenia and schizo-affective disorder: findings from the treatment of early-onset schizophrenia spectrum disorders (TEOSS) study. Am J Psychiatry 2008;165(11):1420-31.

[14] Grundy SM, Hansen B, Smith SC Jr., Cleeman JI, Kahn RA. Clinical management of metabolic syndrome: Report of the American Heart Association/National Heart, Lung, and Blood Institute/American Diabetes Association conference on scientific issues related to management. Circulation 2004;109(4):551-6.

[15] Pilling S, Bebbington P, Kuipers E, Garety P, Geddes J, Orbach G, et al. Psychological treatments in schizophrenia: I. Meta-analysis of family intervention and cognitive behaviour therapy. Psychol Med 2002; 32(5):763-82.

In: Public Health Yearbook 2016
Editor: Joav Merrick
ISBN: 978-1-53610-947-4

Chapter 38

CHILDHOOD AND ADOLESCENCE: PERSPECTIVES ON PERSONALITY DISORDERS

Kathryn White[1], MA, Michelle Stahl[2], MA and Helen D Pratt[1,*], PhD

[1]Western Michigan University Homer Stryker MD School of Medicine, Kalamazoo, Michigan, US

[2]Department of Counselor Education and Counseling Psychology, Western Michigan University, Kalamazoo, Michigan, US

ABSTRACT

Symptoms that are associated with personality disorders (PD) can lead to clinicians diagnosing personality disorders in youth who have not reached full developmental maturity; most symptoms these youth exhibit can often be better explained by other incidents, factors or reactions that a child experiences throughout their stages of development. A personality disorder is defined by the "Diagnostic and statistical manual of mental disorders", fifth edition, as being characterized by enduring patterns of internal experiences and behaviors that markedly deviates from the individual's culture. These stable patterns are pervasive and inflexible and usually begin in adolescence or early adulthood, the results are disruptive and impair the adolescent's a) cognition, b) affectivity, c) interpersonal d) impulse control functions. Personality disorders are commonly diagnosed in adults but apprehensions arise when the children and adolescent population is considered. Trauma, abuse, and exposure to violence during stages of development can result in deviant or maladaptive behavior that significantly impairs children or adolescent's growth and development (cognitive, emotional, and mental). Clinicians are encouraged to examine external influences in the lives of children and adolescent development. Youth who are affected by these disorders should be appropriately diagnosed and provided with early and intensive psychotherapy. Effective treatment involves several treatment modalities including cognitive therapy, dialectical behavior therapy, mode deactivation therapy, and pharmacotherapy.

* Corresponding author: Professor Helen D Pratt, Pediatrics and Adolescent Medicine, Western Michigan University Homer Stryker MD School of Medicine, 1000 Oakland Drive, Kalamazoo, MI 49008-8048, United States. E-mail: helen.pratt@med.wmich.edu.

Keywords: child health, adolescent health, mental health, psychiatry, psychology, personality disorders

Introduction

Youth who exhibit symptoms associated with personality disorders (PD) can result in that person being diagnosed with a personality disorder (1). This is problematic because these youth have not reached full maturity. Most symptoms they exhibit can often be better explained by other incidents, factors or reactions that they experience throughout stages of development (cognitive, emotional, and mental); such as: a) trauma; b) abuse (emotional, physical, verbal); c) violence (domestic between care-providers, abuse from care providers or siblings; d) multiple trauma exposures; e) parents who have a history of uncontrolled mental disorders; and f) a strong familial genetic history of serious psychopathology (such as, depression, personality disorders. Not all youth who are exposed to the above conditions develop personality disorders (1). Some children who are exposed to factors identified in the above list as a neonate, during infancy, childhood, adolescence, or young adulthood can often receive appropriate psychotherapy to alleviate distress and teach effective coping strategies.

Other youth diagnosed with comorbid disorders and exposed multiple traumatic events are at risk for developing deviant or maladaptive behavior patterns that significantly impairs their growth and development. A personality disorder can develop in youth who do not developmental flexibility, resilience, consistent supportive relationships with others, strong connections to their school or community, future orientation, and a sense of hope; they may develop personality traits that are inflexible and maladaptive and cause significant functional impairment or subjective distress (2-5).

Definition

A personality disorder is defined by the “Diagnostic and statistical manual of mental disorders,” fifth edition, as being characterized by enduring patterns of internal experiences and behaviors that markedly deviates from the individual’s culture (3). These stable patterns are pervasive, enduring, inflexible deviant and maladaptive cognitions, perceptions, impulse control, interpersonal relationships, and behaviors that usually begin in adolescence or early adulthood; the outcome for affected youth results in disruptive and impaired function. Their behaviors are exhibited in a wide range of social and personal contexts. There are 10 classifications of personality disorders, divided into three clusters; Cluster A: Odd and eccentric, Cluster B: Dramatic, emotional, and erratic and Cluster C: Anxious and fearful. The reader is referred to the DSM-V or the National Institute of Mental Health (NIMH) website for further information (3, 6-12).

PREVALENCE RATES

The estimated prevalence rate for any personality disorder in the general adult population in the United States is 10-15%; 5.7% in Cluster A disorders; 1.5% for Cluster B and 6% for Cluster C disorders (3, 5, 7-10, 13). Research on prevalence rates of personality disorders in youth is lacking. Research from community samples in primary care estimated that adolescents with at least one personality disorder range from 6%-17%. Prevalence rates tend to peak in early adolescence and then decline steadily during adolescence and early adulthood. Such data is sparse for specific personality disorders. Prevalence of child-onset bipolar is not well established due to debate about the appropriate definition of caseness (or boundaries of diagnosis) among preadolescents (9).

CLINICAL FEATURES

In order to be diagnosed with a personality disorder, an individual must meet certain criteria as established by the DSM-V which include; 1) an enduring pattern of inner experience and behavior that deviates markedly from the expectations of the individual's culture in two or more areas: a) cognition, b) affectivity, c) interpersonal relationships and d) impulse control; 2) The enduring pattern is inflexible, pervasive and stable occurs across a broad range of personal and social situations; 3) the enduring pattern leads to clinically significant distress or impairment in social, occupational or other important areas of functioning (3). Retrospective data shows that onset usually occurs during adolescence or early adulthood with some individuals reporting onset in childhood.

In order to diagnose the problem characteristics are not better accounted for as a manifestation or consequence of another mental disorder and not due to the direct physiological effects of a substance or a general medical condition (3). This NOS (not otherwise specified) diagnosis is used when the patient meets criteria for a personality disorder but fails to meet the criterion set for the ten specific personality disorders that the DSM-IV-TR offers. These ten personality disorders are broken up and divided into three clusters, A, B and C as designated by their general presentations (see Table 1) (1, 3, 6-11).

Expressed human behavior is divided into characteristics and patterns of behavior labeled as traits; those traits are often further used to describe key features of an individual's temperament. Personality traits are consistent ways that people tend to think, behave, and feel across situations and time. These infants'/children's temperament and subsequent personality traits are among the first indications of a person's personality. Theorists contend that temperament is influenced by environmental experiences and genetics. Researchers support that these factors have been linked to observed personality traits in adulthood (2, 13).

However, there is little research that identifies causal relationships between these factors and personality disorders in adulthood. Controversy over the diagnosing of personality disorders prior to adulthood exists. Proponents offer that it is imperative that youth who present with the devastating symptoms of PD, receive early and intense treatment to minimize outcomes and the impact on the adult's life. Opponents reason that prior to adulthood a) youth are not in control of their environments or situations, b) youth under the age of 18 do not control the family finances nor do they have legal standing which means they have limited access to mental health care; and c) current research offers that the human brain does not fully mature until after age 22 years in most human, therefore youth should not be expected to manage the adversities of their situation (4, 14).

Table 1. Personality disorders comparison

Disorder	**Character Traits**	**Differential Diagnosis**	**Co-morbidity**
Cluster A		**Odd and Eccentric**	
Paranoid Personality Disorder	• Extremely suspicious of others • Misinterprets Believes other's intent is malevolent, exploitive, harmful or deceptive in the face of lack of evidence • Holds grudges Problems with close relationships • Does not trust others • Difficult to get along with	• Rule out: • Pervasive developmental disorder • Schizophrenia • Mood disorders with psychotic features • Psychotic disorders • Direct physiological effects of neurological or other medical condition • Medication side effects	• Pervasive developmental disorder • Schizophrenia • Mood disorders with psychotic features • Psychotic disorders • Direct physiological effects of neurological or other medical condition • Medication side effects
Schizoid Personality Disorder	• Restricted range of affect • Indifferent to feedback from others • Emotional coldness • Detached or flattened affect • Not interested in sex or sexual behavior • Misinterprets • Few activities viewed as pleasurable • Solitary		
Schizotypal Personality Disorder	Perceptual and cognitive distortions Eccentric Inappropriate or constricted affect Superstitious or distorted cognition Delusions of Reference Severely impaired interpersonal relationships		
Cluster B	**Dramatic, Emotional and Erratic**		
Antisocial Personality Disorder	• Violate the rights of others • Rationalizes exploitive behavior • Lacks Remorse • Aggressive • Self-indulgent • Does not conform to social norms or ideals • Impulsive • Irresponsible	Rule out: • Schizophrenia and Manic episode	• Conduct Disorder • Dysthymia • Alcohol use disorder • Generalized anxiety disorder
Borderline Personality Disorder	• Unstable interpersonal relationships • Marked reactive • Unstable self-image • Exhibits many symptoms of psychopathology • Exhibits intense episodic emotional reactions • Chronically complains feeling • empty • Frantically avoids abandonment • Marked impulsivity • Very high risk for self-mutilation & suicidal behavior, sex and substance abuse, binging and drinking	Rule out: • Mood disorders • At risk of self-harm and suicidal	• Depression • Anxiety disorders • Substance abuse • Eating disorders • Behaviors, and completed suicides.

Subtype of Disorder	Character Traits	Differential Diagnosis	Comorbidity
Histrionic Personality Disorder	• Highly suggestible • Marked Impulsivity • Easily influences by others • Inappropriate sexually, seductive or provocative • Must be the center of attention or is uncomfortable • Rapid shifts/shallow emotions • Inappropriate attachments • Speech lacks detail • Dramatic	Rule out: • Personality change due to a general medical condition • Symptoms that develop in association with chronic substance abuse	• Substance abuse
Narcissistic Personality Disorder	• Grandiosity • Sense of entitlement • Lacks empathy • Fantasies • Requires excessive admiration • May have some perfectionist qualities • Self-Indulgent but not generous to others • Exploitive • Arrogant • Works hard to prevent others from discovering personal flaws or deficits	Rule out: • Schizotypal personality disorder • Paranoid personality disorder	
Cluster C		**Anxious and Fearful**	
Avoidant Personality Disorder	• Extreme social inhibition (shyness), • Feelings of inadequacy • Acute sensitivity to actual or perceived rejection	Rule out: • Shyness • Developmentally appropriate avoidant behavior Social phobia • Problems with acculturation following immigration	• May share features with social phobia
Dependent Personality Disorder	• Difficulty initiating anything and making decisions • Has trouble doing things • Submissive • Always attempts to get others to assume responsibility Strong feelings of helplessness Fears of abandonment, afraid to disagree with others • Excessive and urgent need for care • Goes to excessive lengths to gain nurturing and support • Most often diagnosed in females and LGBT individuals	Rule Out: • Developmentally appropriate behavior • Mood disorders • Panic disorders • Personality disorders • Agoraphobia • General medical condition	• Mood disorders • Panic disorders • Agoraphobia • Results of general medical condition
Obsessive-Compulsive Personality Disorder	• Life is governed by details, rules • Inflexible in morals and ethics for the behavior of others • Preoccupations with orderliness, perfectionism, control • Rigid, Stubborn, Self-Critical • Not generous • Maybe socially detached	Rule out: • Substance abuse, especially substances that impact the central nervous system • OCD • Personality disorder due to a general medical condition • Narcissistic, antisocial and schizoid personality disorders	• Other personality disorders

Adapted with permission from Pratt HD. Personality disorders and adolescents: A developmental perspective. In: Greydanus DE, Patel DR, Pratt HD, Calles Jr JL, eds. Behavioral pediatrics, 3rd ed. New York: Nova Science, 2009:369-82.

The most prominent theory of PD involves the Five Factor model. Five major traits emerge between the pre-school and the early adolescence developmental year, as a person develops: openness, extraversion/surgency, negative affectivity/neuroticism, effortful control/conscientiousness and affiliativeness/agreeableness. Shriner (14) described each factor in terms of how children experience the world and the traits they exhibit.

Children who experience typical maturation (psychological, physical, cognitive, emotional development), who live in healthy environments, and have strong positive support systems are more likely to develop into young adults who are productive and stable. Those who experience poverty, violence, trauma, or disruptions to their growth and development are a greater risk for impaired personality development. Any form of trauma in a youth's life can disturb a normal healthy development and lead to that youth experiencing problems with their personality development.

Detailed criteria for the ten subcategories are not offered in this chapter but a comparison table for the characteristics is presented in Table 1. Based on the general descriptors applicable to all subtypes of personality disorders, the personality traits are inflexible, maladaptive, persistent, and cause significant functional impairments or subjective distress in the individual who has a personality disorder.

Youth who show symptoms of personality disorders may be described as having bizarre thinking, being suspicious, paranoid, may prefer to be alone, and may often get angry with others for reasons not congruent with the facts. These youth may seem strange, be described as manipulative, self-centered or grandiose. This mixture of descriptors does not represent any one specific disorder.

Research and studies have concluded clinicians agree that when an adult is diagnosed with a personality disorders, it is common that there was pathology of personality precursors that could have been identified in youth. However, most personality disorder traits that appear in childhood will not persist into adulthood (2-14).

DIAGNOSIS

It is an intimidating effort to diagnose personality disorders in adolescents and children. These concerns contemplate that it is difficult to make this diagnosis because: a) personality development continues into adulthood, b) theories regarding the origins and causes of PD's remain controversial, c) the way the DSM IV has categorized PD is confusing, d) this diagnosis is recorded as an Axis II diagnosis, e) this diagnosis is considered enduring and defines who an individual is and finally e) the research surrounding this condition in the child and adolescent population is scarce (2-14).

It is essential that clinicians use caution and carefully interpret and examine the data they use to when making this diagnosis. Clinicians also need to make sure that they understand the influences of a child and adolescents development as it impacts the progression of their personality traits. Child and adolescents learn to behave in a cultural context and exhibit those behaviors in a cultural context requiring clinicians to conduct accurate assessments that allow them to select appropriate interventions.

Diagnosis should follow a comprehensive evaluation that includes a complete mental status exam (MSE); screens for affective disorders and other psychiatric disorders, suicidal ideation, history of attempts, deliberate self-injury; clinical observations the youth's behavior across different settings (i.e., school, home, and social activity settings); consult with the individual's primary care physician and psychiatrist to gather information on medical and treatment history. Include data from other treating clinicians before making a differential diagnosis.

Additionally the clinician should obtain a developmental history for the youth and a thorough family mental health, status of parental and sibling relations. Personality disorders are complex and difficult to diagnose. This will help in developing a chronological time line of the issues presented regarding the child or adolescent. Clinicians should assess if the parents have typical expectations for their youth's behavior that fall within age appropriate developmental and social norms. Ask if there have been any traumatic events or extreme changes within the family (such as death or incarceration of a parent or care provider).

Clinicians also need to take into account a patient's social and cultural group in order to avoid inappropriate diagnoses. It is important that clinician's do not mistake symptoms that are associated with personality disorders with symptoms that can be better explained by other incidents, factors or reactions that a child experiences throughout their stages of development that may not persist into adulthood (2-14).

Co-morbidity

There is an association between mental disorders in childhood and adolescence and adult personality disorders (3). However, symptoms of avoidant personality disorder gradually dissipate as the youth matures. Those who develop this disorder become increasingly shy during adolescence and early adulthood. Disruptive behavior disorder, substance abuse disorder, conduct disorder, juvenile delinquency, severe aggression or violence have all been identified as being co-morbid with personality disorders.

The likelihood of being diagnosed with a personality disorder increases if a person has already been diagnosed with other mental disorders (especially major depressive disorder) or has multiple diagnoses. The presence of symptoms of personality disorders during adolescence is associated with an increased risk for violence behavior that persists into early adulthood. When compared to teens not diagnosed with a personality disorder, adolescents with personality disorders are more likely to engage in heavy alcohol consumption, cigarette smoking and adolescents diagnosed with avoidant personality disorders are also more likely to use illicit drugs.

Treatment

There is minimal research or definite answers about the development personality disorders or on effective evidence-based treatment and prevention of personality disorders in children and adolescents (15-18). Clinicians should be trained in the treatment of children and adolescents with personality disorders and other severe psychopathology. Most youth do not grow up to exhibit pathological behavior. Depending on the age and developmental stage of a young person, their behavior may be viewed as typical or deviant. The clinician that is competent in the treatment of youth and psychopathology can use that information to predict the best therapy and offer predications for prognosis.

Several treatment modalities have been studied and researched as treatment tools: Mode deactivation therapy, cognitive therapy, dialectical behavior therapy, and pharmacotherapy. It is imperative to for clinicians to realize that treatment for these disorders is difficult because of the symptomology that makes up each disorder (see Table 2).

Studies have shown that mode deactivation therapy (MDT) has been successful in reducing both physical aggression and therapeutic holds in personality disorder youths who participate in longer-term residential treatment. MDT has also been shown to reduce sexual aggression and internal and external distress in adolescents and adults.

Cognitive behavior therapy (CBT) is a promising treatment strategy especially for those diagnosed with bipolar disorder and anti-social personality disorder. CBT has been shown to be effective for treating children, adolescents and adults.

Table 2. Treatments for youth with personality disorders

Subtype of Disorder	Forms of Treatment
Paranoid Personality Disorder	Pharmacological Therapy to manage symptoms
Schizoid Personality Disorder	May be resistant to therapy Age appropriate supportive Psychotherapy that emphasizes education and feedback concerning interpersonal skills and communication.
Schizotypal Personality Disorder	Cognitive Behavior Therapy Pharmacological to manage symptoms
Anti-Social Personality Disorder	Most difficult personality disorder to treat Community residential or wilderness programs that provide a firm structure, close supervision and intense confrontation by peers Pharmacological Therapy to manage symptoms Cognitive Behavior Therapy
Borderline Personality Disorder	Cognitive behavioral therapy (CBT). Dialectical behavior therapy (DBT). Schema-focused therapy.
Histrionic Personality Disorder	Group therapy Pharmacological to manage symptoms
Narcissistic Personality Disorder	Cognitive Behavior Therapy Group Therapy
Avoidant Personality Disorder	Group Therapy Social Skills Training Pharmacological to manage symptoms
Dependent Personality Disorder	Cognitive Behavior Therapy Group Therapy
Obsessive Compulsive Personality Disorder	Pharmacological Cognitive Behavior Therapy

Dialectical behavior therapy (DBT) is a form of CBT and was developed to treat bipolar affective disorder. Both therapies address teaching individuals a) to control, modulate and manage their emotions; and b) strategies to address distortions in thinking, perceptions and impulse control (16).

Pharmacological treatments are not designed to treat the personality disorders but had been the most often employed treatment strategy to control or minimizing symptoms of depression, anger, anxiety, and psychosis. Clinicians must remember that the focus of care should be on controlling the aversive outcomes of disturbances in emotional regulation and core beliefs. Impulse control and faulty thinking can result in the manifestation of the maladaptive and sometimes dangerous behaviors that may be symptomatic of personality disorders.

CONCLUSION

Personality traits are developing as a child grows from infancy into adolescents and adulthood. Personality disorders are most often diagnosed in the adult population; since the retrospective research indicates that personality disorders have an onset during adolescence and sometimes during childhood, many clinicians have advocated for early diagnosis so that prevention and treatment interventions can minimize aversive outcome for affected youth. A diagnosis of personality disorder indicates a) there is no cure for these disorders, b) the affected person has an enduring, pervasive and stable set of personality traits and c) will present with the associated accompanying social and emotional deficits. Personality disorders do occur in this population, but caution and care must be exercised in assigning these diagnoses. Youth who manifest symptoms of personality disorders may be responding to abuse, trauma, and chaotic environments or may simply be a product of their specific sub group's cultural norms.

Several concerns arise when a personality diagnosis is considered. Clinicians have to take into account that children are rapidly developing and behaviors will likely transform across different contexts and patterns of behavior will also change. Often times this diagnosis can also cause teachers, clinicians and others involved in the child's or adolescent's care to give up because the stigma attached to these types of diagnoses. These diagnoses will affect the individual for life. Adolescents are in a phase of development that can be characterized as stormy and their personality pathology is transient. Children and adolescents do not have control of their lives, environments, or ability to seek treatment at this time of their development. They are at the mercy of their caregivers who are often times the ones to articulate and relate the child's behavior.

Personality disorders exist in society and are a major mental health problem because of the disability they produce and the cost for treatment. If a personality disorder exists the youth is best served by being diagnosed early and receiving effective treatment intervention. Treatment should be designed to foster the youth's personal strengths and competencies and develop resiliency. Clinicians are cautioned when making this diagnosis in youth to use due diligence. Although the diagnosis of a personality disorder means that the person cannot change the associated deficits, he or she can be helped to learn to manage potential negative outcomes.

References

[1] Pratt HD. Personality disorders and adolescents: A developmental perspective. In: Greydanus DE, Patel DR, Pratt HD, Calles Jr JL, eds. Behavioral pediatrics, 3rd ed. New York: Nova Science, 2009: 369-82.

[2] Calabrese WR, Rudick M., Clark LA, Simms LJ. Development and validation of big four personality scales for the schedule for nonadaptive and adaptive personality—Second Edition (SNAP–2). Psychol Assess 2012; 24(3): 751–63.

[3] American Psychiatric Association. Personality disorders. Diagnostic and statistical manual of mental disorders, fifth ed. Washington, DC: American Psychiatric Association, 2013: 645-84.

[4] Crain W. Theories of development. Upper Saddle River, NJ: Prentice Hall, 2000.

[5] Freeman A, Reinecke MA. Personality disorders in childhood and adolescence. Hoboken, NJ: Wiley, 2007.

[6] Laurenssen EM, Hutsebaut J. Feenstra DJ, Van Busschbach JJ, Luyten P. Diagnosis of personality disorders in adolescents: a study among psychologists. Child Adolesc Psychiatr Mental Health 2013; 7(1): 3.

[7] National Institute of Mental Health (NIMH). Avoidant personality disorder. National Institutes of Health (NIH), 2015. Accessed 2015 Feb 3. URL: http://www.nimh.nih.gov/health/ statistics/ prevalence/avoidant-personality-disorder.shtml.

[8] National Institute of Mental Health (NIMH). Bipolar disorder. National Institutes of Health (NIH), 2015. Assessed 2015 Feb 3. URL: http://www.nimh.nih.gov/ad rhealth/topics/bipolar-disorder/ index.shtml.

[9] National Institute of Mental Health (NIMH). National Institute of Mental Health (NIMH). Bipolar disorder in children and adolescents (fact sheet). National Institutes of Health (NIH), 2015. Assessed 2015 Feb 3. URL: http://www.nimh.nih.gov/health/publications/bipolar-disorder-in-children-and-adolescnts-fact-sheet/index .shtml.

[10] National Institute of Mental Health (NIMH). National Institute of Mental Health (NIMH). Borderline personality disorder. National Institutes of Health (NIH), 2015. Assessed 2015 Feb 3. URL: http:// www. nimh.nih.gov/health/publications/borderline-personality-disorder/index.shtml.

[11] Rey JM, Morris-Yates A, Singh M, Andrews G, Stewart G. Continuities between psychiatric disorders in adolescents and personality disorders in young adults. Am J Psychiatry 1995; 152(6): 895-900.

[12] Vijay NR, Langley J, Links P. Adolescent personality disorders in adolescent medicine. Adolesc Med Clin 2006; 17(1): 115-30.

[13] Snyderman D, Rovner B. Mental status exam in primary care: a review. Am Fam Physician 2009; 80(8): 809-14.

[14] Shiner RL. The development of personality disorders: Perspectives from normal personality development in childhood and adolescents. Dev Psychopathol 2009; 21: 715-34.

[15] Apsche JA, Bass CK, Siv AM. A review and empirical comparison of three treatments for adolescent males with conduct and personality disorder: mode deactivation therapy, cognitive behavior therapy and social skills training. Int J Behav Consult Ther 2005; 1(4): 371-81.

[16] Apsche JA, Bass CK, DiMeo L. Mode deactivation therapy (MDT) comprehensive meta-analysis. Int J Behav Consult Ther 2011; 7(1): 47–54.

[17] Magallon-Neri EM, Canalda G, De la Fuente JE, Forns M, Garcia R, Gonzalez E, et al. The influence of personality disorders on the use of mental health service s in adolescents with psychiatric disorders. Comprehens Psychiatry 2012; 53: 509-15.

[18] National Registry of Evidence-based Programs and Practices (NREPP), US Department of Health and Human Services, Substance Abuse and Mental Health Services Administration. Dialectical behavior therapy, 2014. Assessed: 2015 Feb 3. URL: http://www.nrepp. samhsa.gov/ViewIntervention. aspx?id=36.

In: Public Health Yearbook 2016
Editor: Joav Merrick
ISBN: 978-1-53610-947-4

Chapter 39

PUBLIC HEALTH ASPECTS OF SUBSTANCE USE AND ABUSE IN ADOLESCENCE

Donald E Greydanus[1,*], MD, DrHC (Athens), William J Reed[2], MD and Elizabeth K Hawver[3], MSW

[1]Department of Pediatric and Adolescent Medicine,
Western Michigan University Homer Stryker MD School of Medicine,
Kalamazoo, Michigan, US
[2]Department of Pediatrics, Driscoll Children's Hospital,
Texas A & M University College of Medicine, Corpus Christi, Texas, US
[3]Elizabeth Upjohn Community Healing Center, Kalamazoo, Michigan, US

ABSTRACT

Substance use and abuse remains a major public health issue of adolescents throughout the world, including the United States. Encouragement by the media, peers, and many adults along with easy access to drugs of all types continues to lure countless millions of youth into use and abuse of many drugs. Results of the 2013 US Centers for Disease Control and Prevention Youth Risk Behavior Surveillance notes that there is significant abuse of drugs including illicit drugs but also prescription medications including stimulants, synthetic narcotics, and "recreational" cough syrups. This review considers various drugs, including tobacco, alcohol, marijuana, cocaine, heroin, hallucinogens, inhalants, and designer drugs.

Keywords: adolescence, health, substance abuse, public health, behavior

* Correspondence: Professor Donald E Greydanus, MD, DrHC (Athens), Founding Chair, Department of Pediatric and Adolescent Medicine, Western Michigan University Homer Stryker MD School of Medicine, Oakland Drive Campus, 1000 Oakland Drive, Kalamazoo, MI 49008-1284, United States. E-mail: donald.greydanus@med.wmich.edu.

INTRODUCTION

The United States SAMHSA (Substance Abuse and Mental Health Services Administration) directs a survey every year of the US population (non-military, non-institutionalized) who are 12 years of age and older (1). The publications is called NSDUH (National Survey of Drug Use and Health) and its 2013 report noted that 24.6 million Americans 12 years of age and older used illicit drugs in that they had used an illicit drug during the month prior to the survey (1). Racial disparities in illicit drug use are being identified by various studies (2, 3).

It is important that clinicians who are caring for adolescents be directly involved in teaching their patients how to prevent the use and abuse of drugs (Table 1); clinicians can also remain active in the management of substance abuse disorders, if it develops in their patient (4-11). Adolescent exposure to illicit drugs can lead to a lifetime of medical and psychiatric effects (7). The impact of illicit drugs, when taken during pregnancy, can be devastating to the fetus and the child (12). Drug addiction involves mesocorticolimbic circuitry dysfunction and can be a lifelong problem, especially from cannabis, cocaine, nicotine, alcohol, and ecstasy (13). A number of factors are involved in drug addiction, including the role of serotonin, ghrelin, and other factors that are under study (14, 15). Death from the use of illicit drugs continues, as is seen with the use of heroin, amphetamines, inhalants, and others (16).

Table 1. Drugs of abuse

– Tobacco
– Marijuana
– Alcohol
– Cocaine
– Heroin
– Amphetamine
– Methamphetamine
– MDMA [*Ecstasy]*
– Flunitrazepam [Rohypnol]
– Gamma-hydroxybutyrate [*GHB*]
– Ketamine [Ketalar]
– LSD {*lysergic acid diethylamide}*
– *PCP {phencyclidine}*
– *Tryptamines*
– Barbiturates
– Designer drugs
– *Sports Doping and Performance Enhancing Drugs*

Screening for substance abuse (17) is critical because the neuro-psychiatric changes caused by some drugs (i.e., Ecstasy) may be irreversible and there have been reports of acute psychosis following marijuana and phencyclidine (PCP). One should also consider the likelihood of co-morbid conditions (see Table 2) in any adolescent or young adult with a history of continuing or repeated substance abuse; these conditions include ADHD, especially when associated with or secondary to a learning disorder where treatment is protective. Risk factors for drug abuse are reviewed in Table 3, while Table 4 considers non-specific indicators of drug abuse and Table 5 outlines protective factors for drug abuse. Screening tests may be helpful, such as the CRAFFT questions for alcohol use. The role of prescription medication dependence must be considered also by clinicians (18).

A major contribution that the primary care clinician can provide is to establish a medical home for all youth including those with substance use (19). The success of management is partially based on the underling genetics of addiction for a person, especially with opioid, alcohol, and cocaine dependence (20). Straightforward talk with teens about drug use is important in the screening process, though the teenager's estimates are often lower than the actual use. The clinician can work with the community in supporting community-based drug abuse prevention programs. Models of treatment are available ranging from brief to intensive management (21). Attention to improving sleep dysfunction in those with substance dependence and depression is an important goal in overall management of these person (22).

Table 2. Co-morbid disorders of substance abuse disorder

– ADHD
– Oppositional Defiant Disorder
– Conduct Disorder
– Personality Disorders (antisocial, borderline, narcissistic)
– Mood Disorders
– Anxiety Disorders
– Evolving Psychosis
– Post-traumatic Stress Disorder
– Eating disorders

Adolescents generally progress from initial drug use to more serious drug use behavior in a pattern that is recognizable (see Table 6). At first, there is curiosity about drugs, though no drug use may be occurring. A need for acceptance by some peer group along with a low self-esteem may lead to experimentation with some drugs—often the "gateway" drugs--- tobacco, alcohol and/or marijuana.

At some point the euphoria some drugs deliver is felt by the adolescent, typically at weekend parties or when combined with other substances. In some youth, there develops a state of actively seeking out the euphoria of drug use with widening of the types of drugs used (i.e., cocaine, Ecstasy, heroin, others), using personal drug paraphernalia, buying and/or stealing drugs on a regular basis, and becoming more dependent on one or more drugs. There is often a drop in grades, change of clothes, switching of peer group, and a strong denial of using/abusing any drugs. Seeking the euphoric state becomes the center piece of the individual's life which becomes out of control as the menu of drugs tried increases in scope. There may also be evidence of depression, worsening mood swings, acting out behaviors, suicide, violence, malaise, and lethargy. At this stage, the abuser seeks the euphoric state to feel "normal." This progression from experimenting with drugs to abuse and burnout can be seen over months to years.

Table 3. Risk factors for substance abuse in adolescents*

Genetics	Alcoholism among 1st or 2nd degree relatives Male gender
Self/Individual/Personal	Abuse Early onset of drug use Early sexual activity / homosexuality Attention deficit disorders Antisocial behavior Aggressive temperament Depression Poor self-image Learning disorders Parental rejection Lack of self-control Low self-esteem Euphoric/mood altering effects of drugs Body modification (as cutting)
Family	Dysfunctional family dynamics Permissiveness Authoritarianism Parental conflict, divorce, separation Poor supervision, lack of supervision Poor parental role modeling
Community/Environmental/ Societal	Easy availability of drugs and alcohol Acceptance of drug use behavior Poor general quality of life in the neighborhood Media influence Criminal activities in neighborhood Cultural and religious sanction Low religiosity Employment Increased use of drugs and alcohol in certain ethnic groups
Peer Group Influence	Substance using peers Rebellion Rites of passage of puberty Risk-taking behavior Curiosity Desire to belong Independence Early tobacco use
School/Academic	Poor school performance Poor school environment Truancy

*Modified with permission: Patel DR and Greydanus DE: Substance abuse: a pediatric concern. *Indian J. Pediatrics* 66:557-567, 1999.

Table 4. Non-specific indicators of substance abuse*

Physical indicators	Academic indicators	Behavioral and psychological indicators
Unexplained weight loss Hypertension Red eyes Nasal irritation	Deterioration of short-term memory Poor judgment Falling grades	Risk taking behavior Mood swings Depression, withdrawal Panic reaction
Frequent "colds" or "allergies" Hoarseness Chronic cough Hemoptysis Chest pain Wheezing Frequent unexplained injuries Needle tracks Blank stares into space Scratch marks Tattoos Excessive acne Testicular atrophy Malaise	Frequent absences Truancy Conflicts with teachers Suspensions Expulsion	Acute psychosis Paranoia Lying Stealing Promiscuity Conflict with authorities and family members Runaway behavior Altered sleep pattern Altered appetite Poor hygiene Loss of interest in extracurricular activities Drug using peers Preferences for dress, music, movies, identifying with drug using culture Drug paraphernalia

*Used with permission: Patel DR and Greydanus DE: Substance abuse: a pediatric concern. Indian J Pediatrics 66:557-567, 1999.

Table 5. Factors protective of substance abuse in adolescents*

- Nurturing home environment
- Good communication within family
- Supportive parents, intact family, appropriate adult supervision
- Positive self-esteem
- Assertiveness
- Social competence
- Academic success
- Good schools
- Good general health
- High intelligence
- Positive adult role models
- Peer group with positive personal attributes
- Religious involvement
- A personal sense of morality

*Used with permission: Patel DR and Greydanus DE: Substance abuse: a pediatric concern. Indian J Pediatrics 66: 557-567, 1999.

Table 6. MacDonald's stages of substance abuse*

Stage	1. Learning the mood swing	2. Seeking the mood swing	3. Preoccupation with the mood swing	4. Using drugs to feel normal
Mood Alteration	Euphoria Normal	Euphoria Normal Some pain	Euphoria Normal Definite pain	Euphoria Normal Marked pain
Feelings	Feels good; few consequences	Excitement; early guilt	Euphoric highs; doubts, including severe shame and guilt; depression, suicidal thoughts	Chronic guilt; shame, remorse, depression
Drugs	Tobacco Marijuana Alcohol	All of the above plus inhalants, hashish, depressants, methamphetamine, prescription drugs	All listed plus psilocybin, PCP, LSD, cocaine	Whatever is available
Sources	Peers	Buying	Selling	Any way possible
Behavior	Little detectable change; moderate after-the-fact lying	Dropping extracurricular activities and hobbies; mixed friends (straight and drug users); dress changing; erratic school performance and truancy; unpredictable mood and attitude swings; manipulative behavior	"Cool" appearance; straight friends dropped; family fights (verbal or physical); stealing (police incidents); pathological lying; school failure; truancy, expulsion, jobs lost	Physical deterioration (weight loss, chronic cough); severe mental deterioration (memory loss and flashbacks); paranoia, volcanic anger; school dropout; frequent overdosing
Frequency	Progress to weekend use	Weekend use progressing to four to five times per week; some solo use	Daily; frequent solo use	All day every day

PCP = phencyclidine; LSD = lysersic acid diethylamide.

*Used with permission: Patel DR and Greydanus DE: Substance abuse: a pediatric concern. Indian J Pediatrics 66:557-567, 1999.

DSM-5

The American Psychiatric Association published its 5th edition of the "Diagnostic and statistical manual of mental disorders" (DSM-5) in 2013 (23). Some changes were seen in this 5th edition in contrast to the 4th edition (24) (see the preface). The DSM-5 provided changes in the diagnostic criteria of substance related disorders (SRD). In the previous edition (DSM-IV-TR, 2000), SRDs were classified as substance use disorders (SUD) and substance induced disorders (SID). SUD was also identified as "abuse" and "dependence" disorders according to specific substances (i.e., opioid abuse and dependence, alcohol abuse and dependence, and so forth). SID included such classifications as intoxication, withdrawal, delirium, anxiety and others as induced by specific substances (i.e., opioids, alcohol, others) (25). The diagnoses of "abuse" and "dependence" categories needed their own specific criteria. Abuse could be diagnosed by meeting only one of those criteria while dependence needed at least three of those criteria.

In the DSM-5 SUD and SID terms remain but in SUD the previous diagnostic distinction between abuse and dependence was removed and a single category was developed called "substance use disorder" that ranged from mild to severe. A mild disorder is defiend as meeting 2-3 of the SUD criteria versus 4-5 for moderate and 6 or more for a severe disorder (American Psychiatric Association, DSM-5, 2013).

In the DSM-5 there was an increase in the diagnostic threshold in that at least 2 criteria (versus 1) are required for an SUD. "Craving" is added as a new criterion and refers to an intense desire or urge for a drug. Also, the criteria, "problems with law enforcement" was removed since laws vary from country to country and over time.

A variety of illict drugs are reviewed in this chapter with prevalence mainly based on the US Centers for Disease and Prevention (CDC) 2013 Youth Risk Behavioral Surveillance (YRBS) (2). The reader is encouraged to review this document. A number of other drug issues are considered in this report including taking steroids without a doctor's prescription, taking prescription drugs without a doctor's prescription, and ever injecting any illegal drugs. This survey reveals that 3.2% of US high school students had taken steroid pills or shots without a doctor's prescription; this increased from 2.7% in 1991 to 3.2% in 2013 (2).

The report also notes that 17.8% of students had taken prescription drugs without a doctor's prescription one or more times during their life; these drugs included Oxycontin, Percocet, Vicodin, codeine, Adderall, Ritalin, or Xanax. The prevalence was 20.7% in 2011. Also, 1.7% of students had used a needle to inject any illegal drug into their body one or more times during their life; this prevalence was 2.3% in 2011 (2). The survey also noted that 22.1% of students had been offered, sold, or given an illegal drug by someone on school property during the 12 months prior to the survey; this prevalence was 24.0% in 1993.

Energy drinks

The negative effects of energy drinks often containing large amounts of caffeine is becoming an increasing problem in adolescents and young adults; cardiovascular and neurological adverse effects are particularly seen (26). The DSM-5 lists four caffeine-related disorders: caffeine intoxication, caffeine withdrawal, other caffeine-induced disorders, and unspecified caffeine-related disorders (23).

Designer drugs

Clandestine chemists and surreptitious laboratories are developing a wide variety of designer drugs or "legal highs" which are analogs of such drugs as opioids, cannabinoids, phencyclidine, amphetamine, and others (27-32). Their development can be traced to the

1960s but their production has escalated since 2008. They are used to mimic the effects of these drugs such as synthetic cannabinoids which mimic the psychoactive effects of cannabis and have been called spice drugs or K2 drugs. Cathinone is a natural occurring amphetamine analogue that is found in the Catha edulis plant leaves and synthetic cathinones (such as mephedrone or 3,4-methylenedioxypyro-valerone[MDPV]) are derivatives of phenylalkylamines which as amphetamine-like effects. Some are piperazine derivatives. Designer psychostimulants have been developed to mimic the effects of amphetamines, cocaine, or ecstasy. Methoxydine and methoxetamine are designer drugs with phencyclidine effects.

They may be sold on the internet or elsewhere as "bath salts" or "plant foods" and marked as "not for human consumption" in order to escape legal prosecution. Many adverse side effects may result depending on the exact product, its doses, what impurities it contains and other factors. Their use can lead to negative effects that are cardiovascular, neurological, renal, psychotic and others including death. Management of adverse reactions can be difficult and complicated by lack of knowledge of the patient and clinician what was taken. Negative reactions to synthetic cathinones ("bath salts") for example, focus on lowing the agitation and psychosis that are seen along with supporting renal perfusion; benzodiazepines and antipsychotics are used (33). Persons seeking euphoric experiences, including adolescents and young adults, should be educated about these designer drugs that are increasingly becoming available outside local laws.

TOBACCO

Tobacco remains a widely used and abused drug that enjoys a high level of acceptance by society, including governments that allow it to be grown for profit. In a 1999 national survey conducted by the Centers for Disease Control, one in every eight middle-school students reported using some form of tobacco (cigarettes, cigars, bidis, or kreteks) in the past month. Bidis (or beedies) are brown, hand-rolled, flavored tobacco while Kreteks (clove cigarettes) contain a mixture of tobacco and cloves; both are imported from Indonesia. Electronic cigarettes (E-cigarette) are now available on the market place which also can pose a threat to adolescents, though more research is needed (34, 35). The role of nicotine as a gateway drug has been shown by research (36, 37). The DSM-5 lists a number of tobacco-related disorders: tobacco use disorder (mild, moderate, severe), tobacco withdrawal, other tobacco-induced disorders, and unspecified tobacco related disorders (23).

The 2013 Youth Risk Behavioral Surveillance (YRBS) reports that 41.1% of high school students had ever tried cigarette smoking with a prevalence of 42.5% in males and 39.6% in females (2). The prevalence was higher among white and Hispanic students than black students. The prevalence of ever smoked cigarettes from 70.1% in 1991 to 41.1% in 2013. This survey also revealed that 9.3% had smoked a whole cigarette for the first time before age 13 years and this dropped from 23.8% in 1991 to 9.3% in 2013. Also, 15.7% of students had smoked cigarettes on at least one day during the 30 days prior to the survey and this had dropped from 27.5% in 1991 to 15.7% in 2013. It also noted that 5.6% of students had smoked cigarettes 20 or more days during the 30 days before the survey and this dropped from 12.7% in 1991 to 5.6% in 2013. Among the 15.7% who currently smoke cigarettes,

8.6% had smoked more than 10 cigarettes per day on the days they smoked during the 30 days before the survey; this dropped from 18.0% in 1991 to 8.6% in 2013 (Kann, 2013).

Among the 15.7% who currently smoked cigarettes, 48.0% had tried to quit smoking cigarettes during the 12 months before the survey; this prevalence dropped from 57.4% in 2001 to 48.0% in 2013. Also, 8.8% of students had ever smoked at least one cigarette daily for 30 days and this dropped from 20.0% in 2001 to 8.8% in 2013. The 2013 survey reported that 4.0% of students had smoked cigarettes on all 30 days during the 30 days before the survey; this prevalence dropped from 9.8% in 1991 to 4.0% in 2013. Also, 3.8% had smoked cigarettes on school property on at least one day during the 30 days before the survey; this prevalence dropped from 13.2% in 1993 to 3.8% in 2013.

The 2013 report reveals that 8.8% of students had used smokeless tobacco on at least 1 days during the 30 days before the survey; this dropped from 11.4% in 1995 to 8.8% in 2013. It also notes that 12.6% of students had smoked cigars, cigarillos, or little cigars on at least one day during the 30 days before the survey; this decreased from 22.0% in 1997 to 12.6% in 2013. It also noted that 22.4% of students had reported current cigarette use, current smokeless tobacco use, or current cigar use; this prevalence had decreased from 43.4% in 1997 to 22.4% in 2013 (2).

General

The smoke of cigars is more alkaline than that of cigarettes, dissolves more easily in saliva, and achieves the desired dose of nicotine without the need to inhale smoke into the lungs. Cigars are capable of providing high levels of nicotine at a rate fast enough to produce clear dependence, even if the smoke is not inhaled. The risk of lung cancer for cigar aficionados (well-known to cigarette smokers), is much higher than once thought. This rate increases more for cigar smokers if they were previous cigarette smokers. A class of carcinogenic compounds known as tobacco-specific, N-nitrosamines (TSNA) is present in cigar smoke at significantly higher levels than in cigarette smoke. Examination on a "per gram of tobacco smoke" basis reveals that tar, carbon monoxide, and ammonia are produced at greater quantities by cigars. When equal doses are applied, the tar produced by cigars exerts a greater tumor-producing activity in mice because of higher concentrations of carcinogenic polycyclic aromatic hydrocarbons.

Nicotine, an important component in tobacco, is highly addictive and a number of genes are involved such as the nicotinic receptor gene cluster on chromosome 15q25 (38). Current research shows that adolescents experience symptoms of nicotine dependence long before they become everyday smokers. Early and continued intervention, including the clinical use of such instruments as the HONC (hooked on nicotine checklist), is required because initiation of smoking during adolescence is related to drunkenness-oriented alcohol use and an increased risk for future substance abuse. The most powerful predictor of drunk driving in this research is regular smoking at age 14.

Nicotine is absorbed over various sites: lungs, buccal mucosa, skin, and gastrointestinal tract. Approximately 10 mg of nicotine is found in one cigarette; when smoked, 1.0 to 3.0 mg of nicotine is absorbed by the user. Nicotine is rapidly taken up by the brain's nicotinic acetylcholine receptors that are found in numerous non-cholinergic presynaptic and postsynaptic areas. The tobacco addict has chronic exposure to many dangerous chemicals, including nicotine, tar, carbon monoxide, arsenous oxide, radioactive polonium, benzopyrene, others. The addicted cigarette abuser becomes an adult with significant risks for the many well-known complications of this drug—lung cancer, emphysema, laryngeal carcinoma, other cancers, heart disease, and many other disorders. Lung cancer in female adult smokers is now more common than breast cancer.

A common condition noted in smokers and reverse smokers is keratosis of the mucosal palate posterior to the rugae. This was originally described in 1926 and is caused by the concentrated hot steam of smoke and chemicals producing a nicotine or "smoker's patch." Reverse smoking has been associated with dysplastic and malignant changes over time. Recent research also notes negative effects which occur from smoking during pregnancy, including lower birth weight and attention deficit hyperactivity disorder. Nicotine staining of the teeth, crow's feet from the occlusion of micro-arterioles near the eyes, bad breath, cough, and dyspnea are also well-recognized and widespread stigmata of smoking. Passive smoking is also known to be dangerous to those exposed to the smoking of others. Oral cancer is a serious consequence of using chewing tobacco.

It is important for clinicians caring for adolescents to join the struggle to limit the use of tobacco by adolescents. For example, advertising to youth must be prevented, and efforts to reduce the acceptance of tobacco by society strengthened. The prevention and reduction of adolescent tobacco use and abuse must be encouraged on a national and statewide level. On a local level, a broad range program is recommended that targets the family, community, and schools.

Pharmacologic management

Table 7 reviews current pharmacologic management options for tobacco addicts who are motivated to quit using tobacco products (39). Clinicians should take every opportunity to remind tobacco-addicted teens that their habit is very dangerous and help is available when they are ready to stop. Psychosocial issues in the lives of teen smokers and underlying cues to smoking should be reviewed with the adolescent. Special situations may arise, such as the pregnant adolescent who also smokes. A variety of nicotine replacement (NT) products are produced, as reviewed in Tables 7 and 8; the rate of quitting smoking is doubled by use of these products for the motivated smoker (i.e., 30%), in contrast to those seeking to stop smoking without pharmacologic agents (i.e., 15%). The choice of NT product is patient-driven; teens should not smoke while on NT products, though no overt negative sequelae have been reported in such cases.

The NT patch is prescribed for two months (changed each morning), using a high strength patch for one month, and then the lower dose for one more month (see Table 8). The patch is not placed over a site with hair. Up to half will develop local dermatitis, usually improved with local hydrocortisone application. The patch is applied only while awake if patch-induced secondary vivid dreams or insomnia develop. The NT gum (nicotine polacrilex) has a bitter taste that many teens do not like; some youth feel embarrassed while choosing the nicotine gum. If the tobacco addict smokes over 25 cigarettes a day, prescribe the 4 mg gum; eventually lower the patient to the 2 mg gum. Since acidic liquids reduce nicotine absorption, they should not be used for 15 minutes before gum use and while chewing. Instructions to give patients who chew this gum are provided in Table 9. Adverse effects of this gum, though temporary, include dyspepsia, mouth soreness, jaw ache and hiccups.

Table 7. Pharmacologic products available in the USA to treat tobacco addiction*

Nicotine Medications	
Nicotine gum	– Nicorette OTC – Nicorette DS OTC
Nicotine patch	– Nicoderm CQ(SmithKline Beecham) OTC – Nicotrol Patch (McNeil) OTC
Nicotine inhaler	– Habitrol (Novartis)
Nasal spray	– Prostep (Lederle) – Nicotrol Inhaler (McNeil) – Nicotrol Nasal Spray (McNeil)
Non-Nicotine Medications Bupropion	Zyban SR (Glaxo Wellcome) Sustained-release tablets

*Reprinted with permission from: Patel DR and Greydanus DE: Office interventions for adolescent smokers. State of the Art Reviews: Adolescent Medicine 11 (3): 1-11, 2000.

Table 8. Nicotine patch regimens*

Brand	Duration	Dosage
Nicoderm CQ and Habitrol	4 weeks then 2 weeks then 2 weeks	21 mg/24 hours 14 mg/24 hours 7 mg/24 hours
Prostep	4 weeks then 4 weeks	22 mg/24 hours 11 mg/24 hours
Nicotrol	8 weeks	15 mg/24 hours

*Reprinted with Permission from: Patel DR and Greydanus DE: Office interventions for adolescent smokers. State of the Art Reviews: Adolescent Medicine 11 (3): 1-11, 2000.

Table 9. Recommendations for use of nicotine gum

Chew a piece each hour for 6 weeks.

Then, chew a piece every 2 hours for 3 weeks.

Finally, chew a piece every 4 hours for 3 weeks.

Maximum limit is 30 pieces per day for the 2 mg gum and 20 pieces per day for the 4 mg gum.

Chewing instructions:

- Chew slowly until a peppery taste appears (often after 15 chews)
- Then put the gum between the cheek and buccal mucosa until the peppery taste has disappeared (often one minute)
- Start chewing again and repeat the above cycle
- Get rid of the gum when the peppery taste is gone (often 30 minutes).

The nicotine inhaler is designed to mimic the hand-to-mouth movement of the smoker; 4 mg of nicotine are delivered from the cartridge which contains about 10 mg overall (see Table 7). Low nicotine levels are produced and the user inhales 6-16 cartridges daily. Adequate nicotine absorption is accomplished with 80 inhalations over 20 minutes; absorption is through the oral mucosa. It is prescribed for 3 months and then slowly tapered off over 3 months. Adverse effects that often improve over time include coughing, dyspepsia, irritation of the mouth and throat, and nasal irritation.

The nicotine nasal spray is provided as one to two doses (1 to 2 mg of nicotine) per hour over 3 months; there is a rapid rise in nicotine serum levels (see Table 7). It is prescribed as a minimum of 8 doses per day, not over 40 per day or over 5 inhalations per hour. Bronchospasm may occur and the nasal spray is not used for nicotine addicts with asthma. Other adverse effects include cough, rhinitis, nasal irritation, sneezing, and water eyes. The use of electronic cigarette for the cessation or reduction of smoking in adults remains under active research (40).

Non-nicotine therapy

The use of bupropion (see Table 7) in the nicotine addict who is motivated to quit smoking is helpful in up to 40% of cases; its relative success is attributed to the drug's ability to lower the classic nicotine craving while improving the nicotine-withdrawal problems of weight gain and depression. It was found to be twice as effective as placebo. It is prescribed as Zyban in a sustained-release form that is provided as 150 mg a day for three days; if tolerated, it is increased to 150 mg twice daily. The dose should not exceed 300 mg a day. Additionally, the second dose should not be given less than 8 hours after the first to reduce the incidence of a seizure. Though NT replacement therapies should not officially be started while the adolescent is still smoking, it is acceptable to start the teen smoker on bupropion while still using nicotine; a date of stopping the tobacco should still be negotiated while providing the bupropion. Bupropion is contraindicated in adolescents who have overt seizures and those with factors that increase the risk for seizures; the latter includes those with a history of epilepsy, an eating disorder, central nervous system tumor, and any medications that may lower the seizure threshold. Bupropion is contraindicated in those on MAO inhibitors. Bupropion adverse effects include insomnia, skin reactions, tremors, headaches, and dry mouth.

Clonidine and nortriptyline may be useful to some late adolescents and adult smokers to help them quit using tobacco. Various medications have been studied but not shown to help improve the craving for nicotine; these include buspirone, mecamylamine, naltrexone, doxepin, and oral dextrose. Another smoking cessation product is varenicline tartrate (Chantix®), an alpha-4 beta-2- nicotinic acetylcholine receptor partial agonist that binds to central nervous system receptors with a greater affinity than nicotine. It is FDA approved for adults with nicotine addiction and may be more effective than bupropion. Abstinence rates are 22% versus 16% for bupropion and 8% for placebo. In the short term, 44% of study patients quit smoking v. 30% using Zyban. Starting dose is 0.5 mg per day for three days, twice a day for 4-7 days, then 1 mg twice daily. Chantix® decreases the pleasure of nicotine use and lessens the withdrawal craving. The major side effect is nausea, but weight gain is not a problem. There are reports of suicidality, agitation, hostility, and agitation (7). The use of cytisine, a partial agonist that binds the nicotinic acetylcholine receptor, is under study (41). The use of a nicotine vaccine is also under active research (42, 43).

MARIJUANA

Marijuana (cannabis) remains a popular euphoric and hallucinogenic drug for millions of youth and adults; it has many names, including "pot," "hash," "weed,." "doobs," "BC Bud," "Ganja," "grass," "smoke," and others. It is the most widely used illicit drug in the United States, accounting for up to 85% of the illicit drug trade. The 2013 YRBS reported that 40.7% of high school students had used pot one or more times during their life (2). Previous CDC surveys noted that the category of "ever used marijuana" had increased from 1991-1997 (31.3% to 47.1%); it did then decrease from 1997 to 2013 (47.1% to 40.7%) (2). The survey noted that 8.6% of students had tried pot for the first time before age 13 years and 23.4% of students had used pot one or more times during the 30 days prior to the survey. The prevalence of having ever used pot was higher among males versus females and higher among black and Hispanic youth versus white youth. In the 2013 National Survey on Drug Use and Health marijuana was the most commonly illicit consumed drug with 19.8 million users 12 years of age and older over the past month of the survey (1). From 2006 to 2013 the number of persons using daily cannabis almost doubled in this survey.

This controversial drug is derived from Cannabis sativa or C indica (hemp plant) and the active euphoric chemical is delta-9-tetrahydrocannabinol or THC. It is present in the dried leaves, stems, seeds, flowers (sensimilla) and oil. This major lipophilic drug works on the cannibinoid receptors (ECS) in the mesocortical and limbic systems. The marijuana of the 1960s and 1970s' hippie generation contained only 2% THC, while the Hawaiian sensimilla product was about 3% THC. Today's street pot can vary from 3 to 7%+ THC content, while cultivated sensimilla can contain 7 to 13%+. A popular brand of pot is BC Bud, a product imported by the ton from Canada at $3000- 8,000 dollars per pound; it is grown in British Columbia and may contain up to 24% active ingredients. Many growers, commercial exporter consortiums (Canada), a significant fraction of the public and their elected officials, as well as active pot users are actively advocating for the legalization of marijuana.

Cannabis contains over 60 phytocannabinoids including cannabinol (or CBN--metabolite of THC), cannabidiol (or CBD--isomer of THC), cannabigerol (or CBG-- alpha-2-adrenergic receptor agonist), tetra-hydrocannabivarin (or THCV;THV--TCH homolog), and cannabichromene (or CBC) (8, 11). Many other chemicals are found in this complex plant, including terpenoids, and endocannabinoids (such as 2-AG [2-arachidonoyl glycerol] and anandamide [arachidonoyl ethanolamide]). The role of pot smoking as a gateway drug is well-known and many smokers also use tobacco, alcohol, and other drugs.

Commercial preparations of synthetic cannabinoids include nabilone (schedule II drug), dronabinol (synthetic THC in sesame oil; schedule III drug), and nabiximols (phytocannabinoid marketed in Canada). Dronabinol capsules were approved on May 31, 1985 by the US Food and Drug Administration (FDA) for nausea and emesis management due to cancer chemotherapy; the US FDA also approved dronabinol on December 22, 1992 for persons with AIDS who have anorexia associated with weight loss. Oral nabilone was approved by the US FDA on December 26, 1985 for nausea and vomiting due to cancer chemotherapy. Though these and other cannabis products are suggested for various other medical disorders, they are not approved by the FDA. Smoking marijuana is not approved by the FDA nor leading medical organizations because there is no research to support smoking pot and because of the many potential adverse side effects from cannabis smoking (Greydanus, 2014, 2015). In Canada the oromucosal spray, nabiximols, is indicated for management of cancer pain in addition to neuropathic pain and spasticity seen in persons with multiple sclerosis.

Though usually smoked, marijuana can also be eaten in such homemade concoctions as cookies, brownies, and spaghetti. The typical cannabis cigarette (joint) usually contains approximately 20 mg of THC obtained from about a gram of leaves and buds; however, much variation can be noted. The "blunt" is another popular way to smoke pot and consists of a cigarette with marijuana added to a hollowed cigarette. "Pot" is often combined with other drugs, such as phencyclidine, though glutethimide and methaqualone were also popular in the past as additives. PCP (phencyclidine) is frequently dissolved in an organic solvent, such as formaldehyde, in which a joint or hand-rolled cigarette is first dipped, dried, and then smoked. This preparation is variously referred to as "wet"' "water," or "Sherms"; the latter term refers to the well-known tobacconist Nat Sherman. This is a good reason for doing a urine drug test with informed consent and assent of a using teenager.

Marijuana use results in a potent sensation of euphoria ("buzz") that is noted within minutes of its use, and which can last for hours. Both THC and its metabolites are highly lipid soluble and are stored in fatty tissue. Serum half-life is 19 hours. Marijuana can be found on urine drug screen and stool for as long as one month following regular use, and ten days after a single use. The behavioral effects are mediated by cannibinoid receptors and results in the release of dopamine in the nucleus accumbens. The effects of THC also include relaxation, time and perceptual distortions, and heightened sensory experiences such as listening to music, watching television, or eating ("getting the munchies"). Some drugs (alcohol or diazepam) may potentiate the sedative effects of marijuana, while other drugs (cocaine or amphetamines) worsen the stimulatory effects of marijuana.

A large number of potential adverse effects are seen with smoking cannabis, including cardio-vascular, pulmonary, gastrointestinal (cannabis hyperemesis syndrome), dental, and central nervous system effects (8, 11). Cardiovascular adverse effects cam include arteritis, cardiomyopathy, myocardial infarction, sudden cardiac death, transient ischemic accident (TIA), cardiovascular accident (CVA), and cardiac arrhythmias. Pulmonary side effects can include chronic cough, allergic hypersensitivity, bronchitis, bullous emphysema (COPD: chronic obstructive pulmonary disease), pneumothorax/pneumomediastinum, pulmonary dyplasia, pulmonary tuberculosis, other respiratory infections, and even dust disease (talcosis) in hemp workers.

Potential adverse dental effects can include dental caries, dental dysplasia, gingival enlargement, gingivitis, leukoedema, nicotinic stomatitis, oral infections, periodontal disease, poor dental health, uvulitis, and xerostomia. Potential adverse effects on the offspring of females smoking cannabis while pregnant include low birth weight, preterm labor, small for gestational age, treatment in a neonatal intensive care unit, and various childhood effects such as inattention problems, problem-solving problems, aggression, executive function dysfunction, problems with memory and processing information, and depressive symptoms.

Cannabis poisoning can arise from consuming oral cannabis products and this is increasing being seen in young children whose parents are pot smokers. Cannabis smoking (including Spice drugs) increases risks for MVAs (double or more) and this can be worsened when combined with other drugs (i.e., alcohol, others). If one has smoked cannabis, 8 or more hours should pass before driving a motor vehicle. Pot smoking also increase road rage.

The central nervous system of young adolescents is very sensitive to cannabis and adverse effects may include decline in IQ, decreased coordination, distorted visuospatial perception, impaired executive function, impaired novel learning, impulsivity, inattention, memory loss, neuropsychiatric disorders (i.e., psychosis), and cannabis dependence. The DSM-5 has listed a number of cannabis-related disorders including cannabis use disorder (mild, moderate severe), cannabis intoxication (with or without perceptual disturbances), cannabis withdrawal, other cannabis-induced disorders, and unspecified cannabis-related disorders (23).

Management of cannabis use disorder is very difficult and there is no pharmaceutical agent approved for its management. Research continues to find medications that may be of help to those with cannabis use disorders and these include alpha 2 adrenergic agonists, antipsychotics (atypical), benzodiazepines, cannabidiol, dronabinol, gabapentin, lithium, lofexidine, nabilone, nabiximols, N-acetylcysteine (NAC), N-arachidonoylethanolamine (anandamide), nefazodone, 2-arachidonoyl glycerol (2-AG), and others (11).

Therapy is typically prescribed and its efficacy may be low because of lack of motivation for the person with cannabis dependence to stop their drug of choice. Approximately 25% of the 19.8 million cannabis users in the United States meet the DSM-5 criteria for cannabis use disorders. Many fail to seek treatment and this tends to be due to failure to recognize the severity of their disorder and this denial may reflect their own brain dysfunction. Of the 7.6 million persons aged 12 or older who need treatment for an illicit drug use problem in 2013, only 1.5 million (19.5%) received management in a specialty program (11). Of the 6.1 million persons who needed but did not receive management, only 395,000 (6.4%) reported they were aware of a need for treatment.

ALCOHOL

Alcohol continues to be among the most used and abused "licit" substances (#1 choice of 29% youth) that enjoys a wide range of societal acceptance (44). Alcohol is the leading cause of substance use morbidity and mortality contributing to 8,000 deaths each year. Surveys have revealed that US high school seniors have a lifetime prevalence of over 80%, with over 50% noting alcohol use during the previous survey month, and 4% admitting to daily use The average age that alcohol is first misused is age 12. The prevalence of alcohol use is higher among white and Hispanic youth than among black youth. It is important to ask youth if they drink and if so, what their drinking pattern is; repeated use of alcohol or other substances is not part of normal adolescent defiant behavior. The CRAFFT screening test for adolescent substance abuse is an easy to use instrument for screening drug use (17, 45).

About half of adolescents who are victims of a motor vehicle accident or suicide were drinking before their death. The most common pattern of alcoholic consumption is binge drinking, as defined by 5 drinks in a row in males, and four in females. Blacking out spells are frequently a result of binge drinking behavior. Binge drinking is directly related to drunk driving, increased sexual activity (and teen pregnancy), smoking, dating violence, attempted suicide, and other substance abuse.

The 2013 Youth Risk Behavioral Surveillance (YRBS) revealed that 66.2% of high school students had had at least one drink of alcohol on at least one day during their life (2). This 2013 survey also revealed that 18.6% of students who had drunk alcohol (apart from a few sips) for the first time before age 13 years of age, 34.9% of students had at least one drink of alcohol on at least 1 day during the 30 days before the survey, and among the 34.9% of students who currently drank alcohol - 41.8% had usually obtained the alcohol they drank from someone who gave it to them during the 30 days before the survey. The prevalence of having ever drunk alcohol was higher in females versus males and higher in Hispanic youth than white or black youth.

The survey noted that 20.8% of students had had five or more drinks of alcohol in a row on at least 1 days during the 30 days prior to the survey. Also, 6.1% of students noted the largest number of drinks they had in a row during the 30 days before the survey was 10 or more. In the 2013 YRBS 21.9% of high school students rode in a care at least once with someone who had been consuming alcohol (2). Of the 64.3% of high school students who drove a car or other vehicle during the 30 days before the survey, 10.0% had driven after drinking alcohol during the 30 days prior to the survey.

Alcohol effects

Alcohol is a central nervous system depressant that also induces euphoria in the user; tolerance and psychological dependence may develop, in addition to physiologic dependence in alcoholics. Alcohol drinks vary in their amount of this drug, ranging from 3% to 6% in beer, 12% in wine, and 50% in various liquors. Legal intoxication is usually 0.08 to 0.10 g/dl, though judgment may be impaired at a blood alcohol concentration (BAC) of 0.01 g/dl or lower. Central effects occur at 20-30 ng/dl. Acute intoxication may lead to respiratory depression, coma, and death. Adolescents should be carefully educated about the dangers of alcohol consumption, including the deadly mixture of driving and drinking that kills "innocent" as well as alcohol-consuming victims.

Alcohol dependence is a serious psychiatric disorder in adults, and youth may be involved in this disorder as well. The genetics of alcohol dependence has been studied for decades and its molecular biologic basis is being revealed (46, 47). The abuse of alcohol depletes a number of so-called "comfort" hormones (opioid peptides, serotonin, gamma aminobutryic acid, dopamine) in addition to inducing stress hormone release (i.e., corticotropin releasing factor). Many adolescents do not stop at the social drinking or experimental stage and rapid progression can develop through the later stages of drug abuse. Youth who abuse alcohol tend to come from families where problem drinking occurs as well as families where problem drinking is absent. The DSM-5 lists a number of alcohol-related disorders: alcohol use disorder (mild, moderate, severe), alcohol intoxication, alcohol withdrawal, other alcohol-induced disorders, and unspecified alcohol related disorders (23).

Medical complications of problem drinking include intoxication, pancreatitis, gastritis, worsening of co-morbid medical disorders (i.e., diabetes mellitus, epilepsy), and toxic psychosis. The alcohol withdrawal syndrome presents with such symptoms as tremors, seizures, hallucinations, and even overt delirium tremens. Youth who abuse alcohol may develop anemia, macrocytosis, and elevation in alkaline phosphatase, bilirubin, uric acid, glutamic-oxaloacetic, gamma glutamyl transpeptidase, or pyruvic transaminases. The diagnosis of alcohol abuse disorder is made mainly by a history of excessive alcohol use, and not on the basis of a positive serum or drug screening test. The fetal alcohol syndrome and the effect of alcohol on neuronal migration and pruning (apoptosis) in the unborn fetus exposed to intrauterine alcohol are well recognized consequences of alcohol consumption during pregnancy. The mortality risk to the fetus is 5%, while the accidental risk of harm to family members of alcohol users is increased considerably.

Management of alcohol abuse

Acute alcohol ingestion is treated with gastric emptying, intravenous fluids, glucose, respiratory support, and sometimes, dialysis. The possibility of additional drug use is suggested by respiratory depression greater than that suggested by the available BAC; head injury may also have occurred in this situation. Medications used in the management of alcohol withdrawal syndrome include clorazepate, lorazepam, chlordiazepoxide, diazepam, and various antipsychotics. Medications approved for the management of adults with alcohol dependence include acamprosate, calcium carbimide, naltrexone, tiapride, and disulfiram. Various medications have been used, but have not been approved for use in adults with alcohol dependence; these include buspirone, carbamazepine, nalmefene, selective serotonin reuptake inhibitors, and tricyclic antidepressants (7). Mothers Against Drunk Drivers (MADD) and self-help groups (Alcohol Anonymous [AA] and Alateen) are important programs found in many communities that help with the wide-spread program of alcohol use and abuse in adolescents and adults. Attention to the sleep disruption seen in those abusing alcohol (and other drugs) is important in an overall management strategy (48).

AMPHETAMINES

Amphetamines (Dexedrine, Benzedrine, Desoxyn, chalk, meth, speed, Mollies, black beauties) are classic central nervous system stimulants which lead to a variety of complications, as listed in Table 10.

The DSM-5 lists a number of stimulant-related disorders with regard to amphetamine-type substance: stimulant use disorder- amphetamine-type substance (mild, moderate, severe), stimulant intoxication- amphetamine-type substance, stimulant withdrawal— amphetamine-type substance, other stimulant-induced disorders- amphetamine-type substance, and unspecified stimulant related disorder- amphetamine-type substance (23).

Amphetamines can be taken to develop euphoria, lessen fatigue, improve attention, lose weight, and/or allow continued sports performance. In 2003, high school seniors reported a lifetime use of 14.4%, 9.9% over the past year, and 5.0% over the past 30 days of the survey. In the 2008 MTF, Johnson reported a decline in stimulant use with a prevalence of 4.5% in 8th graders and 6.8% in 12th graders (49). The use of amphetamines has significantly decreased but is next in frequency of abuse to marijuana. Amphetamine can be abused in various forms—oral, subcutaneous, or intravenous. Amphetamine "look alikes" have become more available through mail order sites or from garage production using simple compounds such a phenylpropanolamine, pseudoephedrine, and ephedrine-including the herbal ma huang.

Table 10. Amphetamine adverse reactions

– Anorexia
– Anxiety
– Exhaustion
– Hyperactivity
– Hyperhidrosis
– Hypertension
– Insomnia
– Mydriasis
– Personality changes
– Psychotic experiences
– Tachycardia
– Tolerance
– Weight loss
– Withdrawal syndrome

Table 11. Management of amphetamine overdose

Activated charcoal/magnesium citrate for oral intoxication
Cooling blanket for hyperthermia
Medical control of hypertension and arrhythmias
Haloperidol or droperidol for agitation or delusions
Lorazepam (Ativan®) or diazepam (Valium®) for seizures
Urine acidification with ascorbic acid

While the mechanism of action is not entirely known, amphetamines may act by inhibiting catecholamine re-uptake or facilitating the release of norepinephrine in the presynaptic cleft. Alternatively, they may act as monoxidase inhibitors. They are absorbed through the gastrointestinal tract within 30 minutes and within 5 minutes when used subcutaneously. An initial rush is followed by a prolonged euphoria, alertness, confidence, and excitation. Flushing, sweating, temperature elevation, tachycardia, significant rise in blood pressure, and mydriasis occur. Tolerance is rapid and confusion, irritability, headache, insomnia, seizures, and weight loss may follow. Cerebral hemorrhage and cardiac arrhythmias have been reported. A drug induced psychosis is well known in long time users, but has occurred following a single use. Acute overdose can be life threatening and diagnosis and prompt treatment is necessary (see Table 11).

An infected needle may lead to HIV/AIDS, endocarditis, hepatitis, and other infections (50). An abstinence or withdrawal syndrome is described in amphetamine abusers, with the development of severe apathy, depression, and hypersomnia. Amphetamine abusers develop tolerance and an overdose can lead to hyperthermia, hypertension, cardiac arrhythmias, seizures, and death. Table 11 outlines basic medical support for an amphetamine overdose; avoid the use of phenothiazines, since rapid decrease in blood pressure and increased seizures activity may result.

Clinicians using stimulant medications to manage adolescents with attention deficit hyperactivity disorder (ADHD) should appreciate the potential for abuse of short acting Adderall® (mixed amphetamine salts) and Ritalin® (methylphenidate) (51). Ritalin is also called "the smart drug" and "vitamin R" by abusers, who crush the methylphenidate tablets and snort this chemical to obtain an intense euphoria; large doses can lead to seizure activity, stroke, and psychosis. Published guidelines should be followed carefully when providing stimulant medications to adolescents. This should include the use of the long-acting preparations, such as Concerta®, which have formulations that reduce the risk for dispersion and the quick "buzz." Another stimulant addition with diminished abuse potential is lisdexamfetamine (Vyvanse®) a prodrug formulation The long-acting preparations used for the treatment of ADHD do not produce tachyphylaxis, nor have they lead to addiction.

METHAMPHETAMINE

This illicit drug (meth, ice, crystal, fire, glass, chalk, crank) is an N-methyl homolog of amphetamine and has become the stimulant favored by most adolescents, due to its potent stimulant effect on the central nervous system (52). It is a highly addictive drug prepared by illicit drug laboratories using relatively inexpensive chemicals and sold on the streets and using drug networks. The term "ice" or "crystal" comes from its production as clear, chunky crystals that look like ice; it can also be bought as an odorless, bitter-tasting, white powder that easily dissolves in liquids.

The lifetime use in the 2007 YRBS ranged from 3.7 to 5.3% while the 2013 YRBS noted that 3.2% of students had used this drug one or more times in their lifetime revealing a decreased prevalence of 9.1% in 1999 to 3.2% in 2013 (2). Methamphetamine is now responsible for one-quarter of illicit stimulant use.

This drug can be taken as a pill or its powder can be snorted, leading to a "high" or euphoria; when inhaled via smoking or taken intravenously, methamphetamine hydrochloride induces an immediate, potent euphoria that is described as a "flash" or "rush" lasting a few minutes. It is this intense feeling that abusers seek leading to rapid addiction with increased dosage and frequency of use. This is not the case with the long acting mixed amphetamine salts preparation (Adderall XR®) that is used to manage patients with ADHD.

Users of this drug note that there is increased wakefulness, less need for sleep, and increased physical activity; sometimes extreme anorexia may develop along with weight loss. The temperature, respirations, pulse, and blood pressure are increased; there may be excited speech. Methamphetamine releases high levels of dopamine and thus can affect body movements and mood in these addicts. Central nervous system cells that contain dopamine and serotonin are damaged, eventually leading to low levels of dopamine, thought dysfunction, and a depressed mood ("blue Tuesdays"). Motor impairment or a Parkinsonian-like movement disorder can develop. Adverse reactions are many and some are listed in Table 12. As with other illicit drugs that are taken intravenously, this drug can lead to various infectious diseases, including sexually transmitted diseases, such as hepatitis B and HIV/AIDS. Urine drug testing remains positive 48 hours and may reflect look alike designer drugs or prescription psycho-stimulants.

The treatment of acute toxicity includes the support of cardiac and respiratory function. Orogastric lavage and activated charcoal may be indicated if oral ingestion of other substances is suspected. Droperidal or haloperidol are more effective than the benzodiazepines in blocking the behavioral effects of amphetamines and produce fairly rapid sedation. However, benzodiazepines are indicated for seizure management and thorazine is contraindicated Blood pressure is best managed with labetelol or esmolol. Management of this severe drug addiction is difficult and current research is seeking a medication to block the euphoric effects of methamphetamine to allow the addict to get off the drug, if there is motivation. This antibody-type medication research is part of other addiction research studies seeking to neutralize the euphoric effects of drugs, such as cocaine, heroin, and others. Management of methamphetamine psychosis is difficult but important as is treatment of depression or anxiety related to the use of this drug in order to reduce risks for methamphetamine relapse (53).

Table 12. Adverse effects of methamphetamine

– Irritability
– Anxiety
– Confusion
– Memory loss
– Insomnia
– Tremors
– Convulsions
– Coma
– Hypertension
– Cardiac damage
– Rhabdomyolysis
– Paranoia and psychotic behavior
– Increased aggressiveness with violent behavior
– Cardiovascular collapse and death

COCAINE

This central nervous system stimulant is an alkaloid made from leaves of the South American plant, Erythroxylon coca. There are a number of ways to take this drug: intranasal, intravenous, inhalation, smoking, chewed (coca leaves), or swallowed. Previously, this drug was produced as a crystalline powder that is water soluble and developed from an alkaloidal paste of the plant's leaves. "Free base" and "crack" ("rock") are popular cocaine products used for smoking. Free-base cocaine is vaporized in a water piper (bong) or even a soda can with a hole in it. "Crack" is the street name for cocaine bicarbonate pellets that are pea-sized and produced using ammonia or sodium bicarbonate (baking soda); heating this concoction to remove its hydrochloride component produces a "crackling" sound. Crack may be crushed, tobacco added, and then this "cigarette" is smoked; other chemicals often added include mannitol, quinine, or marijuana. Over half of the cocaine used on the streets is now crack cocaine because cocaine powder is decomposed when ignited to smoke. Crack cocaine has become relatively inexpensive and very popular with adolescents.

The 2013 YRBS noted that 5.5% of students had used any form of cocaine one or more times during their life (2). The CDC surveys noted that the prevalence of ever used cocaine increased from 1991 to 1999 (5.9% to 9.5%) and decreased from 1999 to 2013 (9.5% to 5.5%) (2). The prevalence of ever-used cocaine was higher among male youth versus female youth. Approximately 23% of Americans report they have experience with cocaine before age 30. The DSM-5 lists a number of stimulant-related disorders with regard to cocaine: stimulant use disorder-cocaine (mild, moderate, severe), stimulant intoxication-cocaine, stimulant withdrawal—cocaine, other stimulant-induced disorders-cocaine, and unspecified stimulant related disorder-cocaine (23).

Cocaine is a topical anesthetic, a peripheral sympathomimetic, and a central nervous system stimulant. The drug interferes with neuronal catecholamine reuptake and dopamine reabsorption. The popularity of cocaine is based on its ready availability and the potent euphoric feeling it produces; this high lasts 5 to 10 minutes if cocaine is smoked, in contrast to 10 to 30 minutes if taken intravenously. Because the high is short lived, the usual pattern of use is escalated and dependence is promoted. Urine and blood testing remains positive for 48-72 hours following its use. Once the euphoria is gone, irritability and fatigue set in. Users of this powerful drug develop severe psychological and physiological addiction along with tolerance. Serious physiological complications are infrequent and the death rate is low even in heavy long-term users; but, when they occur, they can be disastrous. A partial list of the serious side effects of cocaine is listed in Table 13.

Table 13. Adverse effects of cocaine

- Anxiety
- Irritability and restlessness
- Confusion
- Peripheral blood vessel constriction
- Pupillary dilation
- Hyperpyexia, tachycardia, and hypertension
- Cardiac complications
- Angina pectoris
- Myocardial infarction
- Ventricular arrhythmia
- Sudden death
- Seizures
- Nasal septum infection and perforation
- Frontal lobe infarction
- Intravenous needle complications (including hepatitis B, HIV/AIDS, endocarditis)
- Increased premature delivery
- Abruption (bleeding between placenta and uterine wall)
- Adverse neurodevelopmental sequelae in infants
- Vascular spasm-induced limb reduction anomalies and strokes

As with other drugs, addicts look to mix various drugs together to intensify the pleasant or euphoric feeling of their drug of choice. When alcohol is mixed with cocaine, cocaethylene is produced in the liver; this chemical heightens the cocaine euphoria (i.e., more potent and lasts longer), blunts some of the stimulant adverse cocaine effects, and increases the risk of sudden cardiac death 25 fold. The term, speedballing, refers to the mixture of cocaine and heroin (or morphine) and this combination also increases the risk for sudden death.

The method of using cocaine leads to various complications, as nasal perforation/infection with snorting and the infectious sequelae from intravenous use. The high abuse rate of cocaine is associated with increased risk of sexually transmitted diseases among adolescents and young adults; this includes HIV/AIDS, lymphogranuloma venereum, and chancroid. Smoking crack may lead to the development of a very aggressive paranoia. Sudden death occurs and is a constant risk, whether it is the first time or the user is very experienced with this drug; such death is probably due to a terminal ventricular arrhythmia. Use of cocaine during pregnancy can lead to a variety of adverse effects on the fetus including preterm-labor, placenta infarction, placental abruption, pre-eclampsia, impaired fetal growth, and neurodevelopmental defects (54).

Management of cocaine addiction

While acute intoxication is usually not severe, it may be complicated by the use of opioids, alcohol, marijuana, and other drugs. Emergency management includes the maintenance of an airway and naloxone if opiate use is suspected. Treatment of arrhythmias may require lidocaine, phenytoin, or cardioversion. Lorazepam or diazepam can be used for severe agitation or seizures. Nitroprusside or labetalol can be used for hypertension. A cooling blanket and intravenous fluids may be used for hyperthermia. Phenothiazines are contraindicated.

Cocaine addiction is a difficult central nervous system disorder to manage. If tachycardia and hypertension develop while on cocaine, short acting beta-blockers and short-acting direct vasodilators (as esmolol) may be helpful; clinicians should avoid long-acting vasodilators, since cocaine intoxication is typically a short, self-limited phenomenon and use of these other drugs (as morphine, propranolol, thorazine) may lead to severe hypotension. Though naloxone is helpful for opioid addiction, it does not help with cocaine addiction.

Cocaine addicts with ADHD may observe that methylphenidate calms them down along with improving their concentration abilities; a reduction in cocaine use has been observed in some cocaine addicts who have ADHD and use methylphenidate.

Current addiction research seeks to find a way to stop the potent euphoric effects of cocaine and enable the motivated abuser to stop this drug. Dependence on cocaine involves various pathways (i.e., noradrenergic and dopaminergic) in the primitive midbrain reward center. Multiple CNS sites are involved with the addiction and thus any drug used to help the addict must work over many CNS areas. Table 14 lists proposed drug mechanisms that are being researched to potentially manage cocaine addiction by blocking this drug's many effects, including the use of vaccine technology (55).

Table 14. Potential mechanism to manage cocaine addiction

– Bind to cocaine molecules and prevent movement into the CNS via the blood-brain barrier
– Change cocaine molecules into harmless (inactive) particles
– Remove the cocaine molecule as a vaccine using an antibody-type response
– “Catalytic” antibodies changing cocaine into inactive fragments

For example, research is looking at drugs called “peripheral blockers,” such as Dopamine D3 Receptor Agonists (D3 agonists), to prevent cocaine-induced CNS stimulation by neutralizing this drug in the blood; such drugs may help with addiction as well as with overdose and cocaine-induced seizures. Oxytocin may be helpful via effects on the glutamate receptor systems (56). N-acetylcysteine is also under active research for the management of cocaine dependence.

If the addict uses other drugs, treatment of dependence on those other drugs may help. For example, naltrexone or disulfiram may help with alcohol abuse and be of benefit to the addict who uses both cocaine and alcohol.

OPIOIDS

A number of opiate narcotics are abused by adolescents and adults, as reviewed in Table 15. The DSM-5 lists a number of opioid-related disorders: opioid use disorder (mild, moderate, severe), opioid intoxication, opioid withdrawal, other opioid-induced disorders, and unspecified opioid-related disorders (23).

Prescribed narcotics have been popular for many years, and are available in many ways, as stealing them from home medicine supplies, obtained from emergency room or office clinicians by faking (exaggerating) injuries or illnesses (i.e., migraine headaches, dysmenorrhea), or simply buying the opiate of choice on the street. Most are obtained free from friends or bought from school mates. The 2008 MTF reports use by 10% of 12th graders with Vicodin being the choice of 9.7% (49). Oxycontin use was reported by 2.1 and 4.7% of 8th and 12th graders respectively. Seven of the top 11 abused prescription medications are opiates.

Table 15. Narcotic opiates

– Codeine
– Fentanyl
– Heroin
– Meperidine
– Methadone
– Morphine
– Oxycodone
– Pentazocine
– Propoxyphene
– Others

Clinicians may forget or not be aware of the addictive potential of such classic analgesics as Darvocet®, Dilaudid®, Percocet®, Stadol®, Vicodin®, or Ultram®. News media have covered the recent increased popularity of Oxycodone (OxyContin®), a narcotic that is abused by some in place of heroin; a variety of ways of abuse are noted, including chewing an oxycodone tablet, crushing the pill and either snorting the contents or intravenous use after boiling the powder. Its acceptance by addicts is reflected in the many street names it has acquired, including OXY, OC, oxycotto, and killers. Fentanyl is a prescribed narcotic that is ten times more potent than heroin and there are a number of reported overdoses from this drug.

HEROIN

Inexpensive and potent heroin (diacetyl morphine hydrochloride) is available and comes from Mexico, Columbia, Afghanistan, and Pakistan. Heroin (junk, smack, Mexican brown, China white) can be abused in a snuff form, intravenously, or subcutaneously (skin-popping). China White is 2000 times more potent than morphine and responsible for some 28 documented fatalities. Speedballing, as noted above, refers to the combination of heroin or morphine with cocaine in an effort to block the sedative effect of heroin. Use of both heroin and morphine is called "New Jack swing." "Cheese" which blends black tar heroin and Tylenol PM® has been associated with 12 deaths in the United States.

The mean age of heroin use dropped from 27 years of age in 1988 to 19 years of age in 1995. There was a doubling of high school seniors who used this drug from 1990 to 1996 at a time when the price of heroin was dropping along with a 40% increase in drug purity. The purity of available heroin has increased from 5% in the 1990s to over 80% presently. The 1999 YRBS noted that 2.4% of high school students had tried heroin on at least one occasion; this was broken down to 3.5% males and 1.3% females. The 2003 Monitor the Future (MTF) Study recorded that 1.5% of high school seniors had a lifetime use of heroin, 0.8% over the past year and 0.4% over the past survey month (49). The lifetime heroin use for these seniors was 1.5% in the 2007 YRBS, and < 1% in the 2008 MTF Study. The 2013 YRBS reported that 2.2% of students had used heroin one or more times during their life and this decreased from 2.9% in 2011 to 2.2% in 2013 (2).

Unfortunately, this use increases as these seniors leave school and also increases in those who drop out of school before graduation of their peers who stay in school. The typical situation is an adolescent who begins to snort this drug, then develops an intense craving for the resultant euphoria, and progresses to smoking or intravenous use (mainlining). An all-consuming addiction with tolerance develops, as noted by the saying: "once is too much, 1000 times not enough;" also classic, is the development of physical addiction, psychological dependence, and a narcotic withdrawal syndrome. This may follow initiation of abuse by as little as several weeks. Approximately 30% of adolescents who smoke heroin become mainlining adults. Those who smoke or snort this drug often mistakenly feel they are bypassing the dangerous effects of heroin by smoking. However, this is not true, and the younger the addiction starts, the greater is the risk for post-cessation relapse.

Opiate overdose presents with the triad of respiratory and CNS depression associated with miotic constriction of the pupils. Mydriasis is seen with withdrawal which presents with flu-like symptoms, lacrimation, irritability, abdominal cramps and diarrhea. Cardiopulmonary failure with bradycardia, hypotension, and pulmonary edema can occur. A rapid response to the opiate antagonist naloxone is diagnostic of opiate overdose. Support of both respiratory and circulatory systems with airway maintenance is imperative. Correction of hypotension is necessary while monitoring for hypoglycemia, pulmonary edema, and arrhythmias. Thin-layer chromatography immunoassay will detect opiate metabolites for 2-3 days.

Table 16 lists some of the medical complications of heroin abuse, including an overdose that leads to death from respiratory depression and pulmonary edema. For example, an increase in heroin overdose deaths in 28 states was reported by the CDC for the period 2010 to 2012 (57). Clinicians should observe for the use of tattoos to obscure puncture wounds or needle-tract marks made by the heroin intravenous abuse; such mainlining and tattooing phenomena increase the infectious complications of needle use. A newborn withdrawal syndrome is described in newborns whose mothers abuse narcotics; heroin withdrawal in utero can lead to meconium aspiration, bile pneumonitis, and severe respiratory distress.

Table 16. Medical complications of heroin abuse

- Amenorrhea
- Endocarditis (from *Staphylococcus aureus*)
- False-positive VDRL
- Fat necrosis
- HIV/AIDS
- Hepatitis (B and C)
- Lipodystrophy
- Osteomyelitis
- Peptic ulcer disease
- Pulmonary edema and pneumonia
- Respiratory arrest
- Skin infections
- Tetanus
- Others

Management of opioid addiction

Addiction research of the last part of the 20th century led to the conclusion that opioid dependence is a neurobiological central nervous system disorder that involves brain receptors. This science looks at reward circuits controlling such processes as hunger, thirst, reproduction, and even drug addiction. Drug-induced alterations in CNS opiate receptors lead to drug dependence and tolerance phenomena. Opiate addiction induces significant social dysfunction with complex biological and psychological components that are not corrected by incarceration. Unfortunately, the majority of such addicts are not in treatment designed to manage their brain disorder. These patients often need acute detoxification measures followed by residential and/or outpatient management of sufficient nature to blunt their often overwhelming need to find the narcotic euphoria. Community programs as the 12-Step groups (i.e., Narcotics Anonymous) can be very helpful to these individuals to stay off the drug (s).

The opioid addict may benefit from the judicious use of various medications that are available as part of the overall management program (see Table 17) (7). Naltrexone (ReVia®, Depade®) is an opiate antagonist that can help many with opiate addiction, including addicts with additional alcohol dependence. Methadone may block classic narcotic effects without giving the user the classic opiate euphoria; it can also remove withdrawal symptomatology and help with on-going desires for additional drugs. Clinicians have used this drug as a substitute agonist for opiate dependence since the 1960s. Pharmacokinetics allow once a day dosing and the patient officially must be at least 18 years of age or older. Daily doses may range from 40 mg to 400 mg and successful patients, while on methadone, are then able to maintain a more normal life, in contrast to the addict's chaotic life of only seeking money for another high.

In search of longer-acting alternatives to methadone, addiction specialists have turned to levomethadyl acetate and buprenorphine, both of which are medications that are effective with narcotic addicts Clinicians can also use the sublingual combination of buprenorphine/naloxone (Suboxone®) that provides benefit at least equal to that of methadone and seems more efficacious than detoxification/counseling. The naloxone part of this dual treatment is used to stop diversion of the buprenorphine to intravenous administration. There have been some reports of ventricular tachycardia with prolonged QT intervals (Torsade de pointes) after taking LAAM and more research is needed to see if this drug is safe enough to be used.

Table 17. Medications available for opioid addiction

–	Naltrexone
–	Methadone hydrochloride
–	LAAM (levo-alpha-acetyl methadol or levomethadyl acetate)
–	Buprenorphine
–	Anti-depressant drugs (as selective serotonin reuptake inhibitors)
–	Anti-stress medications (as buspirone)

HALLUCINOGENIC DRUGS

Both the hallucinogens and dissociative drugs may alter a youth's state of mind and mood. Hallucinogens include Psilocybin, Psilocyn (Shrooms, mushrooms), LSD, and mescaline (peyote); these drugs can cause auditory, visual, and tactile hallucinations. Dissociative drugs, such as Ketamine or PCP, alter a persons' state of mind and mood, causing a "feeling of detachment" or "dissociate reaction," but do not cause hallucinations. The 2013 YRBS noted that 7.1% of surveyed students report having used a hallucinogenic drug one or more times during their lifetime (2). From 2001 to 2013 the prevalence dropped from 13.3% in 2001 to 7.1% in 2013.

The DSM-5 lists a number of hallucinogen-related disorders: phencyclidine use disorder (mild, moderate, severe), other hallucinogen use disorder (mild, moderate, severe), phencyclidine intoxication, other hallucinogen intoxication, hallucinogen persisting perception disorder, other phencyclidine-induced disorders, other hallucinogen-induced disorders, unspecified phencyclidine-related disorder, and unspecified hallucinogen-related disorder (23).

PCP (phencyclidine) and LSD (lysergic acid diethylamide) are taken as pills to induce a potent reality distortion with synesthesias or alterations of sensory perception (involving sight and sound) and emotions (involving euphoria and intense fears), in addition to time and place. Tolerance is described in these individuals as are cases of psychosis and the well-known flashback that can be induced by antihistamines or marijuana. Overdosing can induce respiratory depression with coma and death. A recent addition to the "trip" scene is Salvia divanorum (Virgin Mary's Herb, Mary's leaf). This is a hallucinogenic ethnobiological plant grown in the southwest U.S. which may be smoked, squeezed into water, or steeped into a tea. It is absorbed through the mucus membranes and produces a "euphoric experience with God." It cannot be detected by current urinary drug screens.

PHENCYCLIDINE (PCP)

This drug has many street names, including peace, pill, sternly, peace pill, angel dust, hog, and sheets. PCP is an arylcyclohexalamine that can be made in illicit laboratories; it causes adrenergic potentiation by inhibition of neuronal catecholamines. PCP can be taken as tablets, liquid, or in a powder form, sometimes sprinkled on marijuana or cigarettes (joints) to augment pot's potency. It is a dissociative anesthetic with hallucinogenic, stimulant, and depressive properties. Since it is lipophilic it has a 72 hour half-life. PCP is the active ingredient and can be detected for up to eight days after ingestion. Clinical expression may include frank psychosis, mania, delirium, and late manifestations of depression. Agitation associated with vertical and horizontal nystagmus, miotic but reactive pupils, elevated blood pressure, gait ataxia, and delusions should suggest PCP intoxication.

Diagnosis can be confirmed with gas chromatography/mass spectrometry using blood levels with or without urine testing. Excretion is pH dependent (increased in acid pH) High doses of dextromethorphan, especially when mixed with benzodiazepines, have been associated with a similar toxicity to phencyclidine.

Management of a PCP-induced "trip" (bad reaction) involves keeping the patient in a dark, padded room with the provision of diazepam (10-20 mg orally, or 10 mg intramuscularly every four hours). Lorazepam (1-2 mg) may be used IM/IV for seizures. Haloperidol may be reserved for severe agitation. Death may be caused by PCP because of the development of hypothermia, seizures, trauma, severe hypertension or hypotension, and/or psychotic delirium/coma. However, most deaths are caused by accidental injury occurring during intoxication. Psychosis may be helped with D3 agonists and research seeks chemicals to act as "antibodies" to neutralize PCP molecules.

Lysergic acid diethylamine (LSD)

LSD is the most powerful hallucinogen and has earned many street names, including acid, "L," sugar, dots, cubes, big "D," and blotters. LSD is found in morning glory seeds and rye fungus (Ergot). It is easy to produce by amateur chemists and easy to hide since it is odorless, tasteless, and colorless; because of this, it has become popular at marathon dances ("raves") where it can be given to unsuspecting victims. A dose as low as 20 mcg (placed on small objects as a sugar cube, paper blotter, or postage stamps) can lead to its classic euphoric or hallucinogen effects by increasing serotonin; sympathetic activity is potentiated with resultant tachycardia, fever, conjunctival injection, mydriasis, lacrimation, flushing, dry mouth, blurred vision, tremors, incoordination, and elevated blood pressure. Onset of symptoms following an oral dose is 30-45 minutes. The half-life is 3 hours, but routine urine drug screens do not detect LSD. Most youth with a bad trip or unpleasant flashback respond to a reassurance and calm interaction with the clinician; if necessary, haloperidol has been given for major reactions, including prolonged seizure activity.

Tryptamines

Tryptamines include a number of naturally occurring Schedule I hallucinogenic substances obtained from "magic mushrooms" indigenous to South America, Mexico, and the United States. They can be synthetically produced and include Psilocybin (0-phosphoryl-4-hydroxy-N, N-dimethyltryptamine) and Psilocyn (4-hydroxy-n, n-dimethyltryptamine). These chemicals produce muscle relaxation, mydriasis, vivid auditory and visual distortions, as well as emotional liability. These drug effects are not well predictable and vary by the specific mushrooms used as well as the manner in which they are dried, brewed, and consumed. Users of tryptamines often experience a multitude of effects that include hallucinations, euphoria, dilated pupils, empathy, emotional distress, "feelings of love," and visual-auditory disturbances or distortions. Some experience gastrointestinal effects, as nausea, emesis, and diarrhea.

Dimethyltryptamine (DMT) occurs naturally in a variety of wild plants and seeds. It is usually smoked, sniffed, or injected. DMT is inactivated orally and rapidly metabolized. The drug experience is called a "businessman's trip" because its effects are for only one hour. Diethyltryptamine (DET) is an analogue of DMT and produces the same pharmacologic effects, but is less potent than DMT. Alpha-ethyltryptamine (AET) is another tryptamine class hallucinogen added to the list of Schedule I hallucinogens in 1994.

N,N-Diisopropyl-5-methoxytryptamine (referred as "Foxy-Methoxy") is an orally active tryptamine recently encountered in the United States. Alpha-methyltryptamine (AMT), known as "spirals," was designated a Schedule I drug in 2003. Tryptamines, like "Foxy" and AMT, are very dose dependent, which means that the doubling of a moderate dose could result in effects similar to LSD. The duration of effects from 20 mg of AMT usually last between 12 and 24 hours, while the effects from 6 to 10 mg of Foxy reportedly last from 3 to 6 hours. 5-methoxy-alpha-methyltryptamine (5-MeO-AMT) is also a tryptamine. Other common names for 5-MeO-AMT are "alpha-O," "alpha" and "O-DMS."

Bufotenine (bufagin, bufotenin, 5-hydroxy-N-N-dimethyltryptamine) is a Schedule I substance found in certain mushrooms, seeds, and most notably, the skin glands of the green and red Cane Toad (Bufo marinus). In the 1960s-70s, the "toads milks" in northern Florida were obtained by daring to lick ("suck the toad") which lead to accidental handling of the toads. Historically, these toads were killed and their skin boiled to produce a bitter tasting broth. In Australia, the milk is dried into a powder and smoked. In South America, this substance is used as snuff. A mild, though frightening "trip" occurs as this 3-indoleamine works on serotonergic sites in the amygdale and ventral lateral geniculate. The toad can continuously replace the supply and, in general, most bufotenine preparations from natural sources can be extremely toxic.

MDMA (ECSTASY)

Phenethylamines are a family of over 100 chemicals that are hallucinogenic. MDMA (3,4 methylene dioxymethamphetamine) is a phenethylamine that resembles both a stimulant (methamphetamine) and a hallucinogen (mescaline). The U.S. Food and Drug Administration classified MDMA as a Schedule I drug in 1985. MDEA (3,4-methylenedioxy-N-ethyl-amphetamine) or Eve is a close congener of MDMA. There is also a designer version of the banned decongestant and "diet" drug, phenylpropanolamine; it is referred to as U4ia and is similar in action to MDMA with both stimulant and hallucinogenic effects.

MDMA was developed in 1912 by German scientists and synthesized as an appetite suppressant; it was utilized in the 1970s and 1980s in an attempt to improve psychotherapy. Concern over this drug developed as its severe side effects became evident.

The 2013 YRBS reported that 6.6% of students had used ecstasy (MDMA) one or more times during their lifetime and this dropped from 11.1% in 2001 to 6.6% in 2013 (2).

MDMA produces an intense euphoria and energizing effect in users and thus is popular at dance or club halls (called "raves, trances, or dance parties that last all night); it is also popular with college students. It is a designer drug that abusers feel is safe at 1-2 mg/kg and produces prolonged effects; because of this, its availability and use is more common than cocaine at teenage raves. Its effect is normally 3 to 6 hours, though it may be several days. Its purest form is as a white crystalline powder and if red or brown MDMA is found, this suggests impurities are present. MDMA has many street names, such as ecstasy, XTC, X,hug drug, lover's speed, diamonds, clarity, dex, essence, roll, bean, M, E, and Adam.

MDMA has mescaline like effects, probably due to interaction with and destruction of serotoninergic neurons in the central nervous system that are involved with thought and memory. This may result from the formation of quinones which can combine with glutathione and other thiols. MDMA produces an anxious state of "well-being," changes in perception, moderate derealization and depersonalization without producing psychomotor agitation. MDMA abuse may lead to cognitive dysfunction, memory impairment, and behavioral problems. If taken during pregnancy, the risk for congenital anomalies is increased. Users take MDMA to enhance sensual awareness and augmented psychic or emotional energy. A number of side effects are noted, as listed in Table 18.

Table 18. Side effects of MDMA

– Hypertension and increased pulse
– Dehydration and possible heat stroke
– Fatigue
– Sleep dysfunction
– Muscle spasms
– Sweating
– Organ dysfunction: renal, liver, CNS, muscular
– Intracerebral hemorrhage
– Irreversible CNS damage with memory loss in chronic abuse
– Confusion and paranoia
– Psychosis
– Depression
– Anxiety, including panic attacks

MDMA can hide thirst and eventual death that may be due to dehydration (which is not uncommon and hence its association with water bottles at raves), hyperthermia, hyponatremia, or cerebral edema. High doses can lead to muscle breakdown, breakdown of muscles, malignant hyperthermia, renal failure, and cardiovascular failure at the raves. MDMA and some of the other "designer" drugs have been associated with intracerebral hemorrhage in adolescents and young adults who have undiagnosed vascular malformations. Also, anxiety (including paranoia and panic attacks) may last for weeks after drug cessation. MDMA is a popular date-rape drug (see below). Acute management requires diagnosis, rehydration, cardiovascular support, and the use of benzo-diazapines for sympathomimetic effects.

MDMA users may mix this drug with alcohol, marijuana, LSD, dextromethorphan, and other drugs. Preparations with camphor, menthol, and ephedrine are applied to the nasal mucosa or chest to enhance the desired MDMA effects. MDMA can also be taken in increasing doses in a "stacked" schedule similar to that used with anabolic steroids. The drug user may also take chemicals that are ecstasy-like in appearance, such as ketamine ("special K"), alpha-methyl fentanyl ("synthetic heroin," "china white") and ephedrine tablets ("herbal ecstasy," "Chinese ephedra," "Ma Huang"); large amounts of these chemicals may lead to hypertension, cardiac arrhythmias, myocardial infarction, cerebrovascular accidents, and death. The ephedrine found in Herbal ecstasy products as found in "health" food stores has only recently been banned.

"Date rape" drugs

Novel and more creative uses for previously legitimate pharmaceuticals and "nutriceuticals" continue to emerge "on the street," including familiar drugs as marijuana (i.e., increased THC content), phencyclidine (PCP), crack cocaine (or opium) with Viagra, variations on MDMA described previously, short acting benzodiazepines ("benzos"), and those compounds readily made using recipes available on the internet and concocted by amateur chemists.

Table 19. Club drugs

– Methylenedioxymethamphetamine (*Ecstasy*, MDMA)
– Rohypnol (Flunitrazepam; *Roofies, The Date Rape Drug, Roches, Rope*)
– Gamma-hydroxybutyrate (*GHB, Liquid Ecstasy*)
– Gamma-butryl lactone (*GBL, Blue nitro, Renewtrient*)
– Butanediol (*BD, soap, Revitalize plus*)
– Methamphetamine (*meth, ice, crystal, fire, glass, chalk, crank*)
– LSD (*acid, "L", sugar, dots, cubes, big "D",* and *blotters*)
– Ketamine (Ketalar; *Special K, Cat Valiums*)

A variety of chemicals have been used to lower external and internal inhibitions and/or consciousness, helping to facilitate sexual assault. These so-called "date rape" drugs are named for their strong sedative and hypnotic effects that are enhanced with alcohol. They continue to be popular at all night dance parties or "raves," and thus, have also been called Club Drugs or Party Drugs. Some are sold in "nutrition" stores or via magazine ads as sleep aids, muscle builders, and even as "party drugs." A variety of drugs have been used, as partially listed in Table 19; this list includes MDMA-methylenedioxy-meth-amphetamine (Ecstasy) previously discussed.

FLUNITRAZEPAM (ROHYPNOL®)

This is a potent benzodiazepine with sedative, anxiolytic, and anticonvulsant effects. It belongs to the same group as Halcion, Ambien, Xanax (Z Bars), Klonopin, Sonata, Versed, and Valium. Flunitrazepam is a central nervous system depressant produced commercially in Switzerland that reduces inhibition and results in memory loss (blackouts) with short term anterograde amnesia for activity that takes place while under the influence of the drug.

It can also lead to such adverse effects as urinary retention, drowsiness, confusion, dizziness, gastrointestinal dysfunction, visual disturbances, hypotension and others. It is available by prescription in Europe (not the United States) and used as a sedative for management of insomnia and also as a pre-surgery anesthetic.

Flunitrazepam is a tasteless, odorless, and colorless chemical that can be taken as a pill or dissolved in a beverage; anecdotal reports of snorting are noted as well. One milligram can be secretly placed in a liquid to sedate a victim for 8 to 12 hours with unfortunate amnesia for the sexual assault that may follow the ingestion. The victim is seen voluntarily leaving with the rapist, recalls little if anything of the events, and is unable to testify in any later prosecution. It has become a popular and classic date rape drug used by gang members and even high school or college students operating at local parties. Its many street names include forget-me pills, Rope, Roche, Mexican valium, and roofies. It is also an addictive drug used voluntarily by youth as an alternative or adjunctive drug to marijuana or LSD, as well as the self-treatment of anxiety. Its effects are enhanced with alcohol. If used on a regular basis, increasingly higher doses are needed for the desired euphoric effect. Its use has increased

50% over the past several years. In South Texas, along the United-States-Mexico border, it is frequently replaced by the more readily available Klonopin or Xanax, both of which are associated with blacking-out spells and "withdrawal seizures," especially when abused with alcohol and marijuana.

Gamma-hydroxybutyrate (GHB)

This is a CNS depressant that induces euphoria and lowered inhibition. It has many street names, including: Liquid X, Liquid E, Liquid XTC, Liquid Ecstasy, Natural Sleep-500, Organic Quaalude, G Caps, Gamma Hydrate, Georgia Home Boy, Growth Hormone Booster, Cherry Meth, Sodium oxybutyrate, Somatomax PM, Grievous Bodily Harm, G-Riffick, Oxy-Sleep, Scoop, Fantasy, Easy Lay, Soap, Salty Water, Vita G, Gamma OH, Somsanit, GHB; Liquid Ecstasy; G; Georgia home boy, caps, organic qualude, and goop.

Like Rohypnol, GHB and its analogs are used as "date rape" drugs. It has a soapy or salty taste, and hence the name salt is used until it is mixed with any liquid, including water. Because it is colorless, tasteless, and odorless, it is easily and quietly slipped into an unattended party drink to induce sedation and amnesia. Effects develop in 10-20 minutes, peak in 1 to 2 hours, and last for 4 hours. GHB is rapidly cleared from the body and is undetected in subsequent rape investigations. The clinician providing care in an emergency situation must request that the laboratory specifically look for GHB. Adolescent females need to be warned about the danger of leaving drinks unattended.

It is used by bodybuilders and athletes because of beliefs that GHB will augment endogenous human growth hormone (HGH) release while sleeping. GHB is available in single doses that augment or mimic effects of alcohol; increasingly higher doses are needed for desired effects. The risk of seizures and death caused by GHB-induced respiratory depression is raised when mixing GHB with other drugs, such as alcohol, heroin, LSD, and psilocybin. The CNS depression occurs because of increasing CNS dopamine and GABA (gamma-amino-butyric acid); the endogenous opioid system is also activated. It became a Schedule I substance in March of 2000 and in July, 2002, GHB was approved by an FDA advisory committee for study in the treatment of cataplexy. Most of the GHB used in the United States is illegally manufactured in the US. Law enforcement in every region of the United States reports that GHB has surpassed Rohypnol as the most common substance used in drug-facilitated sexual assaults.

Gamma-butyro-lactone (GBL)

Because the DEA is cracking down on GHB use, some are using GHB precursors, such as GBL as well as BD (1-4 butanediol), an industrial solvent; both are promoted to enhance sexual ability and pleasure. Street names for GHL are many, including Renewtrient, Revivarant, Reivivarant G, Blue Nitro, Blue Nitro Vitality, GH Revitalizer, Gamma G, Remforce, and Soap; it is found in paint thinners and floor stripper products. BD leads to bradypnea and can induce emesis, aspiration, and coma. GBL and BD are both easily changed to GHB in vivo, and in vitro by adding water. Some producers are substituting BD for GHB, even though the FDA has identified BD as a potentially life-threatening drug. It is sold as a dietary supplement in a number of sleep aid and muscle enhancing products; names include SomatoPro, NR63, Thunder Nectar, Enliven, GHRE, Weight Belt Cleaner, Revitalize Plus, and Serenity. The FDA asked that products with GBL be recalled in January, 1999; some states, such as California, have told manufactures that it is illegal to sell these products or market them as a supplement or nutritional substance. GBL-related products have been associated with reports of at least 55 adverse health effects, including one death. In 19 of these cases, the consumers became unconscious or comatose, several requiring intubation for assisted breathing.

Ketamine

This drug has been approved since 1970 in the role of an injectable airway-preserving veterinary anesthetic; it is taken orally to induce dissociative states, described as dream-like and hallucinatory. Street names include K, Cat Valium, Special K, and Vitamin K. It can be obtained as a white powder that can be added to tobacco or marijuana or the powder can be snorted; intramuscular abuse is also described. The effects of ketamine last one half to two hours producing an "out of body" distortion of time and space. Ketamine in low doses can lead to dysfunction of learning ability, memory, and attention span; in high doses, it can lead to myalgia, paranoia, elevated blood pressure, delirium, motor function impairment, amnesia, long term flashbacks, and respiratory depression-induced death. There is no urine metabolite.

Inhalants

Inhalant drugs (see Table 20) are central nervous system depressants typically abused by young (ages 6-8, peaks at 14), often male, and homeless adolescents to induce temporary euphoria and excitement (58, 59). These inhaled chemical vapors are viewed as easily available and as inexpensive substitutes or precursors to other drugs, such as alcohol or marijuana. Delivery is by "sniffing, huffing, or bagging."

In 1995 the lifetime use was 21.6% for 8th graders versus 19.7% in 1999 and 17.3% in 2004 (60). Approximately 5% of adolescent girls (age 12-17) used inhalants that included nitrous oxide vials (19.3%), glue sniffing (34.9%), correction fluid (23.4%), hair spray (23%), and inhalation of paints or sprays (6-16%) (49). The 2013 YRBS reported that 8.9% of students had sniffed glue, breathed the contents of aerosol spray cans, or inhaled any paints or sprays to get high one or more times during their life (2). The prevalence dropped from 20.3% in 1995 to 8.9% in 2013.

The main ingredient in airplane glue and some rubber cements is toluene. Another popular inhalant is gasoline, noted especially in rural areas of the United States and with Native American adolescents. Amyl nitrite, butyl nitrite, and other volatile nitrates are found in room deodorizers and are used by older adolescents to induce "aphrodisiac" effects.

Table 20. Types of inhalant drugs*

Solvents	Gases	Nitrites (Aliphatic nitrites)
Industrial or household solvents or solvent-containing products Paint thinners or solvents Degreasers (dry-cleaning fluids) Gasoline Glues Art or office supply solvents Correction fluids Felt-tip-maker fluid Electronic contact cleaners	Gases used in household or commercial products Butane lighters Propane tanks Whipping cream aerosols or dispensers (whippets) Refrigerant gases Household aerosol propellant and associated solvents Found in spray paints Found in hair or deodorant sprays Found in fabric protector sprays Medical anesthetic gases Ether Chloroform Halothane Nitrous oxide	Cyclohexyl nitrite (available to general public) Amyl nitrite (available only with prescription) Butyl nitrite (Illegal substance)

* Greydanus DE, Patel DR: Substance abuse in adolescents: A complex conundrum for the clinician. Pediatric Clin No Amer 59(5): 1179-1223, 2003. (with permission).

Table 21. Effects of inhalants*

Hearing loss
Toluene (paint sprays, glues, dewaxers)
Trichloroethylene (cleaning fluids, correction fluids)
Peripheral neuropathies or Limb spasms
Hexane (glues, gasoline)
Nitrous oxide (whipping cream, gas cylinders)
CNS or Brain Damage: toluene
Bone Marrow Damage: benzene (gasoline)
Liver and Kidney Damage
Toluene-containing substances
Chlorinated hydrocarbons
Correction fluids
Dry-cleaning fluids
Blood Oxygen Depletion/ Methemoglobinemia
Organic nitrites ("*poppers*," "amyl", "*bold*" and "*rush*")
Methylene chloride
Varnish removers
Paint thinners
Loss of the sense of smell (nitrites)
Thermal burn injury with nebulized alcohol/Robitussin® ("RoboFires")
Death
Kaposi's sarcoma

*adapted from Greydanus DE, Patel DR: Substance abuse in adolescents: A complex conundrum for the clinician. Pediatric Clin North Amer 59(5): 1179-1223, 2003. (with permission).

Inhalant use is usually experimental and may occur as a group activity. Inhalation occurs after these substances are placed in a plastic bag ("bagging"), wrap, or inhaled from a soaked rag ("huffing") to induce the intoxicating (psychoactive) effects. Absorption is rapid and the altered mental state lasts for 5-15 minutes. After a mild stimulatory effect, an inhibition reduction occurs, followed by unconsciousness. Death may occur from cardiac arrhythmias. Tolerance develops after long term use, though withdrawal is rare; dependence may develop (61).

Table 21 lists various complications known to occur with various inhalants. The DSM-5 lists a number of inhalant-related disorders: inhalant use disorder (mild, moderate, severe), inhalant intoxication, other inhalant-induced disorders, and unspecified inhalant related disorders (23).

Most abusers of inhalants discontinue these drugs by stopping substance abuse in general or moving on to other drugs. Management of those who become chronic inhalant abusers is difficult, often being hindered by their many, varied behavioral and social problems. Research on management is focusing on inhalant effects on dopaminergic, glutamatergic and GABAergic systems (61). Unfortunately death from volatile substance misuse may occur as seen, for example, with difluoroethane can occur.

BARBITURATES

These are CNS depressants that are classified as sedative-hypnotic drugs. They act on the CNS by enhancing the neuroinhibitory action of gamma-aminobutyric acid (GABA) and producing relief from anxiety and sedation. They are classified as ultra-short acting (thiopental), short acting (pentobarbital [yellow jackets], secobarbital [reds]), and long acting (phenobarbital). The short acting barbiturates have a higher potential for abuse and are more lipid soluble than the long acting formulations.

They can become addicting in 1 to 2 months and are deadly in high doses or when combined with opioids or alcohol. Abuse of these drugs leads to physical addiction, abstinence, and discontinuation syndrome, similar to that noted with alcohol abuse. The DSM-5 lists a number of "sedative, hypnotic, or anxiolytic"-related disorders: sedative, hypnotic, or anxiolytic use disorder (mild, moderate, severe); sedative, hypnotic, or anxiolytic intoxication; sedative, hypnotic, or anxiolytic withdrawal; other sedative, hypnotic, or anxiolytic -induced disorders; and unspecified sedative, hypnotic, or anxiolytic related disorders (23).

Barbiturates are detoxified in the liver and/or excreted unchanged in the urine. Symptoms of acute use and overdose are similar to those of alcohol and include euphoria, slurred speech, lethargy, miosis, and ataxia. Overdosing leads to low blood pressure, bullous dermatological lesions, respiratory depression, coma, and death. It is not commonly abused at current times and involves less than 3% of high school students. This reduced abuse probably reflects infrequent clinician prescription of these drugs, reduced availability on the streets, and the availability of many other illicit drugs. Barbiturates should usually not be prescribed to adolescents and then, only with extreme caution.

CONCLUSION

Substance abuse continues to be a widespread and very serious phenomenon for our adolescents and young adults in the United States and around the globe. Many factors draw our youth into these deadly drugs, leading to many acute and chronic sequelae, ranging from addiction to death. Youth must be clearly and carefully taught that drug use and abuse comes with considerable complications for their current and future life. They also must be taught that there is no scientific evidence that smoking cannabis is safe nor is medically beneficial. They must also become aware of the dangers of the designer drugs that are being produced in greater amounts.

Clinicians must join with other members of society to educate our patients to the many deadly and dangerous drugs of abuse that are available and work with society (including governments) to reduce the availability of drugs (62-78). The human instinct for pleasure at any cost must be tempered with education and direction from clinicians. Management of those addicted to drugs is a complex, often discouraging process. Psychosocial and behavioral therapies are important that involve a variety of health specialists. Group, family, and individual therapy all have a place in management and many need intensive treatment in drug abuse programs.

REFERENCES

[1] NSDUH-SAMHSA, 2013. URL: http://www.samhsa.gov/data/sites/default/files/NSDUHresults PDFWHTML2013/Web/NSDUHresults2013.pdf.
[2] Kann L, Kinchen S, Shanklin SL, Flint KH, Hawkins J, Harris WA, et al. YRBS: Youth Risk Behavioral Surveillance-United States, 2013. MMWR 2014;63(4): 1-169.
[3] Lui CK, Chung PJ, Ford CL, Grella DE, Mulia N. Drinking behaviors and life course socioeconomic status during the transition from adolescence to adulthood among whites and blacks. J Stud Alcohol Drugs 2015;76(1):68-79.
[4] Greydanus DE, Patel DR. Substance abuse in adolescents: A complex conundrum for the clinician. Pediatr Clin North Am 2003;59(5):1179-1223.
[5] Greydanus DE, Patel DR. Substance abuse in adolescents: current concepts. Disease-a-Month 2005; 51(7):392-431.
[6] Greydanus DE, Calles JR JL, Patel DR. Pediatric and adolescent psychopharmacology: A practical manual for pediatricians. Cambridge: Cambridge University Press, 2008:241-77.
[7] Greydanus DE, Kaplan G, Patel DR, Merrick J. Substance abuse in adolescents and young adults: A manual for pediatric and primary care clinicians. Berlin: De Gruyter, 2013.
[8] Greydanus DE, Hawver EK, Greydanus MM, Merrick J. Marijuana: current concepts. Front Public Health 2013;1(42):1-17.
[9] Greydanus DE, Kaplan G, Patel DR, Merrick J. Special issue: The burden of substance abuse. Int Public Health J 2014;6(3):215-90.
[10] Greydanus DE, Kaplan G, Patel DR, Merrick J. Editorial: Substance abuse. Int Public Health J 2014; 6(3):215-24.
[11] Greydanus DE, Kaplan G, Baxter LE-Sr., Patel DR, Feucht CL. Cannabis: The never-ending, nefarious nepenthe of the 21st century: What should the clinician know? Dis-a Mon 2015;61(4):113-76.
[12] Viteri OA, Soto EE, Bahado-Singh RO, Christensen CW, Chauhan SP, Sibai BM. Fetal anomalies and long-term effects associated with substance abuse in pregnancy: a literature review. Am J Perinatol 2014 Dec 8 [Epub ahead of print].

[13] Naim-Feil J, Zangen A. Addiction. Handb Clin Neurol 2013;116:613-30.
[14] Miller CP, Homberg JR. The role of serotonin in drug use and addiction. Behav Brain Res 2015;277:146-92.
[15] Panagopoulos VN, Ralevski E. The role of ghrelin in addiction: a review. Psychopharmacology 2014; 231(14):2725-40.
[16] Lee D, Delcher C, Maldonado-Molina MM, Bazydlo LA, Thogmartin JR, Goldberger BA. Trends in licit and illicit drug-related deaths in Florida from 2001 to 2012. Forensic Sci Int 2014;245:178-86.
[17] Harris SK, Louis-Jacques J, Knight JR. Screening and brief intervention for alcohol and other abuse. Adolesc Med State Art Rev 2014;25(1):126-56.
[18] Imtiaz S, Shield KD, Fisher B, Rehm J. Harms of prescription opioid use in the United States. Subst Abuse Treat Prev Policy 2014 Oct 27;9:43. doi: 10. 1186/1747-597X-9-43.
[19] Levy S, Williams JF. Adolescent substance use: the role of the medical home. Adolesc Med State Art Rev 2014;25(1):1-14.
[20] Nielsen DA, Nielsen EM, Dasari T, Spellicy CJ. Pharmacogenetics of addiction therapy. Methods Mol Biol 2014;1175:589-624.
[21] Winters KC, Tanner-Smith EE, Bresani E, Meyers K. Current advances in the treatment of adolescent drug use. Adolesc Health Med Ther 2014;5:199-210.
[22] Urrila AS, Paunio T, Palom?ki E, Marttunen M. Sleep in adolescent depression: physiological perspectives. Acta Physiol (Oxf) 2015 Jan 5. doi: 10.1111/apha.12449.
[23] American Psychiatric Association. Diagnostic and statistical manual of mental disorders (DSM-5) Washington, DC: American Psychiatric Association, 2013.
[24] American Psychiatric Association. Diagnostic and statistical manual of mental disorders, Fourth Edition, Text Revision (DSM-IV-TR). Washington DC: American Psychiatric Publications, 2000.
[25] American Psychiatric Association. Substance related and addictive disorders. URL: http://www.psychiatry.org/file%20library/practice/dsm/dsm-5/dsm-5-substanc e-use disorder.pdf.
[26] Ali F, Rehman H, Babayan Z, Stapleton D, Joshi D. Energy drinks and their adverse health effects: a systematic review of the current evidence. Postgrad Med 2015;6:1-15.
[27] Musselman ME, Hampton JP. "Not for human consumption": a review of emerging designer drugs. Pharmacotherapy 2014;34(7):745-57.
[28] Baumann MH, Solis E Jr, Watterson LR, Marusich JA, Fantegrossi WE, Wiley JL. Bath salts, spice, and related designer drugs: the science behind the headlines. J Neurosci 2014;34(46):15150-8.
[29] Urban DJ, Roth BL. DREADDs (Designer receptors exclusively activated by designer drugs): Chemogenetic tools with therapeutic utility. Annu Rev Pharmacol Toxicol 2015;55:399-417.
[30] Smith CD, Robert S. 'Designer drugs': update on the management of novel psychoactive substance misuse in the acute care setting. Clin Med 2014;14(4):409-15.
[31] Castaneto MS, Gorelick DA, Desrosiers NA, Hartman RL, Pirard S, Huestis MA. Synthetic cannabinoids: epidemiology, pharmacodynamics, and clinical implications. Drug Alcohol Depend 2014;144:12-41.
[32] Nelson ME, Bryant SM, Aks SE. Emerging drugs of abuse. Emerg Med Clin North Am 2014;32(1):1-28.
[33] Banks ML, Worst TJ, Rusyniak DE, Sprague JE. Synthetic cathinones ("bath salts"). J Emerg Med 2014; 46(5):632-42.
[34] Hajek P, Etter JF, Benowitz N, Eissenberg T, McRobbie H. Electronic cigarettes: review of use, content, safety, effects on smokers and potential for harm and benefit. Addiction 2014;109(11):1801-10.
[35] Knorst MM, Benedetto IG, Hoffmeister MC, Gazzana MB. The electronic cigarette; the new cigarette of the 21st century? J Bras Pneumol 2014;40(5):564-72.
[36] Rosenberg JM. A molecular basis fro nicotine as a gateway drug. N Engl J Med 2014;371(21):2038. doi:10.1056/NEJMc1411785#SA1.
[37] Kandel D, Kandel E. The gateway hypothesis of substance abuse: developmental, biological and societal perspectives. Acta Paediatr 2014 Nov 6. doi: 10.1111/apa.12851.
[38] Loukola A, Hillfors J, Korhonen T, Kaprio J. Genetics and smoking. Curr Addict Rep 2014;1(1):75-82.

[39] Collins GB, Jerry JM, Bales R. Quitting smoking: still a challenge, but new tools show promise. Cleve Clin J Med 2015;82(1):39-48.
[40] McRobbie H, Bullen C, Hartmann-Boyce J, Hajek P. Electronic cigarettes for smoking cessation and reduction. Cochrane Database Syst Rev 2014;12: CD010216.
[41] Walker N, Howe C, Glover M, McRobbie H, Barnes J, Nosa V, et al. Cytisine versus nicotine for smoking cessation. N Engl J Med 2014;371(25):2353-62.
[42] Jain R, Majumder P, Gupta T. Pharmacological intervention of nicotine dependence. Biomed Res Int 2013;2013:278392. doi: 10.1155/2013/278392.
[43] Wolters A, de Wert G, van Schayck OC, Horstman K. Vaccination against smoking: an annotated agenda for debate. A review of scientific journals, 2001-2013. Addiction 2014;109(8):1268-73.
[44] Gutierrez A, Sher L. Alcohol and drug use among adolescents: an educational overview. Int J Adolesc Med Health 2014 Nov 20. pii:/j/ijamh.ahead-of-print/ijamh-2015-5013/iljamh-2015—5013.xml. doi:10.1515/ijamh-2015-5013.
[45] Knight J, Sherrit L, Shrier L: Validity of the CRAFFT substance abuse screening test among adolescent clinic patients. Arch Pediatr Adolesc Med 2002;156:607.
[46] Samochowiec J, Samochowiec A, Puls I, Bienkowski P, Schott BH. Genetics of alcohol dependence: a review of clinical studies. Neuropsychobiology 2014;70(2):77-94.
[47] Ferraguti G, Pascale E, Lucarelli M. Alcohol addiction: a molecular biology perspective. Curr Med Chem 2014 Dec 28 [Epub ahead of print].
[48] Thakkar MM, Sharma R, Sahota P. Alcohol disrupts sleep homeostasis. Alcohol 2014 Nov 11. pii: S0741-8329(14)20115-7. doi: 10.1016/j.alcohol.2014.07.019.
[49] Johnston L, O'Malley PM, Bachman JG, Sckhlenberg JE. National Survey Results on Drug Use from the Monitoring the Future Study, 2003, 2006, 2007, 2008. Ann Arbor: Institute for Social Research, University of Michigan, 2009.
[50] Tung MK, Light M, Giri R Lane S, Appelbe A, Harvey C, Athan E. Evolving epidemiology of injecting drug use-associated infective endocarditis: a regional centre experience. Drug Alcohol Rev 2014 Dec 29. doi: 10.1111/dar.12228.
[51] Clemow DB, Walker DJ. The potential for misuse and abuse of medications in ADHD: a review. Postgrad Med 2014;126(5):64-81.
[52] Rawson RA. Current research on the epidemiology, medical and psychiatric effects, and treatment of methamphetamine use. J Food Drug Anal 2013;21(4): S77-S81.
[53] Glasner-Edwards S, Mooney LJ. Methamphetamine psychosis: epidemiology and management. CNS Drugs 2014;28(12):1115-26.
[54] Cressman AM, Natekar A, Kim E, Koren G, Bozzo P. Cocaine abuse during pregnancy. J Obstet Gynaecol Can 2014;36(7):628-31.
[55] Alving CR, Matyas GR, Torres O, Jalah R, Beck Z. Adjuvants for vaccines to drugs of abuse and addiction. Vaccine 2014;32(42):5382-9.
[56] Zhou L, Sun W, Young AB, Lee K, McGinty JF, See RE. Oxytocin reduces cocaine seeking and reverses chronic cocaine-induced changes in glutamate receptor function. Int J Neuropsychopharmacol 2014 Oct 31. pii:pyu009. doi: 10.1093/ijnp/pyu009.
[57] Rudd RA, Paulozzi LJ, Bauer MJ, Burleson RW, Carlson RE, Dao D, et al. Increase in heroin overdose deaths, 28 states, 2010-2012. MMWR 2014;63(39):849-54.
[58] Tormoehlen LM, Tekulve KJ, Na?agas KA. Hydrocarbon toxicity: a review. Clin Toxicol (Phila) 2014;52(5):479-89.
[59] Nakawaki B, Crano W. Patterns of substance use, delinquency, and risk factors among adolescent inhalant users. Subst Use Misuse 2015;50(1):114-22.
[60] Grunbaum JA, Kann, L Kinchen S, Ross J, Hawkins J, Lowry R, et al. Youth risk behavior surveillence, United States 2003. MMWR Surveill Summ 2004;53(2):1-96.
[61] Duncan JR, Lawrence AJ. Conventional concepts and new perspectives for understanding the addictive properties of inhalants. J Pharmacol Sci 2013;122(4): 237-43.
[62] Comerci GB, Schwebel R: Substance abuse: Adolesc Med 2000;11(1): 79-101.
[63] Friedman RA: The changing face of teenage drug abuse—the trend toward prescription drugs. N Engl J Med 2006;354:1448-50.

[64] Marasco CC, Goodwin CR, Winder DG, Schramm-Sapyta NL, McLean JA, Wikswo JP. Systems-level view of cocaine addiction: the interconnection of the immune and nervous systems. Exp Biol Med (Maywood) 2014;239(11):1433-42.

[65] Ossiander EM. Volatile substance misuse deaths in Washington State, 2003-2012. Am J Drug Alcohol Abuse 2015;41(1):30-4.

[66] Patel DR, Greydanus DE: Office interventions for adolescent smokers. Adolesc Med 2000;11(3):1-11.

[67] National Institute on Drug Abuse. URL: www.nida.gov/ NIDAHome.html.

[68] National Clearinghouse on Alcohol and Drug Information. URL: www.health.org.

[69] National Institute on Alcohol Abuse and Alcoholism. URL: www.niaaa.nih.gov.

[70] Monitoring the future. URL: http://www.MonitoringTheFuture.org.

[71] Fiore MC, Jaen CR, Baker TB, Bailey WC, Benowitz NL, Curry SJ, et al. Treating tobacco use and dependence: 2008 update. Washington, DC: US Department Health Human Services, 2008.

[72] ancaster T, Stead LF. Individual behavioral counseling for smoking cessation. Cochrane Database Syst Rev 2005;2:CD001292.

[73] Lancaster T, Stead LF. Self-help interventions for smoking cessation. Cochrane Database Syst Rev 2002;3:CD001118.

[74] London ED, Kohno M, Morales AM, Ballard ME. Chronic methamphetamine abuse and corticostriatal defects revealed by neuroimaging. Brain Res 2014 Nov 4. pii: S0006-8993(14)01466-8. doi: 10.1016/j.brainres.2014.10.044.

[75] O'Connor PG: Treating opioid dependence—New data and new opportunities. N. Engl J Med 2000;343(18): 193-5.

[76] Poikolainen K: Ecstasy and the antecedents of illicit drug use. BMJ 2006; 332: 803-4.

[77] World Health Organization. The world health report 1999: Combating the tobacco epidemic. Geneva: WHO, 2000.

[78] Greydanus DE, Kaplan G, Patel DR, Merrick J, eds. Special issue: Management of substance abuse. Int J Child Adolesc Health 2014;7(4):257-380.

In: Public Health Yearbook 2016
Editor: Joav Merrick
ISBN: 978-1-53610-947-4

Chapter 40

FROM THE BATTERED CHILD SYNDROME TO ABUSE AND MALTREATMENT: A PUBLIC HEALTH VIEW

Vincent J Palusci**, MD, MS and Margaret T McHugh, MD, MPH
Department of Pediatrics, New York University School of Medicine,
Frances L Loeb Child Protection and Development Center, New York, US

ABSTRACT

This review serves as a primer for professionals who, regardless of their individual interests and fields of expertise, can improve the growth and development of children by understanding, responding to, and preventing abuse and maltreatment in the child and adolescent. It provides an overview of the types, medical assessment, and treatment of children with potential abuse and maltreatment, and the preventive community services that can be provided to help their families. It outlines areas of current research and highlights issues that still need to be addressed. The experience of the past fifty years has established a solid foundation in preparation for the work that child health clinicians still need to do in the field of child abuse medicine.

Keywords: childhood, adolescence, abuse, neglect, maltreatment, public health

INTRODUCTION

In the fifty years since the publication of C Henry Kempe's (1922-1984) landmark article, "The battered child syndrome" (1), the subject of child maltreatment has become a universal topic, not restricted to one community or to one type of provider. As the field has grown, professionals have had to broaden their intellectual and personal perspectives to not only identify maltreatment but also to provide interventions to prevent further abuse. The current

* Corresponding author: Professor Vincent J. Palusci, MD, MS, Frances L Loeb Child Protection and Development Center, Bellevue Hospital, 462 First Avenue, Rm GC-65, New York, NY 10016, United States. E-mail: Vincent.palusci@nyumc.org.

goal of professionals dedicated to this field is primary prevention, to insure that child abuse, like many infectious diseases of the past century, will be eradicated in the near future.

While each state in the United States (US) defines child maltreatment in its child welfare and criminal statutes, broad definitions have been developed for the Child Abuse Prevention and Treatment Act (2) and by the World Health Organization (see Table 1).

While child abuse overall pertains to the variety of acts committed or omitted by parents or caretakers for children, the quality of the parent-child relationship and nurturing is often left out of state laws. In the broader sense, the WHO (3) adds qualitative definition and context to this relationship and the more broad nature of caring for children.

Table 1. World Health Organization definitions*

Child Abuse - **Child abuse or maltreatment constitutes all forms of physical and/or emotional ill-treatment, sexual abuse, neglect or negligent treatment or commercial or other exploitation, resulting in actual or potential harm to the child's health, survival, development, or dignity in the context of a relationship of responsibility, trust or power.**
Physical Abuse - Physical Abuse of a child is that which results in actual or potential physical harm from an interaction or lack of an interaction, which is reasonably within the control of a parent or person in a position of responsibility, power or trust. There may be a single or repeated incidents.
Emotional Abuse - Emotional abuse includes the failure to provide a developmentally appropriate, supportive environment, including the availability of a primary attachment figure, so that the child can establish a stable and full range of emotional and social competencies commensurate with her or his personal potentials and in the context of the society in which the child dwells. There may also be acts towards the child that cause or have a high probability of causing harm to the child's health or physical, mental, spiritual, moral or social development. These acts must be reasonably within the control of a parent or person in a position of responsibility, power or trust. Acts include restriction of movement, patterns of belittling, denigrating, scapegoating, threatening, scaring, discriminating, ridiculing or other non-physical forms of hostile or rejecting treatment.
Neglect and negligent treatment - Neglect is the failure to provide for the development of the child in all spheres: health, education, emotional development, nutrition, shelter and safe living conditions, in the context of resources reasonably available to the family or caretakers and causes or has a high probability of causing harm to the child's health or physical, mental, spiritual, moral or social development. This includes the failure to properly supervise and protect children from harm as much as is feasible.
Sexual abuse - Child sexual abuse is the involvement of a child in sexual activity that he or she does not fully comprehend or is unable to give informed consent to, or that violates the laws or social taboos of society. Child sexual abuse is evidenced by this activity between a child and an adult or another child who by age or development is in a relationship of responsibility, trust or power, the activity being intended to gratify or satisfy the needs of the other person. This may include but is not limited to: The inducement or coercion of a child to engage in any unlawful activity The exploitative use of a child in prostitution or other unlawful sexual practices The exploitative use of children in pornographic performances and materials
Exploitation - Commercial or other exploitation of a child refers to the use of the child in work or other activities for the benefit of others. This includes, but is not limited to, child labour and child prostitution. These activities are to the detriment of the child's physical or mental health, education, or spiritual, moral or social-emotional development.

*World Health Organization (WHO). (1999). *Report of the consultation on child abuse prevention.* Geneva, Switzerland: Author.

Table 2. International classification of disease codes applicable to child abuse (ICD-9)

ICD-9	*ICD-10*
995.50 Child abuse, unspecified	T74.92 **Unspecified child maltreatment**
995.51 Child emotional/psychological abuse	T74.32 **Child psychological abuse**
995.52 Child neglect (nutritional) Use additional code to identify intent of neglect (E904.0,E968.4)	T74.02 **Child neglect or abandonment**
995.53 Child sexual abuse	T74.22 **Child sexual abuse**
995.54 Child physical abuse Battered baby or child syndrome *Excludes: Shaken infant syndrome (995.55)*	T74.12 **Child physical abuse**
995.55 Shaken infant syndrome Use additional code(s) to identify any associated injuries	T74.4 **Shaken infant syndrome**
E967 Perpetrator of child and adult abuse	
E967.0 By father, stepfather, or boyfriend Male partner of child's parent or guardian	
E967.2 By mother, stepmother, or girlfriend Female partner of child's parent or guardian	
E967.3 By spouse or partner Abuse of spouse or partner by ex-spouse or ex-partner	
E967.4 By child	
E967.5 By sibling	
E967.6 By grandparent	
E967.7 By other relative	
E967.8 By non-related caregiver	
E967.9 By unspecified person	

In the effort to allow diagnostic coding for physicians in medical systems and for medical examiners and coroners for state public health statutes, the International Classification of Disease Codes have been developed applicable to child abuse and neglect. ICD-9 lists individual types as well as external modifiers related to perpetrator relationship ("E codes"). A revised set of codes (ICD-10) is increasingly being used (4), and comparisons of the two systems are listed in Table 2.

EPIDEMIOLOGY

The victimization of children through abuse and neglect remains an all too common occurrence. In the United States, 1-2 per 1,000 children are victimized by physical abuse each year, and young children and infants have the highest rates. Maltreated children suffer from a variety of behavior problems and mental disorders in addition to physical injuries (5, 6). The Adverse Childhood Experiences study has noted the powerful relationship between adverse childhood experiences and several conditions of adulthood, including risk of suicide, alcoholism, depression, illicit drug use, and other lifestyle changes (7-9). While the exact pathways are still being explored, childhood abuse is thought to affect adult health by putting people at risk for depression and post-traumatic stress disorders, difficulties in relationships, and negative beliefs and attitudes towards others through mechanisms of toxic stress (10-11).

Two large administrative sources provide information about the U.S. annual incidence of child maltreatment, the National Child Abuse and Neglect Data System (NCANDS) and the National Incidence Studies of child abuse and neglect (NIS). NCANDS contains aggregate and case-level data on child abuse reports received by state Child Protective Service (CPS) agencies, and almost all US states and territories provide information annually about the outcomes of child abuse reports, types of maltreatment, child and family factors and services being provided (12). National estimates of the overall numbers of victims (substantiated or indicated CPS reports) as well as victims identified with physical and sexual abuse show decline over the 20+ years of nationally collected data in NCANDS (see Figure 1), following similar trends in other national crime statistics (12).

In contrast, NIS samples sentinel counties to identify maltreatment under two standards: the harm standard (relatively stringent in that it generally requires that an act or omission result in demonstrable harm in order to be classified as abuse or neglect) and the endangerment standard (which allows children who were not yet harmed by maltreatment to be counted if the CM was confirmed by CPS or identified as endangerment by professionals outside CPS, either by their parents or other adults) (13). The Fourth National Incidence Study of Child Abuse and Neglect (NIS–4) also shows an overall decrease in the incidence of maltreatment since the NIS–3, as well as decreases in some specific maltreatment categories and increases in others. Using the stringent Harm Standard definition, more than 1.25 million children (an estimated 1,256,600 children) experienced maltreatment during the NIS–4 study year (2005–2006). A large percentage (44%) or an estimated total of 553,300 were abused, and most of these abused children experienced physical abuse (58%).

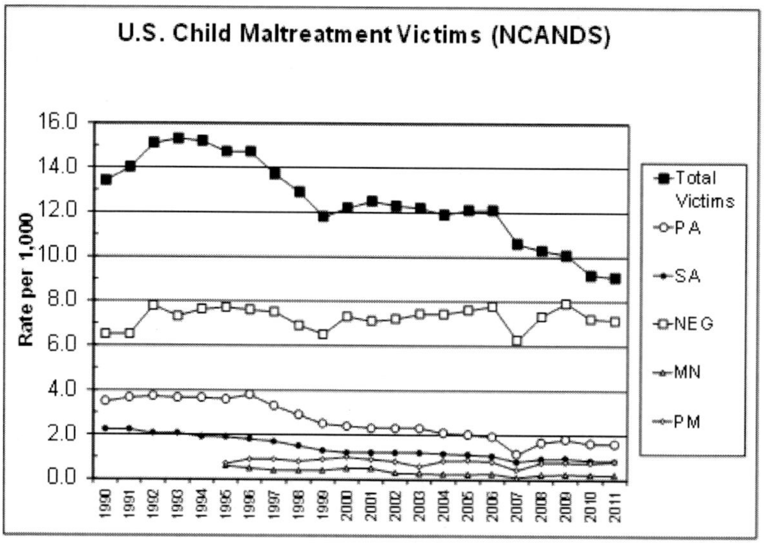

MN = Medical Neglect; NEG = Neglect; PA = Physical Abuse; PM = Psychological Maltreatment; SA = Sexual Abuse (6).

Figure 1. United States child maltreatment victims (NCANDS), 1990-2011.

Smaller independent samples offer additional information. In the Carolinas, the incidence of harsh physical discipline was found to be 4.3% of respondents (with 2.4% shaking infants), and a retrospective prevalence survey, reported 24% of adolescents being physically assaulted (14, 15). The range of incidence rates of abusive head trauma (AHT) has been found to be 27.5-32.2 per 100,000 in a large U.S. inpatient database, with an estimates rising during 1997 to 2009 (16). Lane et al. (17) noted hospital discharge rates of 1.8 per 100k, with 25% of head trauma in infants being abusive.

Unlike the reported incidence of sexual abuse, in which it has been suggested that at least some of the decrease is real, it is not clear if or why physical abuse rates have actually declined (18, 19). While economic indicators improved in the 1990's during the decline, the number of cases continued to fall in NCANDS in 2008-2011 during an economic recession (20). This may indicate that states are changing how they count child maltreatment fatalities or how they are delivering that information to NCANDS as could occur with differential response systems (12). Further studies are needed to ascertain whether the number of physical abuse cases is continuing to decline and the causes why this is occurring. A number of smaller samples have suggested a rise in more serious child physical abuse associated with the U.S. economic recession.

It has been noted that the abusive head trauma rate increased from 8.9 to 14.7 per 100,000 and a doubling from 0.7 to 1.4 per month during the recession (20). Wood et al. (21) noted increasing rates of children admitted to hospitals for physical abuse over 10 years 2000-2009, rising from 0.8 to 3% annually. Rates of physical abuse reportedly also fell in the UK during 1974 to 2008 (22). Neglect continues to affect more than 50% of those children reported to child protective services, and the parents of young neglected children were less likely to have completed high school, had more preschool children and had less parenting skills and social support (23). Disabled children also have increased risk (24). When broken down by age and type of child maltreatment, it is apparent that most CM occurs in very young children and most CM is neglect (see Figure 2). This pattern continues with older children, but the number falls dramatically. For sexual abuse, older children are more affected. Medical neglect, in contrast, affects mostly infants.

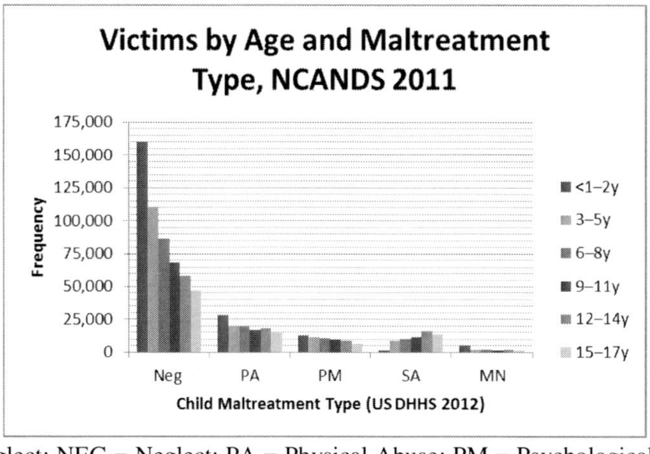

MN = Medical Neglect; NEG = Neglect; PA = Physical Abuse; PM = Psychological Maltreatment; SA = Sexual Abuse (6).

Figure 2. Victims by age and maltreatment type, NCANDS 2011 (12).

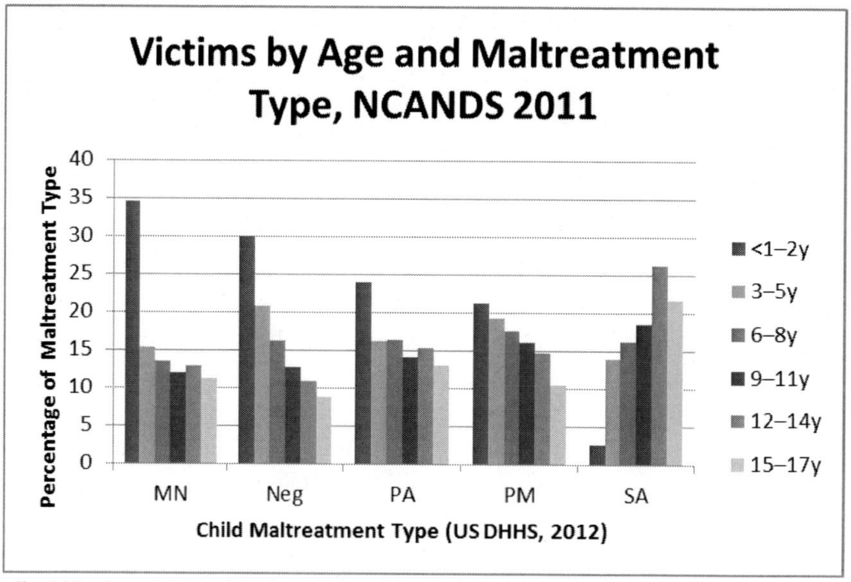

MN = Medical Neglect; NEG = Neglect; PA = Physical Abuse; PM = Psychological Maltreatment; SA = Sexual Abuse (6).

Figure 3. Victims by age as a percentage of child maltreatment types, NCANDS 2011 (20).

Similar relationships hold as a proportion of the total number of victims identified in NCANDS. Younger children are the highest proportion for all CM types, except sexual abuse (see Figure 3).

Although the focus of concern about maltreatment is usually the younger child, statistics show that 30 to 50% of all reported cases involve adolescents (12). In New York State in 1985, for example, there were 84,119 child maltreatment reports with substantiation rate of 35%. Within the adolescent reports, 19% were for physical abuse, 42.4% for sexual abuse, and the remainder for neglect (25). In 2002, there were 153,603 reports of child maltreatment in New York with a substantiation rate of 31.1%. Of those, children from ages 10-17 years accounted for 47.9% (21,727 children) of the cases. Almost half (47%) of children entering foster care were over 10 years of age, and approximately 75% remained in care for longer than one year. In the same year in New York City, there were 10,922 children ages 10 to 17 years placed in foster care. Alarmingly, 15% of those in foster care were adolescents who had been in the system more than one year. These child maltreatment cases can only reflect those that come to the attention of the child protection system. Based on other sources of information regarding adolescent behaviors, maltreatment is given as a comorbid factor in a spectrum of adolescent problems, such as substance abuse, truancy, runaways and psychiatric disorders (26-28).

While there are varying schools of thought on the origins of maltreatment, most theories of child maltreatment recognize that the root causes can be divided into four principal systems: (1) the child, (2) the family, (3) the community, and (4) society. While children are certainly not responsible for the abuse inflicted upon them, there are certain characteristics that have been found to increase the risk for maltreatment. Children with disabilities or mental retardation, for example, are significantly more likely to be abused (24). Evidence also suggests that age and gender are predictive of maltreatment risk. Younger children are more likely to be neglected, while the risk for sexual abuse increases with age. Female children and adolescents are significantly more likely than males to suffer sexual abuse.

Several factors have been associated with physical abuse. Unlike previous NIS cycles, NIS–4 found strong and pervasive race differences in the incidence of maltreatment with rates of maltreatment for Black children significantly higher than those for White and Hispanic children. Under the Harm Standard, children with confirmed disabilities had significantly lower rates of physical abuse and of moderate harm from maltreatment, but they had significantly higher rates of emotional neglect and of serious injury or harm (13). NIS-4 also confirmed findings from other studies which associated increased physical abuse in poor, larger, unemployed families, and one parent and an unrelated caregiver present. Zhou, Hallisey, & Freymann (29) found that infant maltreatment can best be predicted when there are young mothers less than 20 years, who are unmarried, with inadequate prenatal care, are poor, who smoke during the pregnancy, or when there are three or more siblings. In an NCANDS sample, parent emotional problems, alcohol abuse and other family violence were found to be associated with the recurrence of physical abuse before age three years (30).

Community and social factors also play a role in child maltreatment. Poverty, for example, has been linked with maltreatment, particularly neglect, in each of the national incidence studies (13), and has been associated with child neglect, a strong predictor of substantiated child maltreatment (31). The following factors have been linked to child maltreatment: fewer friends in their social support networks, less contact with friends, and lower ratings of quality support received from friends (32). Violence and unemployment are other community-level variables that have been found to be associated with child maltreatment.

Perhaps the least understood and studied level of child maltreatment is that of society. Ecological theories postulate that factors such as the narrow legal definitions of child maltreatment, the social acceptance of violence (as evidenced by video games, television and films, and music lyrics), and political or religious views that value noninterference in families above all may be associated with child maltreatment (6).

Clinical features

Several health effects of child maltreatment have been identified. While there is considerable overlap, specific health effects and injuries are often related to a major subtype of child abuse, and the medical diagnostic evaluation varies with the type of child maltreatment and the injuries of concern (see Table 3).

Table 3. Medical diagnostic evaluation in child victimization emphasizing identification of cause and sequelae of physical injury

History- Questions asked by healthcare professionals of the child and caretakers during medical encounter
Chief Complaint (Why are you here today?)
History of Present Illness Circumstances surrounding injury Physical symptoms such as pain, bleeding, sensory problems, etc. Events leading to seeking medical care Timing
Prior medical treatments, surgery, medications, hospitalizations, mental health services
Prior evaluations for victimization
Chronic medical conditions, particularly bleeding, neurologic, metabolic, growth disorders
Immunizations received
Known allergies
Psychosocial history (caretakers, school attendance, housing, income, family structure)
Physical Examination- done by the physician, nurse, or other practitioner based on history Vital signs (pulse, respiration rate, height, weight, head circumference, Glasgow Coma Scale, pain scale) Skin (bruising, burns, pattern marks, contusions, tenderness) Head (presence of skin swelling, bruising, skull deformity, fontanels) Eyes (pupillary response, sclera, retina, periorbital tissues) Ears (earlobes, canals, tympanic membranes) Nose (bleeding, nares, deformity) Mouth, throat (condition of teeth, tonsils, pharynx, frenula) Neck (flexibility, lymph glands, thyroid) Chest (rib deformities, air movement and congestion, tenderness) Heart (heart sounds, rhythm) Abdomen (tenderness, organ swelling, bowel sounds) Genitals (penis, scrotum, testes, urethra in males; labia, hymen, urethra, vagina in females) Anorectal (perineum, internal and external anal sphincters, ruggal folds, tone) Extremities (movement, tenderness, swelling, joint involvement, pulses, ambulation) Neurological (alertness, reflexes, muscular strength and tone, cranial nerves, sensation)
Laboratory – Tests performed as indicated by history and physical findings Complete blood count (white and red blood cells, hematocrit, platelet counts) Coagulation studies (prothrombin, partial thromboplastin times, fibrinogen, platelet function) Blood chemistries, liver function tests X-rays of affected areas or skeletal survey of all bones for children less than three years Computer-assisted tomography (CT) scan of brain or other affected part Magnetic Resonance Imaging (MRI) of head or other affected part Specialized metabolic tests (collagen, organic and amino acids, others) Microbiologic cultures and tests for sexually transmitted infections Collection of forensic trace specimens (less than 72 hours after contact) Pregnancy testing (depending on sexual development and potential contact)
Diagnosis and Treatment- Identification of disease or sequelae of trauma Hospitalization for further diagnostic assessment or treatment (based on severity of illness/injury and/or need for surgical or supportive care) Reassurance and emotional support Referral for ongoing medical and mental health treatment CPS reporting and provision for immediate safety needs and protection

Physical abuse

The most common injury from physical abuse affects the skin by bruising or burning. Recognition and documentation of bruises, burns and other skin lesions requires complete undressing of the child and comprehensive physical examination. Skin lesions should describe location, size, color, depth, and integrity of the epidermis and may be documented using notes, hand-drawn diagrams or photographs; law enforcement and child protection workers often have resources to assure high quality photo documentation. Even if photographs are taken, the pediatrician should also contemporaneously document skin injuries identified (33). Additionally, specific statements by the family and child should also be copied verbatim in the medical chart for potential use later in the legal system.

In the case of bruising, standard coagulation tests should be ordered to objectively assess platelet count and function as well as coagulation factors. Any skin lesion beyond temporary reddening should be considered as potential physical abuse when (1) the injury is inflicted and non-accidental, (2) the pattern of injury fits biomechanical models of abusive trauma, (3) the pattern corresponds to infliction with an instrument that would not occur through play or in the environment, (4) the history provided is not in keeping with the child's development, or (5) the history does not explain the injury (33).

The aging of bruises in children has received considerable attention and current guidelines are severely limited in their ability to precisely time when an injury occurred. Pattern, depth (degree), and healing of burns helps in determining their specificity for maltreatment. Developmental and other considerations need to be entertained as there are a host of potential confounders or 'mimics' which need to be reviewed when coming to a diagnosis. Some children as young as 10 months of age, for example, have been shown to have the developmental capability to climb into the bath, suggesting that nonspecific burn patterns could be attributed to actions by the child rather than the parent in some cases (34).

The distribution of lesions can be a critical factor in determining if a child has been abused. Certain sites are highly correlated with abuse, such as buttocks, the lower back, the posterior aspects of the extremities and the ears (35). Bruising at other sites, such as the bony prominences of the forehead, the elbows and lower legs, are consistent with the normal childhood trauma seen in mobile children. Sugar et al. (36) noted "those who don't cruise rarely bruise," signaling we should be concerned when non-walking infants or motor delayed children have bruising. Inflicted bruising may have clear patterns or may be non-specific.

When an object is used, the pattern of the injury may clearly show the outline of the object. Another form of patterned bruising comes from biting. A careful inspection and measurement of the lesion can determine if a bite is human or animal, adult or child, or self-inflicted. Since the most common skin manifestation of physical abuse is multiple bruises in different stages of healing, it is imperative to use a diagram and appropriate imaging to document the color, distribution and pattern of these injuries. A burn is the destruction of skin and underlying tissue caused by the application of a physical agent. These agents may be chemicals, heat, cold, or electrical in nature. Since the spectrum of burns can range from a simple isolated injury to the involvement of major portions of the child's body, the clinician should assess the type of agent, the distribution and extent of the burn, and the history given of how the burn occurred (37). Many burns in childhood are accidental but are also the result of poor judgment or the failure of the caretaker to provide adequate supervision. Here, as in other forms of abuse, the developmental age and the size of the child are very important. Inflicted burns often have very specific patterns such as those seen with immersion or dunking. Burns may result from splash, immersion, or contact with a heated instrument or utensil, a flame, a chemical/caustic agent or an electrical source.

Accidental burns/scalds commonly involve hot liquids in contact with a child's face, neck, and upper chest (38). If a child pulls down a cup of hot water, this will produce a different pattern than if he had pulled a cup of thick liquid. The action may be modified by the height from which the hot liquid fell, the vehicle that contained the hot substance, and the child's size. Immersion burns present with distinctive patterns that result from placing the child in hot water. The patterns include stocking/glove burns that are symmetrical burns of the extremities. Forced immersion of the child in a tub can produce a burn pattern with well-demarcated lesions and little or no evidence of splash.

Contact burns can present with identifiable object patterns such as an iron or a cigarette lighter. A child can easily have contact with the iron left on the floor or by pulling the cord. Other sources of contact burns are room heaters, hair curling irons, electric cooking utensils, and radiators which can each produce distinctive lesions. Lit cigarettes can produce lesions that can be difficult to distinguish from chicken pox or impetigo given the similarity of the size and shape.

A variety of diagnostic issues await further study. As the Institute of Medicine (6) pointed out, there is a great deal of additional data needed by clinicians on the frontlines to assist in determining which children need evaluation for abuse, when subspecialists should be called, and what tests should be done. There are still issues on how to fund training for physicians to recognize and report abusive bruises and how to best train case workers, social workers and other investigators about medical issues. More research is needed to study innovative systems-level changes that may address challenges associated with decision making on medical issues by frontline workers.

Acute fractures may be clinically apparent as soft tissue swelling over a fracture site, a deformity of the involved limb, or as a decrease in movement with or without external bruising. Infants may present with irritability and/or not using an affected limb. Healing fractures may sometimes be identified as palpable lesions consistent with callus formation, especially over the ribs (39). The absence of swelling or bruises near a fracture site is not uncommon in fractures of the extremities and ribs. A case series of 703 consecutive skeletal series reported 11% fractures, with higher rates in infants less than 6 months old, apparent life threatening events, seizures and abusive head trauma. 79% had healing fractures seen (40). One study reported that when skeletal surveys were done, 23% identified additional fractures, 10% in the hands, feet or spine and follow-up x-rays in 1-2 weeks have been found to identify additional fractures in 8.5% of children (41).

There is no fracture type that is pathognomonic for abuse, and all fracture types can potentially result from inflicted injury. The diagnosis of inflicted fracture must be made through careful correlation of the history provided by the caregiver with the child's developmental level and physical and radiographic findings. Classic metaphyseal lesions, rib fractures (particularly posteriorly), scapular fractures, vertebral spinous process fractures, and sternal fractures all have a high specificity for abuse (42). Common, nonspecific injuries include subperiosteal new bone formation, clavicular fractures, diaphyseal fractures of long bones, and linear skull fractures. There are some fracture types and findings of intermediate specificity that are concerning but may be accidental if a clearly plausible mechanism is provided. This group includes multiple fractures (particularly when bilateral), fractures of different ages, epiphyseal separation, digital fractures, vertebral body fractures and subluxations, and complex skull fractures.

The age of fractures can be helpful in assessing the plausibility of the history, and multiple fractures of different ages raise the suspicion of abuse. Fracture healing manifests as periosteal reaction, also called callus, which is radiographically apparent after 10–14 days, and can be seen earlier in infants (43, 44). Subperiosteal new bone formation can be a normal finding in infants under 6 months of age when it is found along the shafts of long bones and is symmetrical on both sides of the body. Skull fractures cannot be dated with accuracy, however, when non-accidental trauma is suspected, appropriate skeletal studies should be done as outlined by the American College of Radiology (45) and the American Academy of Pediatrics Section on Radiology (46).

Skeletal survey is the standard diagnostic investigation when there is concern for physical abuse of infants and toddlers under two years old (46). It includes anterio-posterior (AP) views of the extremities including feet, with the exception of the hands which are imaged in the posterior-anterior view; AP and lateral skull; AP and lateral views of the thorax and oblique ribs; AP pelvis; and lateral views of the spine. Radiologic evaluation is necessary to assess both the fracture itself and overall status of the bony skeleton to identify any metabolic/genetic process that might produce bone fragility. A discussion of the various metabolic bones diseases associated with fractures is beyond the scope of this chapter, and a pediatric radiologist should be utilized since familiarity with the presentation of growth variables in the pediatric patient is very important in determining if the findings are consistent with non-accidental trauma or other explanations.

Several areas of continuing medical research include the delineation of the diagnosis, pathophysiology and injury mechanics of fractures, head trauma and other abuse injuries. Further research is indicated, and physicians should appropriately search and test for alternate explanations while appropriately weighting the strong available evidence to ensure that a child remains protected from harm. CT, for example has been suggested to be a more sensitive test for rib fractures, yet the increased radiation exposure may not warrant it for screening (47). While it has been noted that vitamin D deficiency does not predispose to fracture in the absence of clinical rickets (48, 49), additional studies regarding the quantitative effects of such deficiencies could be helpful.

The leading cause of abusive mortality and morbidity is inflicted traumatic brain injury (50). With mortality rates of 10–50% and more than 90% of survivors having significant developmental sequelae, physical abuse to the head has been noted to have patterns of injuries that are distinct from accidental or medical causes. At least 1,400 cases of fatal abusive head trauma occur annually in the United States, and there is growing sophistication in our ability to differentiate these fatalities from those from non-abusive causes. Prior to 1974, the presence of subdural hematomas in infants who had no apparent history or evidence of trauma was given the diagnosis of "idiopathic subdural hematoma of infancy". With the publication of the article by Caffey in 1974 based on interviews of caretakers, this entity became known as the "Shaken Baby Syndrome" and later the "Shaken Baby/Impact Syndrome" as the awareness of this clinical entity grew and applied to related clinical situations (51). New diagnostic technologies developed in the last century, from radiographs to sophisticated computer-assisted imaging techniques, have proved invaluable in visualizing internal bleeding and injury.

The mechanism for the injury has been described as the violent shaking of an infant resulting in the movement of the brain within the skull and related hemorrhage within the eye and optic nerve. Subdural bleeding is thought to be caused by the disruption of the bridging veins within the subdural space. Rib fractures are attributed to the compression of the chest by the caretaker as the infant was shaken. This mechanism of injury is consistent with the histories given by providers over the years in which the caretaker sought to silence the crying infant by grabbing the child around the thorax and shaking the child until the child stopped crying. Alternative terms for this clinical entity are now being used, including Abusive Head Trauma or Non-Accidental Head Injury, to indicate head trauma without reference to the mode of injury. Infants and children under 3 years with interhemispheric subdural hemorrhage were found to have a greater than 99% probability of intentional trauma, and predictive values of a variety of injuries have been calculated (52). However, a pattern of head crush injuries increasingly seen after TV falls reminds us that these finding are not always pathognomonic for abusive head trauma (53). Whether external hydrocephalus or "benign extra-axial fluid of infancy" predisposes to subdural bleeding is still not clear. The potential contribution of birth and other factors such as maternal anti-Ro antibodies is also provocative (54). Newer imaging modalities, such as diffusion tensor imaging, offer valuable ways to detect the effects of AHT, but further studies are needed to help us integrate them into clinical practice (55-57).

Approximately 4%-6% of abused children have ocular findings. Any ocular injury can be the result of abuse, and all forms of abuse may have ophthalmic manifestations (58). The incidence of retinal hemorrhages (RH) in shaken-baby syndrome (SBS) is 85%, but higher in children who have died versus unimpaired survivors. There is an association between severity of brain injury and RH severity, and RH can rarely occur without intracranial hemorrhage or cerebral edema (59). Approximately two-thirds of victims have RHs that are too numerous to count and are multilayered. These RHs extend out to the retinal periphery, with no particular anatomic pattern, and cover the majority of the retinal surface. Macular retinoschisis also indicates trauma. RH cannot be dated with precision. Massive numbers of superficial or small-dot hemorrhages can resolve within 24 hours.

There is some evidence that mild increases of RH, or the appearance of RH not previously present, can occur early during hospitalization in very ill children, which underscores the need for prompt ophthalmology consultation and retinal evaluation (60). A small number of infants have been noted to have RH after birth that resolve within two weeks. It is also known that RHs in the posterior pole are associated with non-abusive causes. The overwhelming body of literature supports a conclusion that severe hemorrhagic retinopathy in otherwise previously well children without obvious history to the contrary (e.g., head crush or high velocity impact) suggests that the child has been submitted to repetitive acceleration-deceleration trauma with or without head impact (58).

There is a growing body of knowledge about abusive abdominal and chest trauma which are often 'silent' injuries with potentially devastating consequences. Abdominal injuries are the second leading cause of death after abusive head trauma but are difficult to assess given their occult nature, relative lack of bruising, and potential for significant delay in symptoms. Even with a history of a severe blow to the abdomen, bruising of the skin is often not seen.

Examination may reveal guarding and change/loss of bowel sounds. Lab studies must address injuries to all the abdominal organs including the kidneys. CT scans of the abdomen are very useful in determining the extent of these injuries when the physical findings are diffuse and non-specific. Direct blows to the abdomen such as a punch, kick or use of an object can injure both solid and hollow organs which are both impacted and compressed against the vertebral column (61).

One study demonstrated that solid organ injuries were most common in both accidental and inflicted trauma. Hollow viscus injuries, alone or in combination with solid organ damage, were more common in cases of inflicted injuries (62). Recent studies suggest that abdominal CT imaging and liver function and pancreatic testing should be carried out in all abusive head trauma victims to identify occult abdominal trauma given that 25% or more of even fatal abdominal trauma cases can have few or no visible external bruises (61). Inflicted chest injuries in children are uncommon as a single episode of trauma but are often seen in conjunction with other non-accidental injuries such as inflicted head trauma with compression fractures of the ribs. Direct blows to the chest wall rarely present with damage to the heart or the thoracic duct (63). Many of these injuries are fatal and only identified at post mortem exam. Cardiac troponins have been found to be increased after abusive chest trauma, and the time course and screening evaluation of serologic markers for abusive abdominal trauma need further study (64).

Sexual abuse

Sexual abuse has been defined as sexual contacts or exploitation of children by adults, which cannot be consented to, and which violate social laws or taboos. Sexual assault is a comprehensive term encompassing several types of forced sexual activity, while the term molestation means non-coital sexual activity between a child and an adolescent or adult. Rape is defined as forced sexual intercourse with vaginal, oral or anal penetration by the offender. Acquaintance or "date rape" apply when the assailant and victim know each other. Statutory rape involves sexual penetration of a minor by an adult as defined in varying state laws, regardless of assent (65).

A prime injury of sexual abuse is emotional. While most young children with proven sexual abuse have few physical injuries, patterns of anogenital injury and sexually transmitted diseases have been identified (66). Several large case series have been published highlighting the normalcy of most examinations (66-68). Assessing sexual abuse requires detailed knowledge of anogenital anatomy and sexually transmitted infections (STIs) in children, both of which have important differences from adults, and specialized skills and examination techniques have had to be developed (69, 70). It has become apparent that most physicians have little knowledge about prepubertal genital anatomy and cannot identify key landmarks. This is compounded by the paucity of studies clearly documenting the differences between abusive and non-abusive injury and the changing interpretation over time. When confronted with concerns of potential sexual abuse, the pediatrician should obtain key elements of the history such as type, frequency and timing of contact and physically assess the child for gross injuries and infection (65). Definitive assessment and treatment is increasingly handled by referral to pediatricians with specialized experience in testing, interpretation, and documentation of anogenital findings (71).

The issues surrounding sexual abuse are compounded during adolescence (25). In surveys of high school students, over 25% reported that they have experienced unwanted sexual contact; in clinical populations, the rates are even higher (72). A recent prospective study demonstrated that child maltreatment is an independent predictor of later adolescent pregnancies, with birth rates highest for sexually abused and neglected females when compared to a matched cohort (73). Repeated sexual contact and pregnancy places teenagers at increased risk for several health harms. Repeated sexual contact has been associated with younger ages of sexual initiation, higher rates of depression, anxiety, substance abuse and delinquency.

Most adolescent rape and sexual assault is perpetrated by an acquaintance or relative of the adolescent, with younger adolescents having assailants more likely from the extended family. Increased rates of sexual assault are seen in adolescents with disabilities, alcohol use and other family dysfunction (74). Males are less likely to report sexual assault, less likely to receive treatment, and more likely to become perpetrators themselves after being victimized than are female adolescents (75).

Clinicians caring for sexual abuse victims should be trained in the procedures required for documentation and collection of evidence and the steps to minimize the child from further victimization (65, 76-78). They should inquire about psychological traits and behaviors; also, there should be specific inquiry about the types and timing of reported sexual contact (72). The examination begins with a comprehensive general examination followed by detailed visualization of the genitals, anus and oral cavity.

Procedures such as colposcopy and video-colposcopy offer ways to document and record trauma, to allow the child to be more relaxed and cooperative during examination, and to begin the process of emotional healing (79). While it is beyond the scope of this chapter to detail all of the findings associated with sexual abuse, recent research suggests that only limited findings have high specificity, such as lacerations and transections of the hymen and bruising or other injury to the anus and genitals. Several findings which were once thought to indicate trauma are now considered non-specific, accidentally acquired, or congenital variations (66). Follow-up exams can be vital for evaluating certain lesions, determining the course of healing, and treatment efficacy (80).

While all STIs should raise the suspicion of possible sexual contact, infections with Neisseria gonorrhea and Treponema pallidum are most specific for mucosal sexual contact and must generally be reported (65, 69). The presence of STIs needs to be evaluated on a case-by-case basis, and the possibility of non-sexual or vertical transmission considered. Other infections to be considered include chlamydia trachomatis, Trichomonas species, human immunodeficiency virus and hepatitis B and C viruses. The clinician should be knowledgeable about the potential sources of infection, body sites, types of contact and testing strategies before treatment eradicates microbiologic evidence. There are several new methods being used to detect STIs, not all of which have acceptance in legal proceedings (81-84). The clinician needs to carefully consider the types and timing of any prophylaxis for STI or pregnancy based on the age and development of the child, the type and timing of contact, and the risk factors for disease in the alleged perpetrator (69).

Psychological maltreatment

Psychological maltreatment (PM) is commonly associated with other forms of abuse but may also occur in isolation in a small number of cases. By definition, PM is a repeated pattern of interaction between a parent and child that harms the child's emotional well-being. Spurning, belittling, degrading, ridiculing, or shaming a child is considered harming a child's self-worth. Terrorizing and otherwise exploiting the child increases the harm further. The shear denial of emotional closeness leads to physical and developmental delays in young children and failure to thrive in infants. Rejection, isolation, and inconsistent parenting styles lead children to feel insecure in their home and relationships. An emerging form of PM occurs when a child witnesses violence in the home, including spousal violence, community violence, or even violence on television or movies (84). PM is seldom the focus of CPS investigation and has increasingly been coupled with other forms of CM in CPS reports (85, 86).

PM is associated with a variety of negative and lasting effects. Shaffer et al. suggested that the effects of emotional maltreatment are disabling and enduring, with adjustment outcomes varying according the type of psychological maltreatment (i.e., emotional abuse, emotional neglect), gender, and other factors (87). PM is strongly linked to depression and problems with relationships and attachment, and it predicts more rapid onset of major and minor mental illness in a dose-dependent manner (88-92). PM and recurrent PM in childhood and adolescence represent important risk factors for increased victimization, and children with high levels of co-occurring internalizing and externalizing symptoms are particularly likely to experience increased exposure to peer victimization, maltreatment, and sexual victimization, thereby escalating physical and mental harm (93).

Psychological neglect and failure to thrive have been significantly associated with behavior problems and poor cognitive development, even while controlling for poverty (94, 95) and services put in place (96, 97). The psychological effects of maltreatment may be very difficult to recognize in the medical office. Sometimes the poor parent-child relationship is seen and the verbal stigmata of PM exposed, but often there are little or no physical findings demonstrating the emotional harm, other than weight loss or excessive weight gain. The quiet, depressed child is not often identified as a victim of neglect as readily as is the hyperactive, aggressive child (98). The pediatrician needs to evaluate the harm or potential harm to the child's mental health, while realizing that it may take several years for such harm to become apparent and the effects are often confounded with exposure to other violence (85).

Documentation must be objective, with appropriate use of psychological tests and mental health referrals in the evaluation. Behavioral changes in the child are early but non-specific events, and assessment should include multiple domains, including function at home, school and at play. The psychological effects of malnutrition are further modified by the intensity, type, frequency, and severity of exposure as well as the developmental stage and resiliency of the child (84, 96). A recent study noted that fewer than 25% of families received counseling, mental health or other services after PM, and service referrals varied significantly based on family race, ethnicity, poverty and co-occurring child maltreatment. When offered, counseling was associated with a 54% reduction in PM recurrence, and other services were not associated with significant reductions (99).

Neglect

Child neglect is the most common form of child maltreatment, affecting 50% or more of children reported annually to Child Protective Services (12). Dr. Ray Helfer reminded pediatricians about the significant harms caused by the 'litany of smoldering neglect' and the de-emphasis of neglect that has caused mandated reporters to have second thoughts about reporting neglect because little, if anything, could supposedly be done by overwhelmed, understaffed child protective services agencies (100). Neglect is the omission or lack of a minimal level of care by the parents or caretakers that results in actual or potential harm to the child. Neglect is often associated with poverty, but poor families are not necessarily neglectful (13).

Many subtypes of neglect often occur concurrently, but our understanding of its outcome is often aided by identifying subtypes that can direct potential interventions. Physical neglect is the lack of food, clothing or shelter; emotional neglect is a form of psychological maltreatment, and educational neglect refers to the lack of proper educational resources. Pediatricians are most likely to identify and treat medical care neglect and failure to thrive resulting in illness (101-103).

The morbidity and mortality associated with neglect are substantial. Although poorly identified on death certificates, child death review teams consistent identify supervisional and other forms of neglect as causing as many or more deaths as physical abuse (104). Physical conditions caused by neglect include injuries, ingestions, inadequately treated illnesses, dental problems, malnutrition, and neurological and developmental deficits. Manifestations in neglectful families include noncompliance or non-adherence to medical recommendations, delay or failure in seeking appropriate health care, hunger, failure to thrive and unmanaged morbid obesity, poor hygiene and physical and medical conditions contributing to poor cognitive and educational achievement (101).

Poor supervision is less defined but has been broken down into broad categories, consisting of not watching the child closely enough, inadequate substitute child care, failure to protect from third parties, knowingly allowing the child to participate in harmful activities, and driving recklessly or while intoxicated (105). A comprehensive response requires that the pediatrician address the actual or potential harms that have occurred to the child and to make appropriate referrals to a myriad of community services to address a variety of social and economic issues in the family, including reporting (102, 106).

Management of neglect first centers on properly identifying the sources contributing to neglect. For example, while malnutrition is medically addressed through proper provision of fluids, calories, and protein as dictated by commonly accepted parameters, the pediatrician must also assess the lack of appropriate food, the provision of that food to the child, and the explanation, if any, as to why it was not provided. Important screening questions that can elicit further avenues of intervention include inquiring about the family's access to food, their access to appropriate medical and dental services and medicines, substance abuse during and after pregnancy, homelessness, housing and environmental safety, depression, domestic violence, and degree of supervision (101).

Failure to thrive, otherwise coded as the lack of normal physiological development, is associated with malnutrition in infancy, and has historically been grouped into organic, non-organic (NOFTT), and mixed varieties. NOFTT is more realistically called malnutrition due to neglect. To the extent that many cases fall into the mixed category, it is important to sort out the contribution of neglect in a particular case (96, 103). While a full discussion of the evaluation of NOFTT is beyond the scope of this chapter, it is important to emphasize that the findings on a comprehensive history and physical examination should guide management and initial laboratory testing. In the face of normal basic metabolic measurements, a careful observation of parental feeding practices and the child's intake and output is often illuminating. Height and weight need to be precisely measured over multiple visits and compared to currently accepted norms, some of which are modified by race, prematurity or other medical conditions. With acceptable weight gain under direct observation and lack of significant medical cause for malnutrition, a presumptive diagnosis of NOFTT can be made and community resources activated.

Challenges for research on child neglect remain, including the changing demographics of the nation and health disparities. Evidenced-based early interventions and treatments may be an opportunity for prevention of child neglect and improving child welfare services, particularly in an era of health care reform. Developmental researchers across the translational pipeline are encouraged to integrate child neglect research into future studies to inform prevention, treatment and policy efforts for the improved health and well-being of children, families and communities (101).

Special issues for adolescents

Pediatricians should be knowledgeable about legal definitions and reporting requirements; they also should provide preventive counseling and screen adolescents for a history of assault and potential emotional effects. They should be knowledgeable about the physical findings associated with sexual assault and testing for STIs and pregnancy and be able to provide these services or refer the adolescent to other providers in the community. There has been considerable growth in treatments available for victims of child abuse and neglect, but adolescents face the additional burdens of developing risk-taking behaviors, paraphilias, and becoming perpetrators as the result of their victimization if not appropriately treated (72, 75). Sexual abuse, in particular, appears to be a strong risk factor for subsequent perpetration, influencing adolescents and young adults to develop an orientation that is abusive to other children (107). An adolescent's exposure to a pervasive atmosphere of violence in the home is a key risk factor of future perpetration and suggests the need to address the specific behaviors and risks in the child as well as the overall environment.

There is a proper focus on the need to confront offending behavior while taking into account the developing cognitive and social abilities of the adolescent. Sex offenders report more histories of maltreatment, both physical and sexual, compared to conduct-disordered young people in general. Thus, any treatments must take into account the adolescent's victimization as well as their developing patterns of perpetration and their environment. When young people are identified as being responsible for committing abusive acts against others, it is essential to assess and intervene in their own victimization experiences to prevent post-traumatic stress and other emotional effects. Pediatricians need to be sensitive to the psychological needs of the adolescent and provide initial psychological support after sexual assault while making referrals to appropriate mental health professionals and community resources for longer-term assessment and counseling (74).

Diagnosis

At a minimum, the clinician caring for children should be able to recognize and report potential child maltreatment, using standard methods for obtaining history, physical examination and selected laboratory and imaging tests. This clinician must also be cognizant that multiple forms of maltreatment may co-exist, understand the importance of certain risk factors, assist in choosing the appropriate location and timing of evaluation, and appropriately refer children and families to specialized medical and social services. In health care, a clinical assessment of child victimization begins with a medical encounter that usually follows information-gathering, physical assessment, testing, and clinical diagnosis followed by treatment and referral (see Table 3).

Medical diagnosis of child abuse and neglect follows commonly-accepted practices for other medical diagnosis. Pediatricians should consult current Clinical Procedural Terminology for coding for encounters and International Classification of Disease codes for diagnosis (see Table 2). While the use of such coding does not guarantee reimbursement, it highlights the standard approach to maltreatment as a concern of the health care system and allows collection of population data from hospital discharge and emergency department databases (4).

Medical history, a cornerstone of medical diagnosis, plays the most important part in the diagnosis of child abuse and neglect. It is the history, taken with the physical examination findings and imaging studies, that offers a sound basis for diagnosis and treatment recommendations for the child and family. Inquiring and recording the specific complaints and disclosures of maltreatment by the child and parent, if any, in their own words is vitally important to the ultimate protection of the child. Behavioral and emotional issues are important in this assessment. Certain non-specific behaviors, developmental delays, and history of abuse should be recorded as part of the medical history; this history aids in assessing harm and planning for appropriate treatment (66). A simple set of screening questions for use during the general pediatric encounter has been developed but has yet to be widely implemented (108). In cases of child victimization, the content and methods used to obtain the patient's history and the techniques used for physical examination are further specialized to concentrate on areas of increased risk and the types of suspected maltreatment (109).

The practitioner then arrives at an assessment or diagnosis, usually utilizing schema of diagnostic categories, such as the International Classification of Disease (4) or a specialized diagnostic scheme for certain types of abuse (66). Unique to child maltreatment diagnosis is a determination of certainty. A low level of certainty is required to meet general standards of a 'reasonable cause to suspect' that maltreatment has occurred for mandated reporting.

This presumptive diagnosis leads the practitioner to request diagnostic tests for the child, such as x-rays, blood work, or microbiologic cultures, if such tests are indicated. The presumptive diagnosis also leads the practitioner at the time of the encounter to begin treatment of any acute injury, ensure protection of the child from further harm, and arrange referrals to appropriate physical or mental health specialists for further evaluation and treatment (110).

Treatment, reporting, and court appearance

Pediatricians have historically had an important role in the assessment and reporting of suspected child abuse and neglect, and now have an increasingly important role with mental health professionals, community, and government services in treatment and prevention activities (111). Medical professionals have had a long history of evaluating children and participating as team members in the interdisciplinary assessment of child maltreatment (112). Abraham Jacobi, a forefather of modern pediatric medicine, joined the New York Society for the Prevention of Cruelty to Children in New York City in 1881 (113), and multidisciplinary hospital committees were created to address this multidimensional problem (114). These "child protection teams" consist of social workers, physicians, nurses, and other child advocates.

A key element is the pediatrician's understanding of child development, how injuries occur accidentally and non-accidentally, basic concepts of good parenting, and other family violence, such as intimate partner violence and elder abuse. In a recent survey, two-thirds of pediatricians reported treating injuries from child abuse, two-thirds had treated injuries from other community violence, and one-half had treated injuries related to domestic violence (115). Pediatricians assist the community response by collaborating with community agencies (such as child advocacy centers and social services agencies) and governmental entities (such as police and child protective services) that have the resources, responsibility, and authority to protect and improve the lives of child victims.

Nurses have been increasingly called upon to perform more than routine nursing services in the evaluation of suspected abuse. For example, "Sexual Assault Nurse Examiners" or "SANE" nurses have provided medical examinations for the collection of forensic evidence of suspected sexual and physical assault (116). In addition, some nurses also visit homes of new parents to help reduce the risk of child maltreatment (117, 118).

Physicians have legal responsibilities to report their concerns of child abuse and neglect to appropriate state agencies in all fifty states in the US (12, 119). Although the forms of the legislation vary from state to state, these "child protection laws" stipulate that certain professionals must report their concerns of child abuse and neglect to appropriate governmental agencies. The reporting requirements of these laws supersede the confidentiality of medical records and the patient-provider relationship. The "mandated reporters" generally include physicians, nurses, and other professionals working in hospitals, in addition to a variety of other licensed professionals who include teachers, counselors, law enforcement officers, and mental health professionals.

Specific protections are usually given for reports made "in good faith," and certain penalties are listed for the failure to report when child maltreatment would "reasonably" have been suspected. It is important to note that child abuse reporting is one of the few instances in which health care professionals are required to contact a governmental agency in the routine course of their practice. While disease reporting has traditionally existed within public health (particularly when a contagious infection may pose a hazard to the community's health), reporting actions that are deemed to be "crimes" have historically been less accepted by the medical community. Less clear statutory requirements have been enacted in the United States for the reporting of victimization of elderly, vulnerable adults, and domestic violence.

Physicians have historically underreported suspected maltreatment (120, 121). Several reasons have been identified for this failure, such as fear of losing patients, distaste for the legal system and liability concerns (115, 122). Penalties for not reporting range from fines in some states to criminal charges in others, but also include civil penalties so that the child and/or the child's family may litigate to redress financial losses sustained because maltreatment was not reported. Recent federal legislation in the United States specifically allows child abuse reporting and exempts such state reporting laws from HIPAA requirements.

Reporting child victimization to governmental agencies begins an investigation to identify the presence or absence of "evidence" to support or "substantiate" the suspicions. Requirements vary from state to state, and no national criteria exist for determining whether to report suspected abuse or neglect. General guidelines have been suggested that include the patient meeting the definition of being a child, the act or omission having been committed by the parent or caretaker, the acts or omissions lead to harm or the risk of harm, or the features of an episode fulfill other criteria for abuse or neglect in the medical record (123).

Multiple missed medical appointments, unreasonable delay in seeking medical treatment, abandonment, illnesses that could be prevented by routine medical care and inadequate care have been identified as potential minimal criteria for a neglect report (106). Fractures, soft tissue injuries of normally protected body parts, inflicted traumatic brain injury and witnessed physical injury caused by the caretaker indicate cause to suspect physical abuse. Statements made by the child or parent disclosing potential sexual contact with a caretaker or contrary to state law, certain anogenital injuries, and sexually-transmitted infection are generally a basis for diagnosing suspected sexual abuse.

The ultimate and perhaps most important action to protect a child from further victimization may involve going to court. Physicians and other health care providers are routinely called to provide information regarding their medical evaluation of children, particularly with regard to statements made by the child, the medical history obtained, and any findings of physical examination. While giving testimony in court, physicians and other health care professionals are often asked their opinion, "within a reasonable degree of medical certainty," concerning the diagnosis of child abuse and neglect or victimization. Significant differences exist between standards for medical diagnosis and those for civil or criminal adjudication. Medical diagnosis is defined as "the act of distinguishing one disease from another" or "the determination of the nature of a case of disease" (124).

A constellation of the patient's history, physical examination, and laboratory findings may result in multiple diagnoses, which may lead the practitioner to a treatment plan without 100 percent or even probable certainty after diagnosis. These criteria differ significantly from legal standards, by which a level of certainty must be carefully crafted to include "credible" evidence, a "preponderance" of evidence, "clear and convincing" evidence, or evidence "beyond a reasonable doubt." Differences in interpretation of certainty lead to difficulty in communication between legal and medical practitioners.

Court appearance and testimony, while often inconvenient, is vital to provide the evidence and opinion for the state to take action to protect children. Recently, testimony provided by physicians has been considered part of medical practice, and providing "irresponsible testimony" may have negative repercussions for a physician's practice (125). Despite the legal system's need for health care professionals to provide evidence in maltreatment cases, it is relatively uncommon for health care professionals to be required to attend court hearings, even if they specialize in caring for maltreated children (126).

Training and prevention

Health care professionals have a unique role in the training of child welfare professionals, law enforcement, child protection services workers, and all professionals who manage the day-to-day care of children. To fulfill their mandatory roles in reporting child abuse and neglect, teachers, child development specialists, mental health workers and others who provide daycare, education, and counseling services need to understand the medical manifestations of child victimization. They also need to identify the physical as well as emotional signs of abuse and neglect so that they can provide the optimal treatment for children in their care. Professionals from a variety of health care disciplines provide specialized training at a national level for medical and nonmedical providers through multidisciplinary organizations such as the American Professional Society on the Abuse of Children (www.APSAC.org) or medical organizations such as the American Academy of Pediatrics (www.AAP.org). Additionally, various child protective service agencies and university programs render services to nonmedical providers and offer information about medical issues related to child victimization.

The prevention of child abuse and neglect ultimately rests with the family, but pediatricians and the community can still play important roles preventing abuse from occurring (127). The economic burden, estimated at over $80 billion annually, calls for prevention (128). Local county councils for the prevention of child abuse and neglect sponsor programs, social service agencies provide childcare or foster care, and state departments of social services have the legal authority to investigate suspected child maltreatment. Community approaches, such as home visitation, parenting classes, certain cognitive behavioral therapies for children, and parent-child interaction therapy, have been shown to be effective in changing parents' behavior, and reducing social isolation and stress, particularly in families at risk for maltreatment (129, 130).

Preventing child abuse and neglect spares children physical and psychological pain and improves their long-term health. Dubowitz (131) noted that prevention "is intuitively and morally preferable to intervening after the fact." There is increasing evidence supporting the effectiveness of several universal and selective prevention interventions the effectiveness of most programs is still not known (132, 133). Robert Caldwell (134) estimated that the costs of a home visitor program in Michigan would be 3.5% of the $823 million estimated cost of child abuse, and small reductions in the rate of child maltreatment were thought to make prevention cost effective. However, home-visiting programs are not uniformly effective, parenting programs appear to improve parenting but not necessarily reduce child maltreatment, and some family programs are successful in reducing physical abuse but not neglect.

Ray Helfer (135) noted the "window of opportunity" that is present in the perinatal period to enhance parent-child interactions and prevent physical abuse. Several program models have shown promise based upon key periods, including pre-pregnancy planning, early conception, late pregnancy, pre-labor and labor, immediately following delivery, and at home with the child. Opportunities for prevention include teaching parents and caregivers to cope with infant crying and how to provide a safe sleep environment for their infant. A meta-analysis of several early childhood interventions concluded that the evidence for their preventing child maltreatment is weak, but longer-term studies may show reductions in child maltreatment similar to other programs such as home visiting, when longer follow-up can be achieved (136).

Several parent education programs have been evaluated for their association with decreases in physical abuse and neglect. Family Connections, a multifaceted, home visiting community-based child neglect prevention program, showed "cost effective" improvements in risk and protective factors and behavioral outcomes (137). To address a specific form of physical abuse, Mark Dias and colleagues devised a hospital-based parent education program implemented immediately after birth that has been shown to decrease the incidence of shaken baby syndrome (138, 139). Barr and colleagues (140) have devised a program of parent education in late pregnancy, delivery, and early infancy to change maternal knowledge and behaviors relevant to infant shaking. Using a randomized controlled trial, they were able to demonstrate how "The Period of Purple Crying" was able to increase maternal knowledge scores, knowledge about the dangers of shaking, and sharing that information with other caretakers.

A randomized trial of the "SEEK" program in an inner-city clinic with high-risk families was able to show lower rates of maltreatment, CPS reports, harsh punishment, and improved health services after an intervention of pediatric resident education (141). Several barriers (time, training, culture, sensitive issues) to widespread implementation could be addressed by identifying potential strategies, such as the use of handouts and local news stories, to begin a dialogue during routine pediatric visits (142).

With the generosity of the Doris Duke Charitable Foundation, the American Academy of Pediatrics launched a program called Practicing Safety: Connected Kids aimed at decreasing child abuse and neglect by enhancing anticipatory guidance and increasing screening provided by pediatric practices to children ages 0-3y, focusing on helping parents and families to raise resilient children (143). Anticipatory guidance has significant potential for decreasing violence, and each counseling topic discusses the child's development, the parent's feelings and reactions in response to the child's development and behavior, and specific practical suggestions on how to encourage healthy social, emotional, and physical growth in an environment of support and open communication. Practices screened for maternal depression and improved their discussion of coping with crying, maternal bonding, toilet training and discipline (143).

Sexual assault and rape prevention strategies begin with the child and family being able to identify and avoid high-risk situations and immediately reporting potential sexual contact. Pediatricians and others can provide screening for victims of domestic violence during routine medical care and can provide guidance and strategies to prevent or minimize abuse (such as avoiding late night use of alcohol or drugs or seeking immediate medical care after assault). Finkelhor (2007) has concluded that the available evidence supports providing high quality child-focused prevention education programs because children are able to acquire the concepts, the programs promote disclosure, there are lower rates of victimization, and children have less self-blame. Parent education and media campaigns have also demonstrated some positive effects (144).

A review confirmed the effectiveness of school-based sexual abuse prevention (145). Pediatricians have the ability to explain child development and the special health needs of children, particularly those with chronic medical conditions, to the community and to provide the scientific background and structure for the implementation and evaluation of community programs. Prenatal clinics and other services for high-risk adolescents need to provide primary care interventions to prevent future maltreatment.

CONCLUSION

Pediatricians and other clinicians play a vital role in the assessment, identification, care, and treatment of victims of child abuse and neglect. Physicians, nurses, and other health professionals have developed increasingly sophisticated techniques for diagnosing and documenting physical abuse, head trauma, fractures, anogenital trauma, and sexually transmitted infections. They have integrated such diagnostic findings with referral to specialized services. They are important members of the crew of the 'lifeboat' needed to save children in the sometimes turbulent 'ocean of life' (146).

While C. Henry Kempe first taught us about the battered child in 1962 and Ray E. Helfer showed the importance of understanding a child's perspective in 1984, we still have a long way to go in solving the problems of child neglect and victimization in our communities. Many segments of our population do not understand the impact of higher rates of poverty, unique health concerns, and other special circumstances of children. Our response to the needs of abused and neglected children requires earnest dedication by all medical professionals in clinical care, training, research, and advocacy to identify, treat, and prevent the devastating physical and emotional consequences of child abuse and maltreatment.

REFERENCES

[1] Kempe CH, Silverman FN, Steele BF, Droegemueller W, Silver HK. The battered child syndrome. JAMA 1962; 181: 17-24.

[2] Child Abuse Prevention and Treatment Act, 42 U.S.C. § 5101 et seq; 42 U.S.C. § 5116 et seq, 1974.

[3] World Health Organization. Report of the consultation on child abuse prevention. Geneva: World Health Organization, 1999. URL: http://whqlibdoc.who.int/hq/1999/WHO_HSC_PVI_99.1.pdf.

[4] US Department of Health and Human Services, Centers for Disease Control and Prevention, & National Center for Health Statistics. ICD-10: International statistical classification of diseases and related health problems, Tenth revision. Washington, DC: US Government Printing Office, 1998.

[5] Kaplan SJ, Labruna V, Pelcovitz D, Salzinger S, Mandel F, Weiner M. Physically abused adolescents: Behavior problems, functional impairment, and comparison of informants' reports. Pediatrics 1999; 104: 43-49.

[6] Institute of Medicine and National Research Council. Child maltreatment research, policy, and practice for the next decade: Workshop summary. Washington, DC: The National Academies Press, 2012.

[7] Centers for Disease Control and Prevention. Adverse Childhood Experiences (ACE) Study: Major findings by publication year, 2012. URL: http://www.cdc.gov/ace/year.htm.

[8] Felitti VJ, Anda RF, Nordenberg D, Williamson DF, Spitz AM, Edwards V, et al. The relationship of adult health status to childhood abuse and household dysfunction. Am J Prevent Med 1998; 14: 245–258.

[9] Palusci VJ. Adverse childhood experiences and lifelong health. JAMA Pediatrics 2013; 167(1): 95-6.
[10] Kendall-Tackett K. The health effects of childhood abuse: Four pathways by which abuse can influence health. Child Abuse Negl 2002; 26: 715-29.
[11] Shonkoff JP, Garner AS, and The Committee On Psychosocial Aspects of Child and Family Health, Committee on Early Childhood, Adoption and Dependent Care, and Section on Developmental and Behavioral Pediatrics. The Lifelong Effects of Early Childhood Adversity and Toxic Stress. Pediatrics 2012; 129(1): e232-46.
[12] US Department of Health and Human Services. Child Maltreatment 2011: Reports from the States to the National Child Abuse and Neglect Data System. Washington, DC: US Government Printing Office, 2012.
[13] Sedlak AJ, Mettenburg J, Basena M, Petta I, McPherson K, Greene A, Li S. Fourth National Incidence Study of Child Abuse and Neglect (NIS–4): Report to Congress. Washington, DC: Department of Health and Human Services, Administration for Children and Families, 2010.
[14] Hussey JM, Chang JJ, Kotch JB. Child maltreatment in the United States: prevalence, risk factors and adolescent health consequences. Pediatrics 2006; 118: 933-42.
[15] Theodore AD, Chang JJ, Runyan DK, Hunter WM, Bangdiwala SI, Agans R. Epidemiologic features of the physical and sexual maltreatment of children in the Carolinas. Pediatrics 2005; 115: e331-7.
[16] Leventhal JM, Gaither JR. Incidence of serious injuries due to physical abuse in the United States: 1997 to 2009. Pediatrics 2012; 130(5): e847-52.
[17] Lane WG, Dubowitz H, Langenberg P, Dischinger P. Epidemiology of abusive abdominal trauma hospital-izations in United States children. Child Abuse Negl 2012; 36: 142–8.
[18] Finkelhor D, Jones L, Shattuck A. Updated trends in child maltreatment, 2011. Durham, NH: University of New Hampshire crimes Against Children Research Center, 2013. URL: http://www.unh.edu/ccrc/pdf/ CV203_Updated%20Trends%20in%20Child%20Maltreatment%202008 _8-6-10.pdf.
[19] Finkelhor D, Jones L. Why have child maltreatment and child victimization declined? J Soc Issues 2006; 62: 685-716.
[20] Huang MI, O'Riordan MA, Fitzenrider E, McDavid L, Cohen AR, Robinson S. Increased incidence of nonaccidental head trauma in infants associated with the economic recession. J Neurosurg Pediatr 2011; 8: 171-6.
[21] Wood JN, Medina SP, Feundtner C, Luan X, Localio R, Fieldston ES, Rubin DM. Local macroeconomic trends and hospital admissions for child abuse, 2000–2009. Pediatrics 2012; 130: e358-64.
[22] Sidebotham P, Atkins B, Hutton JL. Changes in rates of violent child deaths in England and Wales between 1974 and 2008: An analysis of national mortality data. Arch Dis Child 2012; 97: 193–9.
[23] Brayden RM, Altemeier WA, Tucker DD, Dietrich MS, Vietze P. Antecedents of child neglect in the first two years of life. J Pediatr 2012; 120: 426-9.
[24] Crosse S, Kaye E, Ratnofsky A. A report on the maltreatment of children with disabilities. Washington, DC: National Clearinghouse on Child Abuse and Neglect Information, 1993.
[25] New York State Office of Children and Family Services. 1998-2002 Monitoring and analysis profiles. Albany, NY: New York State Office of Children and Family Services, 2003.
[26] Powers JL, Eckenrode J. The maltreatment of adolescents. Child Abuse Negl 1988; 12: 189-200.
[27] Cohen J, Mannarino R, Zhitova A, Capone M. Treating child abuse-related posttraumatic stress and comorbid abuse in adolescents. Child Abuse Negl 2003; 27: 1345-65.
[28] Ferguson D, Horwood LJ, Lynskey M. Childhood sexual abuse, adolescent sexual behaviors and sexual revictimization. Child Abuse Negl 1997; 21: 789-803.
[29] Zhou Y, Hallisey EJ, Freymann GR. Identifying perinatal risk factors for infant maltreatment: An ecological approach. Int J Health Geo 2006; 5: 53-63.
[30] Palusci VJ, Smith EG, Paneth N. Predicting recurrence of child maltreatment in young children using NCANDS. Child Youth Serv Rev 2005; 27(6): 667-82.
[31] Black DA, Heyman RE, Smith AM. Risk factors for child physical abuse. Aggress Viol Behav 2001; 6: 121-88.

[32] Brown J, Cohen P, Johnson JG, Salzinger S. A longitudinal analysis of risk factors for child maltreatment: Findings of a 17-year prospective study of officially recorded and self-reported child abuse and neglect. Child Abuse Negl 1998; 22: 1065-78.
[33] Christian CW, Committee on Child Abuse and Neglect. The evaluation of suspected child physical abuse. Pediatrics 2015; 133(5): 1337-54.
[34] Allasio D, Fischer H. Immersion scald burns and the ability of young children to climb into a bath tub. Pediatrics 2005; 115: 1419-21.
[35] Maguire S, Mann MK, Siebert J, Kemp A. Can you age bruises accurately in children? A systematic review. Arch Dis Child 2005; 90: 187-9.
[36] Sugar NF, Taylor JA, Feldman KW. Bruises in infant and toddlers: those who don't cruise rarely bruise. Arch Pediatr Adolesc Med, 1999; 153: 399-403.
[37] Toon MH, Maybauer DM, Arceneoux LL, Fraser JF, Meyer W, Runge A, Maybauer MO. Children with burn injuries-assessment of trauma, neglect, violence and abuse. J Inj Viol Res 2003; 3(2): 98-110.
[38] Drago DA. Kitchen scalds and thermal burns in children five years and younger. Pediatrics 2005; 115: 10-6.
[39] Jenny CJ and the Committee on Child Abuse and Neglect. Evaluating infants and young children with multiple fractures. Pediatrics 2006; 118: 1299-1303.
[40] Duffy SO, Squires J, Fromkin JB, Berger RP. Use of skeletal surveys to evaluate for physical abuse: Analysis of 703 consecutive skeletal surveys. Pediatrics 2011; 127: e47-e52.
[41] Bennett BL, Chua MS, Care M, Kachelmeyer A, Mahabee-Gittens M. Retrospective review to determine the utility of follow-up skeletal surveys in child abuse evaluations when the initial skeletal survey is normal. BMC Res Note 2011; 4: 354.
[42] Kleinman PK. Diagnostic imaging of child abuse (2nd ed). St. Louis, MO: Mosby, 1998.
[43] Halliday KE, Broderick NJ, Somers JM, Hawkes R. Dating fractures in infants. Clin Radiol 2011; 66: 1049-54.
[44] Prosser I, Lawson Z, Evans A, Harrison, S, Maguire S. Kemp AM. A timetable for the radiologic features of fracture healing in young children. Am J Radiol 2012; 198: 1014-20.
[45] American College of Radiology. ACR–SPR practice guideline for skeletal surveys In Children. Reston, VA: American College of Radiology, 2011. URL: http://www.acr.org/~/media/9BDCDB EE99B84E87BAAC2B1695BC07B6.pdf.
[46] American Academy of Pediatrics, Section on Radiology. Diagnostic imaging of child abuse. Pediatrics 2009: 123(5): 1430-5.
[47] Berdon WE. A modest proposal: Thoracic CT for rib fracture diagnosis in child abuse (letter). Child Abuse Negl 2012; 36: 200– 201.
[48] British Paediatric and Adolescent Bone Group. British Paediatric and Adolescent Bone Group's position statement on vitamin D deficiency. BMJ 2012; 345: e8182.
[49] Slovis TL, Strouse PJ, Coley BD, Rigsby CK. The creation of non-disease: an assault on the diagnosis of child abuse. Pediatr Radiol 2012; 42(8): 903-5.
[50] Christian CW, Block R, and the Committee of Child Abuse and Neglect. Abusive head trauma in infants and children. Pediatrics 2009; 123: 1409-11.
[51] Caffey J. The whiplash shaken baby syndrome: A manual shaking by the extremities with whiplash-induced intracranial and intraocular bleeding linked with residual permanent brain damage and mental retardation. Pediatrics 1974; 54: 396-403.
[52] Kemp AM. Abusive head trauma: recognition and the essential investigation. Arch Dis Child Educ Pract Edit 2011. doi:10.1136/adc.2009.170449.
[53] Deisch J, Quinton R, Gruszecki AC. Craniocerebral trauma inflicted by television falls. J Forensic Sci 2011; 56(4): 1049-53.
[54] Edwards RJ, Allport RJ, Stoodley NG, O'Callaghan O, Lock RJ, Carter MR. External hydrocephalus and subdural bleeding in infancy associated with transplacental anti-Ro antibodies. Arch Dis Child 2012; 97: 316–9.
[55] Hart H, Rubia K. Neuroimaging of child abuse: A critical review. Front Hum Neurosci 2012; 52(6): 1-24.

[56] Xu D, Mukherjee P, Barkovich J. Pediatric brain injury: Can DTI scalars predict functional outcome? Pediatr Radiol 2013; 43: 55–9.

[57] Yoshida S, Oishi K, Faria AV, Mori S. Diffusion tensor imaging of normal brain development. Pediatr Radiol 2013; 43: 15–27.

[58] Levin AV. Retinal hemorrhage in abusive head trauma. Pediatrics 2010; 126: 961-70.

[59] Levin AV. Ocular complications of head trauma in children. Pediatr Emerg Care 1991; 7: 129-30.

[60] Gilles E, McGregor M, Levy-Clarke G. Retinal hemorrhage asymmetry in inflicted head injury: a clue to pathogenesis? J Pediatrics 2003; 143(4): 494–9.

[61] Herr S, Fallat ME. Abusive abdominal and thoracic trauma. Clin Pediatr Emerg Med 2006: 7: 149-52.

[62] Wood J, Rubin DM, Nance ML, Christian CW. Distinguishing inflicted versus accidental abdominal injuries in young children. J Trauma 2005; 59: 1203-8.

[63] Guleserian KJ, Gilchrist BF, Luks FL, et al. Child abuse as a cause of traumatic chylothorax. J Pediatr Surg 1986; 31: 1696-7.

[64] Bennett BL, Macabee-Gittens MS, Chua M, Hirsch R. Elevated cardiac troponin I level in cases of thoracic nonaccidental trauma. Pediatr Emerg Care 2011; 10: 941-4.

[65] Kellogg N, American Academy of Pediatrics. The evaluation of sexual abuse in children. Pediatrics 2005; 116: 506-12.

[66] Adams JA, Kaplan RA, Starling SP, et al. Guidelines for medical care of children who may have been sexually abused. J Pediatr Adolesc Gynecol 2007; 20: 163-72.

[67] Adams JA. Harper K, Knudson S, Revilla J. Examination findings in legally-confirmed child sexual abuse: It's normal to be normal. Pediatrics 1994; 94: 310-7.

[68] Heger A, Ticson L, Velasquez O, Bernier R. Children referred for possible sexual abuse: Medical findings in 2384 children. Child Abuse Negl 2002; 26: 645-59.

[69] Centers for Disease Control and Prevention. Sexually transmitted diseases treatment guidelines. MMWR 2010; 59(RR-12): 1-110.

[70] Palusci VJ, Reeves MJ. Testing for genital gonorrhea infections in prepubertal girls with suspected sexual abuse. Pediatr Infect Dis J 2003; 22(7): 618-23.

[71] Block RW, Palusci VJ. Child abuse pediatrics: A new pediatric subspecialty. Pediatrics 2006; 148(6): 711-2.

[72] Adams JA. Sexual abuse and adolescents. Pediatr Ann 1997; 26: 299-304.

[73] Noll J, Shenk C. Teen birth rates in sexually abused and neglected females Pediatrics 2012; 131: e1181-e1187.

[74] Kaufman M, Committee on Adolescence. Care of the adolescent sexual assault victim. Pediatrics 2008; 122: 462–470.

[75] Pratt HD, Greydanus DE. Violence: concepts of its impact on children and youth. Pediatr Clin North Am 2003; 50: 963-1003.

[76] Palusci VJ, Cox EO, Cyrus TA, Heartwell SW, Vandervort FE, Pott ES. Medical assessment and legal outcome in child sexual abuse. Arch Pediatr Adolesc Med 1999; 153(4): 388-92.

[77] Thackeray JD, Hornor G, Benzinger EA, Scribano PV. Forensic evidence collection and DNA identification in acute child sexual assault. Pediatrics 2011; 128(2): 227-32.

[78] Palusci VJ, Cox EO, Shatz EM, Schultze JM. Urgent medical assessment after child sexual abuse. Child Abuse Negl 2006; 30(4): 367-80.

[79] Palusci VJ, Cyrus TA. Reaction to videocolposcopy in the assessment of child sexual abuse. Child Abuse Negl 2001; 25(11): 1535-46.

[80] Gavril AR, Kellogg ND, Nair P. Value of follow-up examinations of children and adolescents evaluated for sexual abuse and assault. Pediatrics 2010; 129(2): 282-9.

[81] Hammerschlag MR, Guillén CD. Medical and legal implications of testing for sexually transmitted infections in children. Clin Microbiol Rev 2010; 23(3): 493-506.

[82] Whaitiri S, Kelly P. Genital gonorrhoea in children: determining the source and mode of infection. Arch Dis Child 2011; 96(3): 247-51.

[83] Adams JA, Starling SP, Frasier LD, Palusci VP, Shapiro RA, Finkel MA, Botash AS. Diagnostic accuracy in child sexual abuse medical evaluation: role of experience, training, and expert case review. Child Abuse Negl 2012; 36: 383-392

[84] Adams JA, Kellogg ND, Farst KJ, Harper NS, Palusci VJ, Frasier LD, Levitt CJ, Shapiro RA, Moles RA, Starling SP. Updated guidelines for the medical assessment and care of children who may have been sexually abused. J Pediatr Adolesc Gyn. Published online March 2015. DOI: 10.1016/j.jpag.2015.01.007.

[85] Kairys SW, Johnson CF, Committee on Child Abuse and Neglect. The psychological maltreatment of children- Technical report. Pediatrics 2002; 109: e68.

[86] Trickett PK, Mennen FE, Kim K, Sang J. Emotional abuse in a sample of multiply maltreated, urban young adolescents: Issues of definition and identification. Child Abuse Negl 2009; 33: 27–35.

[87] Shaffer A, Yates TM, Egeland BR. The relation of emotional maltreatment to early adolescent competence: Developmental processes in a prospective study. Child Abuse Negl 2009; 33(1): 36-44.

[88] Allen B. An analysis of the impact of diverse forms of childhood psychological maltreatment on emotional adjustment in early adulthood. Child Maltreat 2008; 13(3): 307-12.

[89] Liu RT, Alloy LB, Abramson LY, Iacoviello BM, Whitehouse WG. Emotional maltreatment and depression: Prospective prediction of depressive episodes. Depress Anxiety 2009; 26(2): 174-81.

[90] Reyome ND. The effect of childhood emotional maltreatment on the emerging attachment system and later intimate relationships. J Aggress Maltreat Trauma 2010; 19(1): 1-4.

[91] Steinberg JA, Gibb BE, Alloy LB, Abramson LY. Childhood emotional maltreatment, cognitive vulner-ability to depression, and self-referent information processing in adulthood: Reciprocal relations. J Cogn Psychother 2003; 17(4): 347-58.

[92] Uhrlass DJ, Gibb BE. Childhood emotional mal-treatment and the stress generation model of depression. J Soc Clin Psychol 2007; 26(1): 119-30.

[93] Turner HA, Finkelhor D, Ormrod R. Child mental health problems as risk factors for victimization. Child Maltreat 2010; 15: 132-143.

[94] Dubowitz H, Papas MA, Black MM, Starr RH. Child neglect: Outcomes in high-risk urban preschoolers. Pediatrics 2002; 109: 1100-7.

[95] Liu J, Raine A, Venables PH, Dalais C, Mednick SA. Malnutrition at age 3 years and lower cognitive ability at age 11 years. Arch Pediatr Adolesc Med 2003; 157: 593-600.

[96] Block RW, Krebs NF. Failure to thrive as a manifestation of child neglect. Pediatrics 2005; 116(5): 1234-7.

[97] Wright CM. Identification and management of failure to thrive: A community perspective. Arch Dis Child 2000; 82(1): 5-9.

[98] Palusci VJ, Bliss R, Crum P. Outcomes for groups for children exposed to violence with behavior problems. Trauma Loss 2007; 7(1): 27-38.

[99] Palusci VJ, Ondersma SJ. Services and recurrence after CPS confirmed psychological maltreatment. Child Maltreat 2012; 17(2): 153-63.

[100] Helfer RE. The neglect of our children. Pediatr Clin North Am 1990; 37: 923-42.

[101] Dubowitz H. Child neglect: Guidance for pediatricians. Pediatr Rev 2000; 21: 111- 6.

[102] Jenny C, American Academy of Pediatrics. Recognizing and responding to medical neglect. Pediatrics 2007; 120(6): 1385-9.

[103] Black MM, Dubowitz H, Casey PH, Cutts D, Drewett RF, Drotar D, et al. Failure to thrive as distinct from child neglect. Pediatrics 2006; 117(4): 1456-9.

[104] Palusci VJ, Wirtz SJ, Covington TM. Using capture-recapture methods to better ascertain the incidence of fatal child maltreatment. Child Abuse Negl 2010; 34(6): 396-402.

[105] Coohey C. Defining and classifying supervisory neglect. Child Maltreat 2003; 8: 145-56.

[106] Paradise JE, Bass J, Forman SD, Berkowitz J, Greenberg DB, Mehta K. Minimum criteria for reporting child abuse from health care settings. Pediatr Emerg Care 1995; 11: 335-9.

[107] Bentovim A. Preventing sexually abused young people from becoming abusers, and treating the victimization experiences of young people who offend sexually. Child Abuse Negl 2011; 26, 661-78.

[108] Palusci VJ, Palusci JV. Screening tools for child sexual abuse. J Pediatr (Rio J) 2006; 82(6): 409-10.

[109] Council of the American Academy of Child and Adolescent Psychiatry. Statement: Practice parameters for the forensic evaluation of children and adolescents who may have been physically or sexually abused. J Am Acad Child Adolesc Psychiatry 1997; 36: 423-42.

[110] Blythe MJ, Orr DP. Childhood sexual abuse: Guidelines for evaluation. Indiana Med 1995; 88, 11-8.

[111] Myers JEB, ed. The APSAC handbook on child maltreatment, 3rd ed. Thousand Oaks, CA: Sage, 2010.
[112] Bross DC, Krugman R D, Lenherr MR, Rosenburg DA, Schmitt BD, eds. The new child protection team handbook. New York: Garland, 1988.
[113] Burke EC. Abraham Jacobi: The man and his legacy. Pediatrics 1998; 101: 309-312.
[114] Krugman SD. Multidisciplinary teams. In: Krugman RD, Korbin JE, eds. C Henry Kempe: A fifty year legacy to the field of child abuse and neglect. New York: Springer, 2013: 71-8.
[115] Flaherty EG, Sege R, Price LL, Christoffel KK, Norton DP, O'Connor KG. Pediatrician characteristics associated with child abuse identification and reporting: results from a national survey of pediatricians. Child Maltreat 2006; 11(4): 361-9.
[116] Little K. Sexual assault nurse examiner (SANE) Programs: Improving the community response to sexual assault victims (NCJ 186366). Washington, DC: US Department of Justice, Office of Justice Programs, 2001.
[117] American Academy of Pediatrics. The role of home visitation programs in improving health outcomes for children and families. Pediatrics 1998; 101: 486-9.
[118] Olds DL. Home visitation for pregnant women and parents of young children. Am J Dis Child 1992; 146: 704-8.
[119] Fontana VJ. Child abuse: The physician's responsibility. NY State J Med 1989; 89: 152-5.
[120] Johnson CF. Physicians and medical neglect: Variables that affect reporting. Child Abuse Negl 1993; 17: 605-15.
[121] Palusci VJ, Marshall J. An open letter to Michigan physicians. Mich Med 2003; 102(2): 6.
[122] Morris JL, Johnson CF, Clasen M. To report or not to report: Physicians' attitudes toward discipline and child abuse. Am J Dis Child 1985; 139: 194-7.
[123] Hymel KP, American Academy of Pediatrics. When is lack of supervision neglect? Pediatrics 2006; 118: 1296-8.
[124] Dorland's Illustrated Medical Dictionary (25 ed). Philadelphia, PA: WB Saunders, 1974; 435.
[125] Chadwick D, Krous HF. Irresponsible medical testimony by medical experts in cases involving the physical abuse and neglect of children. Child Maltreat 1997; 2(4): 313-21.
[126] Palusci VJ, Hicks RA, Vandervort FE. "You are hereby commanded to appear": Pediatrician subpoena and court appearance in child maltreatment. Pediatrics 2001; 107(6): 1427-30.
[127] Palusci VJ, Haney ML. Strategies to prevent child maltreatment and integration into practice. APSAC Advisor 2010; 22(1): 8-17.
[128] Fang X, Brown DS, Florence CS, Mercy JA. The economic burden of child maltreatment in the United States and implications for prevention. Child Abuse Negl 2012; 36: 156-65.
[129] Flaherty EG, Stirling J, American Academy of Pediatrics Committee on Child Abuse and Neglect. Clinical report—The pediatrician's role in child maltreatment prevention. Pediatrics 2010; 126(4): 833-41.
[130] Centers for Disease Control and Prevention. First reports evaluating the effectiveness of strategies for preventing violence: early childhood home visitation and firearms laws. Findings from the Task Force on Community Preventive Services. MMWR 2003; 52 (RR-14): 1-9.
[131] Dubowitz H. Preventing child neglect and physical abuse: A role for pediatricians. Pediatr Rev 2002; 23(6): 191–196.
[132] MacMillan HL, Wathen CN, Fergusson DM, Leventhal JM, Taussig HN. Interventions to prevent child maltreatment and associated impairment. Lancet 2009; 373:250–66.
[133] Mikton C, Butchart A. Child maltreatment prevention: A systematic review of reviews. Bull WHO 2009; 87: 353–61.
[134] Caldwell RA. The costs of child abuse vs. child abuse prevention: Michigan's experience, 1992. URL: https://www.msu.edu/~bob/cost1992.pdf.
[135] Helfer RE. The perinatal period, a window of opportunity for enhancing parent-infant communication: An approach to prevention. Child Abuse Negl 1987; 11(4): 565–79.
[136] Reynolds AJ, Mathieson LC, Topitzes JW. Do early childhood interventions prevent child maltreatment? Child Maltreat 2009; 14(5): 182–206.

[137] DePanfilis D, Dubowitz H, Kunz, J. Assessing the cost effectiveness of family connections. Child Abuse Negl 2008; 32(3): 335–51.

[138] Dias M S, Smith K, deGuehery K, Mazur P, Li V, Shaffer ML. Preventing abusive head trauma among infant and young children: A hospital-based, parent education program. Pediatrics 2005; 115(4): 470–7.

[139] Altman RL, Canter J, Patrick PA, Daley N, Butt NK, Brand DA. Parent education by maternity nurses and prevention of abusive head trauma. Pediatrics 2011; 128(5): e1164-72.

[140] Barr RG, Rivara FP, Barr M, Cummings P, Taylor J, Lengua LJ, et al. Effectiveness of educational materials designed to change knowledge and behaviors regarding crying and shaken baby syndrome in mothers of newborns: A randomized, controlled trial. Pediatrics 2009; 123(6): 972–80.

[141] Dubowitz H, Feigelman S, Lane W, Kim J. Pediatric primary care to help prevent child maltreatment: The Safe Environment for Every Kid (SEEK) model. Pediatrics 2009; 123(3): 858–64.

[142] Sege RD, Hatmaker-Flanigan E, De Vos E, Levin-Goodman R, Spivak H. Anticipatory guidance and violence prevention: Results from family and pediatrician focus groups. Pediatrics 2006; 117: 455–63.

[143] American Academy of Pediatrics. Connected Kids: Safe Strong Secure, A new violence prevention program from the American Academy of Pediatrics. Elk Grove Village, IL: AAP, 2005.

[144] Finkelhor D. Prevention of sexual abuse through educational programs directed toward children. Pediatrics 2007; 120(3): 640-5.

[145] Barron I, Topping K. School-based child sexual abuse prevention programs: Implications for practitioners. APSAC Advisor 2010; 22 (2/3): 11-9.

[146] Myers JEB. Keep the lifeboat afloat. Child Abuse Negl 2002; 26: 561-7.

In: Public Health Yearbook 2016
Editor: Joav Merrick
ISBN: 978-1-53610-947-4

Chapter 41

PUBLIC HEALTH ASPECTS OF YOUTH SEXUAL OFFENDERS

Helen D Pratt,* PhD
and Donald E Greydanus, MD, DrHC (Athens)
Department of Pediatric and Adolescent Medicine,
Western Michigan University
Homer Stryker MD School of Medicine,
Kalamazoo, Michigan, US

ABSTRACT

Children and adolescents under the age of 18 years account for one-fifth of arrests for all sexual offenses (excluding prostitution). These young perpetrators can be found among all socio-economic groups and live in all regions of the United States. They often come to the attention of primary care clinicians when their parents bring them to the office for protection from the authorities and help with addressing their maladaptive behavior. Clinician-collected information may get used as a part of criminal investigations or to facilitate initial evaluation and coordination of services. Frequently, parents will bring their child or adolescent in for an office visit once the parents have caught them engaging in some form of sexual activity. The parent's concern is typically whether or not this is normal or abnormal behavior. Physicians who are aware of adolescent sexual offending can increase their ability to detect adolescents who have aberrant or deviant sexual behavior patterns allowing for *early* referral and comprehensive intervention.

Keywords: childhood, adolescence, behavior, crime, sexual offense, sexual offenders

* Correspondence: Helen D Pratt PhD, Professor, Department of Pediatric and Adolescent Medicine, Western Michigan University Homer Stryker MD School of Medicine, 1000 Oakland Drive, Kalamazoo, MI 49008-8048, United States. E-mail: helen.pratt@med.wmich.edu.

INTRODUCTION

Most of the sexual abuse literature focuses on adult perpetrators or child/teen victims. In the past five years, only a few new articles have been published discussing adolescent sexual offenders (1-4). Most of those articles consisted of meta-analyses of previous studies. The office of Juvenile Justice Delinquency and Prevention, National Center on Sexual Behavior of Youth (NCSBY) has published statistics (2009-2011) on youth sexual offenders (1-4). Otherwise there has not more current data since the original article by the authors of this chapter who have published on adolescent sexual offending (5-7). There is still a paucity of data available in the literature on adolescent sexual offenders who are involved in sexual abuse of younger children. Primary care clinicians must be prepared to act in a manner that does not contaminate forensic evidence nor alter the testimony of either the perpetrator or victims in a legal trial. Clinicians may encounter these youth in their practices under several circumstances: adolescent revelation, parental report, or at the request of legal representatives.

What we know about sexual offenders, in general, is based only on those individuals who are caught or prosecuted. Even youth who are caught, arrested, and convicted frequently receive minimal punishments (i.e., probation, community service). The costs to society for the crimes of juvenile sex offenders are considerable, not only for those inflicted on crime victims and society as a whole, but also for those imposed on offenders and their families. The rehabilitation focus of interventions for those youth referred to treatment programs is considered to be controversial because the interventions are not evidenced-based for the adolescent sexual offender population. Most adjudicated adolescents live and are treated in community settings and often reoffend. Unfortunately, there remains little empirical evidence of the long-term effects of different interventions with adolescent sexual offenders (5-7).

DEFINITION

Adolescent sex offenders are defined as youth between the ages of 13 and 17 years who commit illegal sexual behavior as defined by the sex crimes statues of the legal jurisdictions in which they reside. Legal meanings of sexual offenses vary from state to state (10). However, statutes typically define sexual offenses in terms of: a) penetration offenses, which include penetration of virtually any body orifice for a sexual purpose, and are felonies; and b) crimes not involving physical contact (e.g., voyeurism, exhibitionism, obscene phone calls). Such offenses progress from privacy issues at the misdemeanor level to the felony level, depending on the specific circumstances of each case. The addition of physical force or coercion will almost always result in a felony life offense. Most adolescents are not sexual predators, nor do they meet the accepted criteria for pedophilia (9).

EPIDEMIOLOGY

The incidence of sexual victimization of children by adolescents has become a serious problem in our society. Juveniles account for more than one-third (35.6 percent) of those known; less than 1 percent of all arrests of youth 17 years of age and younger were for sex offenses (3). Each year, there are approximately 2,200 arrests of juveniles for forcible rape and this includes an additional estimated 9,200 arrests of juveniles for other types of sex offenses. The percentages of adolescents arrested for sexual offending in 2010 were for youth in the following age groups: younger than 9 years (5%); younger than 12 years (16%); between ages 12 and 14 (~13%), and between ages 15 and 17 (46%) (10-12). The vast majority (93 percent) were male. The number of arrests of juveniles in 2010 was 21% fewer than the number of arrests in 2001.

CLINICAL FEATURES

Adolescents do not typically commit sex offenses against adults, although the risk of offending against adults increases slightly after an adolescent reaches age 16. Sexual offenses against other children are more likely to offend in groups, at school, have more male victims, and have younger victims. Sexual offenses against young children are typically committed by boys between the ages of 12 to 15 years of age. In 2011, 53% youth arrested for sexual offences involved youth younger than 16 and 28% involved females (14-16). Most females adolescents sex offenders were mainly younger than their male peers, had more multiple-victim and multiple-perpetrator episodes, and their victims were primarily family members or males.

Researchers generally agree that there are *multiple* factors (psychological, biological and sociological) that interact in complex and poorly understood ways; these factors include the adolescent's temperament, cognitive abilities, impulse control, family variables, and socioeconomic factors as well as access to potential victims and opportunities to offend. A number of factors have been found to be associated with a higher prevalence of adolescent sexual offending and these include a history of prior physical or sexual abuse, impaired family functioning, alcohol and substance abuse, exposure to erotica, neurobiological factors, and psychiatric co-morbidity.

However, we do not know specific and direct causation. Adolescent sex offenders are considered to be more responsive to treatment than adult sex offenders and do not appear to continue re-offending into adulthood, especially when provided with appropriate treatment. Across a number of treatment research studies, the overall sexual recidivism rate for adolescent sex offenders who receive treatment is low in most US settings as compared to adults. Adolescents who offend against young children tend to have slightly lower sexual recidivism rates than adolescents who sexually offend against other adolescents. Adolescent sex offenders' rates for sexual re-offenses (5-14%) are substantially less than their rates of recidivism for other delinquent behavior (8-58%) (12).

Presentation in the office

The serious psychosocial and legal implications for the offender and his or her family often prevent parents from seeking help. More often the offender will be brought to the physician by an appropriate agency in the course of a child abuse investigation for a) assistance with medical and psychological evaluation, b) to facilitate further expert evaluation, c) specialized referral, or d) to co-ordinate on-going care.

Sometimes parents may bring their teen in with concerns about his or her social development and provide indirect or non-specific indicators of an adolescent being involved in the sexual abuse of younger children. The parent may express concern about their teen's sexual activities with a younger child (i.e., sibling, other relative, or acquaintance); they may also ask if such activities are "normal." Also, the parents of victims may report fear of the offender or incidences of sex play between their young child with an older teen to the offender's parents; then the offender's parents presents that information to the physician. The goal of the parent is for the physician to tell them how to help their offending adolescent.

Most offenses are committed by a small number of adolescents who repeatedly reoffend and account for the molestation and sexual abuse of half of the male victims and one quarter of the female victims. Juveniles who have committed sex offenses are males who represent a heterogeneous mix, commit multiple offenses, usually have more than one victim, and usually offend against females; if they violate very young children, then their victims are usually male. Unfortunately, they may have several types of victims. The juvenile offenders differ according to victim and offense characteristics and a wide range of other variables, including types of offending behaviors, histories of child maltreatment, sexual knowledge and experiences, academic and cognitive functioning, and mental health issues. They usually have not been victims of childhood sexual abuse. Also, very little data are available on female sexual offenders (10-16).

Adolescent sex offenders rarely have previous convictions for sexual assault, but are likely to have committed nonsexual offenses. Those who have been physically abused were 7.6 times more likely to rape or sodomize other children when compared to adolescents who were sexually abused or neglected (5-7). One in two adult sex offenders began their sexually abusive behavior as a juvenile. Adolescents who commit incest offenses do so in the victim's home and often when providing child care services. Adolescent rapists, on the other hand, tend to victimize strangers. As the age of the victim increases, sexual intercourse becomes a part of the offense.

The families of adolescent sexual offenders tend to be two parent families, have at least one sibling living with them, and more closely resemble those of youth with severe emotional or behavioral problems. Their parents often deny sexual tensions and exhibit a paucity of sexual knowledge or education; also, one quarter of their parents have known sexual pathology. Adolescent sexual offenders who had committed sexual homicides experienced exaggerated personal and family dysfunction (5-7).

Diagnosis

A significant percentage of reported criminal sexual acts against children are various types of paraphilias. The *paraphilias* represent a diagnostic category in the 2013 *Diagnostic and statistical manual of mental disorders, Fifth edition (DSM-V)* and consists of the following subcategories: exhibitionism, fetishism, frotteurism, sexual masochism, sexual sadism, transvestic fetishism, voyeurism, and pedophilia (8). The victimization is by perpetrators who have intense sexually arousing urges, fantasies, or behaviors; also, a number of other issues are involved in adult perpetrators, though this discussion involves children and adolescents. The reader is referred to the *DSM-V* for further details in this regard. A psychiatric diagnosis is made if the behaviors have occurred for at least six months and caused distress or impairment that impedes social, occupational, or other important areas of functioning (8). Pedophilia is the diagnosis of our focus and involves sexual activity with a prepubescent child or children (generally ages 13 years or younger). Perpetrators should be age 18 years or older and be at least 5 years older than their victims.

Sexual exploitation versus normal sexual play

When a parent presents with a teen who was accused or caught engaging in sexual play with a younger child or a developmentally younger child, the physician may be asked to tell the parent if this is normal or not. The physician who understands the differences between sexual *exploration* and *exploitation* will be better prepared to make that distinction when faced with a report of adolescent sexual behavior. "Normal" or *developmentally sexual curiosity* and exploration are a normal part of the developmental play and should meet the criteria listed (5-7, 16):

1) The two involved individuals who are age and developmental peers.
2) Children and pre-pubertal adolescents may engage in exploratory behaviors.
    - The play or exploration usually involves only mutual genital display, touching, and fondling.
    - Curiosity about the differences and similarities in anatomy is normal.
    - Exploratory sexual play is not coercive.
    - Mutual consent is typical of exploratory behaviors.

- Does not include multiple participants.
    - Observers or additional participants are not acceptable.
- Manifestations of anger, fear, sadness, or other strongly negative responses are not present.

Exploitation involves the absence of the factors listed above and the inclusion of the following:

- If one of the individuals is cognitively impaired, then a peer relationship does not exist.
- Attempted intercourse is atypical among preschoolers and is rare in the young school-aged child (6-9 years).
- Abusive behavior often involves elements of pressure, misrepresentation, force, threat, secrecy, or other forms of coercion. Although some of the threat or coercion is obvious and violent, the evaluator must take care to recognize subtle emotional pressure or the use of implied authority by an older child or adolescent in some cases.

- If the sexual contact has been arranged for the pleasure of another older individual, it is exploitative. One of the participants manifests feelings anger, fear, sadness, or other strongly negative responses.
- The victim views the experience in negative terms; however, some abused children will appear to have a neutral or positive emotional response to this abuse.

Regardless of whether or not the sexual play is normal or abnormal, parents and adult caregivers need to be vigilant and give children other healthy outlets. Parents should be encouraged to always keep young children under surveillance, especially when older individuals are around.

If the "sex play" is determined to be experimental or exploratory, the physician should discuss normal childhood and adolescent sexual behavior with parents and outline measures to minimize inappropriate sexual stimulation in the home. Parents should be advised to provide closer supervision of the adolescent. Older adolescents can be instructed to stay away from compromising situations with younger children (16).

Co-morbid disorders

Adolescent sexual offender can have concurrent diagnoses of psychopathology. They rarely exhibit behavior problems; they are more likely to be shy, and more comfortable with younger children. The most common psychiatric diagnoses, respectively, are conduct disorder, substance abuse disorders, adjustment disorders, attention-deficit/hyperactivity disorder, specific phobia, and mood disorder. They frequently engage in distorted thinking to make their offenses more socially acceptable to themselves and others; much like other delinquents, their distorted thinking allows them to excuse their offenses. Male offenders are more often diagnosed with paraphilias and antisocial behavior. Female offenders are more likely to be diagnosed with mood disorders and engage in self-mutilation (8, 11, 13, 14).

INTERVENTION

In most states adolescent sexual offenders can be adjudicated for criminal behavior as young at 6 years old. However, most states set 10 years as the lowest age of criminal responsibility. Victim consent is not always considered important. Once there is sufficient evidence to identify an offender, a decision regarding prosecution is often made at the juvenile court level. If the child or adolescent goes to trial, the setting in the juvenile justice system is usually less formal and hearings are often conducted in private without the use of a jury. Juveniles in this system are more likely to receive efforts at rehabilitation and less likely to be held fully accountable for their actions, than if they were adjudicated in the adult courts. However, in the case of rape, sodomy or sexual homicide, most states have moved to address adolescent offending in the adult criminal justice system, which can impose harsher punishments.

Local statutes usually govern physician-patient privileges (i.e., the right to respect the confidentiality of all communications). Thus, the development of such privileges in each state is subject to *local* interpretation and state-by-state case law developments. Physicians should explain, at the outset, to all adolescents and their families the limits of confidentiality. If the adolescent's behavior must be reported to the authorities or potential victims warned, the physician should inform the patient and the family.

Professionals, who deal with children, have an *enforceable* mandate to report *suspected* child abuse. All fifty states have "mandated reporting" laws which require professionals to report "reasonable suspicions" that abuse or neglect has occurred. Professional obligations pertaining to confidentiality may be seriously challenged by the requirements of the law and the local community, particularly when it involves sexual conduct. It is helpful to explain to the parents and the patient that reporting any crime changes the status of the act from private to criminal; however, this is required as part of mandatory reporting laws.

No clinician should consider serving as a witness or expert witness in sexual abuse cases involving adolescent offenders without *specific* training in this area. A more definitive treatment may not be within the purview of all clinicians and generally, the adolescent offender will be referred to professionals and programs specializing in such treatment (3, 14, 18).

RECIDIVISM

The most beneficial treatment program identified in the treatment literature is multi-systemic therapy (MST) (19). Outcome studies contend that MST has its best effects on youth who engage in antisocial and deviant sexual behaviors. This treatment showed that interventions increased caregiver follow-through on discipline practices as well as decreased caregiver disapproval of their child's behavior. When compared to recidivism rates between adults and juvenile sex offenders, the juvenile sex offenders appeared to have lower recidivism rates and perform better in treatment than (5-14%). Those adolescents who offend against young children tend to have slightly lower sexual recidivism rates than adolescents who sexually offend against other teens. Adolescent sex offenders' rates for sexual re-offenses are substantially less than their rates of recidivism for other delinquent behavior (8-58%). Research has shown that a young person who commits a sex offense is unlikely to commit another one (1-4, 11, 14).

In the event that the physician determines that sexual abuse has occurred, he or she should follow the guidelines from the governing child protective services organizations and medical oversight organizations; also, medical examination and documentation should be performed as required by state child abuse laws. The family should be referred to the appropriate agency for further evaluation. If the adolescent has access to other children, especially very young ones, the physician should assess the level of risk posed to those children.

When it is determined that the child or adolescent is at high risk of sexually offending, then the physician should inform the family and the appropriate persons. Furthermore, the family should be advised to:

- ***STOP*** all baby-sitting and childcare activities under all circumstances!
- Parents must provide enhanced/additional supervision of their offender.

- The youth offender should not have access to young children or potential victims without direct supervision by a responsible adult who is aware of the problem---especially in school, churches or other related activities.
- The child or adolescent offender should not have access to, possession of or use of sexually explicit, "x-rated," media or pornographic materials.

The physician can encourage parents/care-providers to allow their youth sexual offenders to engage in most ordinary daily activities, such as going to school, church, stores, or restaurants with family, or involvement in age-appropriate and appropriately supervised peer activities. However, caution that one of the parents'/care-givers' major responsibilities is to limit the child/adolescent offender's opportunity to re-offend.

Conclusion

Children and adolescents under the age of 18 years account for one-fifth of arrests for all sexual offenses (excluding prostitution). They commit multiple offenses, usually have more than one victim, and may not limit their offenses to one type of victim. These young perpetrators can be found among all socio-economic groups and live in all regions of the United States. They often come to the attention of primary care clinicians when their parents bring them to the office for protection from the authorities and help with addressing their maladaptive behavior. Because most offenders are not detected, and those who are discovered are not often adjudicated, the physician can help to prevent and minimize the occurrence of sexual offending by educating parents about the importance of close supervision and seeking appropriate professional help for deviant sexual behavior in children and adolescents.

References

[1] Finkelhor D, Ormrod R, Chaffin M. Juveniles who commit sex offenses against minors. Office of Juvenile Justice Delinquency and Prevention (OJJDP), 2009. Accessed 2015 Mar 22. URL: https://www.ncjrs.gov/pdffiles1/ojjdp/227763.pdf.

[2] Puzzanchera C. Juvenile Arrests, 2010. US National Report Series. Department of Justice, Office of Justice Programs, Office of Juvenile Justice and Delinquency Prevention 2013. Accessed 2015 Mar 22. URL: http://www.ojjdp.gov/pubs/242770.pdf U.S. Department of Justice.

[3] Puzzancher C. Juvenile Arrests, 2011. National Report Series. US Department of Justice, Office of Justice Program, Office of Juvenile Justice and Delinquency Prevention. 2013. Accessed 2015 Mar 22. URL: http://www.ojjdp.gov/pubs/244476.pdf.

[4] Hockenberry S, Puzzanchera C. Juvenile Court statistics 2011 Report. Pittsburgh, PA: National Center for Juvenile Justice 2014:1-116.

[5] Pratt HD, Patel DR, Greydanus DE. Dannison L, Walcott D, Sloane MA. Adolescent sexual offenders: Issues for pediatricians. Int Pediatr 2001;16(2):1-8.

[6] Pratt HD, Greydanus DE, Patel D. The adolescent sexual offender. Prim Care Clin Office Pract 2007; 34:305–16.

[7] Pratt HD, Patel D. Greydanus DE. Sexual offenders. In: DE Greydanus, DR Patel, HD Pratt, JL Calles, Jr, eds. New York: Nova Science, 2009:485-93.

[8] Kole SM. Statute protecting minors in a specified age range from rape o other sexual activity as applicable to defendant minor within protected age groups. Am Law Rep (ALR5th) Annotations and Cases 18 ALR 5th: 1994:856-90.

[9] American Psychiatric Association. Diagnostic and statistical manual of mental disorders, Fifth edition (DSM-V). Arlington, VA: American Psychiatric Association, 2013:685-708.

[10] Snyder HN. Juvenile arrests, 2004. Washington, DC: US Department of Justice, Office of Justice Programs, Office of Juvenile Justice and Delinquency Prevention, 2006:1-12.

[11] Justice Policy Institute. Youth who commit sex offenses: Facts and fiction. Washington, DC, No date: 1-2. Accessed 2015 Mar 22. URL: http://www.justice policy.org/images/upload/08-8_FAC_SORNA Fact Fiction_JJ.pdf.

[12] Righthand S, Welch C. Juveniles who have sexually offended: A review of the professional literature: Report. Washington, DC: US Department of Justice, Office of Justice Programs, Office of Juvenile Justice and Delinquency Prevention, 2001:NCJ 184739.

[13] Akakpo TF, Burton DL. Emergence of nonsexual crimes and their relationship to sexual crime characteristics and the deviant arousal of male adolescent sexual offenders: An exploratory study. J Child Sex Abus 2014;23(5):595-613.

[14] Hockenberry S, Puzzanchera C. Juvenile Court Statistics, 2011. Pittsburgh, PA: National Center for Juvenile Justice, 2014:1-119.

[15] Pullmana LE, Lerouxb EJ, Motaynec G, Setoda MC. Examining the developmental trajectories of adolescent sexual offenders. Child Abuse Negl 2014;38:1249–58.

[16] De Jong AR. Sexual interactions among siblings and cousins: Experimentation or exploitation? Child Abuse Negl 1989;13:271-9.

[17] Pereda N, Guilera G, Forns M, Gomez-Benito J. The international epidemiology of child sexual abuse: A continuation of Finkelhor (1994). Child Abuse Negl 2009;33:331-42.

[18] Seto MC, Lalumie`re ML. What is so special about male adolescent sexual offending? A review and test of explanations through meta-analysis. Psychol Bull 2010; 136(4):526–75.

[19] Henggeler SW, Letourneau EJ, Chapman JE, Borduin CM, Schewe PA, McCart MR. Mediators of change for multisystemic therapy with juvenile sexual offenders. J Consult Clin Psychol 2009;77(3): 451–62.

In: Public Health Yearbook 2016
Editor: Joav Merrick

ISBN: 978-1-53610-947-4

Chapter 42

DETERMINANTS ASSOCIATED WITH CONTRACEPTIVE USE AMONG CHINESE YOUNG MIGRANTS

Xiaoming Yu[1,*], MD, MPH, Xiaomei Zhou[2], MD, Shuping Zhang[3], MD and Suhong Gao[4], MD, MPH

[1]The Institute of Child and Adolescent Health, School of Public Health, Peking University, Beijing, China
[2]Futian District Traditional Chinese Medicine Hospital, Shenzhen City, Guangdong Province, China
[3]Jinan Municipal Maternal Care Hospital, Shandong Province, China
[4]Haidian District Maternal Care Hospital, Beijing, China

ABSTRACT

The aim of this study was to understand contraceptive use and relevant determinants, further to explore the direct and mediating effects on contraceptive use amongst young rural-to-urban migrants in China. 6,266 migrants (2,478 male and 3,788 female) aged at 16-24 years were recruited and completed anonymous and self-administered questionnaire in four Chinese cities. 61.4% of the participants admitted to having sex recently, and one-fourth did not use contraception. Condom, withdrawal, and rhythm method were ranked as the top three choices with no difference identified in sex and marital status. Path analysis revealed that individual education level, marriage status, number of sex partners and knowledge on HIV/AIDS prevention are direct factors affecting young migrants' contraceptive use. The study suggested that inconsistent and less reliable forms of contraception remain widespread among Chinese young migrants. Special attention should be paid to their lower education and risk perception regarding HIV/AIDS prevention to improve contraceptive use for young migrants.

Keywords: contraception, young migrants, determinants, HIV/AIDS prevention, unplanned pregnancy

---

* Correspondence: Professor. Xiaoming YU MD, MPH, The Institute of Child and Adolescent health, School of Public Health, Peking University, No. 38, Xueyuan Road, Haidian District, Beijing, 100191, China. E-mail: yxm@bjum.edu.cn

INTRODUCTION

Since the 1980s the rural-to-urban migrant population in China has increased dramatically. According to the 6th China National Census conducted in 2010, the total number of rural-to-urban migrants reached about 260 million, with an 81% increase compared to the 5th China National Census (in the year 2000). 26.7% of the total migrants are youth aged between 15-24 years (1-2).

Previous studies conducted in other countries have showed that there is a relation between the movement of rural-to-urban population and an increased risk of HIV/AIDS infection around the world. These studies indicate that migration has emerged as a risk factor for the spread of HIV/AIDS, and demonstrated that migrant population are highly vulnerable to HIV/AIDS infection. Furthermore, the increasing proportion of HIV/AIDS cases amongst migrant people is related to cross-cultural variation in people's ideas, partner choice, sexual behaviors etc. (3-6).

Over the past decades the number of Chinese young people engaging in premarital sexual relationships has sharply increased, with a high percentage not taking the necessary precaution to prevent unwanted pregnancies and the transmission of HIV/AIDS. The prevalence of sexual intercourse among young people out of school is higher than those in school (23.3% versus 7.2%) (7). A study from 4 cities in China showed that 38.7% of the young unmarried female migrants investigated had a previous induced abortion, with a prevalence of reproductive tract infections (RTIs) and STDs of 56.1% and 9.7% respectively (8). Other research found that 35.1% of male migrants suffered from reproductive health problems, such as phimosis, cryptorchidism, and 17.4% of the female migrants experienced unwanted pregnancies and suffered from RTIs such as vaginitis, cervical erosion, pelvic inflammatory disease (9). In China, the epidemic of HIV/AIDS is experiencing fast growth. The official estimated number of persons infected with HIV exceeded 780,000 by the end of 2011. Sexual transmission has become the most important transmission route of HIV infection in China (10). More than 80% of new infections were caused from both heterosexual and homosexual transmission in 2014 (11). Researchers who have explored the trends in the HIV/AIDS epidemic among the Chinese migrant population have found that rural-to-urban migrants have a strong impact on the continued spread of HIV/AIDS in China. The migrant population acts as an important bridge spreading HIV/AIDS from high risk groups to the general population (12).

The regular use of condom and/or other contraceptive methods have been acknowledged as effective measures to prevent HIV/AIDS infections and unwanted pregnancies (13, 14). But many studies also suggest that the decision for young people to use condoms and/or other contraceptive methods for unwanted pregnancy or HIV/AIDS prevention is the result of different factors including age, gender, cultural values, sexual orientation, and personal attitudes towards contraceptive use. Other relevant factors are also the use of alcohol and drugs, the duration of intimate relations, peer norms, knowledge of HIV/AIDS and awareness on preventing unwanted pregnancy (15-17). Previous studies applied the Health Belief Model (HBM) to explain and predict the practice of condom or contraceptive use among young people (18-20). Hall (21) reviewed the contraceptive research describing HBM-guided between January 1966 and February 2011 and confirmed that the HBM was the most comprehensive social cognitive framework including perceived threat of pregnancy(e.g., knowledge, beliefs), modifying and enabling factors (e.g., demographic, psychological and social aspects etc.) as well as contraceptive cost-benefit analysis (e.g., knowledge of and beliefs about efficacy etc.) can guide modern contraceptive behavior research and practice.

Young migrants are a complex and diverse group. Due to their temporary urban household registration, they do not have access to social welfare benefits available to urban residents, such as housing, education, long-term employment contracts and health care systems and are, therefore, more vulnerable to health problems including HIV/STDs infection (22).

The study has two purposes. The first was to investigate and better understand young migrants' sexual behavior and contraceptive use, as well as their relevant determinants. The second to find the direct and mediating effects of these factors on consistent contraceptive use, and to develop a causal model to examine their relationship and relevant predictors. Our study explores the interaction among these factors aiming to find the cues to positive actions and determine priorities in developing strategies culturally appropriate to increasing the use of contraceptive among Chinese young rural-to-urban migrants who are vulnerable to HIV/AIDS and unwanted pregnancies.

METHODS

The study conducted in four cities of China, namely Beijing, Guangzhou, Shenzhen and Jinan city, they are all bigger and more representative locations attracting immigrants from rural areas in China. Young migrants aged 16-24 years, who are legally on hire, were selected for this study. The sampling was undertaken with a stratified sampling design according to the demographic information of rural-to-urban immigrants (23). The samples investigated were mainly recruited from four occupational groups in urban areas: 1) house-building workers, 2) workers in manufacturing, such as automobile, garment factory, 3) attendants in hotels, waiters and waitress in restaurants and 4) others, such as market venders. For each of the stratified samples, a sufficient number of participants were selected and recruited to ensure the study was representative.

Data collection

The questionnaire used in the study was developed by researchers on the base of considerable literature review. The Health Belief Model (HBM) provided the theoretical framework of the study design and variables measured. According to the HBM, the determinants of performance mediate the relation between antecedents and components of behaviors. The HBM configuration contained two main components: threat perception (perceived susceptibility and anticipated severity), behavioral evaluation. The component of our questionnaire based on this model and relevant reviews included three parts:

1) *Socio-demographic information:* age, gender, monthly income, education level, marital status, employment and length of employment in the urban area.

2) *Threat perception:* i.e., perceived susceptibility to risk including HIV infection and unwanted pregnancy as measured by knowledge of prevention, attitudes toward sex and unwanted pregnancies, etc. It consisted of 18 items (nine items for HIV/AIDS using UNGASS indicators and nine items for general sexual development). Each correct response was given a point value of 1. The total knowledge score was computed from the correct responses, with a higher score indicating a better knowledge level. In addition, two questions were asked regarding attitudes toward premarital sex and pregnancies in the context of Chinese cultural background. They were given the 5-point Likert-type score with ranging from 4 to 0.
3) *Behavioral evaluation related to sex and contraception:* age at the first intercourse, pregnancy or becoming pregnant, experience with abortion, the number of sexual partners, condom and other contraceptive use, and access to services. The actual use of contraceptive was measured by seven questions including 1) How old were you when you first had sexual intercourse with your partner? 2) Did you or your partner use condoms or any form of contraceptive during your first sexual intercourse? 3) Did you or your partner use a condom or any form of contraceptive during your most recent sexual intercourse? 4) In general, when you have sex with your current partner, which kind of contraception do you use? 5) If no contraception was used, why did you not use during the most recent sex? 6) What did you do when your partner wanted to have sex with you but you didn't want? and 7) What did you do when your partner insisted on using a condom or other contraceptive but it happened not to be available to you? Meanwhile, Behavioral Attributes of Psychosocial Competence Scale-Condensed Form (BAPC-C) was used aiming to assess the respondents' self-efficacy to action. The shortened version of BAPC (24), which has been applied in China, consisting of 13 forced-choice items, the total score ranging from 0 to 13 with a higher score indicating more active behavior intention and higher confidence.

The anonymous self-administered questionnaires were dispensed to the sampled participants in a separated and quiet room at each survey site to ensure privacy. All the participants were provided a clear and detailed explanation of the study purpose, and the confidentiality of data administration. Verbal and written consent was obtained from the participants before they were enrolled to fill in the questionnaire of the study. The questionnaire took approximately 20 to 30 minutes to complete.

Data analysis

The software program EpiData 3.0 was used to build a database, coding the collected questionnaires with a parallel double entry. All data was analyzed using Statistical Package for the Social Sciences version 13.0 for Windows SPSS (SPSS Inc., Chicago) after excluding unqualified questionnaires.

Descriptive statistics including mean, standard deviation, percentage, and frequency distribution were performed in describing the sample. Logistic regression was used to explore the influencing factors of actual use of contraceptives among young migrants. The significance level was set at $p = 0.05$.

To identify the relationship among different factors influencing contraceptive use among young migrants, path analysis was conducted using AMOS software 7.0. First, establishing a rudimentary model according to a hypothesized relationship between contraceptive use and social-demographic characteristics, the score of knowledge, attitude and behaviors related to HIV/AIDS infections and unwanted pregnancies, and then using the AMOS software to fit the model.

RESULTS

The final effective respondents were 6,266 with 2,478 male and 3,788 female. These young migrants came from 34 provinces all over China and the average age was at 20.3 ± 2.1 years. The majority (88.4%) were unmarried. 43.2% had a middle school education and 44.8% reported having worked in the city more than two year since leaving from their rural hometown. About 28.6 percent had monthly income of less than 1,000 RMB (equal to $166). The most popular forms of employment were bellhop and restaurant services, accounting for 37.1%, following manufacturing accounting for 41.4% (see Table 1).

Table 1. General demographic and social information of subjects

Classify		N	%
Sex	Male	2478	39.5
	Female	3788	60.5
	Total	6266	100.0
Marriage status	Unmarried	5537	88.7
	Married	675	10.8
	Divorce/Widowed	24	0.5
	Total	6236	100.0
Education level	Primary School	192	3.1
	Junior Middle School	2685	43.2
	High Middle School	3339	53.7
	Total	6216	100.0
Occupation	Services	2325	37.1
	Manufacturing	2594	41.4
	House-building	251	4.0
	Others	1096	17.5
	Total	6266	100.0
Monthly income (RMB: Yuan)	<1000	1779	28.6
	1000~1599	3095	49.7
	≥1600	1351	21.7
	Total	6225	100.0
Length of employed in urban	<6months	1120	17.9
	6months-1year	973	15.6
	1-2years	1352	21.7
	>2years	2792	44.8
	Total	6237	100.0

Sexual behaviors and contraceptive use

35.2% (2,191/6,231) of the respondents reported having had sex, with 41.1% of males and 31.3% of females, and the difference was of significance ($P < 0.001$). 88.7% among the total sexual active young migrants were unmarried. The average age of sexual debut was 19.29 years of age, some respondents (2.35%) had sex at 15 or even younger.

In the last month before the investigation, 61.4% of young migrants reported having sex, those unmarried higher than the married (57.2% vs.32.9%), and about one-fourth (24.4%) reported not using any contraceptive method. Concerning their options amongst various contraceptive methods, condom, withdrawal and safe period contraception ranked as the top three choices. No difference was shown according to gender and marriage status. 29.4% (468/1,593) of unmarried sexually active migrants reported to have experienced a pregnancy or to have made their partner do so. Whether married or not, 62.0% of the pregnancies ended with an induced abortion, with a significantly higher proportion of unmarried immigrants compared to married immigrants (85.9% vs. 30.1%) (see Table 2).

The reasons why young migrants felt it difficult to use condoms or other contraceptive are the following: lack of preparation when having sex (25.7%); unaware that pregnancy can occur after having sex only once (23.5%); shyness in buying contraceptive (19.9%); worrying that using contraceptive can have a bad influence on sex (19.9%); didn't know how to use condoms and other contraceptives (14.%); unaware of having sex can lead to pregnancy (13.9%); partner dislike in using a condom or contraceptive (13.6%); did not know where to get/buy contraceptive (8.3%), and not minding having an abortion in case of pregnancy (3.95%).

Table 2. Sexual activity and contraceptive use in Chinese young rural-to-urban migrants, by marriage

	Total (%)	Unmarried Subjects (%)	Married Subjects (%)
Had sexual activity	35.2	28.8	88.6
Recently sexual activity	61.4	57.2	32.9
Contraceptive use at first sex	45.4	45.8	42.3
Contraceptive use at most recent sex (among sexual active individuals)	75.4	79.1	68.0
Pregnancy (among sexual active individuals)	38.9	29.4	61.3
Abortion (among pregnant individuals)	62.0	85.9	30.1
Contraceptive methods at sex			
Condom	41.0	40.2	43.3
Withdrawal	16.2	16.0	17.3
Rhythm	9.6	8.1	13.7
Urgent prophylactic	5.1	5.2	5.1
Oral pills	5.1	5.0	5.6
Diaphragm	0.9	1.0	0.7
Intrauterine device	4.0	0.9	12.6

Influent factor analysis for contraceptive use

The result through multiple regression analysis found that individual education level, marriage status, individual incomes, number of sex partners, and knowledge on HIV/AIDS prevention were relative determinants for contraceptive use. A higher education level and knowledge on HIV/AIDS were protecting factors. On the contrary, being unmarried, having a lower monthly income and multiple sex partners were regarded as risk factors (see Table 3).

Table 3. Logistic regression of influencing factors of contraceptive use

Factors	β	Standard error	P-value	OR	95% CI of OR Lower-upper
Education level (1 = junior school and below; 2 = high school and above)	0.399	0.139	0.004*	1.490	1.136-1.955
Marital status (1 = unmarried; 2 = married)	-0.729	0.153	0.000*	0.482	0.357-0.651
Monthly income (1 = < 1000 yuan/month; 2 = > 1000 yuan/month)	-0.371	0.180	0.040*	0.690	0.485-0.983
Sexual partner number (1 = only one sexual partner; 2 = sexual partner > 1)	-0.618	0.145	0.000*	0.539	0.406-0.717
STD prevention knowledge (1 score < 60; 2 score > 60)	0.572	0.151	0.000*	1.772	1.319-2.382

* P-value <0.05.

The path analysis was further applied to explore causal relationships between contraceptive use and determinants. Figure 1 shows the final path analysis model. The values between variables are standardized regression coefficients at a 0.05 significant level. The model fit indices are used to evaluate the applicability of the model. The indices in the study showed that the final model fits the data well (Comparative Fit Index = 0.992, Bentler's Goodness of Fit Index = 0.997, Normal Fit Index = 0.975 (recommended to be > 0.90) and the Root Mean Square Error of Approximation = 0.019 (recommended to be < 0.08).

The results of path analysis as shown in figure 1 indicating educational level, marital status, number of sex partners, and the knowledge level of HIV/AIDS prevention. All except monthly income were identified as direct factors. The leading factor affecting contraceptive use is educational level with total effect value at 0.108. A positive standardized regression coefficient indicates that those migrants who have a higher education level tend to adopt contraceptive methods when having sex. The second direct factor is the number of sex partners. The more sexual partners a person has, the less likely to use a contraceptive. In addition, the unmarried migrants who have higher score of HIV/AIDS prevention knowledge were more likely to use contraceptive. Contrarily, sex, age, residence region at present, salary and length of employed in urban were all indirect factors. They can influence contraceptive use through sexual partners and HIV/AIDS cognition. But some factors designed in the survey, such as current employment, score of BAPC-C were not entered to the final model of path analysis.

DISCUSSION

Our study was conducted among 6,266 young rural-to-urban migrants originating from 34 provinces in China through stratified cluster sampling. The large sample provided good representation. Results indicate a high rate of sexual intercourse among young rural-to-urban migrants. However, contraceptive use was low regardless of sex, and both in their first and most recent time having sex. This is consistent with the results of our previous research (7).

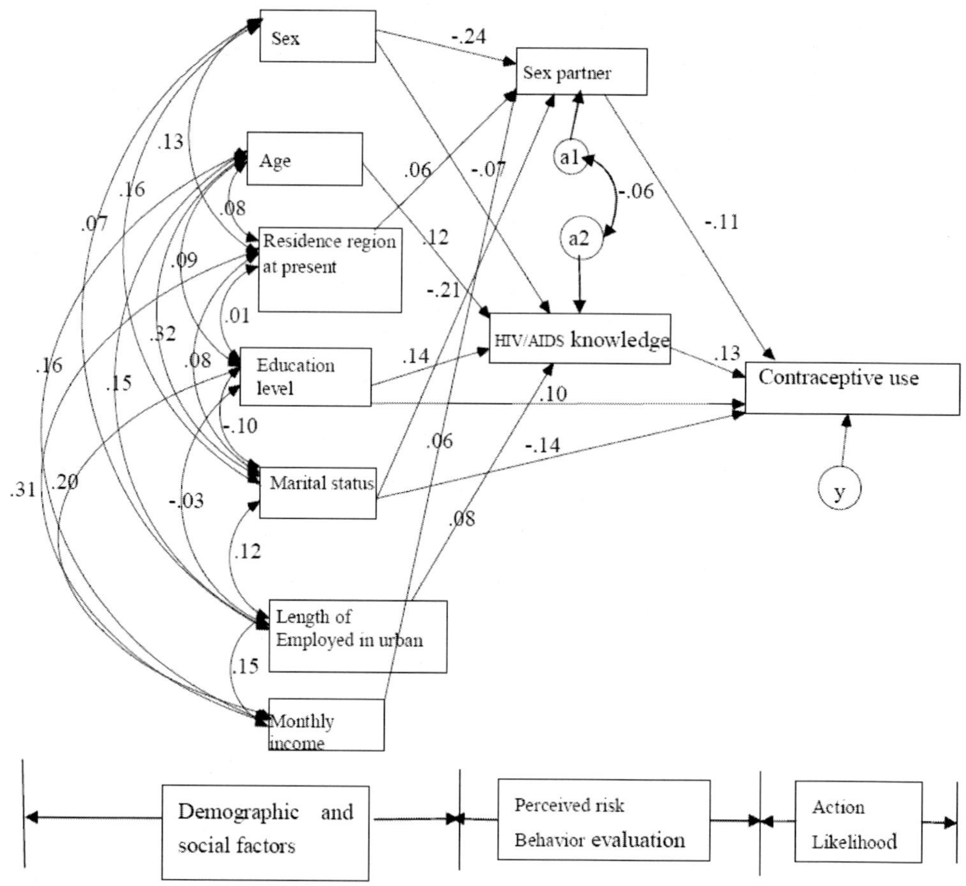

Figure 1. The final model of contraceptive use among Chinese young migrants.

Of all the contraceptive methods, condoms were the first choice for both groups regardless of their marital status. However, the research also found that natural contraceptive methods such as coitus interruptus and the rhythm method were frequently used among migrant young people. This finding is disturbing because such methods are of low security and more likely to fail in preventing HIV/AIDS and unwanted pregnancy which has been proven in previous studies (15). A research report on Global Burden of Disease indicated that the main risk factors for incident DALYs in 10–24-year-olds were unsafe sex (4%), lack of contraception (2%) especially in late adolescence and early adulthood for unsafe sex and lack of contraception leading to pregnancy and HIV/STDs (25). Our study identified a high rate of unwanted pregnancy and abortion among participants, proving that young migrants lack awareness of safe sex and contraception. They suffer from many unexpected results due to unprotected sex. Early sexual exposure and inconsistent contraception use among Chinese young migrants further suggests their vulnerability and the importance of advocating for safe and effective use of contraceptives.

Role and relationship of individual and social factors with contraception use

Previous studies conducted in China only paid attention to what were considered influencing factors associated with contraceptive use but did not focus on their relationships and mutual interactions. Our study utilized multivariate analysis and path analysis that reveals that education background, marriage status, numbers of sex partners and knowledge of HIV/AIDS prevention are the main factors affecting the use of contraception among young migrants. This means that those who have higher education levels, and who have better HIV/AIDS prevention knowledge tended to use contraceptive when sexual intercourse. However, those with multiple sexual partners were less likely to use contraceptive. This study distinctly proved that the risk perception on unwanted pregnancy and HIV/AIDS prevention were associated with the use of contraceptives.

Furthermore, the study results based on the path analysis indicated the role and interactive relationship of various determinants. According to HBM, people's behaviors are generally associated with three parts: individual character, their perception to the threat and the behavior evaluation within them. The final model of contraceptive use among young migrants in our study indicated that some sub-factors among the three parts have played different roles. The knowledge level on HIV prevention involving in threat perception and the number of sex partners involved in behavior evaluation were leading factors that directly affected the contraceptive adoption among young migrants. Contrarily, most of individual factors, such as sex, age, income, excluding educational level and marital status were all indirect factors influencing contraceptive use in virtue of the direct factors. In other words, the number of sexual partners and the knowledge on HIV prevention played a mediating role in individual contraception adoption. While educational level is correlated with the obtaining and understanding of information and knowledge, marital status correlated with sex and partner choice, thus we can find these two social factors effect on contraceptive use either directly or indirectly. Young migrants are often marginalized and have limited access to health care system in urban. They are continuously challenged to make many decisions that can have an impact on their health and how they live within society. Some studies have proved that young people encountered difficulties and misunderstanding in rejecting unwanted sex and/or negotiating contraceptive use with their partners. In some cases, having a pregnancy can even be sought as a way to remain in an intimate relationship with the partner (26, 27). As a consequence, decision making related to contraceptive use depends on their partners, marital status, and relevant sexual and reproductive health knowledge.

Our study provided an empirical support for the theoretical model identifying that antecedents and determinants affecting contraceptive use among young migrants are closely associated. The study demonstrated lack of risk perception on unprotected sexual behavior and HIV/AIDS prevention, and some social factors(mainly educational level and marriage status) can possess a predictive power for using contraceptive practices of young migrants. These findings suggest the priority in our development strategy of HIV/AIDS prevention and sexual health for young migrants. In terms of the practical significance, that special attention regarding to programs or policies should be paid to the direct factors, such as improving education level and increasing risk awareness, to reduce the vulnerability of young migrants.

This study has several limitations. Firstly, we used self-reported retrospective questionnaires to collect data. Although the researcher ensured privacy during the completion of the questionnaire to minimize this bias, naturally some information was missed due to the particularity of the target group and the sensitivity of personal issues. Secondly, in our study we used BAPC-C (24) to assess participants' coping ability regarding sex and contraception matters. However, this psychosocial competence factor was not found in the final model. Therefore, further research should be well designed and developed.

Conclusion

Our study verified that it was common among sexually active migrants to choose lower protective contraceptive methods. Also, it identified their direct and indirect determinants along with relevant causal relationship. It suggests that particular attention should be paid to the significance of contraception guidance and improvements in the accessibility to contraceptives to young migrants in China, especially considering their lower education level. Programs targeted at migrant young people should aim at the promotion of safer sex practices and risk awareness regarding HIV/AIDS prevention.

Acknowledgments

This study was supported by WHPR/WHO and China MOH corporation project (grant number 01.01.01.AW.04.2). The authors thank all the investigators in the study for their contributions and efforts in data collection. Also we thank all the participants in our study. We specially appreciate Dr. Alessandra Aresu, specialist in the field of gender, education and sexuality in China, for her support in revising the manuscript and her invaluable insights.

References

[1] National Bureau of Statistics of China. Communique (No.1) of the sixth census data in 2010. URL: http:// www.stats.gov.cn/tjgb/rkpcgb/qgrkpcgb/t20110428_402722232.htm.

[2] National Bureau of Statistics of China. The fifth census data in 2000. URL: http://www.stats.gov.cn/tjsj/ndsj/renkoupucha/2000pucha/html/t0301.htm.

[3] Ford K, King G, Lucila N, Chris R. AIDS knowledge and risk behaviors among midwest migrant farm workers. AIDS Educ Prev 2001;13(6):551-60.

[4] Ford K, Chamrathrithirong A. Sexual partners and condom use of migrant workers in Thailand. AIDS Behav 2007;11:905-14.

[5] Hirsch JS, Higgins J, Bentley ME, Nathanson CA. The social constructions of sexuality: Marital infidelity and sexually transmitted disease–HIV risk in a Mexican migrant community. Am J Public Health 2002;92(8): 1227-37.

[6] Puri M, Cleland J. Sexual behavior and perceived risk of HIV/AIDS among young migrant factory workers in Nepal. J Adolesc Health 2006; 38: 237-46.

[7] Yu XM, Guo SJ, Sun YY. Sexual behaviors and associated risks in young Chinese people: a meta-analysis. Sex Health 2013;10:424-33.
[8] Zhao GL, Zhang XS, Wang LH, Wu JL, Xenos, P. Analysis of reproductive health situation of unmarried non-resident young women sought abortion in cities. J Reprod Med 2005;14(5):268-71. [Chinese].
[9] Gao SH, Yu XM, Gong LX, Wang B, Yu M, Xu L. Gender difference in sexual and reproductive health among young migrant workers. Chin J Public Health 2009;25(8):913-5. [Chinese].
[10] Ministry of Health of the People's Republic of China, UNAIDS, World Health Organization. 2011 Estimates for the HIV/AIDS epidemic in China. Chin J AIDS STD 2012;18(1):1-5. [Chinese].
[11] National Center for AIDS/STD Control and Prevention of China. Update on the AIDS/STD epidemic in China and Main response in control and prevention in the second quarter of 2014. Chin J AIDS STD 2014; 20(8):555. [Chinese].
[12] Meng XJ, Wang L, Chan S, Reilly KH, Peng ZH, Guo W, Ding ZW, Qin QQ. Estimation and projection of the HIV epidemic trend among the migrant population in China. Biomed Environ Sci 2011;24(4):343-8.
[13] UNAIDS interagency task team on HIV and young people (WHO/UNAIDS/UNFPA/UNICEF). Preventing HIV/AIDS in young people: A systematic review of the evidence from developing countries. Geneva: WHO technical report series 938, 2006.
[14] Santelli JS, Lindberg LD, Finer LB, Singh S. Explaining recent declines in adolescent pregnancy in the United States: the contribution of abstinence and improved contraceptive use. Am J Public Health 2007; 97(1) :150-6.
[15] Khumsaen N, Gary FA. Determinants of actual condom use among adolescents in Thailand. J Assoc Nurs AIDS Care 2009;20(3):218-29.
[16] Leigh BC. Alcohol and condom use: A meta-analysis of event-level studies. Sex Transm Dis 2002;29(8):476-82.
[17] Villarruel AM, Jemmott JB III, Jemmott LS, Ronis D. Predictors of sexual intercourse and condom use intentions among Spanish-Dominant Latino Youth: A test of the planned behavior theory. Nurs Res 2004; 53(3):172-81.
[18] Mahoney CA, Thombs DL, Ford OJ. Health belief and self-efficacy models: Their utility in explaining college students' condom use. AIDS Educ Prev 1995;7(1):32-49.
[19] Laraque D, Mclean DE, Brown-Peterside P, Ashton D, Diamond B. Predictors of reported condom use in central Harlem youth as conceptualized by the health belief model. J Adolesc Health 1997;21: 318-27.
[20] Lollis CM, Johnson EH, Antoni MH. The efficacy of health belief model for predicting condom usage and risky sexual practices in University students. AIDS Educ Prev 1997;9(6):551-63.
[21] Hall KS. The health belief model can guide modern contraceptive behavior research and practice. J Midwifery Women's Health 2012; 57(1):74–81.
[22] Shi XY, Yu XM, Duan CM, You X, Wang J. The research on the factors in the utilization of AIDS services among adolescents outside school. Modern Prev Med 2007;34([11):2031-4. [Chinese].
[23] Study group of China State Council. Survey report on rural-to-urban migrant workers in China. Beijing: China Yanshi Publishing House, 2006. [Chinese].
[24] Wei W, Yu XM, Qiu M, Du W, Yuan W, Yue M. The application of N-S locus of control scale and behavioral attributes of psychosocial competence scale in college students. Chin J Behav Med Sci 2007;16(10):945-7. [Chinese].
[25] Gore FM, Bloem PJ, Patton GC, Ferguson J, Joseph V, Coffey C, et al. Global burden of disease in young people aged 10-24 years: a systematic analysis. Lancet 2011;377(9783): 2093-2102.
[26] Baele J, Dusseldorp E, Maes S. Condom use self-effiicacy: effect on intended and actual condom use in adolescents. J Adolesc Health 2001;28:421-31.
[27] Marston C, King E. Factors that shape young people's sexual behavior: A systematic review. Lancet 2006; 368(4),1581-6.

In: Public Health Yearbook 2016
Editor: Joav Merrick
ISBN: 978-1-53610-947-4

Chapter 43

TERRITORIAL DISTRIBUTION OF MEDICAL DIAGNOSTIC LABORATORIES IN OUTPATIENT CARE IN VARNA REGION, BULGARIA

Emilia Georgieva, MSc, PhD, Galina Petrova*, MSc, PhD, Minko Milev, MSc, PhD and Todorka Kostadinova, MSc, PhD
Medical University "Prof. Dr. Paraskev Stoyanov", Varna, Bulgaria

ABSTRACT

Changes in population and territorial distribution are important for healthcare, because they directly affect the pool of manpower, the number of users and the opportunities for natural population. In recent years, there is a noticeable trend of deterioration of the performance of health-demographic status of the population in Varna district and observed changes in the regional health care system related to an imbalance of the geographical distribution of medical structures, unequal access of the population to medical care, and uneven inefficient spending of public resources and as a result, poor quality of medical services and growing dissatisfaction of the population.

Keywords: territorial distribution, medical diagnostic laboratories, outpatient care

INTRODUCTION

Ensuring the population with universality, equality, accessibility and quality of medical care with maximum efficiency of the public resources is a primary goal of the national and regional health policies. This aims for an increase in efficiency of the health care system, by providing the citizens with equality and access to a well-timed and sufficient in volume and

* Correspondence: Galina Petrova, PhD, Assistant-in-chief, Department of Economics and Management of Health, Faculty of Public Health, Medical University "Prof. Dr. Paraskev Stoyanov" Varna, 55, Marin Drinov St, Varna, Bulgaria. E-mail: galina.petrova@mu-varna.bg.

quality non-hospital care, along with diagnostic laboratory activity. The territorial distribution and planning of the clinics and medical laboratories for non-hospital, emergency and hospital medical care, introduced with the regional health map, ensures equality in treatment accessibility for the patients.

The territorial distribution of the diagnostic laboratories must depend on the health and demographic status of the population in the Varna region, as well as in compliance with the most socially significant diseases. With the application of the European standards and indicators of health service, there will be an opportunity to determine the actual needs of the regional population for the corresponding volume of hospitals, laboratories and medical services and to ensure the adequate access of the people. The clinical laboratory is an integral part of the diagnostic process and the reliable diagnosis as well as successful treatment, depend on it (control of the diseases). One of the main problems for the clinical laboratory is the constant increase in volume of the different laboratory tests. According to BMA (Bulgarian Medical Association), it has doubled during the last five years. The main purpose of the medical diagnostic services, is the timely assistance for achieving an accurate diagnosis. According to the regulations in our country, every citizen has the right of medical help under the conditions, stated in the "Law for healthcare" and the "Law for health insurance."

The purpose of this paper is to reveal and analyze the main problems in the territorial distribution and ensuring the population with universality, equality, accessibility and quality of the medical diagnostic laboratories in Varna region.

METHODS

The opinion of 569 respondents was investigated in this research. Based on an anonymous individual survey, we researched the opinion of patients, as well as physicians with general practice, laboratory scientists and clinical laboratory physicians, working in non-hospital care settings in the Varna region, in the timeline between August and October 2014, which statistically includes 90% of all laboratory experts in non-hospital care and 64.3% of the physicians with general practice. Documentary, statistical and sociological methods were used. Quantitative and qualitative methods, as well as comparison analysis of the condition of the regional medical diagnostic laboratories for non-hospital care, were applied during the data processing and situation analysis.

RESULTS AND DISCUSSION

Sociodemographic data analysis shows, that the patients in the survey have different socio-demographic profile, which impacts the opinion. The availability of laboratory units in non-hospital care, is essential for effective medical care. The main negative result of the laboratory deficiency in the remote areas is the delay in the required laboratory tests and objectifying the diagnosis that prevents the medical process. Of research interest, we studied the distance between patient location and the closest laboratory, required for the necessary tests.

The results showed, that the majority of the patients (30.4%), lived between 500 meters and 3 kilometers from the closest medical laboratory, followed by those, living more than 10 kilometers away. The patients, living within a short distance, are those in the 100m – 500m range (21.5%). They are followed by, with a small difference, the respondents (20.9%), in the 3-5 kilometers range. The smallest percentage are those, living in close proximity (100 meters or less) to the required laboratory (4.7%) (see Figure 1).

By analysis of variance, a connection was found between the distance to the closest laboratory and the populated areas, by municipalities (F e 3,25; $p<0,05$). According to the correlation analysis, it is weak and reverse, but still existent ($r = - 0,169$; $p = 0,01<0,05$). The connection between the distance and whether they live in Varna, or in the area, is expected to be interesting. Data analysis made it clear, that it is stronger and straight ($r = 0,31$; $p<0,01$).

In Varna, most of the patients are located either in the range between 500 meters and 3 kilometers from the laboratory, or in the 100 to 500 meters range, in contrast with the respondents from the area, where most live more than 10 kilometers away. The cities in the area – Byala and Dolni Chiflik, being the ones with the most respondents, gave that answer. In the cities of Devnya, Aksakovo and Valchi Dol, most of the respondents were located in the range between 500 meters and 3 kilometers from a medical diagnostic laboratory. Only in the cities of Dolni Chiflik, Beloslav and Varna, there are patients, living within 100 meters from the laboratory.

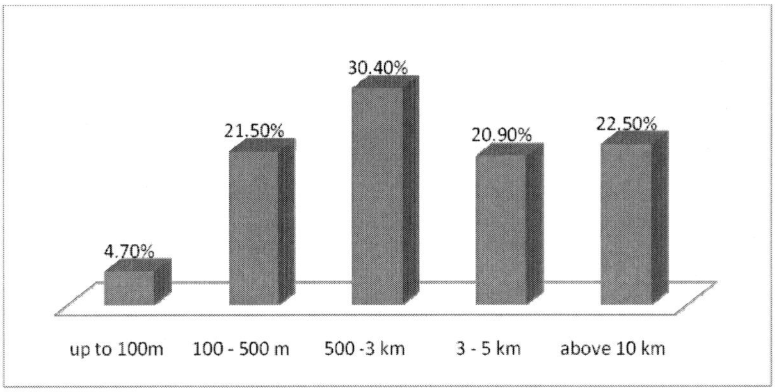

Figure 1. Distance between the home of the patients and the closest laboratory.

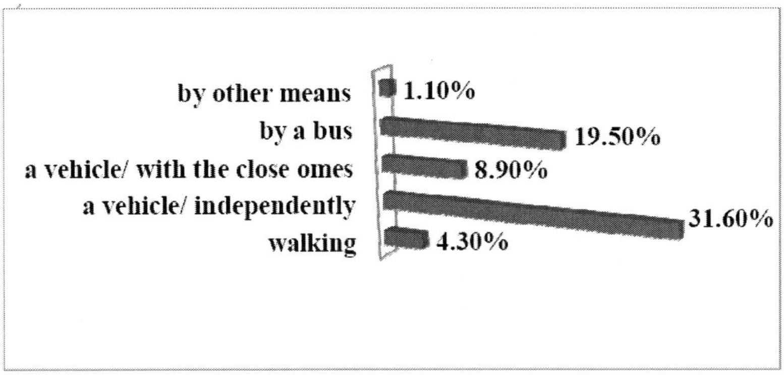

Figure 2. Patient preferences for transportation to a medical laboratory.

Analysis of the data about the transportation of the patient to the laboratory, show that, although the distances are long, most patients prefer to walk to the required place (38.9%) and those, using a private vehicle are 31.6%. Those, who prefer a bus, are only one quarter. Significantly less, are the patients, that prefer transportation with their close ones (8.9%) (Figure 2).

By ANOVA (analysis of variance), a connection is found between distance and means of transportation (Fanalysis = 44,669; $p < 0,05$). With the help of the correlation analysis, it is revealed, that the connection is strong and straight ($r = 0,62$). By analysis of the connection between the populated area and the means of transportation, a dependence is found, but it is not statistically significant. If the means of transportation and populated area, with it being Varna city or Varna region, then the existing connection is statistically significant. The correlation analysis reveals a weak reverse connection between the choice of transportation to the laboratory and residence in municipalities separately ($r = -0,14$; $p < 0,05$). If that connection is viewed as a connection between transport and residence within the main city of the area or the other area cities, it is slightly stronger and straight ($r = 0,24$; $p < 0,01$).

According to research data, the cabinets of the general practitioners are fairly close to the laboratories. 52.7% of the general practitioners indicated the presence of a laboratory in the same building. 1/3 are located within 500 meters from the closest medical diagnostic laboratory, followed by those, practicing in the distance between 600 meters and 3 kilometers (12.5%). The smallest part are those practicing more than 5 kilometers away from the laboratory (6.2%) and those, whose cabinets are in the 3 to 5 kilometers range from the laboratory (0.9%). The percentage of the remote practices is low, because of the fact, that the working general practitioners are not a lot and there are some unfilled medical practices. The general practitioner availability for a population of 10 000 is 9,4. One general practitioner works with roughly 920 people (Figure 3).

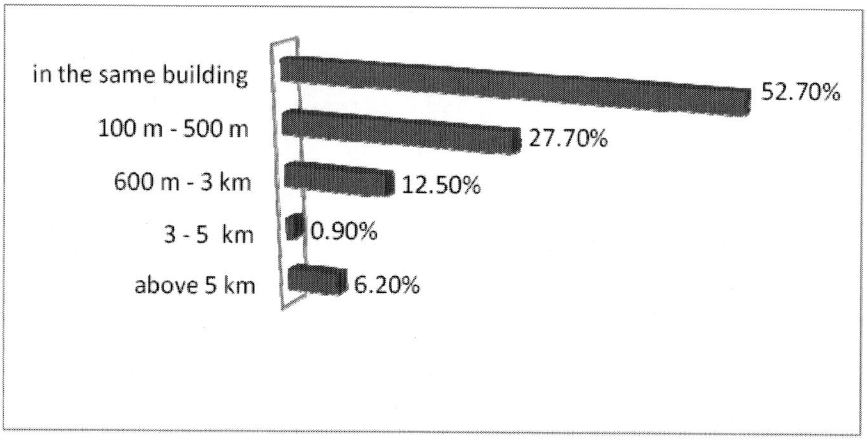

Figure 3. Distance between a general practitioner and the closest laboratory.

Data showed, that half of the physicians were comparatively satisfied from the territorial distribution, and also pointed out that the medical laboratories cover the needs of the area population. The unsatisfied respondents (those, answering "mostly not" – 13.5% and those, giving "no" as an answer – 5.4%), were from remote areas. By analysis of variance, a connection is found between the distance from the general practitioner's cabinet to the closest medical laboratory and the satisfaction from the number of the laboratories in the area (Fanalysis 43,340; $p < 0,05$). The link is straight and moderate ($r = 0, 437$; $p < 0,01$). The respondents, thinking that the number of laboratories does not cover the needs of the area population, are located more than 5 kilometers away from them.

With a X^2 test, a link was found, although not statistically significant, between the populated area, with it being either the regional city, or the area as a whole and the satisfaction from the number of laboratories in Varna region in total (X^2 e 36,364; $p < 0,05$), that dependency is moving from moderate towards significant ($r = 0,55$; $p < 0,01$).

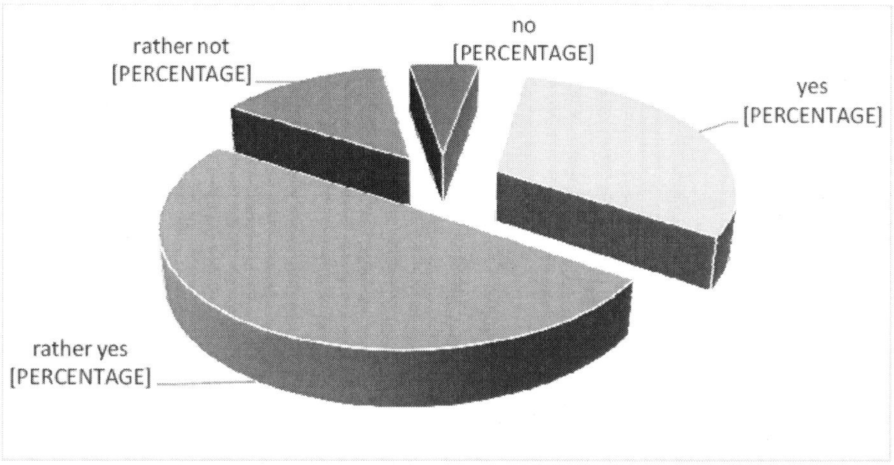

Figure 4. Satisfaction of general practitioners from the territorial distribution of medical diagnostic laboratories in the Varna region.

Most of the general practitioners, concerning the sufficiency of the regional medical diagnostic laboratories, have answered "mostly yes," with them being from Varna or the area, and amongst those from the city, none have answered negatively. From the region, those, that are completely satisfied with the number of laboratories, are significantly less. The specialists, giving the answer "mostly not," are mostly from the region, rather than the regional city. The mostly unsatisfied ones are from the smaller populated areas: the towns of Staro Oryahovo, Byala, Kichevo, Dolni Chiflik. The most satisfied from the territorial distribution of the medical laboratories, besides the ones in Varna, are in the cities Devnya and Zornitsa, and those, giving "mostly yes" as an answer, are the satisfied ones from Provadiya, Suvorovo, Vaglen and Aksakovo (see Figure 4).

CONCLUSION

The medical laboratories in Varna region are unevenly distributed, with most of them being concentrated in the regional city. The rest of the area has a serious deficiency of laboratory units. The current condition of the non-hospital care in Varna region is characterized mainly with the uneven distribution of the general practitioners and their concentration in the regional city, inequality of the population in terms of availability of non-hospital care mainly in the remote towns and the lack of well-organized emergency assistance.

The infrastructure of non-hospital care in Varna region, the availability of medical diagnostic laboratories and the increasing number of the providers of laboratory services, gives opportunities for providing equal access to the population, and also creates a favorable and competitive setting, aiming for laboratory cervices of higher quality.

REFERENCES

[1] Bulgarian Health Act, 2014 Jan 03.
[2] Health Insurance Act, 2014 Mar 04.
[3] Order of the Bulgarian Health Minister, NRD09-115, 2009 Mar 10.
[4] Country health map. URL: www.blsvarna.org/uploaded/ 1.doc.
[5] Bulgarian Society of Clinical Laboratory. URL: http:// www.bscl.eu/

Section Five – Acknowledgments

In: Public Health Yearbook 2016
Editor: Joav Merrick
ISBN: 978-1-53610-947-4

Chapter 44

About the Editor

Joav Merrick, MD, MMedSci, DMSc, born and educated in Denmark is professor of pediatrics, child health and human development, Division of Pediatrics, Hadassah Hebrew University Medical Center, Mt Scopus Campus, Jerusalem, Israel and Kentucky Children's Hospital, University of Kentucky, Lexington, Kentucky United States and professor of public health at the Center for Healthy Development, School of Public Health, Georgia State University, Atlanta, United States, the medical director of the Health Services, Division for Intellectual and Developmental Disabilities, Ministry of Social Affairs and Social Services, Jerusalem, the founder and director of the National Institute of Child Health and Human Development in Israel. Numerous publications in the field of pediatrics, child health and human development, rehabilitation, intellectual disability, disability, health, welfare, abuse, advocacy, quality of life and prevention. Received the Peter Sabroe Child Award for outstanding work on behalf of Danish Children in 1985 and the International LEGO-Prize ("The Children's Nobel Prize") for an extraordinary contribution towards improvement in child welfare and well-being in 1987. E-mail: jmerrick@zahav.net.il

In: Public Health Yearbook 2016
Editor: Joav Merrick

ISBN: 978-1-53610-947-4

Chapter 45

About the National Institute of Child Health and Human Development in Israel

The National Institute of Child Health and Human Development (NICHD) in Israel was established in 1998 as a virtual institute under the auspices of the Medical Director, Ministry of Social Affairs and Social Services in order to function as the research arm for the Office of the Medical Director. In 1998 the National Council for Child Health and Pediatrics, Ministry of Health and in 1999 the Director General and Deputy Director General of the Ministry of Health endorsed the establishment of the NICHD.

Mission

The mission of a National Institute for Child Health and Human Development in Israel is to provide an academic focal point for the scholarly interdisciplinary study of child life, health, public health, welfare, disability, rehabilitation, intellectual disability and related aspects of human development. This mission includes research, teaching, clinical work, information and public service activities in the field of child health and human development.

Service and academic activities

Over the years many activities became focused in the south of Israel due to collaboration with various professionals at the Faculty of Health Sciences (FOHS) at the Ben Gurion University of the Negev (BGU). Since 2000 an affiliation with the Zusman Child Development Center at the Pediatric Division of Soroka University Medical Center has resulted in collaboration around the establishment of the Down Syndrome Clinic at that center. In 2002 a full course on "Disability" was established at the Recanati School for Allied Professions in the Community, FOHS, BGU and in 2005 collaboration was started with the Primary Care Unit of the faculty and disability became part of the master of public health course on "Children and society". In the academic year 2005-2006 a one semester course on "Aging with disability" was started as part of the master of science program in gerontology in our collaboration with the Center for Multidisciplinary Research in Aging. In 2010 collaborations with the Division of Pediatrics, Hadassah Hebrew University Medical Center, Jerusalem, Israel around the National Down Syndrome Center and teaching students and residents about intellectual and developmental disabilities as part of their training at this campus.

Research activities

The affiliated staff have over the years published work from projects and research activities in this national and international collaboration. In the year 2000 the International Journal of Adolescent Medicine and Health and in 2005 the International Journal on Disability and Human Development of De Gruyter Publishing House (Berlin and New York) were affiliated with the National Institute of Child Health and Human Development. From 2008 also the International Journal of Child Health and Human Development (Nova Science, New York), the International Journal of Child and Adolescent Health (Nova Science) and the Journal of Pain Management (Nova Science) affiliated and from 2009 the International Public Health Journal (Nova Science) and Journal of Alternative Medicine Research (Nova Science). All peer-reviewed international journals.

National collaborations

Nationally the NICHD works in collaboration with the Faculty of Health Sciences, Ben Gurion University of the Negev; Department of Physical Therapy, Sackler School of Medicine, Tel Aviv University; Autism Center, Assaf HaRofeh Medical Center; National Rett and PKU Centers at Chaim Sheba Medical Center, Tel HaShomer; Department of Physiotherapy, Haifa University; Department of Education, Bar Ilan University, Ramat Gan, Faculty of Social Sciences and Health Sciences; College of Judea and Samaria in Ariel and in 2011 affiliation with Center for Pediatric Chronic Diseases and National Center for Down Syndrome, Department of Pediatrics, Hadassah Hebrew University Medical Center, Mount Scopus Campus, Jerusalem.

International collaborations

Internationally with the Department of Disability and Human Development, College of Applied Health Sciences, University of Illinois at Chicago; Strong Center for Developmental Disabilities, Golisano Children's Hospital at Strong, University of Rochester School of Medicine and Dentistry, New York; Centre on Intellectual Disabilities, University of Albany, New York; Centre for Chronic Disease Prevention and Control, Health Canada, Ottawa; Chandler Medical Center and Children’s Hospital, Kentucky Children’s Hospital, Section of Adolescent Medicine, University of Kentucky, Lexington; Chronic Disease Prevention and Control Research Center, Baylor College of Medicine, Houston, Texas; Division of Neuroscience, Department of Psychiatry, Columbia University, New York; Institute for the Study of Disadvantage and Disability, Atlanta; Center for Autism and Related Disorders, Department Psychiatry, Children’s Hospital Boston, Boston; Department of Pediatric and Adolescent Medicine, Western Michigan University Homer Stryker MD School of Medicine,

Kalamazoo, Michigan, United States; Department of Paediatrics, Child Health and Adolescent Medicine, Children's Hospital at Westmead, Westmead, Australia; International Centre for the Study of Occupational and Mental Health, Düsseldorf, Germany; Centre for Advanced Studies in Nursing, Department of General Practice and Primary Care, University of Aberdeen, Aberdeen, United Kingdom; Quality of Life Research Center, Copenhagen, Denmark; Nordic School of Public Health, Gottenburg, Sweden, Scandinavian Institute of Quality of Working Life, Oslo, Norway; The Department of Applied Social Sciences (APSS) of The Hong Kong Polytechnic University Hong Kong.

Targets

Our focus is on research, international collaborations, clinical work, teaching and policy in health, disability and human development and to establish the NICHD as a permanent institute at one of the residential care centers for persons with intellectual disability in Israel in order to conduct model research and together with the four university schools of public health/medicine in Israel establish a national master and doctoral program in disability and human development at the institute to secure the next generation of professionals working in this often non-prestigious/low-status field of work.

Contact

Joav Merrick, MD, MMedSci, DMSc
Professor of Pediatrics and Public Health
Medical Director, Health Services, Division for Intellectual and Developmental Disabilities, Ministry of Social Affairs and Social Services, POB 1260, IL-91012 Jerusalem, Israel.
E-mail: jmerrick@zahav.net.il

SECTION SIX – INDEX

INDEX

A

B

C

D

E

F

G

N

O

P

Q

R

S

T

U

V

W

Y

Z